SIGNS AND SYMPTOMS
IN CLINICAL PRACTICE

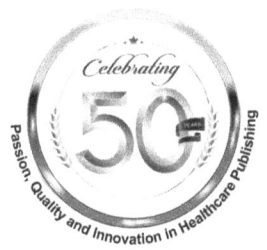

SIGNS AND SYMPTOMS IN CLINICAL PRACTICE

Editor

Devendra Richhariya
MBBS MD FICM
Associate Director
Emergency and Trauma Care
Medanta—The Medicity
Gurugram, Haryana, India

Co-Editors

Jesus Daniel López Tapia
MD
Master in Research and Education
President of Mexican Society of Emergency Medicine
Dean of Medicine School in Universidad de Monterrey
Nuevo León, Mexico

Khusrav Bajan
MD EDIC
Head, Emergency Department
PD Hinduja Hospital and Medical
Research Centre
Mumbai, Maharashtra, India

Bhawana Sharma
MBBS DNB (Respiratory Medicine)
Classified Specialist
Department of Critical Care
Artemis Hospital
Gurugram, Haryana, India

Forewords

Naresh Trehan
Yatin Mehta
Praveen Aggarwal

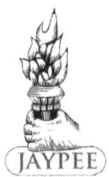

JAYPEE BROTHERS MEDICAL PUBLISHERS
The Health Sciences Publisher
New Delhi | London

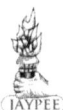 **Jaypee Brothers Medical Publishers (P) Ltd**

Headquarters

Jaypee Brothers Medical Publishers (P) Ltd
4838/24, Ansari Road, Daryaganj
New Delhi 110 002, India
Phone: +91-11-43574357
Fax: +91-11-43574314
E-mail: jaypee@jaypeebrothers.com

Overseas Office

JP Medical Ltd
83 Victoria Street, London
SW1H 0HW (UK)
Phone: +44 20 3170 8910
Fax: +44 (0)20 3008 6180
E-mail: info@jpmedpub.com

Website: www.jaypeebrothers.com
Website: www.jaypeedigital.com

© 2020, Jaypee Brothers Medical Publishers

The views and opinions expressed in this book are solely those of the original contributor(s)/author(s) and do not necessarily represent those of editor(s) of the book.

All rights reserved. No part of this publication may be reproduced, stored or transmitted in any form or by any means, electronic, mechanical, photocopying, recording or otherwise, without the prior permission in writing of the publishers.

All brand names and product names used in this book are trade names, service marks, trademarks or registered trademarks of their respective owners. The publisher is not associated with any product or vendor mentioned in this book.

Medical knowledge and practice change constantly. This book is designed to provide accurate, authoritative information about the subject matter in question. However, readers are advised to check the most current information available on procedures included and check information from the manufacturer of each product to be administered, to verify the recommended dose, formula, method and duration of administration, adverse effects and contraindications. It is the responsibility of the practitioner to take all appropriate safety precautions. Neither the publisher nor the author(s)/editor(s) assume any liability for any injury and/or damage to persons or property arising from or related to use of material in this book.

This book is sold on the understanding that the publisher is not engaged in providing professional medical services. If such advice or services are required, the services of a competent medical professional should be sought.

Every effort has been made where necessary to contact holders of copyright to obtain permission to reproduce copyright material. If any have been inadvertently overlooked, the publisher will be pleased to make the necessary arrangements at the first opportunity. The **CD/DVD-ROM** (if any) provided in the sealed envelope with this book is complimentary and free of cost. **Not meant for sale.**

Inquiries for bulk sales may be solicited at: jaypee@jaypeebrothers.com

Signs and Symptoms in Clinical Practice

First Edition: **2020**

ISBN: 978-93-89188-56-1

Dedicated to

My Parents, Family and Friends

Contributors

Aditya Agarwal MBBS MS MCh (Plastic Surgery) DNB (Plastic Surgery) MNAMS
Director
Department of Plastic, Esthetic and Reconstructive Surgery
Medanta—The Medicity
Gurugram, Haryana, India

Ajay Singh Thapa MD DM (Emergency Medicine)
Chief Consultant and Head
Department of Emergency Medicine and
Emergency Medical Services
Grande International Hospital
Kathmandu, Nepal

Akanksha Rastogi MBBS DNB (Medicine) MNAMS
Consultant
Department of Internal Medicine
Medanta—The Medicity
Gurugram, Haryana, India

Akshat Taneja MBBS MEM
Senior Resident
Emergency Department
Max Super Speciality Hospital
Patparganj, New Delhi, India

Aldo Emigdio Bartolini Salinas MD
Medical Surgeon and Midwife
Medicine School
Universidad de Monterrey
Nuevo León, Mexico

Aldo Tua MD
Faculty, Emergency Department
Sant'Andrea Hospital
Vercelli, Italy

Ali Abdolrazaghnejad MD
Assistant Professor
Department of Emergency Medicine
Tehran University of Medical Sciences
Tehran, Iran

Alireza Baratloo MD
Associate Professor
Department of Emergency Medicine
Tehran University of Medical Sciences
Tehran, Iran

Aman Sharma MD (Physician) Dip EM MEM
Senior Resident
Department of Emergency Medicine
Apollo Hospital
Bilaspur, Chhattisgarh, India

Amit Mittal MBBS DNB (Medicine), DNB (Gastroenterology), MNAMS
Senior Consultant
Department of Gastroenterology
Paras Hospital
Gurugram, Haryana, India

Amit Nabar MD DA FCPS MBBS LLB
Head
Department of Accident and Emergency
SL Raheja Hospital
Mumbai, Maharashtra, India

Anukalp Prakash MBBS MD (Medicine) DNB (Gastroenterology)
Senior Consultant
Department of Gastroenterology
Paras Hospital
Gurugram, Haryana, India

Apurva Arora MBBS MS MCh (Pediatric Surgery)
Senior Fellow
Department of Pediatric Surgery
Medanta—The Medicity
Gurugram, Haryana, India

Ashok Mishra MBBS MD PhD FIAPSM
Professor and Head
Department of Community Medicine
Gajara Raja Medical College and JA Groups of Hospital
Gwalior, Madhya Pradesh, India

Ashok Puranik MBBS MS Fellowship Trauma RACS
Professor and Head
General and Trauma Surgery
All India Institute of Medical Sciences
Jodhpur, Rajasthan, India

Ashok K Taneja MD DIP CARD FRCP (UK) FACP (USA) FICP FIAE FDI FAPSC (Taiwan)
Medical Director
Taneja Heart—Diabetes Centre
Gurugram, Haryana, India

Asit Misra MD (Physician)
Simulation Fellow
Ohio Health Learning
Columbus, Ohio, USA

Attique Vasdev MBBS MS (Ortho)
Director
Medanta Bone and Joint Institute
Medanta—The Medicity
Gurugram, Haryana, India

Au Kin Heng Constantine MBBS (HK) DPD (Wales) PG Dip SEM (Bath) Dip Clin Tox (HKPIC & HKCEM) PgDip–Medical Toxicology (Cardiff) MSc in Infectious Diseases (LSHTM, London External Program) MRCS (Ed) FHKCEM FHKAM (Emergency Medicine) FRCEM
Medical Director
Emergency Care Training (HK) Rescue Products Limited
Hong Kong

Avdi Tahiri MD
Specialist of Emergency Medicine
General Hospital Ferizaj
University Clinical Centre of Kosova
Ferizaj, Republic of Kosova

Ayesha Musabbah Almemari MD
Royal College of Physicians of Canada Certification in Emergency Medicine and Critical Care
Master in Quality and Safety in Health Care Management
Chair of Emergency Department and Program Director
Mafraq Hospital
Abu Dhabi, UAE

Ayşegül Bayır MD
Professor
Department of Emergency Medicine
Faculty of Medicine
Selçuk University
Konya, Turkey

Azza Omar Yousif MBBS
Arab Board in Emergency Medicine
European Board in Emergency Medicine
Emergency Physician
Rashid Hospital Trauma Centre
Dubai, UAE

Behcet Al MD
Professor
Emergency Department
Sahinbey Education and Application Hospital
University of Gaziantep
General Secretary of Emergency Medicine Physician Association of Turkey
Gaziantep, Turkey

Bhawana Sharma MBBS DNB (Respiratory Medicine)
Classified Specialist
Department of Critical Care
Artemis Hospital
Gurugram, Haryana, India

Carreen Pakrasi MBBS MD
Director
Department of Ophthalmology
Medanta—The Medicity
Gurugram, Haryana, India

Chintan Thanki MD (EU) MPH (Aus) DEM
Registrar, Emergency Department
Care Institute of Medical Sciences Hospital
Ahmedabad, Gujarat, India

Chitra Mehta DNB (Respiratory Medicine) DNB (Critical Care)
Associate Director, Critical Care
Medanta—The Medicity
Gurugram, Haryana, India

Deepak Dalmia MBBS MS (ENT) DNB (ENT)
Head, Department of ENT
Dr BAM Central Railway Zonal Hospital
Mumbai, Maharashtra, India

Deepika Gupta DNB (Plastic Surgery)
Resident
Department of Plastic, Esthetic and Reconstructive Surgery
Medanta—The Medicity
Gurugram, Haryana, India

Devendra Richhariya MBBS MD FICM
Associate Director
Emergency and Trauma Care
Medanta—The Medicity
Gurugram, Haryana, India

Dheeraj Kapoor MD DM
Head
Department of Endocrinology
Artemis Hospital
Gurugram, Haryana, India

Eric Revue MD
French Society of Emergency Medicine (SFMU)
Co-Chair of the Prehospital Section of the
European Society of Emergency Medicine (EuSEM)
Head of the Prehospital EMS (SMUR) and
Emergency Department
Chartres, France

Evith Pereira MD
Consultant
PD Hinduja Hospital and Medical Research Centre
Mumbai, Maharashtra, India

Faiz Ahmad MD FAAP
Division Chief
Pediatric Emergency Department
Tawam Hospital
Al Ain, Abu Dhabi, UAE

Goma Bali Bajaj MBBS MEM (GWU, USA)
Head, Emergency Department
Medical College
Ambala, Haryana, India

Govind Sharma MBBS MS (Ortho)
Associate Consultant
Medanta Bone and Joint Institute
Medanta—The Medicity
Gurugram, Haryana, India

Hanan Salah Al Hajri MBBS
Resident of Emergency Medicine
Mafraq Hospital
Abu Dhabi, UAE

Hardeep Singh MBBS MS MCh
(Plastic Surgery)
Consultant
Department of Plastic, Esthetic and Reconstructive Surgery
Medanta—The Medicity
Gurugram, Haryana, India

Harshil Mehta MD MRCEM FACEE
Consultant
Department of Emergency Medicine
Shalby Hospital
Ahmedabad, Gujarat, India

Hatinderjeet Singh Sethi
MBBS MD (Internal Medicine)
Consultant Internal Medicine and Preventive Health
Medanta—The Medicity
Gurugram, Haryana, India

Irene Oriaifo MD FAAP
Assistant Professor of Pediatrics
Department of Pediatric Emergency Medicine
Cardinal Glennon Children's Hospital
Saint Louis University
Saint Louis, Missouri, USA

Jasvinder Singh Anand MD
(Internal Medicine)
Senior Consultant
Department of Internal Medicine and Preventive Health
Medanta—The Medicity
Gurugram, Haryana, India

Jesus Daniel López Tapia MD
Master in Research and Education
President of Mexican Society of Emergency Medicine
Dean of Medicine School in Universidad de Monterrey
Nuevo León, Mexico

Kamal Lashkari MD IDCCM EDIC
Specialist
Department of Critical Care Medicine
Thumbay Hospital
Ajman, UAE

Khusrav Bajan MD EDIC
Head, Emergency Department
PD Hinduja Hospital and Medical Research Centre
Mumbai, Maharashtra, India

Kishalay Datta MBBS MD MRCP MACEP MHA
Associate Director and Head
Emergeny Department
Max Super Speciality Hospital
New Delhi, India

Lumturije Njazi Asllani-Hashani MD
Specialist of Parodontology and Oral Medicine
Main Family Health Centre UBT Higher Education Institution QKMF
Ferizaj City, Ferizaj, Republic of Kosovo

M Sai Surendar MD DEM FICM
Head, Emergency Department
Dr Rela Hospital
Chennai, Tamil Nadu, India

Madhusoodan Gupta DNB
(Plastic Surgery)
Resident
Department of Plastic, Esthetic and Reconstructive Surgery
Medanta—The Medicity
Gurugram, Haryana, India

Maninder S Dhaliwal MD
(Pediatrics) FIAP (Pediatric Intensive Care)
Associate Director, Pediatric Intensive Care Unit
Medanta—The Medicity
Gurugram, Haryana, India

Mariana Patricia Valdez Rodríguez MD
Medical Surgeon and Midwife
Medicine School
Universidad de Monterrey
Nuevo León, Mexico

Maryam Hasan Darwish Alshehhi MD FRCPC
Consultant Hematologist
Sheikh Khalifa Specialty Hospital
Ras al Khaimah, UAE

Mayank Tripathi MDS
Director
Ojam Orthodontic Centre
Raipur, Chhattisgarh, India

Meera Luthra MBBS MS MCh DNB (Pediatric Surgery)
Senior Consultant
Department of Pediatric Surgery
Medanta—The Medicity
Gurugram, Haryana, India

Mohammed Moizuddin Qureshi MD
PGY II Emergency Medicine
Penn State Health Milton S Hershey Medical Center
Hershey, Pennsylvania, USA

Mohsen Banaie MD
Assistant Professor
Department of Emergency Medicine
Tehran University of Medical Sciences
Tehran, Iran

Mustafa Sabak MD
Faculty, Emergency Medicine
Department of Medicine
Nizip State Hospital
University of Gaziantep
Gaziantep, Turkey

Nadeem Uddin Qureshi MD FAAP FCCM
Associate Professor of Pediatrics
Department of Pediatric Emergency Medicine
Cardinal Glennon Children's Hospital
Saint Louis University
Saint Louis, Missouri, USA

Neha Dubey MD
Visiting Consultant
Dermatologist
Department of Dermatology
Medanta—The Medicity
Gurugram, Haryana, India

Nikhil Tambe MBBS
Associate Consultant
Department of Emergency Medicine
Fortis Hospital
Mumbai, Maharashtra, India

Nilu Sunil MBBS
Fellowship in Emergency Medicine and Trauma Care
Diploma in Medicolegal Systems and Hospital and Healthcare Management
Consultant
Emergency Department
Bangalore Baptist Hospital
Bengaluru, Karnataka, India

Nimarpreet Kaur MBBS MD
Assistant Professor
Department of Physiology
SGT Medical College and Research Institute
Gurugram, Haryana, India

Nisreen Hamza Maghraby
MBBS FRCPC (EM) MM
Emergency Medicine, Trauma and Disaster Consultant
Head of ED Clinical Services
King Fahd University Hospital
KSA, Saudi Arabia

Omar Ghazanfar MBBS EBBEM EMDM
Independent Medical Appraiser (General Medical Council, UK)
Associate Member of the Royal College of Emergency Medicine, UK
Emergency Physician
Zayed Military Hospital
Abu Dhabi, UAE

Pooja Kataria MBBS
Postgraduate Resident
Department of Community Medicine
Maharaja Agrasen Medical College
Agroha, Haryana, India

Pooja Sharma MD
Senior Scientist
Medanta—The Medicity
Gurugram, Haryana, India

Prafull Mishra MBBS MS DNB
Urology (2nd year)
Senior Resident
Medanta—The Medicity
Gurugram, Haryana, India

Prashant Kumar MD FNB (Critical Care), EDIC
Senior Consultant
Department of Critical Care
Medanta—The Medicity
Gurugram, Haryana, India

Praveen Aggarwal MD DNB
Professor and Head
Department of Emergency Medicine
All India Institute of Medical Sciences
New Delhi, India

Praveen Saraogi MS
Professor
Department of Orthopedics
Jhansi Medical College
Jhansi, Uttar Pradesh, India

Puneet Ahluwalia MBBS MS MCh (Urology)
Senior Consultant
Division of Uro-Oncology
Department of Surgical Oncology
Max Institute of Healthcare
New Delhi, India

Rahul Mehrotra MD (Medicine) DNB (Cardiology)
Associate Director and Head
Noninvasive Cardiology
Max Super Speciality Hospital
Saket, New Delhi, India

Rajeev Agarwal MBBS MS
Fellowship (Surgical Oncology)
Director, Breast Surgery
Medanta—The Medicity
Gurugram, Haryana, India

Rajeev Kapur MD
Principal Consultant
Aviation Medicine and Hospital Management
Medanta—The Medicity
Gurugram, Haryana, India

Rakesh K khazanchi MBBS MS MCh (Plastic Surgery)
Chairman
Department of Plastic, Esthetic and Reconstructive Surgery
Medanta—The Medicity
Gurugram, Haryana, India

Rakesh Khera MBBS MS (Surgery) MCh (Urology) DNB (Urology)
Director
Urology, Robotics and Kidney Transplant
Medanta—The Medicity
Gurugram, Haryana, India

Ramanjit Singh MD
Visiting Consultant
Dermatologist
Department of Dermatology
Medanta—The Medicity
Gurugram, Haryana, India

Ranjana Bhatt MBBS DNB (Medicine)
Registrar
Department of Endocrinology
Artemis Hospital
Gurugram, Haryana, India

Ravindra Kale MD DM (Gastroenterologist)
Senior Consultant
CHL Hospital
Indore, Madhya Pradesh, India

Rekha Gadiparthi MD FAAP
Fellow
Department of Pediatric Emergency Medicine
Cardinal Glennon Children's Hospital
Saint Louis University
Saint Louis, Missouri, USA

Rigenjyoti Kalita MBBS MEM
Attending Consultant
Emergeny Department
Max Super Speciality Hospital
New Delhi, India

Ritin Mohindra MD
Assistant Professor
Department of Emergency Medicine
All India Institute of Medical Sciences
New Delhi, India

Roberta Petrino MD
Faculty, Emergency Department
Sant'Andrea Hospital
Vercelli, Italy

Rohan N Shah MEM DEM FACEE
Emergency Physician
Mediclinic Parkview Hospital
Dubai, UAE

Ronak Mankodi MD (Anesthesia)
Senior Resident
Department of Emergency and Trauma Care
Medanta—The Medicity
Gurugram, Harayana, India

Ruchi Kapoor MD (Pathology)
Chief Consultant Pathologist
Oncquest Diagnostics
New Delhi, India

Saleh Fares MD MPH FRCPC (EM) FACEP FAAEM
Consultant
Emergency, Emergency Medical Services and Disaster Medicine
Zayed Military Hospital, Abu Dhabi
Founder and President
Emirates Society of Emergency Medicine
Abu Dhabi, UAE

Sandeep B Gore MBBS MRCEM (UK) FAEM (CMC, Vellore)
Head
Department of Emergency Medicine
Fortis Hospital
Mumbai, Maharashtra, India

Sandeep Jain MS FNB (Trauma Care) PGDMLS MEM
Senior Consultant and Head
Emergency Department
Max Super Speciality Hospital
Saket, New Delhi, India

Sandip Kumar MBBS DCh IDPCCM
Pediatric Intensivist
Dr Mehta's Children's Hospital
Chennai, Tamil Nadu, India

Sanjay Kumar MD DM (Gastroenterology) FACG
Director and Chief Gastroenterologist
Bhopal Institute of Gastroenterology

Gastrocare Liver and Digestive Disease Center
Bhopal, Madhya Pradesh, India

Sanjay Mahendru MBBS MS DNB MCh (Plastic Surgery)
Associate Director
Department of Plastic, Esthetic and Reconstructive Surgery
Medanta—The Medicity
Gurugram, Haryana, India

Sanjay Shah MBBS MS DNB (Surgery) FNB (Trauma Care)
Head, Emergency Department
Director, Trauma Center
Care Institute of Medical Sciences Hospital
Ahmedabad, Gujarat, India

Sanjaya Bahera MBBS MS (ENT) DNB (ENT)
Department of ENT
Dr BAM Central Railway Zonal Hospital
Mumbai, Maharashtra, India

Sanjukta Dutta MBBS PGFEM MEM
Consultant and Head
Department of Emergency Medicine
Fortis Hospital
Kolkata, West Bengal, India

Sara Nooruddin Kazim MD FRCPC (EM) MSc (Health Care Management)
Clinical Pharmacology and Medical Toxicology Fellowship
Consultant and Head
Emergency Department
Rashid Hospital Trauma Center
Dubai, UAE

Saurabh Garg DNB (Plastic Surgery)
Resident
Department of Plastic, Esthetic and Reconstructive Surgery
Medanta—The Medicity
Gurugram, Haryana, India

Saurabh Patil MBBS MS MCh
(Urology)
Fellow, Uro-Oncology
Max Institute of Healthcare
New Delhi, India

Sayuri Enriquez Saenz MD
Consultant
Department of Emergency
Medicine and Disaster
Cayetano Heredia Hospital
Lima, Peru

Seema Sharma MD
Associate Professor
Department of Community
Medicine
Maharaja Agrasen Medical
College
Agroha, Haryana, India

Sharad Bedi MBBS MD MRCP (UK)
Associate Consultant
Department of Preventive
Cardiology
Medanta—The Medicity
Gurugram, Haryana, India

Shashank Karale DNB (3rd year)
Emergency and Trauma Care
Medanta—The Medicity
Gurugram, Haryana, India

Shubham Chelawat MBBS MD
(Medicine) DNB
Senior Resident
Department of Cardiology
Max Super Speciality Hospital
Saket, New Delhi, India

Shweta Tyagi MRCEM (UK), FAEM
(CMC Vellore)
Consultant
Department of Emergency
Medicine
Sir HN Reliance Foundation
Hospital and Research Centre
Mumbai, Maharashtra, India

Sourabh Malviya MD
Fellowship in Rheumatology
Senior Consultant and Head
Division of Rheumatology
Medanta Super Speciality
Hospital
Indore, Madhya Pradesh, India

Srinivas Monanga MD
(Anesthesia) FNB (Critical Care)
Attending Consultant
Department of Critical Care
Medanta—The Medicity
Gurugram, Haryana, India

Sudipto Pakrasi MBBS MD
Chairman
Department of Ophthalmology
Medanta—The Medicity
Gurugram, Haryana, India

Sukhdeep Singh MBBS MS MCh
(Plastic Surgery)
Consultant
Department of Plastic, Esthetic
and Reconstructive Surgery
Medanta—The Medicity
Gurugram, Haryana, India

Suman Thakur MBBS MD
Microbiologist
Culture and Drug Sensitivity
Lab Microbiology
Indira Gandhi Medical College
Shimla, Himachal Pradesh, India

Thiagrajan Jaiganesh MS DNB
FRCS (Surg) FRCS (A&E) DCH FRCEM
PGCHCL
Chairman and Consultant
Emergency Department
Tawam Hospital
Al Ain, Abu Dhabi, UAE

Uday Sanglodkar MBBS DNB
(Gastro)
Senior Resident
Global Hospital
Chennai, Tamil Nadu, India

Veena Raghunathan MD
(Pediatrics) DNB (Pediatrics) FNB
(Pediatric Intensive Care)
Senior Consultant, Pediatric
Intensive Care Unit
Medanta—The Medicity
Gurugram, Haryana, India

Veerottam Tomar MD FCCP
EDRM
Director
Dr Shivraj Memorial Chest and
Allergy Centre
Meerut, Uttar Pradesh, India

Vimlendu Brajesh MBBS MS
MCh (Plastic Surgery)
Consultant
Department of Plastic, Esthetic
and Reconstructive Surgery
Medanta—The Medicity
Gurugram, Haryana, India

Vivek Chauhan MBBS MD
Assistant Professor
Department of Medicine
Indira Gandhi Medical College
Shimla, Himachal Pradesh,
India

Vivekanshu Verma MBBS
Diploma in Forensic Medicine
and Toxicology
Associate Consultant
Department of Emergency and
Trauma Care
Medanta—The Medicity
Gurugram, Haryana, India

Yatin Mehta MD MNAMS FRCA
FAMS FIACTA FICCM FTEE
Chairman
Medanta Institute of Critical
Care and Anesthesiology
Medanta—The Medicity
Gurugram, Haryana, India

Foreword

It is a commonly accepted truth that real knowledge illustrates the extent of our ignorance. The more we learn, the more we realize how little we know, and how much more remains unknown. In the clinical field, this never-ending quest to acquire knowledge, share it widely and retain its currency is our most vital attribute.

Devendra Richhariya practices this principle and it finds expression in his medical writings. I am delighted to introduce his second book entitled *'Signs and Symptoms in Clinical Practice'*. I am certain it will be received with the same enthusiasm, as his earlier work 'Textbook of Emergency and Trauma Care' This too is written with great attention to detail. With comprehensive approach and easy reference. *'Signs and Symptoms in Clinical Practice'* covers varied aspects of medicine. The content offers therapeutic approaches to critically ill patients besides a coherent understanding of primary and secondary syndromes. It should be readily accessible to everyone concerned with forming a differential diagnosis to rendering care.

A laudable effort, for which I extend my best wishes to Devendra Richhariya, his co-authors and medical students.

Naresh Trehan
Diplomate, American Board of Cardiothoracic Surgery
Chairman and Managing Director, Medanta—The Medicity
Chairman, Medanta Heart Institute
Gurugram, Haryana, India

Foreword

It is a pleasure to write the foreword for Devendra Richhariya's *Signs and Symptoms in Clinical Practice*. After editing his previous book 'Textbook of Emergency and Trauma Care', he has followed with this in quick succession! With FNB in emergency medicine starting in many major hospitals, it is important that we have adequate academic resources not only for the aspiring/trainee emergency physicians but also for practicing doctors.

This book has 91 chapters on all practical aspects of signs and symptoms of various case scenarios which are useful for any young or practicing emergency physician, general physicians or DNB/MD students and obviously undergraduate medical students. The chapters are contributed by more than 100 renowned physicians/surgeons of various specialties.

When I was in UK, the first thing which I noticed that their trainees did not read the standard textbooks like Bailey and Love, Harrison's, etc. but only read 'lecture notes' in all specialties! They were written in very simple sequence from the time patient presents to, how to deal with him subsequently and so on. These were actual case scenarios which one would see daily in ER. The standard textbooks which we read in undergraduates studies they read only at postgraduate (PG) level! Their fresh medical graduates were better equipped to deal with actual everyday case scenarios, although we had more theoretical knowledge!

So this book is in the right direction to close this gap. It will be a very useful too for undergraduates/emergency physicians/PG students or general practitioners.

I wish you all enjoyable reading!

Yatin Mehta
MD MNAMS FRCA FAMS FIACTA FICCM FTEE
Chairman
Medanta Institute of Critical Care and Anesthesiology
Medanta—The Medicity
Gurugram, Haryana, India

Foreword

The book '*Signs and Symptoms in Clinical Practice*' is for every acute care unit as well as various departments including emergency medicine, surgery, pediatrics, gynecology, orthopedics, psychiatry, cardiology, neurology, pulmonology and gastroenterology. It is also well-suited for the nursing students. The book will be an asset to the medical and nursing libraries. In fact, it should be on the most easily reached shelf for anyone interested in or who comes in contact with medical illness or injury. This compilation of information has many attributes, among which are:

- Evidence-based, well-referenced information
- Editors and authors who are experts in their fields
- Concise and clear presentation
- Tables that convey critical data
- Figures and diagrams that are clinically relevant
- Paragraph headers that allow focused access to information
- Calculations and formulas that are fully explained
- Lists of treatment materials to be obtained in advance with contact information of unusual items
- Therapeutic dosages that are detailed enough to be utilized without additional references.

The quality of this book should come as no surprise after looking at the impressive listing of authors. The editor, Devendra Richhariya, also the editor of 'Textbook of Emergency and Trauma Care', have selected national and international experts whose credibility is unmatched. They represent the best of our profession of medical science and have written a large percentage of the most important and ground breaking publications in our field.

Knowledge of clinical signs and symptoms are the ABCs of the medical education. Thorough knowledge of the signs and symptoms is the key to diagnosis of any disease. I am sure that the '*Signs and Symptoms in Clinical Practice*' will be helpful to all the medical students.

Praveen Aggarwal
Professor and Head
Department of Emergency Medicine
All India Institute of Medical Sciences
New Delhi, India

Preface

The practice of medicine would be simple if each symptom or sign indicated a single disease, but there are enormous number of signs and symptoms (we covered only a hundred of them) and they can occur in nearly infinite number of combinations and temporal patterns. The physician's goal in performing a clinical examination and history taking is to generate diagnostic hypothesis based on signs and symptoms since medicine evolved as an art to practice, this was true since ancient times of Hippocrates, Charaka, Suśruta, Hamilton Bailey, Osler, and remains true today, even after complete digitalization and globalization of medical information. Ancient Indian Physician and Father of Indian Surgery—The Suśruta's Sanskrit name, literally means "well-heard", which is the most important and difficult skill to learn, requiring years of experience and practice during examining patient for hearing his history of past and present illness, hearing his heart sounds, breath and bowel sounds. By reading this book on and signs and symptoms, which are indexed in alphabetical order, just like the rough fibers for cloth weaver, from which the physician will be able to weave a clinical narrative, anatomically and pathophysiologically explicit, to form the accurate diagnostic hypotheses.

Devendra Richhariya

Acknowledgments

I am grateful to all my teachers and friends who supported me during this project.

I am thankful to each and every member of the Medanta family.

I would like to sincerely thank all the authors for providing manuscripts in spite of their busy schedules.

Special thanks to Shri Jitendar P Vij (Group Chairman), Mr Ankit Vij (Managing Director), Mr MS Mani (Group President), Ms Chetna Malhotra Vohra (Associate Director—Content Strategy), Ms Pooja Bhandari (Production Head), Ms Nikita Chauhan (Senior Development Editor) and all members of M/S Jaypee Brothers Medical Publishers (P) Ltd, New Delhi, India for invaluable contribution.

Contents

1. **Abdominal Pain (Adult)** — 1
   Roberta Petrino, Aldo Tua

2. **Abdominal Pain (Acute) in Children** — 13
   Meera Luthra, Apurva Arora

3. **Abdominal Pain (Chronic) in Children** — 18
   Faiz Ahmad, Thiagrajan Jaiganesh

4. **Anal Fissure** — 24
   Ashok Puranik

5. **Anemia** — 27
   Khusrav Bajan, Evith Pereira

6. **Ankle Sprain** — 36
   Sanjay Shah, Chintan Thanki

7. **Ascites** — 45
   Jesus Daniel López Tapia, Mariana Patricia Valdez Rodríguez

8. **Bleeding Disorders** — 52
   Ayesha Musabbah Almemari, Hanan Salah Al Hajri, Maryam Hasan Darwish Alshehhi

9. **Bell's Palsy** — 72
   Ali Abdolrazaghnejad, Mohsen Banaie

10. **Breast Problems** — 77
    Rajeev Agarwal

11. **Bowel Obstruction** — 83
    Jesus Daniel López Tapia, Aldo Emigdio Bartolini Salinas

12. **Cervical Sprain (Whiplash Injury)** — 93
    Chintan Thanki, Sanjay Shah

13. **Chest Pain** — 99
    Rahul Mehrotra, Shubham Chelawat

14. **Clubbing** — 111
    Vivek Chauhan, Suman Thakur

15. **Clavicle Fracture** — 118
    Sandeep Jain

16.	**Concussion** Mustafa Sabak, Behcet Al	123
17.	**Coma** Saleh Fares, Omar Ghazanfar	128
18.	**Constipation in Adult** Rohan N Shah	137
19.	**Convulsions in Adults** Amit Nabar	141
20.	**Convulsion in Children** Sanjukta Dutta	152
21.	**Cough in Adult** Bhawana Sharma	162
22.	**Cough in Children** Maninder S Dhaliwal	167
23.	**Crying in Infant and Children** Shweta Tyagi	174
24.	**Cyanosis** Suman Thakur, Vivek Chauhan	181
25.	**Deafness** Deepak Dalmia, Sanjaya Bahera	188
26.	**Dental Problems** Mayank Tripathi	193
27.	**Diarrhea in Adult and Travelers** Sanjay Kumar	207
28.	**Diarrhea in Children** Veena Raghunathan	212
29.	**Dysmenorrhea** Nilu Sunil	220
30.	**Dyspepsia** Ravindra Kale	225
31.	**Dysphagia** Amit Mittal, Anukalp Prakash	229
32.	**Dyspnea** Chitra Mehta, Srinivas Monanga	235

33.	**Earache** *Deepak Dalmia, Sanjaya Bahera*	242
34.	**Ear Discharge** *Sanjaya Bahera, Deepak Dalmia*	252
35.	**Epistaxis** *Sandeep B Gore*	256
36.	**Eye Problems** *Carreen Pakrasi, Sudipto Pakrasi*	262
37.	**Emergency Contraception** *Goma Bali Bajaj*	277
38.	**Facial Swelling** *Ashok K Taneja, Akshat Taneja*	279
39.	**Fatigue** *Au Kin Heng Constantine*	284
40.	**Fever** *Akanksha Rastogi, Amit Mittal*	294
41.	**Fever in Infants and Children** *Sandip Kumar*	299
42.	**Fingers and Nail Problems** *Aditya Agarwal, Vimlendu Brajesh, Sukhdeep Singh, Hardeep Singh, Sanjay Mahendru, Pooja Sharma, Madhusoodan Gupta, Saurabh Garg, Deepika Gupta, Rakesh K Khazanchi*	307
43.	**Gait Abnormalities** *Nikhil Tambe, Sandeep B Gore*	316
44.	**Goiter** *Dheeraj Kapoor, Ruchi Kapoor, Ranjana Bhatt*	323
45.	**Gum Disorders** *Avdi Tahiri, Lumturije Njazi Asllani-Hashani*	330
46.	**Heat Illness** *Omar Ghazanfar, Saleh Fares*	334
47.	**Heel Pain** *Vivekanshu Verma*	342
48.	**Hematemesis** *Sanjay Kumar*	345
49.	**Hematuria** *Asit Misra*	348

50.	Hemoptysis Veerottam Tomar	355
51.	Hemorrhoids Ashok Puranik	365
52.	Headache Alireza Baratloo	369
53.	Hiccups Hatinderjeet Singh Sethi, Nimarpreet Kaur	374
54.	Hyperventilation Bhawana Sharma	379
55.	Inflight Medical Problems Rajeev Kapur	382
56.	Immunization for Adults and Travelers Sara Nooruddin Kazim, Nisreen Hamza Maghraby, Azza Omar Yousif	386
57.	Immunization in Pregnancy and Children Ashok Mishra	407
58.	Insect Bite (Arthropods: Bites, Stings, and Other Contacts) Au Kin Heng Constantine	423
59.	Jaundice in Adult Anukalp Prakash, Amit Mittal	440
60.	Jaw Dislocation Harshil Mehta	448
61.	Joint Pain Sourabh Malviya	453
62.	Knee Problems Attique Vasdev, Govind Sharma	464
63.	Lower Extremity Pain, Edema, and Ulcers Ayşegül Bayır	468
64.	Low Back Pain Devendra Richhariya	481
65.	Lymphadenopathy Ritin Mohindra, Praveen Aggarwal	485
66.	Melena Shashank Karale, Uday Sanglodkar	495

67.	**Muscle Cramps** *Sayuri Enriquez Saenz*	**499**
68.	**Muscle Wasting** *Praveen Aggarwal, Ritin Mohindra*	**501**
69.	**Multiple Trauma** *Behcet Al, Mustafa Sabak*	**508**
70.	**Oral Problems (Oral Candidiasis, Oral Herpes Simplex)** *Aman Sharma*	**520**
71.	**Palpitations** *Aldo Tua, Roberta Petrino*	**530**
72.	**Pedal Edema** *Ajay Singh Thapa*	**540**
73.	**Penile Problems** *Puneet Ahluwalia, Saurabh Patil*	**545**
74.	**Procedural Sedation and Analgesia** *Ronak Mankodi*	**556**
75.	**Rabies Prophylaxis** *Pooja Kataria, Seema Sharma*	**565**
76.	**Rashes in Newborn and Infants** *Nadeem Uddin Qureshi, Irene Oriaifo, Mohammed Moizuddin Qureshi, Rekha Gadiparthi*	**570**
77.	**Rib Fractures** *Sandeep Jain*	**579**
78.	**Scrotum (Acute)** *Rakesh Khera, Prafull Mishra*	**584**
79.	**Shoulder Dislocation** *Praveen Saraogi*	**593**
80.	**Skin Problems** *Ramanjit Singh, Neha Dubey*	**596**
81.	**Smoke Inhalation** *Eric Revue*	**618**
82.	**Sore Throat (Pharyngitis)** *Akanksha Rastogi, Amit Mittal*	**625**
83.	**Stridor** *Yatin Mehta, Kamal Lashkari, Prashant Kumar*	**631**

84.	**Tetanus Prophylaxis** *M Sai Surendar*	639
85.	**Torticollis (Wryneck)** *Harshil Mehta*	641
86.	**Tremor** *Devendra Richhariya*	647
87.	**Vertigo (Dizziness)** *Kishalay Datta, Rigenjyoti Kalita*	650
88.	**Voice Disorders** *Deepak Dalmia*	657
89.	**Vomiting in Adults** *Ravindra Kale*	664
90.	**Weight Gain (Obesity)** *Jasvinder Singh Anand*	669
91.	**Weight Loss** *Sharad Bedi*	674

Index   *681*

CHAPTER 1

Abdominal Pain (Adult)

Roberta Petrino, Aldo Tua

■ INTRODUCTION

Abdominal pain is a very common symptom of presentation for patients admitted to the emergency department (ED) and represents a strong challenge for physicians and nurses involved in diagnosis and treatment. Incidence and clinical manifestations are both influenced by many demographic variables (age, gender, geography, etc.).

Although in most of the cases, it is not related to a serious disease, in some cases, it can be the only symptom of a potential rapidly evolved situation.

■ ETIOLOGY/CAUSES

Many intra-abdominal disorders cause abdominal pain and also several extra-abdominal diseases can present with abdominal pain. Some of these are immediately life-threatening, requiring rapid diagnosis and surgery. The knowledge of abdominal anatomy and its innervation helps for differential diagnosis, however, a systematic and logic approach, with a careful medical history and clinical evaluation, is fundamental. Focused clinical history and physical examination are able to place a right diagnostic hypothesis in 80% of patients with abdominal pain (**Table 1**). There are some alert signs and symptoms that must always be taken into careful consideration, because they probably underlie a serious condition (**Table 2**). Often a definitive diagnosis is impossible in the ED but the emergency physician has always to identify and rule out life-threatening clinical conditions. These include ruptured abdominal aortic aneurysm (AAA), perforated viscus, mesenteric ischemia, and ruptured ectopic pregnancy. Other diseases (e.g. acute appendicitis, acute diverticulitis, severe acute pancreatitis, and intestinal obstruction) are also serious and nearly as urgent.

■ PATHOPHYSIOLOGY OF THE CONDITION

The abdominal viscera are innervated by nociceptive fibers on the mesenteric surface and inside the wall of the hollow organs. These fibers are sensitive both to mechanical, mainly stretching, and chemical stimuli. They can produce deaf, subcontinuous, crampy, or violent pain.

Table 1: Correlation between anatomical site of abdominal pain and the differential diagnosis.

RIGHT HYPOCHONDRIUM PAIN	EPIGASTRIC PAIN	LEFT HYPOCHONDRIUM PAIN
Biliar: cholecystitis, cholangitis, cholelitiasis **Colic:** colitis, diverticulitis, ileitis, retrocecal appendicitis, perforated duodenal ulcer **Haepatic:** abscess, haepatitis, masses, haepatic congestion **Pulmonary:** pneumonia, pulmonary embolism **Renal:** nephrolithiasis, pyelonephritis	**Biliar:** cholecystitis, cholangitis, cholelitiasis **Cardiac:** acute myocardial infarction, angina, pericarditis **Gastric:** esophagitis, gastritis, peptic ulcer **Pancreatic:** pancreatitis or tumors **Vascular:** aortic dissection, mesenteric ischemia	**Cardiac:** acute myocardial infarction, angina, pericarditis **Gastric:** esophagitis, gastritis, peptic ulcer **Pancreatic:** pancreatitis or tumors **Pulmonar:** pneumonia, pulmonary embolism **Renal:** nephrolithiasis, pyelonephritis **Splenic:** rupture/infarction/distension **Vascular:** aortic dissection, mesenteric ischemia

RIGHT LUMBAR PAIN	UMBLICAL PAIN	LEFT LUMBAR PAIN
Colic: colitis, diverticulitis, ileitis, appendicitis, constipation **Haepatic:** abscess, haepatitis, masses, haepatic congestion **Renal:** nephrolithiasis, pyelonephritis, ureteral calculi Fitz-Hugh-Curtis syndrome	**Colic:** appendicitis **Gastric:** esophagitis, gastritis, peptic ulcer, small bowel obstruction **Vascular:** aortic dissection, mesenteric ischemia **Cardiac:** acute myocardial infarction	**Colic:** colitis, diverticulitis, constipation **Splenic:** abscess, rupture/infarction/distension **Renal:** nephrolithiasis, pyelonephritis, ureteral calculi

RIGHT ILLIAC FOSSA PAIN	HYPOGASTRIC PAIN	LEFT ILLIAC FOSSA PAIN
Colic: appendicitis, colitis, diverticulitis, Inflammatory bowel disease, irritable bowel syndrome, regional enteritis, epiploic appendagitis, Meckel's diverticulum, Chron's disease, inguinal hernia **Gynecological:** pelvic inflammatory disease, ectopic pregnancy, endometriosis, mittelschmerz, ovarian torsion **Muscolar:** Psoas abscess **Renal/Urinary:** nephrolithiasis, pyelonephritis. Testicular torsion, ureteral calculi **Vascular:** aortic aneurysm (leaking, ruptured)	**Colic:** appendicitis, colitis, diverticulitis, Inflammatory bowel disease, irritable bowel syndrome **Gynecological:** pelvic inflammatory disease, ectopic pregnancy, endometriosis, Mittelschmerz **Renal/Urinary:** cystitis, nephrolithiasis, pyelonephritis	**Colic:** appendicitis, colitis, diverticulitis, Inflammatory bowel disease, irritable bowel syndrome, regional enteritis, epiploic appendagitis, inguinal hernia **Gynecological:** pelvic inflammatory disease, ectopic pregnancy, endometriosis, mittelschmerz, ovarian torsion **Muscolar:** psoas abscess **Renal/Urinary:** nephrolithiasis, pyelonephritis. Testicular torsion, ureteral calculi **Vascular:** aortic aneurysm (leaking, ruptured)

DIFFUSE ABDOMINAL PAIN

Vascular: aortic aneurysm, aortic dissection
Intestinal: appendicitis (early), bowel obstruction, peritonitis (all causes), perforated bowel, mesenteric ischemia. Volvulus, gastroenteritis, peritonitis. Inflammatory bowel disease, strangulated, incarcerated hernia
Miscellaneous: herpes zoster (any single localization, not diffuse), muscular, diabetic gastric paresis, familial Mediterranean fever, sickle cell crisis, narcotic withdrawal, heavy metal poisoning, metabolic disorders (diabetic ketoacidosis, porphyria), hereditary angioedema, malaria

Table 2: Alarm signs and symptoms in abdominal pain.

History: • Extreme ages • Impossibility to feed • Vomiting in jet • Hematemesis • Syncope • Pregnancy • Recent surgical or endoscopic treatment • Fever • Severe pain of rapid onset • Caustic ingestion or foreign bodies
Physical examination: • Abnormal vital signs • Rectorrhagia and melena • Incarcerated or strangulated hernia • Mental deterioration
Laboratory testing: • Renal insufficiency • Metabolic acidosis, ABG lactates • Hyper-hypoglycemia • Anemia, leukocytosis, polyglobulia • High levels of lipases and amylases • High levels of bilirubin, alkaline phosphatase and transaminases
Imaging: • Free air in the abdomen • Thickening of the walls of the gallbladder and pericholecystic fluid • Dilatation of the biliary tract • Hydro-air levels • Intra-abdominal abscess • Air in the portal venous system

The abdominal pain is divided into:
- *Visceral*: Usually secondary to stretching of hollow organs, twist or spastic contraction. It can be dull and continuous or colic, often located in the median site, as visceral innervation is bilateral, and it corresponds to the dermatome relative to the involved organ. Therefore, for the organs located above the Treitz ligament, it will be epigastric, for those between the Treitz and the hepatic flexure of the colon, it will be umbilical, and for the most distal organs, it will be hypogastric.
- *Parietal*: It is usually acute, due to direct irritation of peritoneum located above the involved organ. The parietal innervation is monolateral, so the pain will be well localized. Only when there is a widespread involvement of peritoneum, as for leak of gastric contents, blood, pus, or other, the pain will be extended to all the abdomen. The peritoneal irritation may cause a reflex contracture of abdominal muscles whereby the abdomen will become stiff and untreatable. The irritant reaction to organic or chemical substances is different, so that the peritonitic pain will be much more striking during gastric perforation with spreading of gastric acid than during colic perforation, with leaking of stool or blood.

- *Referred*: Appears when the afferent fibers from an injured abdominal organ enter the spinal cord at the same level of somatic fibers coming from distant regions (for example, the gallbladder pain can be referred to the right shoulder).

CLINICAL PRESENTATION

Major diseases that cause acute abdomen of immediate surgical interest.

Acute Appendicitis

The *inflammatory process* is due to appendicular lumen obstruction, which can cause an increase in pressure within the lumen with consequent local circulatory dysfunction with ischemia of the wall (catarrhal or phlegmonous form) and necrosis. If perforation of the necrotic bowel wall occurs, appendicitis becomes complicated by perforative peritonitis, localized or diffuse (gangrenous or perforated form), generally caused by aerobic (*Escherichia coli*, *Streptococcus*, and *Staphylococcus*) and anaerobic (*Bacteroides*) bacteria superinfection.

In case of acute inflammation, there will be spontaneous, dull pain, which arises in the epi-mesogastric or periumbilical area. Later, when serosa involvement and peritoneal irritation develop, the pain is localized in the right lower abdominal quadrant. In addition, the pain is exacerbated by the cough and is not modified by body position changes. Vomiting is sometimes present and a low-grade fever (37–38°C) can be detected. Steadily, the patient loses appetite, so that the evaluation of this data is very important for diagnostic exclusion of appendicitis. At the physical examination, pain is evoked by palpating the right lower quadrant (RLQ), or more commonly, Blumberg's sign can be present, but Markle's sign is more sensitive to define a peritoneal irritation. Markle's sign, or jar tenderness, consists in the evocation of pain in RLQ by dropping from standing on the toes to the heels with a jarring landing. In case of suspicion, a white blood cell (WBC) count and C-reactive protein (CRP) detection should be tested since the concomitance of neutrophilic leukocytosis and elevated CRP significantly increases the possible diagnosis of appendicitis.

In the presence of a striking clinical picture, no further tests are necessary, but surgical advice must be activated as soon as possible. In less obvious cases, it is necessary to study the diagnosis more in depth. With an expert operator, ultrasonography (US) has a good specificity, but if this examination is not diagnostic or not reliable, a computed tomography (CT) scan of the abdomen and pelvis must be performed. Then, based on the evidence of direct examination, the radiologist will decide whether to complete CT using intravenous or oral contrast agent.

Intestinal Ischemia

Intestinal ischemia can present itself with three distinct syndromes, of which the first two generally have a favorable prognosis. The first syndrome is *chronic mesenteric ischemia*, determined by gradual reduction of blood supply to the affected intestinal tract, generally due to mesenteric vessels atherosclerosis. This condition is present with postprandial intermittent abdominal pain (angina abdominis). The patient is ill when he eats and consequently tends to reduce food intake and may appear debilitated to medical examination, also considering that elderly subjects are the most affected by the disease.

Ischemic colitis is caused by inadequate vascularization of some colon fragments, not necessarily on atherosclerotic basis, and generally starts as rectorrhagia rather than abdominal pain.

Acute mesenteric ischemia is due to acute thromboembolic occlusion of the celiac tripod, superior or inferior mesenteric artery, which leads to rapid necrosis of a no longer vascularized intestinal region, with subsequent development of a systemic toxic syndrome and exitus if not operated immediately.

The syndrome occurs more often in the presence of risk factors for ischemia. Most frequently, the symptom of onset is a severe periumbilical pain with an abdominal physical examination not proportional to the pain described by the patient. When the intestinal infarction has already been established, signs of peritoneal involvement are present. Rectal bleeding is rare.

Blood tests show signs of dehydration, metabolic acidosis, and multiorgan involvement when the situation is advanced, while in earlier stages, it is possible to detect leukocytosis or increase in D-dimer, but with little specificity. It is important to consider the risk factors and the onset symptoms, as the mortality once the intestinal infarction has been established is approximately 90%.

Acute Diverticulitis

About 30% of people over 50 years and 60% of those over 80 years of age have a diverticular disease that mainly affects the sigmoid colon. Diverticulitis is caused by the inflammation and perforation of the diverticulum, which can be circumscribed and buffered by the mesentery or can be opened with abscess formation or frank peritonitis. The patient presents with cramping abdominal pain, more frequently located in the left lower quadrant (LLQ), but in case of dolichocolon or diverticulosis of the ascending colon, the RLQ can also be affected. Nausea, vomiting, and anorexia are frequently associated. The diagnostic workup, in case of clinical suspicion of diverticular disease, involves a CT scan with intravenous or oral contrast medium (**Fig. 1**), while the colonoscopy is contraindicated when diverticular perforation is suspected. Uncomplicated diverticulitis can be managed at home with antibiotic therapy and liquid diet, while perforation with abscess or peritonitis requires immediate surgical evaluation.

Bowel Obstruction

Intestinal occlusion occurs when a mechanical block prevents progression of intestinal contents. This causes a bowel distension upstream from the obstruction due to the ingested air, the gases produced by the bacteria, and the endoluminal secretions. If the occlusion is not recognized and treated rapidly, ischemia and subsequent necrosis of the intestinal tract will develop. **Table 3** lists the main causes of intestinal obstruction.

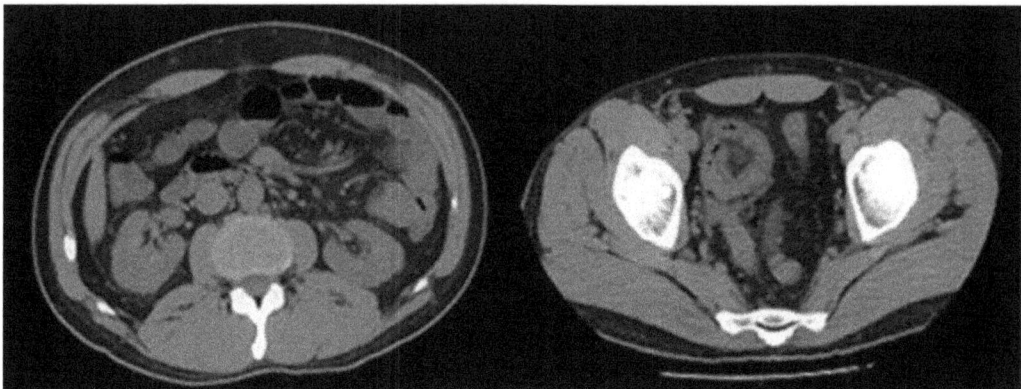

Fig. 1: Contrast enhancement CT scan that highlights the presence of loose ileal loops and with hydroaerial levels, thickening of the wall of the sigma with air bubbles in its context, the surrounding liquid flap. The findings are compatible with a perforated diverticulitis.

Table 3: Main causes of intestinal occlusion*.

• Post laparotomy adhesions
• Incarcerated or strangulated hernia
• Tumors
• Crohn's disease
• Volvulus
• Intussusception
• Calculations
• Ischemia

*The most common causes of obstruction, is constipation with fecalomas.

The abdominal pain is widespread and intermittent, the passage of feces and gases is absent but in the initial stages, diarrhea may be present, caused by the irritation of the mucosa. In advanced stages, vomiting will occur, which may be fecaloid due to bacterial activity.

At the physical examination, the abdomen is distended and painful and the bowel sounds could be increased with metallic sound, reduced or absent. If peritonitis occurs, the abdomen will be rigid with rebound tenderness present. Laboratory tests show hemoconcentration with possible electrolytic imbalances and renal insufficiency. The abdominal plain X-ray makes evident the presence of hydro-air levels, intestinal distention, and absence of air in the rectum (**Figs. 2 and 3**). The diagnostics can be completed with a CT-scan if the clinical condition allows it, which can identify the cause of the occlusion with an approximate sensitivity of 100%. In the event of intestinal obstruction, the surgical evaluation must be timely; however, it is essential to correct fluids and electrolytes imbalances and to decompress the bowel with a nasogastric tube.

Chapter 1: Abdominal Pain (Adult)

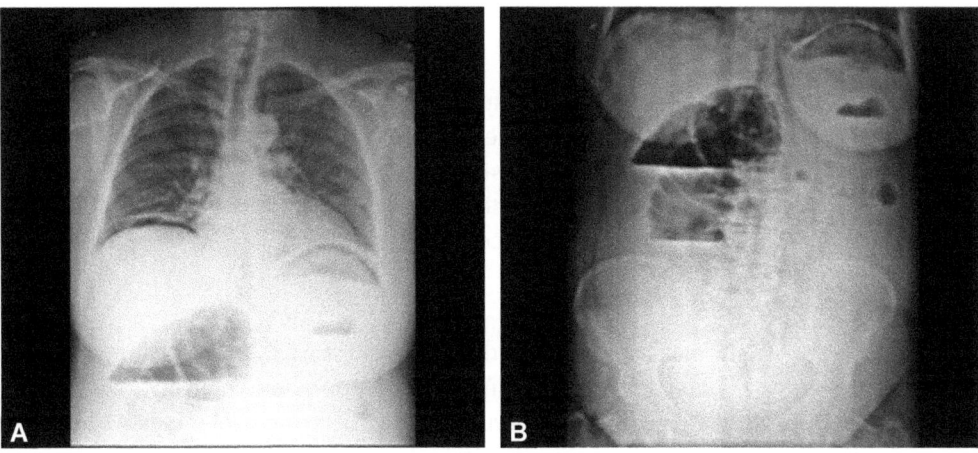

Figs. 2A and B: Plain X-ray of the chest and of the abdomen with evidence of perforation, with typical free gas between the hemidiaphragm and the bowel wall, and hydro-air levels.

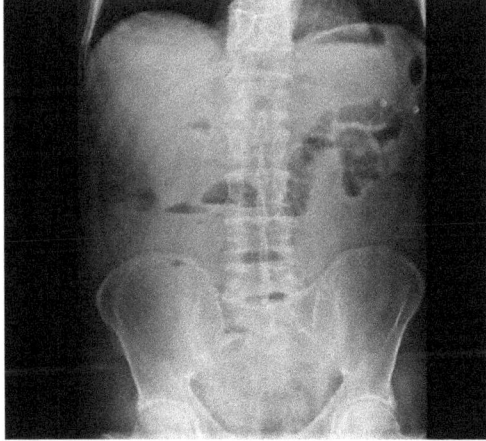

Fig. 3: Plain X-ray of the abdomen with evidence of the classic signs of intestinal occlusion distension of ileal loops, presence of hydro-air levels, absence of air in the rectum.

RED FLAGS

- Signs of shock (e.g. tachycardia, hypotension, diaphoresis, and confusion)
- Severe pain
- Signs of peritonitis
- Abdominal distention
- Attention to nonabdominal diseases that present with abdominal pain (*see* **Table 1**)

■ EVALUATION

Evaluation of mild and severe pain follows the same process, although with severe abdominal pain or important systemic impairment, therapy must precede the other steps, and includes early surgical consultation. Life-threatening conditions should always be ruled out before focusing on less serious diagnoses. In seriously ill patients with severe abdominal pain, an early surgical exploration may be appropriate. In less critical patients, observation and a diagnostic workup are generally the right choice.

History

A thorough history usually suggests the diagnosis. It is necessary to promptly investigate the symptomatology in particular with regard to onset, quality, duration, intensity, radiation, and relationship with meals, causes triggering or attenuating the symptomatology. Of particular importance are characteristics and pain location, associated symptoms, and duration. Concomitant symptoms such as fever, melena, mucus or blood in the stools, hematuria, vomiting, hematemesis, heartburn, nausea, diarrhea, constipation, jaundice, and weight loss help direct subsequent evaluation. Past medical history and medications are essential, taking care that anticoagulants can increase the chances of bleeding and hematoma formation and alcohol predisposes to pancreatitis. Use of nonsteroidal anti-inflammatory drugs is also associated to epigastric pain. Recent antibiotic use if patient experiencing diarrhea. Collect information on the known allergies, on the date and time of the last meal, on any travel and activity employment, and on the use of drugs of abuse.

It is necessary to consider that while in most of cases, an acute abdominal inflammatory process, so as an acute bleeding causes tachycardia, if the process affects the diaphragm wall and therefore, the terminations of the vagus nerve, the patient may have a normal or bradycardic heart rate.

Physical Examination

Vitals signs must be evaluated in all patients as well as level of consciousness. General appearance is important: a sick patient is anxious, pale, diaphoretic, or in obvious pain. The abdomen must be evaluated starting with inspection to evaluate skin color, palpation to check distention of obvious masses, and auscultation of bowel sounds. Decreased bowel sounds suggest functional ileus or mesenteric infarction while hyperactive bowel sounds are present in small bowel obstruction. Palpation starts gently, away from the area of referred pain, detecting areas of particular tenderness, as well as the presence of guarding, rigidity, and rebound (all suggesting peritoneal irritation) and any masses. Voluntary guarding can be diminished by asking patients to flex the knees. Distracting the patient with conversation may divert attention from the examination. The inguinal area and all surgical scars should be palpated for hernias. It is important to look for typical signs like Murphy sign, or stopping the breathing because of the intense pain evoked by palpation of the gallbladder; rebound, or Blumberg sign, indicative of peritoneal irritation, which consists in evoking release pain after

Table 4: Extra-abdominal diseases that can present with abdominal pain.

Cardiac: • Acute myocardial infarction • Aortic aneurysm • Aortic dissection
Dermatological: • Herpes zoster
Endocrinological and metabolic: • Diabetic ketoacidosis • Other acidosis • Addison crisis • Porphyria
Gynecological and obstetric: • Ectopic pregnancy • PID • Ovarian cyst rupture • Ovarian torsion
Hematologic • Familiar mediterranean fever • Sickle cell crisis

deep palpation; the characteristics of the bowel signs. There are controversial opinions on the indication in literature to perform rectal exploration routinely in the patient with abdominal pain. In fact, sensitivity and the specificity of this maneuver are rather low, but the presence of blood in ampoule can suggest diagnosis such as diverticulitis, tumor, and intestinal ischemia, while rectal tenderness poses in differential diagnosis anal fissures, perirectal abscess, and prostatitis.

It is important to consider all the extra-abdominal conditions that can present with abdominal pain (**Table 4**).

INTERPRETATION OF FINDING

Abdominal distention, vomiting, dullness at percussion, and high-pitched peristalsis strongly suggests bowel obstruction.

Severe pain in a patient with a silent abdomen who is lying as still as possible suggests peritonitis; whereas a patient who cannot sit or stand still suggests renal colic.

Back pain and migrant pain with shock suggests ruptured AAA, particularly if there is a tender, pulsatile mass.

Previous abdominal surgery makes obstruction caused by adhesions more likely. Advanced age, generalized atherosclerosis, and hypertension increases the possibility of myocardial infarction, aortic abdominal aneurysm, and mesenteric ischemia.

Shock and vaginal bleeding in a pregnant woman suggest ruptured ectopic pregnancy.

INVESTIGATIONS

Laboratory Tests

Blood tests in abdominal pain should be focused according to clinical evaluation, keeping in mind that specificity and diagnostic accuracy are low.

Among laboratory tests, it is important to include glucose, electrolytes, creatinine, and liver function tests.

A dangerous approach is to rely on "normal" blood test rather than to clinical evidence and avoid observation and reevaluation.

In case of women of childbearing age, pregnancy must be considered, both as cause of the pain (ectopic pregnancy) and for the treatment to use.

Finally, urinalysis, tested by multitask or laboratory, is a routine test: it provides data in suspicion of renal colic, urinary tract infections, or porphyria, to test ketonuria and glycosuria, and to define urine specific gravity.

Arterial blood gas analysis is essential for critically ill patients with abdominal pain: metabolic acidosis and hyperlactatemia, if combined with high levels of creatine phosphokinase and creatinine, must create the suspicion of a systemic involvement, a widespread and advanced pathologic process.

Role of Abdominal X-ray

A standing chest radiograph remains the primary investigation of choice for the detection of free intraperitoneal gas, and may detect lower lobar pneumonia.

Plain abdominal radiography should be used selectively in the event of suspected intestinal obstruction or perforation (*see* **Figs. 2A and B**).

In several studies, the use of abdominal X-ray as first diagnostic step for abdominal pain has shown a very low diagnostic power, being significant only for intestinal obstruction (*see* **Figs. 2 and 3**). In this situation, the sensitivity of abdominal X-ray is 65–90% while specificity is 50–80%. Therefore, even if the CT scan sensitivity and specificity are higher, in the suspicion of intestinal obstruction, the abdomen X-ray is a first level test.

Ingestion of foreign body is another indication for abdomen X-ray, that allows to evaluate the shape, the size, and the position in order to establish the subsequent procedures.

Several studies have shown a higher sensitivity of ultrasound in the suspicion of hollow organ perforation (US 90% vs abdominal X-ray 70%). The only limit is the operator skill.

Role of Ultrasonography and Computed Tomography

Abdominal, contrast enhancement CT scan is the examination with the highest specificity and sensitivity, but bedside ultrasound is now considered the first diagnostic approach in the ED. In most cases, the ultrasound abdominal examination is sufficient to diagnose diseases of the upper right abdominal quadrant (cholecystitis, cholangitis) and in the diagnosis of renal colic, urinary tract infections, and ectopic pregnancy. It is also the fundamental in the diagnosis of aortic syndrome, it is also the fundamental in diagnosis of aortic syndrome and also in diagnosing perforation and intestinal obstruction.

If the ultrasound examination is negative or nondiagnostic but the clinical presentation is persistently altered, it is necessary to perform an abdominal CT scan, generally with the contrast medium, except there are absolute contraindications (history of anaphylactic shock or severe renal impairment). In literature, it is shown that using this method of approach (CT execution to patients with nonconclusive ultrasound), it is possible to reduce the number of CT scan to less than 50%.

TREATMENT

It is still not uncommon to think that treating abdominal pain with analgesic can mask the clinical evidence. On the contrary, it has been widely demonstrated that a correct analgesia facilitates clinical evaluation because it makes the patient better and more collaborative to examination, thus reducing possible complications, increasing the sensitivity of instrumental investigations, without altering the objective framework.

The class of drugs most indicated in the treatment of acute abdominal pain is that are effective, almost without side effects and have an antidote if necessary. Nonsteroidal anti-inflammatory drugs, used extensively in past because considered "safer," are actually burdened from important cardiovascular, gastrointestinal, and renal side effects, particularly in elderly patients. In mild-moderate abdominal pain can be used paracetamol as a first-choice drug.

Antibiotics are indicated in diseases such as peritonitis and abdominal sepsis, urinary tract infections, and pelvic inflammatory disease (PID). Particular attention must be reserved for spontaneous bacterial peritonitis due for gram-positive aerobes.

Remember two nonpharmacologic treatments: (1) nasogastric tube to decompress a bowel obstruction or to confirm a gastrointestinal bleeding and (2) urinary catheter in presence of bladder obstruction or to monitor urinary output in critically ill patient.

SUMMARY

Although patients with abdominal pain in most cases do not have a severe pathology, the symptom may accompany very serious and potentially deadly clinical conditions, if not recognized promptly. Approach to patient with abdominal pain is summarized in **Flowchart 1.**

The knowledge of abdominal anatomy and the careful evaluation of clinical signs and symptoms, together with a precise focused medical history, allows to correctly orient in the diagnosis in 80% of cases.

There are no specific laboratory tests for the various morbid conditions, but the laboratory investigation serves mainly to quantify the degree of systemic involvement of the disease.

The most cost-effective diagnostic-instrumental approach in terms of cost/benefit is represented by the execution of an abdominal focused ultrasound in all patients; abdominal CT scan must be performed only in case of nonconclusive ultrasound.

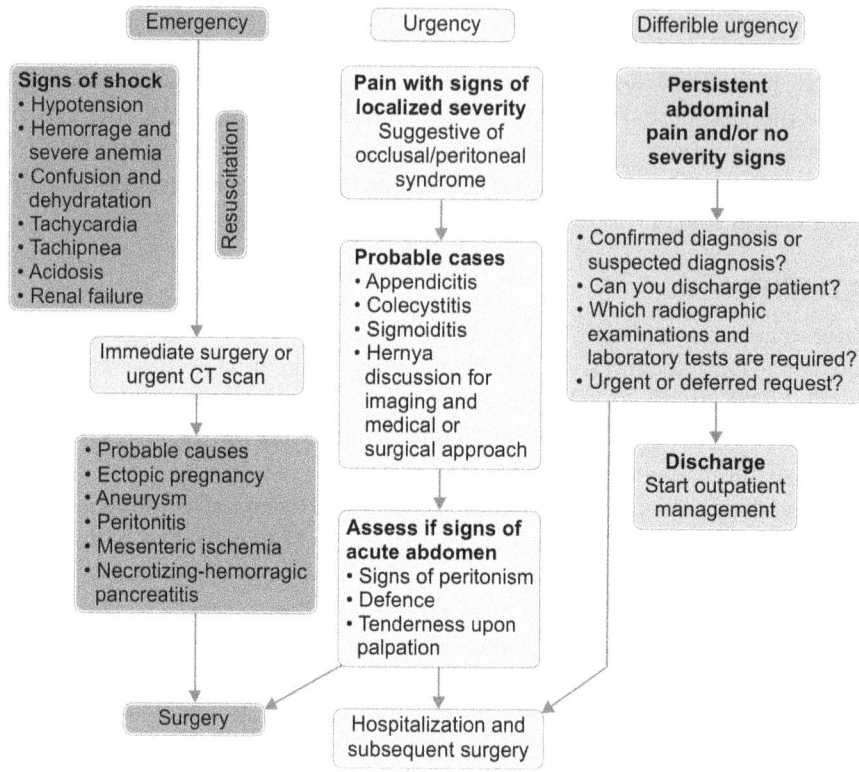

Flowchart 1: Summary of approach to patient with abdominal pain.

Abdominal pain must be treated even before diagnosis, and the use of opioids is safe and recommended.

Also, fluids and electrolytes imbalance must be treated promptly while making the diagnostic workup.

When the diagnosis is uncertain but the patient is still symptomatic, it is often advisable and safe to keep patients under observation to evaluate the possible evolution. Keeping in mind that normal examinations do not exclude an abdominal serious process.

A plain X-ray of the abdomen, which is significant only in the suspicion of intestinal obstruction or perforation.

CHAPTER 2

Abdominal Pain (Acute) in Children

Meera Luthra, Apurva Arora

INTRODUCTION

In children, acute abdominal pain can be the harbinger of acute appendicitis or a presentation of Hirschsprung's disease or can be presentation of a child with pneumonia or a life-threatening illness requiring urgent surgical intervention. Therefore, it is very important to differentiate the cause of the acute abdominal pain in children. This chapter addresses the common causes, red flags, evaluation, and treatment guidelines for a pediatric acute abdomen in the emergency room.

ETIOLOGY

There are numerous medical and surgical causes of acute abdomen in children, out of which only 6% require surgical intervention. In the emergency room, it is a diagnostic challenge to accurately gather all the key signs in a child with severe pain. The most common causes of acute abdominal pain in children are gastroenteritis, mesenteric adenitis, acute appendicitis, colic, obstructed inguinal hernia, ovarian/testicular torsions, intestinal obstruction, and constipation. Various causes of acute abdominal pain are listed in **Table 1**.

PATHOPHYSIOLOGY OF ABDOMINAL PAIN

Essentially, abdominal pain can have three origins. It is more commonly visceral pain or parietal pain and rarely it is referred pain.

Table 1: Causes of acute abdominal pain in children.

Hemodynamically stable (medical causes)	Gastroenteritis Constipation Early stage of acute appendicitis Hemolytic uremic syndrome Acute pneumonia
Hemodynamically unstable (surgical causes) Children are usually in severe pain, sick and signs of shock may be present.	Perforated bowel or appendicitis Intestinal obstruction (volvulus, bands) Intussusception > 24 hours Ovarian/testicular torsion Obstructed and strangulated hernia Trauma

Visceral pain occurs when noxious stimuli affect bowel. Tension, stretching, and ischemia stimulate visceral pain fibers. Tissue congestion and inflammation tend to sensitize nerve endings and lower the threshold for stimuli. Visceral pain fibers are bilateral and unmyelinated and enter the spinal cord at multiple levels, visceral pain usually is dull, poorly localized, and felt in the midline. Pain from foregut structures (e.g. lower esophagus, stomach) generally felt in the epigastrium. Midgut structures (e.g. small intestine) cause periumbilical pain, and hindgut structures (e.g. large intestine) cause lower abdominal pain.

Parietal pain originates from noxious stimulation of the parietal peritoneum. Pain due to ischemia, inflammation, or stretching of the peritoneum is transmitted through myelinated afferent fibers to specific dorsal root ganglia on the same side and at the same dermatomal level as the origin of the pain. Parietal pain usually is sharp, intense, discrete and localized, and coughing or movement can aggravate it.

Referred pain has many of the characteristics of parietal pain but is felt in remote areas supplied by the same dermatome as the diseased organ. It results from shared central pathways for afferent neurons from different sites. A classic example is a patient with pneumonia who presents with abdominal pain because the T9 dermatome distribution is shared by the lung and the abdomen. Pain due to laparoscopic surgeries can be felt in the left shoulder.

CLINICAL PRESENTATION

The challenge for clinician is to identify patient with abdominal pain due to potentially life threatening conditions such as appendicitis, Bowel obstruction (due to volvulus, intussuseption or adhesions) Pancreatitis hepatitis myocartitis or intra-abdomininal mass. Extra-abdominal infections that require specific treatment (such as streptococcal pharyngitis, urinary tract infection, or pneumonia), this is very important to note serious life-threatening signs (red flags) in the early stage (**Table 2**).

If these red flag signs are noted, urgent surgical consult should be obtained and rapid radiological confirmation of the diagnosis is needed before surgical intervention.

EVALUATION

Assess general condition, vitals, and hydration status.

History Taking

It is extremely vital to get an accurate history, although it can sometimes be hearsay in children. The clues we can obtain by simple questioning are—length of current illness, similar episodes in the past, periodicity, colicky nature of pain, aggravating factors. Which came first, pain or vomiting? For example, in surgical causes of acute abdomen, the pain comes before the vomiting, but vice versa in medical causes. Nature of vomiting, whether bilious, also carries significance, as it indicates intestinal obstruction.

Table 2: Red flags of acute abdomen in children.

Red flags	Interpretation
Acute abdomen with septic shock (hypotension, lethargy, tachycardia)	In generalized abdominal sepsis
Bilious vomiting with scaphoid abdomen	Malrotation with volvulus
"Red currant jelly" stools	Classical in intussusception
Generalized guarding/peritonism	Bowel perforation
Irreducible groin swelling	Obstructed inguinal hernias
Testis pulled up into upper scrotum/inguinal region, firm and tender	Testicular torsion
Abdominal distention, tenderness with shock (history of blunt trauma abdomen)	Internal hemorrhage due to solid organ/bowel injury secondary to trauma
Feculent vomitus/obstipation	Intestinal obstruction
Palpable tender abdominal mass	Appendicular mass/abscess
Inability to walk due to abdominal pain	Appendicular/psoas abscess
Hematemesis	Bowel gangrene/portal hypertension
Incessant cry	Bowel strangulation/ischemia/obstruction

Physical Examination

The examiner's technique should be gentle and patient, with both the parent and the child. The examination should end in the area of interest while trying to engage the child in conversation or distraction. A per rectal examination is a must, as it adds diagnostically relevant information regarding the stool, melena, hematochezia, and sphincter tone. Evaluation should be completed by examining the genitalia, testes, and spine of the child. The differential of acute abdominal pain in children is shown in **Table 3**.

INVESTIGATIONS

- X-ray of abdomen—erect/lateral decubitus (in case patient is not ambulatory) and supine
- Ultrasonography (USG) of abdomen
- Computed tomography (CT) of abdomen

X-ray of abdomen is a good diagnostic tool in children with abdominal pain, signs like football sign or Rigler's sign (pneumoperitoneum), multiple air fluid levels indicating bowel obstruction, or the pneumatosis intestinalis gas cysts in bowel wall paucity of bowel gas in volvulus, paucity of rectal gas in Hirschsprung's disease, all are good diagnostic markers of specific disease. X-ray can be used in adjunction with oral contrast also when feasible to confirm certain diagnosis.

Table 3: Differential diagnosis of acute abdomen with regards to the age.

0–1 year	2–5 years	6–10 years	11–15 years
Medical			
Infantile colic	Gastroenteritis	Gastroenteritis	Gastroenteritis
Gastroenteritis	Lower lobe pneumonia	Constipation	Pancreatitis
Constipation	Urinary tract infection	Mesenteric lymphadenitis	Constipation
Urinary tract infection	Henoch-Schönlein purpura	Urinary tract infection	Mittelschmerz
	Constipation	Pneumonia	Pelvic inflammatory disease
	Mesenteric adenitis	Inflammatory bowel disease	Inflammatory bowel disease
	Sickle cell crisis		
Surgical			
Intussusception	Intussusception	Appendicitis	Appendicitis
Obstructed inguinal hernia	Appendicitis	Trauma	Ovarian/testicular torsion
Midgut volvulus	Trauma	Testicular torsion	Trauma
Hirschsprung's disease	Volvulus	Cholecystitis	Hollow viscus perforation
	Ovarian/testicular torsion	Ovarian/testicular torsion	Intestinal obstruction
	Obstructed inguinal hernia	Intestinal obstruction	
	Intestinal obstruction	Hollow viscus perforation	

Ultrasound of abdomen is the standard investigation for the common appendicitis, mesenteric adenitis and intussusception seen in the pediatric emergency room every day. A finding of a nonperistaltic blind ending dilated more than 6 mm in the region of the right iliac fossa is diagnostic of appendicitis. In intussusception, the pseudokidney sign or target sign is the classical finding. When Doppler is added to the USG, malrotation and volvulus can also be picked up, if we see the whirlpool sign. Important modalities of investigation are listed in **Table 4**.

TREATMENT

Treatment should be aimed at the underlying cause of the acute abdomen once the diagnosis is made, till the resuscitative measure should be carried out, for example, intravenous (IV) fluids should be started for dehydrated children according to the metabolic deficit. Urine output assessment can be done by catheterizing the bladder. Nasogastric decompression is advisable

Table 4: Important investigations helpful in acute abdominal pain in children.

Modality	Radiological sign	Interpretation
X-ray abdomen	Football sign/Rigler's sign Multiple air fluid levels Paucity of bowel gas Paucity of rectal gas Pneumatosis intestinalis	Pneumoperitoneum/bowel perforation Intestinal obstruction Midgut volvulus Hirschsprung's disease Necrotizing enterocolitis
USG abdomen	Nonperistaltic blind ending dilated bowel loop > 6 mm in the right iliac fossa (RIF)	Appendicitis
	Pseudokidney sign/target sign	Intussusception
USG abdomen with color Doppler	Whirlpool sign	Midgut volvulus

in children with bilious or feculent vomiting to prevent aspiration of vomitus. Analgesics can be avoided in some situations till the diagnosis is clear, as nature of tenderness can guide the physician. Occasionally an irritable infant may not allow optimal examination unless sedated with oral/nasal/IV sedatives.

CHAPTER 3

Abdominal Pain (Chronic) in Children

Faiz Ahmad, Thiagrajan Jaiganesh

INTRODUCTION

Chronic abdominal pain is defined as at least three episodes of pain over at least 3 months interfering with a child's normal function. In clinical practice, abdominal pain that is more than 2 months in duration is considered chronic abdominal pain.

The term "chronic abdominal pain" encompasses "recurrent abdominal pain" classically defined by four criteria: (1) More than and equal to three episodes of abdominal pain; (2) Pain sufficiently severe to affect activities; (3) Episodes occur over a period of more than and equal to 3 months; and (4) No known organic cause. The prevalence of recurrent abdominal pain in children ranges from 9% to 15%.

Mucosal receptors respond primarily to chemical stimuli (e.g. substance P, bradykinin, serotonin, histamine, and prostaglandins), which are released in response to inflammation or ischemia. Sometimes pain arising in viscera is perceived to originate at a distant site and is called referred pain. This type of pain is due to the sharing of the same spinal cord level by the affected viscera and the affected dermatome. As an example, nociceptive stimuli from the inflamed appendix may be initially perceived in the umbilical area because both the appendix and umbilical area share the same spinal cord level (T10). Actual localization of the pain to the right lower quadrant in patients with acute appendicitis usually occurs when the overlying parietal peritoneum is inflamed.

Chronic abdominal pain in children could result in poor social and education development while placing a significant burden on local health care resources. Therefore, our aim is summarize a variety of childhood disorders that could lead to chronic abdominal pain and provide some diagnostic and treatment strategies.

ETIOLOGY

The two main categories of causes of chronic abdominal pain in children are:
- *Organic disorders*:
  - *Gastrointestinal:* Celiac disease, chemical gastritis, constipation, eosinophilic esophagitis, erosive esophagitis, gallbladder disease, gastroenteritis/colitis, gastroesophageal reflux disease (GERD), helicobacter pylori infection, hiatal hernia, inflammatory bowel disease (IBD), irritable bowel syndrome, pancreatitis, and peptic ulcer.

- *Genitourinary:* Imperforate hymen, menstrual cramps, mittelschmerz, ovarian cyst, endometriosis, pelvic inflammatory disease, recurrent urinary tract infection (UTI), testicular pain, ureteropelvic junction obstruction, and urolithiasis.
- *Metabolic:* Adrenal crisis, diabetic ketoacidosis, and porphyria.
- *Musculoskeletal:* Anterior cutaneous nerve entrapment.
- *Neurologic:* Spinal tumor and transverse myelitis.
- *Other:* Familial Mediterranean fever, lead poisoning, lymphoma, peritoneal abscess/tumor, pneumonia, sickle cell disease, polyarteritis nodosa/vasculitis, and immunoglobulin E (IgE)-mediated food allergy.

- *Functional disorders*: Functional abdominal pain in children can be classified based on recognizable patterns of symptoms.
  - *Functional dyspepsia:* Dyspepsia is pain or discomfort in the epigastric region. Children with dyspepsia and alarm findings should be evaluated for an organic disorder (e.g. peptic ulcer disease).
  - *Irritable bowel syndrome (IBS):* It is characterized by chronic abdominal pain and altered bowel habits (diarrhea or constipation) in the absence of any alarm findings.
  - *Abdominal migraine:* It is characterized by recurrent episodes of abdominal pain for at least 6 months, usually in the midline or poorly localized, moderate to severe in intensity and is associated with at least two more features including anorexia, nausea, vomiting, headache, photophobia, and pallor. A family history of a migraine headache is common.

PATHOPHYSIOLOGY

The pathophysiology of functional abdominal pain is likely due to the involvement of the enteric nervous system (ENS), also known as "gut brain." Pain receptors in the abdomen respond to mechanical or chemical stimuli. Stretch is the major mechanical stimulus involved in visceral pain which is induced by distension, contraction, traction, compression, and torsion.

CLINICAL PRESENTATION

The clinical presentation could be varied, but one should pay attention to the *"red flags"* as they may indicate an organic cause. Organic pathology is identified in approximately 1 in 10 children who present with chronic and or recurrent abdominal pain. The signs and symptoms that could suggest underlying organic pathology are:
- Nocturnal or chronic diarrhea
- Deceleration of linear growth
- Delayed puberty
- Dysphagia
- Family history of inflammatory bowel, celiac or peptic ulcer disease
- Gastrointestinal blood loss
- Genitourinary tract symptoms
- Involuntary weight loss

- Pain that wakes the child from sleep
- Persistent right upper or lower quadrant pain
- Significant vomiting
- Recurrent unexplained fevers.

EVALUATION

The initial evaluation of chronic abdominal pain includes history, physical examination, and stool guaiac for occult blood to determine if the child has any *"red flags"* that can help in distinguishing organic from functional abdominal pain and direct the need for additional evaluation.

History

It is important to ask specifically about the alarm findings:
- Unexplained fever or weight loss
- Painful swallowing or difficulty swallowing
- Vomiting—bilious, protracted, projectile, or worrisome
- Diarrhea—severe and chronic (lasting > 2 weeks and > 20 mL/kg/day), bloody or nocturnal
- Back pain
- Urinary symptoms
- Family history of IBD, celiac disease, or peptic ulcer disease
- Skin changes (e.g. hives, eczema, and rash).

Asking the patient/family to keep the pain diary regarding the time of the day the pain started, pain location and severity, pain duration, triggering factors, and interventions if any and if they were helpful.

Physical Examination

A thorough physical examination may help in the diagnosis of chronic abdominal pain. General appearance and level of discomfort may indicate the severity of abdominal pain. Alarm findings on examination include:
- Deceleration in linear growth
- Anemia
- Oral ulcers or perianal skin tag, fissure or fistula
- Localized abdominal pain, suprapubic tenderness, or costovertebral angle tenderness
- Delayed puberty
- Hepatosplenomegaly
- Guaiac-positive stool
- Joint swelling or tenderness
- Hypertension
- Carnett sign—helps to differentiate visceral from abdominal wall pain. With the child in a supine position, ask him or her to cross the arms and sit halfway forward. A focal

tenderness that increases and or remains the same during abdominal wall contraction (i.e. positive Carnett sign) suggests pain originating in the abdominal wall (e.g. hematoma, hernia, muscular pain, and anterior cutaneous nerve entrapment syndrome).
- Psoas sign—pain on hyperextension of the hip is suggestive of inflammation of psoas muscle (e.g. psoas abscess).
- Delayed puberty may be a clue to organic disease (e.g. IBD); absence of menarche despite sexual maturity may be a clue to hematocolpos.

INVESTIGATIONS

Careful and detailed history and physical examination in combination with judicious and selective use of diagnostic studies is required to delineate the underlying cause of chronic abdominal pain in children. Routine testing in patients with chronic abdominal pain without any *"red flag or alarm findings"* is not useful, though it may be reassuring for the parents. A 2005 systematic review found little or no evidence to suggest that laboratory, ultrasonography, endoscopy or esophageal pH monitoring increases the yield of organic disease in the absence of "red flags/alarm findings."

Laboratory tests to consider in patients with alarm findings are:
- Complete blood count with differential for anemia or infection
- C-reactive protein or erythrocyte sedimentation rate for inflammation or infection
- Metabolic panel
- Liver function test
- Lipase
- Pregnancy test
- Tissue transglutaminase antibody for screening celiac disease
- Thyroid stimulating hormone and free thyroxine (T4) to evaluate for hypothyroidism as a cause of chronic constipation
- Urinalysis and culture for UTI
- Stool guaiac test for gastrointestinal bleeding, stool ova, and parasite
- Helicobacter pylori stool antigen or urea breath test
- The fecal calprotectin test had a pooled sensitivity of 92% and a pooled specificity of 76% for IBD
- A child with weight loss, anemia, and blood in the stool should be evaluated for Crohn disease because these conditions have a cumulative sensitivity of 94% for Crohn disease in children
- Abdominal radiography may be helpful in the diagnosis of obstruction, foreign body or constipation
- Abdominal ultrasound—abnormalities are found in about 10% of children who have jaundice, persistent fever, urinary symptoms, significant weight loss, back or flank pain, vomiting, abnormal abdominal examination findings, abdominal pain away from midline, and gastrointestinal bleeding, compared with less than 1% of those without these findings
- Pelvic ultrasonography—to evaluate ovarian masses or pregnancy

- Upper gastrointestinal series—to assess bowel obstruction
- Computed tomography of the abdomen with contrast to evaluate retroperitoneal or intraperitoneal abscess; usually reserved for urgent evaluation because of the risk of exposure to radiation in young children
- Magnetic resonance enterography if IBD is suspected
- Endoscopy—esophagogastroduodenoscopy and colonoscopy with ileoscopy (if Crohn's disease is suspected).

Diagnosis of functional abdominal pain can be made without additional diagnostic testing in children with chronic abdominal pain who meet the following criteria:
- No alarm findings
- Normal physical examination
- Stool sample negative for occult blood.

TREATMENT

Treatment depends on the cause of pain and whether the abdominal pain is organic or functional. The primary goal of therapy is improving quality of life, reducing parent and child concern about the seriousness of the condition, and reducing disability associated with pain rather than complete resolution of pain. In children with functional abdominal pain, use of probiotics, such as lactobacillus, reduces the intensity and frequency of abdominal pain and is safe for children.

Cognitive behavior therapy is an evidence-based psychosocial method that focuses on changing the patterns of thinking that cause unwanted behaviors. Hypnotherapy is another promising psychological therapy in which a hypnotized child visualizes relaxing images to ease symptoms such as pain and anxiety. Gut-directed hypnotherapy demonstrates sustained long-term effects, with continued pain relief 5 years after treatment in 68% of the patients.

Following interventions may be beneficial as supportive management in the following situations
- Acid reflux—antacid and H_2 receptor antagonists.
- Dyspepsia—proton pump inhibitors, including lansoprazole and pantoprazole, are safe and effective for the treatment of dyspepsia in children, with the improvement of pain in more than 70% of patients.
- Celiac disease—a gluten-free diet should be initiated.
- Inflammatory bowel disease—children should be referred to a pediatric gastroenterologist for anti-inflammatory medications and biologics.
- Chronic constipation—treatment includes dietary interventions, such as increased fluids, fiber, and prune, pear, and apple juices; behavioral interventions, including regular toilet time for five or 10 minutes after meals and use of stool diaries; reward system; and parental education. Polyethylene glycol is the first-line therapy for children. Magnesium hydroxide is another option. Severe constipation may require manual disimpaction, enemas (e.g. saline, mineral oil, and polyethylene glycol), suppositories (e.g. bisacodyl and glycerin) or other laxatives (e.g. magnesium citrate, lactulose, sorbitol, docusate, and mineral oil).

SUMMARY

- Chronic abdominal pain is defined as intermittent or constant abdominal pain that has been present for at least 2 months.
- Two major categories of chronic abdominal pain are organic disorders and functional disorders.
- The initial evaluation of chronic abdominal pain includes history, physical examination, and stool guaiac test. If there are no "alarm findings," no further evaluation is necessary in most cases.
- Patients with alarm findings require additional laboratory and imaging studies to look for organic causes.

CHAPTER 4

Anal Fissure

Ashok Puranik

INTRODUCTION

Anal fissure is a tear in anoderm distal to the dentate line, which may be acute or chronic. Acute fissure is a simple laceration, whereas a chronic anal fissure is an ulceration with scarred edges and visible internal sphincter muscles at its base with anal tag and hypertrophied papilla at the dentate line. Anal fissure almost always occurs in mid-line with posterior location predominance (90% in women and 99% in men). Fissures located at other than these sites often indicate some serious systemic pathology like Crohn's disease, human immunodeficiency viruses (HIV), leukemia, and other immune-deficiency syndromes.

ETIOLOGY

Etiology of fissure-in-ano is probably trauma because of passing hard stool or prolonged diarrhea. Prior anal injury or surgery leading to stenosis, stricture, or scarring is a predisposing factor. Various theories about the cause have been proposed, among them theory of vascular anatomy of internal anal sphincter is most compelling.

In 1989, Klosterhalfen et al. reported the anatomical detail of branches of inferior hemorrhoidal artery. In this study, they found that in 85% of cadaveric specimens, the posterior commissure of anal canal was not directly perfused, rather they received blood supply from end arterioles. So, there is poor perfusion of mucosa in posterior mid-line along with this sphincteric spasm and hypertonicity which is common in this disease may further decrease blood flow in posterior mid-line. Schouten et al. have shown correlation between increased anal tone and decreased vascularity by using laser Doppler flowmeter.

Infections also cause fissure-in-ano over the last century. Syphilis and tuberculosis were seen frequently in United States, but are currently uncommon. Today, sexually transmitted infections (STIs) and infections associated with immunocompromised state may be a cause of fissure-in-ano like chancroid, herpes simplex virus (HSV), and CMV-HSV usually present as multiple superficial ulcers, while syphilitic ulcers have purulent discharge with granulation at the base. So, it is very important to properly diagnose the disease because treatments of these conditions are different.

DIAGNOSIS

A burning pain or tearing pain while defecation is the most common symptom of anal fissure. Bleeding is usually only detected on toilet paper. Pain may last for minutes to hours. The examination should be gentle by separating the buttocks. Patients are often intolerant to digital rectal examination (DRE) and proctoscopy. Topical anesthesia do not provide free examination. Atypical location of fissure requires more intensive history taking and investigation to rule out Crohn's disease, HIV, and other immunodeficiency diseases.

MANAGEMENT

Nonsurgical

Conservative Management

First-line treatment for simple acute fissure-in-ano is warm sitz bath with stool softeners. Warm water lowers the discomforts by muscle relaxation, while stool softeners prevent trauma to the mucosa by loosening the stool. Stool softeners like Psyllium, bran, and fiber draws water and retains them in stool making it soft. Furthermore, bran has been shown to be effective in preventing recurrence of acute anal fissure. Topical creams and steroids have limited role in management and not routinely recommended. These conservative managements successfully heal 90% of acute fissures and 40% of chronic fissures.

Nitroglycerine

Nitroglycerine is a nitric oxide donor and nitric oxide is a potent smooth muscle relaxant, leading to vasodilatation and as the suggested etiology of anal fissure is increased anal tone and poor vascularity in posterior anal canal. So, nitric oxides promote healing of fissure and immediate relief (5 minutes) of pain and spasm.

Headache is a significant side effect of nitroglycerine, which limits its use. Other side effects are orthostatic hypotension, syncopal attack, and tachyphylaxis. These are uncommon side effects.

Calcium Channel Blockers

Nifedipine and diltiazem can be used as agents of "chemical sphincterotomy." Topical nifedipine reduces sending anal tone and then facilitates healing and relieves pain. 2% topical diltiazem is equally effective as nitroglycerine. Topical diltiazem can heal up to 75% of anal fissure that have failed to heal by nitroglycerine alone. This class of drug supersedes nitroglycerine in treatment of chronic anal fissure because of better effectiveness and better side-effect profile.

Botulinum Toxin (Botox)

Another alternative for "chemical sphincterotomy" is botulinum toxin A, an exotoxin produced by *Clostridium botulinum* that prevents the release of acetyl choline from presynaptic vesicles leading to muscle paralysis. It is an effective treatment option for chronic anal fissures. In one study, 75% of chronic anal fissures healed at 8 weeks with no recurrence in 16 months follow-up.

Complication of this form of treatment are infrequent and includes transient incontinence mainly flatus and perianal hematoma formation.

Surgical Management

Lateral internal anal partial sphincterotomy (LIS) is done in patients who fail to respond to nonsurgical management option. This procedure was originally described by Eisenhammer in 1951 as a mid-line posterior incision through the fissure. But subsequent studies found problems with wound healing and formation of a "keyhole" deformity. "Keyhole" deformity is a persistent groove in the mid-line after posterior division of sphincter, it causes problems like anal seepage and incontinence. Subsequent modification to this procedure lead to repositioning of the incision to the right or left lateral position, which has effectively eliminated the complication of this deformity.

Fissurectomy is the excision of the anal fissure. This procedure results in defect in anoderm which can be covered with a rotational or advancement flap to avoid "keyhole" deformity.

Calibrated balloon dilation is also an effective technique for the management of chronic anal fissures. In a study comparing LIS with pneumatic balloon dilation, they found fissures healing rate 83.3% in pneumatic balloon dilation group and 92% in LIS group. At 24 months follow-up, incontinence was zero in pneumatic balloon dilation group and 16% in LIS group. So, pneumatic balloon dilation is also a safe and efficacious method.

CHAPTER 5

Anemia

Khusrav Bajan, Evith Pereira

INTRODUCTION

Anemia (French for an—not and haem—blood) is considered to present, if the hemoglobin concentration or hematocrit is below the lower limit of 95% reference interval for the individual's age, sex, and geographical location.

The Papyrus Ebers (ancient treaties of therapeutics) dating 1550 BC recognized pallor, edema, and breathlessness as a clinical entity. "Panduroga" described by Charak in Charak Samhita way back in 1000 BC describes pallor, emaciation, fatigue, and skin changes.

DEFINITION

Anemia is defined as a reduction of the total circulating red cell mass below normal limits. It is also defined as a hemoglobin concentration in the blood below the lower limit of the normal range for the age and sex of the individual. In adults, the lower extreme of the normal hemoglobin is taken as 13.0 g/dL for males and 11.5 g/dL for females.

A World Health Organization (WHO) categorized anemia in various population subgroup as per **Table 1** given below

CLASSIFICATION OF ANEMIA

Various classification of anemia are proposed on the basis of etiology, cell morphology and hemoglobin.

Table 1: WHO criteria for anemia.

	Hb (g/dL)	Hematocrit
Adult males	13	39
Adult females (nonpregnant)	12	36
Adult female (pregnant)	11	33
Children (12–14 years)	12	36
Children (5–11 years)	11.5	34
Children (6–59 months)	11	33

(Hb: hemoglobin; WHO: World Health Organization)

Etiological Classification

Blood Loss
- *Acute blood loss*: Trauma
- *Chronic blood loss*: Gastrointestinal tract lesions and gynecologic disturbances.

Increased Red Cell Destruction
- *Inherited genetic defects:*
    - Red cell membrane disorders: Hereditary spherocytosis and hereditary elliptocytosis.
    - Enzyme deficiencies:
        * Hexose monophosphate shunt enzyme deficiencies—glucose-6-phosphate dehydrogenase (G6PD) deficiency and glutathione synthetase deficiency
        * Glycolytic enzyme deficiencies—pyruvate kinase deficiency and hexokinase deficiency.
- *Hemoglobin abnormalities*:
    - Deficient globin synthesis—thalassemia syndromes
    - Structurally abnormal globins (hemoglobinopathies)—sickle cell disease and unstable hemoglobins.
- *Acquired genetic defects:*
    - Deficiency of phosphatidylinositol-linked glycoproteins—paroxysmal nocturnal hemoglobinuria.
- Antibody-mediated destruction—hemolytic disease of the newborn, transfusion reaction, drug-induced, and autoimmune disorders.
- *Mechanical trauma*:
    - Microangiopathic hemolytic anemia—hemolytic uremic syndrome, disseminated intravascular coagulation, and thrombotic thrombocytopenic purpura.
    - Cardiac traumatic hemolysis—defective cardiac valves
    - Repetitive physical trauma—bongo drumming, marathon running, and karate chopping
- Infections of red cells—malaria and babesiosis
- Toxic or chemical injury—clostridial sepsis, snake venom, and lead poisoning.
- Membrane lipid abnormalities—abetalipoproteinemia and severe hepatocellular liver disease
- Sequestration—hypersplenism.

Decreased Red Cell Production
- *Inherited genetic defects*:
    - Defects leading to stem cell depletion—Fanconi anemia and telomerase defects
    - Defects affecting erythroblast maturation—thalassemia syndromes.
- *Nutritional deficiencies:*
    - Deficiencies affecting deoxyribonucleic acid (DNA) synthesis—B_{12} and folate deficiencies
    - Deficiencies affecting hemoglobin synthesis—iron deficiency anemia.

- Erythropoietin deficiency—renal failure and anemia of chronic disease
- Immune-mediated injury of progenitors—aplastic anemia and pure red cell aplasia
- Inflammation-mediated iron sequestration—anemia of chronic disease
- Primary hematopoietic neoplasms—acute leukemia, myelodysplasia, and myeloproliferative disorders
- Space-occupying marrow lesions—metastatic neoplasms and granulomatous disease
- Infections of red cell progenitors—parvovirus B_{19} infection
- Unknown mechanisms—endocrine disorders and hepatocellular liver disease.

Morphological Classification (Table 2)
- Microcytic hypochromic anemia—mean corpuscular hemoglobin (MCV) < 80 fL and mean corpuscular hemoglobin concentration (MCHC) < 30 g/dL
- Normocytic normochromic anemia—MCV and MCHC within normal range

Table 2: Morphological types of anemia and its causes.

Morphological types	Causes
Microcytic (MCV < 80 fL): • Decreased Hb • Decreased Hct • Decreased MCV • Decreased MCH • Increased RDW	• Iron deficiency • Anemia of chronic disorder • Thalassemia • Sideroblastic anemia
Macrocytic (MCV > 100 fL): • Decreased Hb • Decreased Hct • Increased MCV • Increased MCH • Increased RDW	• B_{12} deficiency • Folic acid deficiency • Pernicious anemia • Alcoholism • Chronic liver disease • Hypothyroidism • *Drugs*: Methotrexate, etc.
Normocytic (MCV 80–100 fL): • Decreased Hb • Decreased Hct • Normal MCV • Normal MCH • Normal RDW	• Hemolytic anemia • Aplastic anemia • Acute blood loss • *Chronic disease*: RA, SLE

(Hb: hemoglobin; Hct: hematocrit; MCH: mean corpuscular hemoglobin; MCV: mean corpuscular volume; RA: rheumatoid arthritis; RDW: red cell distribution width; SLE: systemic lupus erythematosus)

Table 3: Hemoglobin levels to diagnose anemia at sea level (g/dL).

Population	Nonanemia	Anemia		
		Mild anemia	Moderate anemia	Severe anemia
Children 6–59 months	>11.0	10.0–10.9	7.0–9.9	<7.0
Children 5–11 years	>11.5	11.0–11.4	8.0–10.9	<8.0
Children 12–14 years	>12.0	11.0–11.9	8.0–10.9	<8.0
Nonpregnant women (15 years of age and above)	>12.0	11.0–11.9	8.0–10.9	<8.0
Pregnant women	>11.0	10.0–10.9	7.0–9.9	<7.0
Men (15 years and above)	>13.0	11.0–12.9	8.0–10.9	<8.0

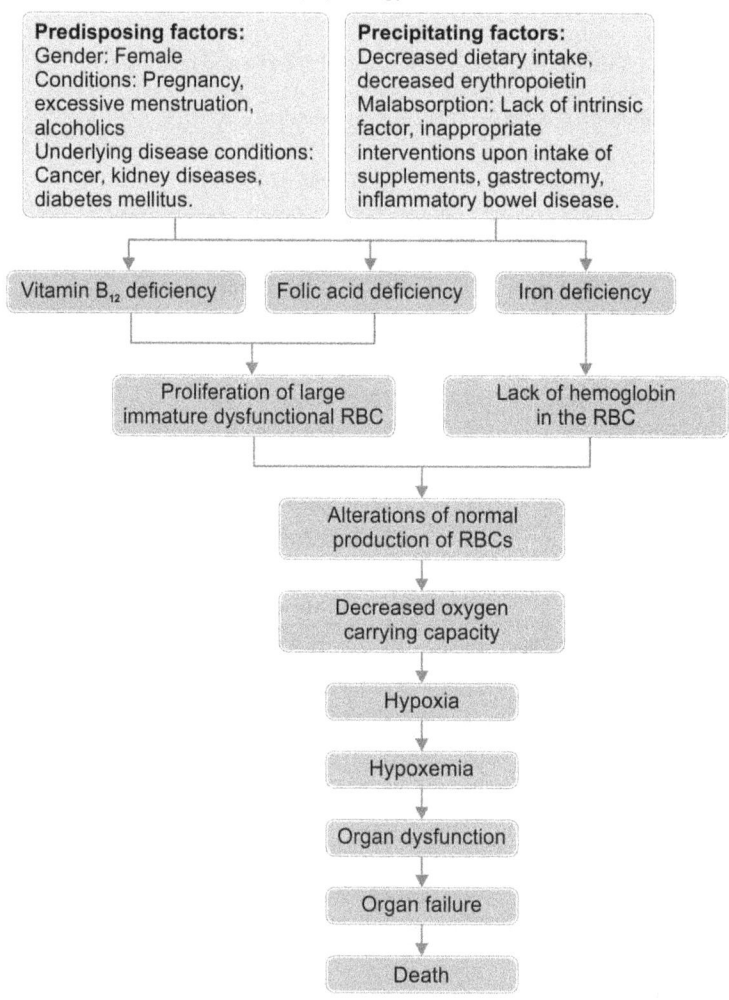

Flowchart 1: Pathophysiology of nutritional anemia.

- Macrocytic anemia—MCV > 96 fL
- Dimorphic anemia.

Classification depending on Hemoglobin

WHO has further classify anemia as mild, moderate, and severe in various age groups (**Table 3**).

▌PATHOPHYSIOLOGY OF ANEMIA

Aanemia is basically due to nutritional deficiency and acute blood loss. **Flowchart 1** describes the pathophysiology of nutritional anemia.

The clinical manifestations of acute blood volume loss reflect adjustments in cardiac output and vascular tone that helps in preventing circulatory collapse and maintaining oxygen supply to vital organs (**Table 4**).

▌APPROACH TO ANEMIA

In a clinical setting evaluation of anemia starts with simple blood test such as complete blood count (**Flowchart 2**),further anemia can be differentiated on the basis of MCV and RDW (**Table 5**).

▌INVESTIGATIONS

Initial investigations to define the underlying cause of anemia include examination of the peripheral blood smear, reticulocyte count and red cell indices. Depending upon these studies further specialized laboratory procedures may be carried out to arrive at definitive diagnosis such as bone marrow examination, determination of serum iron and total iron binding capacity, hemoglobin electrophoresis, biochemical investigations, etc. (**Flowchart 3**).

Table 4: Reaction to acute blood loss of increasing severity.

Total blood volume	Volume lost up to	
	mL	Clinical signs
10	500	None. Rarely vasovagal syncope in blood bank donors.
20	1,000	Impossible to detect volume loss with patient at rest. Tachycardia and postural drop in blood pressure may be evident.
30	1,500	Neck veins are flat when patient is supine. Postural hypotension and exercise tachycardia is present, but resting, supine blood pressure and pulse can be normal.
40	2,000	Central venous pressure, cardiac output, and arterial blood pressure are below normal even when patient is in supine position. Patient usually demonstrates air hunger, a rapid, thready pulse and cold, clammy skin.
50	2,500	Severe shock and death.

Flowchart 2: A simplified approach for evaluation of anemia based on complete blood count.

```
                     Complete blood count
                              ↓
                      Low hemoglobin
                              ↓
                          Anemia
                      ↙            ↘
    Associated abnormalities of     Abnormalities restricted
    white cells and platelets present   to red cell series
              ↓                             ↓
    Bone marrow examination          Reticulocyte count
    (Megaloblastic anemia, aplastic      ↙        ↘
    anemia, myelodysplasia,           Raised    Not raised appropriate
    hematological malignancies)                 to degree of anemia
                                        ↓              ↓
                            Investigate for blood loss,  Red cell Indices
                            hemolytic anemia
                                             ↙     ↓     ↘
                              Microcytic anemia  Normocytic anemia  Macrocytic anemia
```

Table 5: Differential diagnosis of anemias on the basis of MCV and RDW.

MCV	RDW	*Causes*
Low	Normal	Thalassemia carrier, anemia of chronic disease
Low	High	Iron deficiency anemia, hemoglobin H disease, sickle cell-β thalassemia
High	Normal	Myelodysplastic syndrome, aplastic anemia
High	High	Megaloblastic anemia, immune hemolytic anemia
Normal	Normal	Anemia of chronic disease, sickle cell trait, hereditary spherocytosis
Normal	High	Early iron deficiency anemia or megaloblastic anemia, sickle cell anemia, myelofibrosis, sideroblastic anemia.

(MCV: mean corpuscular volume; RDW: red cell distribution width)

Flowchart 3: Investigations to define causes of anemia.

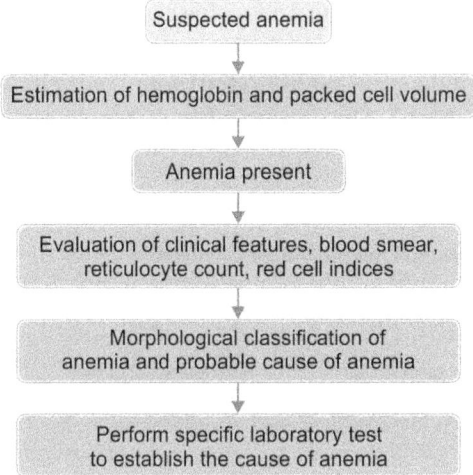

Flowchart 4: Evaluation and treatment of anemia due to blood loss.

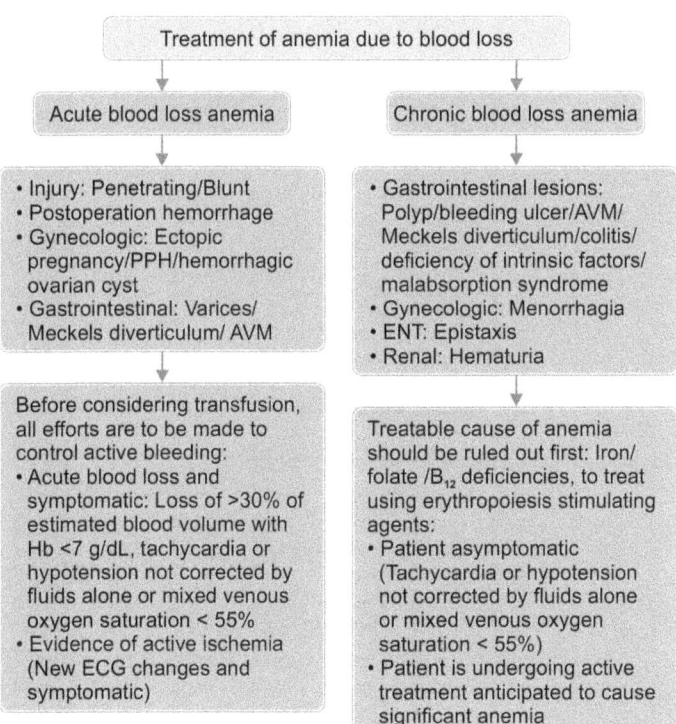

(AVM: arteriovenous malformation; ECG: electrocardiogram; ENT: ear, nose, and throat; Hb: hemoglobin; PPH: postpartum hemorrhage)

TREATMENT

Treatment of anemia varies according to underlying cause. Iron suppliment are prescribed for iron defficiency anemia.Vitamin B is prescribed in patient with low vitamin levels. Anemia due to blood loss should be evaluated as per **Flowchart 4** and red cell should be transfused as per guidelines shown in **Flowchart 5**. Any adverse effect of blood transfusion (**Flowchart 6**) must be treated promptly.

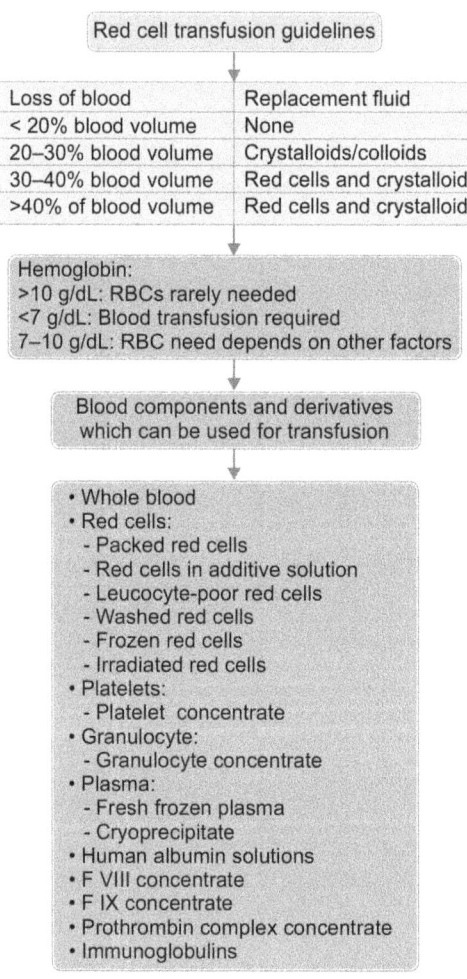

Flowchart 5: Blood transfusion guidlines

Flowchart 6: Overview of adverse events of blood transfusion.

```
                    Adverse effects of blood transfusion
                                    │
                ┌───────────────────┴───────────────────┐
                ▼                                       ▼
    Immediate complications:                Delayed complications:
    • Immunological:                        • Immunological:
      - Febrile nonhemolytic                  - Hemolytic transfusion
        transfusion reactions                   reactions
      - Hemolytic transfusion                 - Post-transfusion
        reactions                               purpura
      - Allergic reactions                    - Graft vs host
      - Anaphylactic reaction                   disease
      - Transfusion associated              • Nonimmunological:
        lung injury                           - Transmission of
    • Nonimmunological                         infectious organisms
      - Circulatory overload                  - Iron overload
      - Bacterial contamination
        of donor blood unit
                │
                ▼
    Complications associated with massive transfusion protocol:*
    • Dilution of platelets causing thrombocytopenia
    • Dilutional coagulopathy
    • Prolonged prothrombin time
    • Prolonged activated partial thromboplastin time
    • Hyperkalemia
    • Hypocalcemia
    • Hypothermia
    • Microaggregates of platelets and leucocytes causing
      respiratory distress syndrome
```

*Massive transfusion protocol (MTP) as per the 10th edition ATLS manual is defined as a need for 10 units of packed cells in 24 hours or 4 units of packed cells in one hour.

SUMMARY

Anemia is a common presenting feature in the ER. Although it has protean etiology, a single Hb report is of no significance. A trend in the Hb, its association with the other complete blood count parameters, and its correlation with the clinical condition of the patient needs to be evaluated in a concerted manner.

CHAPTER 6

Ankle Sprain

Sanjay Shah, Chintan Thanki

INTRODUCTION

Plantar flexion and dorsiflexion are the two basic movements of the ankle joint as a hinge joint. However along with other joints around the ankle, with inversion, eversion, internal rotation and external rotation, its range of motion (ROM) becomes similar to that of a ball and socket joint. With several possible movements, and supporting several ligaments, the ankle joint remains a complex region to understand. In patients with ankle sprain, a common history is that of twisting of the foot with ankle pain. Usually patients are able to walk, thereby ruling out fracture. Absence of paresthesias and cold limb would rule out neurovascular damage.

The most common injury is at the lateral ankle complex involving the anterior talofibular, calcaneofibular, and posterior talofibular ligaments. The most commonly injured ligaments are the anterior and the posterior talofibular ligaments. The most common type of sprain is inversion sprain of the lateral ligaments comprising up to 85% of sprains.

Up to 30% of sports injuries are ankle sprains thereby making it the most common reported musculoskeletal injury. This number may be lesser than the actual number of cases since it is also common that ankle sprains frequently go unreported due to the patients' ability to bear weight and the possibility of self-treatment. Studies have shown that ankle sprains are associated with sports such as football, volleyball, basketball, and soccer. Ankle sprains are more common in females among general population and are more common in males among athletes.

ETIOLOGY

Ankle sprain is a result of mechanical injury beyond the tensile limits of the surrounding ligaments. There are several factors that may lead to ankle sprain. These include poor muscular strength, shortened joint capsule, overweight/obesity, inexperience in a complex physical act and/or mechanical accidents.

Some patients have a tendency for recurrent ankle sprains. There is no specific etiology; however, it is believed that frequent physical activity that puts ankle ligaments at risk in an incompletely healed condition, and the lengthening of the previously injured ligaments due to scar tissue may be responsible. Studies have suggested that recurrent sprains are secondary to reduced proprioception. Furthermore, patients with previous ankle sprains exhibit delayed peroneal reaction time.

PATHOPHYSIOLOGY

Forced internal rotation and/or plantar flexion can cause rupture to the anterior talofibular ligament (ATFL), while forced dorsiflexion can lead to posterior talofibular ligament injury. Forced external rotation can lead to calcaneofibular ligament (CFL) injury. The deltoid ligament with its superficial and deep components is usually the strongest of all ligaments and before its rupture usually the medial malleolus is already fractured. The syndesmotic ligament with its deep and superficial anterior and posterior portions is also uncommonly injured. However, once injured, this ligament should be repaired surgically.

There are three grades of ankle sprains based on severity:
1. *Grade I ankle sprains*: They have the ligament stretched with no macroscopic tearing. There is no inability to bear weight.
2. *Grade II ankle sprains*: They have partial tearing of the ligament with risk of joint instability and difficulty to bear weight.
3. *Grade III ankle sprains*: They have complete tearing of the ligament with swelling, inability to bear weight, and risk of joint instability. Grade III sprains lead to impaired foot reflexes and foot gives way easily.
   This grading system cannot be used when more than one ligament is injured.

Biological ligament healing is described into three different phases:
1. *Inflammatory phase*: until 10 days after trauma
2. *Proliferation phase*: 4–8 weeks
3. *Remodeling or maturation phase*: until 1 year after trauma.

CLINICAL PRESENTATION AND RED FLAGS

Common signs and symptoms of ankle sprain are pain, swelling, paresthesias, and coldness of the affected limb. Details regarding history and clinical examination have been described here under "Evaluation." Further, grade III sprains lead to impaired foot reflexes.

Effective patient education can be a useful strategy in preventing ankle sprains. Keywords for patient education in preventative self-care for ankle sprain include PRICES: protection, rest, ice, compression, elevation, and support. Furthermore, certain red flags should be explained to the patients in order to encourage them for prompt review and early management.
- Movement of joint beyond its normal ROM
- Abnormal bending or deformity of joint or bone
- Excessive pain and/or severe swelling
- Non-weight-bearing beyond 3 days
- Coldness, bluish discoloration, and/or numbness of distal extremity.

■ EVALUATION: HISTORY AND PHYSICAL EXAMINATION

History

The typical history for ankle sprain is twisting of the foot followed by pain and swelling. Patient should be asked about past ankle injuries, mechanism of the injury, rapidly worsening pain, swelling and bruising, paresthesias or coldness of the limb. As with any case of trauma, a targeted history should be applied to rule out any evidence of head injury, headache, loss of consciousness, seizure, vomiting, ear, nose and throat (ENT) bleed, amnesia, and any injury elsewhere in the body. Patient should be asked regarding any comorbidities, ongoing medications, any significant illnesses in the past and related complicating conditions such as arthritis or any joint-related conditions, diabetes, vascular, and connective tissue diseases.

Physical Examination

Physical examination can help in diagnosing ankle sprain and ruling out fracture; and the classic look-feel-move approach can be implemented. The ATFL and CFL ligaments may be really tender. Generally, the degree of swelling may be directly proportional to the probability of fracture, whereas the location of ecchymoses may not necessarily correlate with the site of injury since blood may have flown and settled elsewhere. Bony tenderness should be assessed at medial and lateral malleoli, base of 5th metatarsal and midfoot, along with any deformity or crepitus in order to rule in favor of a fracture. Furthermore, the ROM should be assessed. Neurovascular damage of the limb should also be assessed. This includes palpation of the dorsalis pedis and the posterior tibial arteries. Sensation is tested over distribution of the sural nerve.

The following special tests are included in physical examination:
- Anterior drawer test
- Talar tilt test
- Squeeze test
- External rotation test and the Kleiger test.

Anterior Drawer Test (Fig. 1)

The patient's knees should be flexed and the foot freely suspended with 10° plantar flexion. The examiner would grasp the heel and pull it forward while giving counter-pressure over the distal end of tibia and fibula at the level of ankle joint using the other hand. Several millimeters of lateral bilateral movement indicate a negative ankle anterior drawer test. This test should be checked on both limbs. Prone anterior drawer test can also be performed with the patient lying prone with feet extending from the bed. A positive test result is indicated by excessive anterior movement and dimpling over the skin on both sides of the Achilles tendon.

Talar Tilt Test (Fig. 2)

The talar tilt test is also called inversion stress maneuver. Again, here the patient's knees should be flexed and the foot freely suspended. In this test, the talus is tilted into adduction

Chapter 6: Ankle Sprain

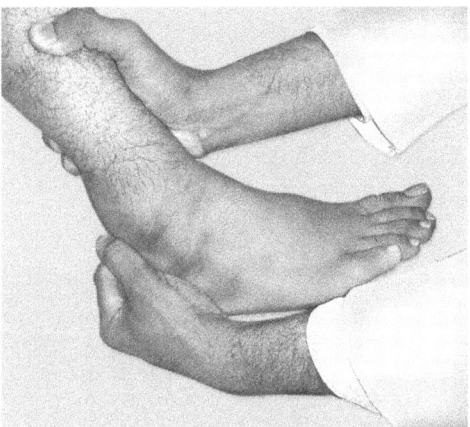

Fig. 1: Anterior drawer test for ankle.

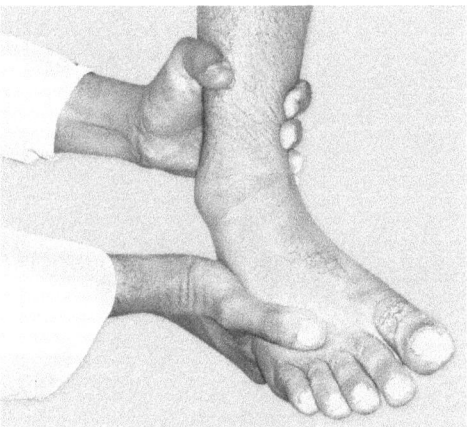

Fig. 2: Talar tilt test.

and abduction, and findings are compared on both feet. Injury to the CFL is suspected when a firm end is absent.

Squeeze Test (Fig. 3)

The squeeze test is also known as the fibular compression test. The examiner's thumb is placed on the tibia with fingers on the fibula at the midpoint of the lower leg and squeezed. Alternatively, examiner's both hands can be encircled for the same. Pain along the fibula indicates a positive test and high ankle sprain involving syndesmosis and tibiofibular ligaments.

External Rotation Test (Fig. 4) and the Kleiger Test

Again here the patient's knee should be flexed and the foot freely suspended. With ankle in neutral position, the foot is externally rotated and if the patient has pain over syndesmosis,

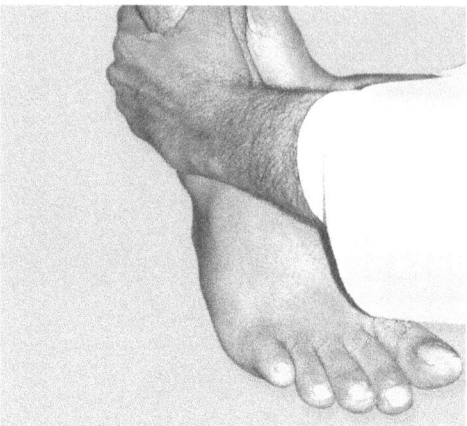

Fig. 3: Squeeze test for ankle.

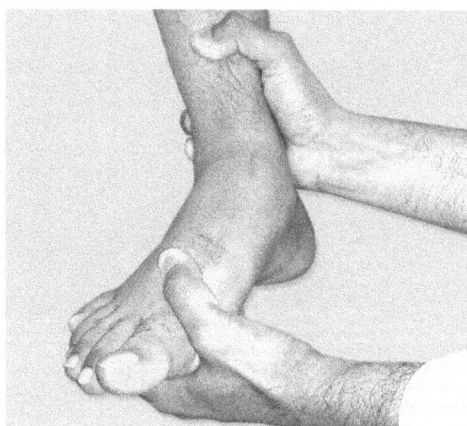

Fig. 4: External rotation test.

the test is considered positive. The Kleiger test is a variation of this and performed in the same manner; however, here a test is considered positive when the patient has pain medially and laterally, and the injury to the deltoid ligament is indicated when the talus displaces from the medial malleolus.

INTERPRETATION OF FINDINGS

The appropriate approach toward the diagnosis of ankle sprain involves detailed history taking, performance of physical examination as described above including the special tests and ruling out of fractures and distal neurovascular damage. Patients' ability to bear weight should exclude fracture. The absence of bony tenderness especially at both malleoli, base of

5th metatarsal and midfoot, and the absence of crepitus should also exclude fracture. Absence of coldness over the foot, absence of paresthesias, the presence of sensation and good pulses over the dorsalis pedis and the posterior tibial arteries should rule out neurovascular damage. Any other injury at any other part of the body should be excluded.

When ankle sprains continue to remain painful despite early rehabilitation, missed fracture of the talar dome or that of the anterior process of calcaneus should be suspected since they can occur with eversion and inversion injuries. Some other injuries that mimic ankle sprain include: Achilles tendon injury or tendonitis, distal fibula fracture, fracture of the tarsals or the metatarsals, gout and pseudogout and certain peroneal tendon syndromes. These should be the differential diagnoses.

INVESTIGATIONS

Plain X-rays and computed tomography (CT) scans are nowadays readily available at most centers. Magnetic resonance imaging (MRI) and bone scans are other useful imaging investigations. An anterior posterior view, a lateral view and a 45° oblique view with ankle in dorsiflexion are useful X-rays for ankle injuries. Some experts ask for stress X-rays to judge the severity of the sprain.

The Ottawa ankle rules are useful guidelines for using X-rays in patients presenting with ankle pain. They are applicable in children aged more than 5 years and within 10 days of the ankle injury. The following findings ask for X-rays in accordance with the Ottawa rules:
- Bone tenderness at the posterior tip of lateral malleolus
- Bone tenderness at the posterior tip of medial malleolus
- Inability to bear weight immediately after the injury and in the emergency department.

Further as per the Ottawa ankle rules a foot X-ray is required only in any of the following conditions:
- Bone tenderness at the base of 5th metatarsal
- Bone tenderness at the navicular bone
- Inability to bear weight immediately after the injury and in the emergency department.

Computed tomography scanning, MRI, and bone scanning may be useful in imaging of soft tissues and that of bones when X-rays alone are inconclusive. Arthroscopy serves as a good technique for diagnosis and treatment of chronic ankle sprain.

TREATMENT

Important aspects of treatment include pain management and restoration of the normal ROM and adequate muscle strength. According to the American National Athletic Trainers' Association guidelines, grade I and II ankle sprains require early functional rehabilitation, whereas grade III ankle sprains require immobilization for at least 10 days. However, grade III injuries may be advised for prolonged immobilization (up to 6 weeks), followed by mobilization. Furthermore, nonsteroidal anti-inflammatory drugs (NSAIDs) should be used for pain and inflammation management. For patients at high risk of ankle sprains, preventive measures should be taken for up to 3 months.

As a general rule for most musculoskeletal injuries, PRICES remain the basis of initial management. A variety of protective braces are available commercially and they can be applied until the pain and swelling have subsided. Resting the limb is very important since it reduces the pain, promotes healing, and protects against abnormal movements. Application of ice is equally important as it alleviates the pain and inflammation. Ice should be applied over a napkin or protective clothing and never directly over the injury and not more than 30 minutes at a stretch. Ankle sleeves, tapes, Velcro straps, modified shoes, and lace-ups are commercially available for compression to reduce the swelling as well as for support. Generally, lace-up ankle support has provided better results when compared with semirigid ankle support, which in turn has given better results than with elastic bandage or tape. Elevating the limb is explained and encouraged with pillows' support while lying down. Nevertheless, instead of complete bed rest, weight-bearing is encouraged as tolerated.

Conservative therapy is useful for recurrent ankle sprains with a view to provide protection and to improve the strength and ROM of ankle. Further in recurrent sprains the use of peroneal strengthening, Achilles tendon stretching, ankle stirrups, orthoses and casts have shown benefits. Chronic instability of the subtalar joint may need surgery.

Medical Management

Pain management is an important therapeutic outcome in the management of ankle sprain. NSAIDs and paracetamol are useful for alleviating pain and inflammation. NSAIDs should be used cautiously in patients with renal dysfunction and are avoided on empty stomach. Some theories have suggested that NSAIDs may actually increase the risk of bleeding and the degree of swelling while many studies have shown their benefit in reducing the patients' pain and swelling.

Apart from pain management, it is very important to improve and prevent any loss of ROM and any distal neurovascular damage.

Surgical Management and Rehabilitation

There are very few indications of surgery in ankle sprain. Firstly, surgery may be required for young patients with sports-related injuries and competitive sport efficiency requirements. Secondly, chronic recurrent ankle sprains and consequent subtalar instability may require surgical correction. Deltoid ligament injury with widened ankle mortise is an indication for surgical intervention. Another indication is when the patient's distal talofibular ligament's third-degree injury leads to a widened ankle mortise. A study showed that surgery decreased the prevalence of reinjury of the lateral ligaments; however, there was a higher rate of osteoarthritis detected by MRI postoperatively. Moreover, an acute surgical reconstruction is advisable for competitive sportspersons, since increased ankle instability is a predictor for recurrent ankle sprains.

The postoperative return to normal activity is allowed only when the patient has no tenderness, near-normal muscle strength and physical examination and full passive ROM. This may take anywhere from 1 week to 6 weeks from the injury. During the rehabilitation and recovery period, physiotherapy is aimed at strengthening the basic movements of ankle joint, i.e. dorsiflexion, plantar flexion, eversion and inversion, making use of a variety of equipment such as elastic bands and balance boards. Apart from isometric muscle strengthening exercises and balance boards, patients are also encouraged for proprioception rehabilitation. One test before allowing return to normal activity is asking the subject to maintain balance on the affected leg for at least 30 seconds with closed eyes. Initially simple physiologic movements such as walking and jogging are encouraged and gradually forward-backward and side-to-side movements are allowed.

Isolated simple ankle sprains carry a very good prognosis when compared with that for other musculoskeletal injuries. Recurrent ankle sprains with early treatment and rehabilitation also have very good prognosis. Post-traumatic osteoarthritis is a common complication arising from ankle sprains. Furthermore, complex regional pain syndrome or reflex sympathetic dystrophy may occur as a complication of ankle sprains. Both the complications may be averted by early diagnosis and rehabilitation of ankle sprain. There remains the possibility of chronic long-term symptoms leading to pain and ankle joint instability in around 10% of acute ankle sprains.

Awareness toward the fact that certain sports carry a higher risk for ankle sprains can help in prevention of the same. The use of braces reduces the incidence of acute ankle injuries in athletes and hence can be a useful measure for preventing ankle sprains. Furthermore, a decrease in body mass, use of adequate ankle protective footwear, ample warm up followed by gradual transition toward strenuous physical activity and development of good muscle strength are other factors that may help prevent ankle sprains.

SUMMARY

Ankle sprain is one of the most common musculoskeletal injuries. The common history in ankle sprain is twisting of the foot. The common symptoms in ankle sprain include pain and swelling. Physical examination plays a role in diagnosis and ascertaining severity of ankle sprain and some special tests are used for assessing injury to specific ligaments. This is summarized in **Flowchart 1**. The Ottawa rules guide for determining the requirement of imaging and imaging in turn helps ruling out fractures. CT, MRI, bone scanning, and arthroscopy serve as additional resources. Distal neurovascular damage has to be ruled out clinically. Initial management comprises of PRICES, pain management and expert opinion. Recurrent ankle sprains may require conservative management and in some cases surgery is indicated followed by adequate rehabilitation and physiotherapy.

Flowchart 1: Summary of approach to patient with ankle sprain.

```
Do you have?
History of twisting of the foot
Presence of pain and swelling
            │
            ▼
Proceed to physical examination
Rule out other injuries, co-morbidities, fracture, DNVD
The anterior and prone anterior drawer tests assess for ankle instability
The Talar tilt test assesses for calcaneofibular ligament injury
The squeeze test and the external rotation test assess for syndesmotic ligaments' injury
The Kleiger test assesses for deltoid ligament injury
            │
            ▼
Proceed to imaging
The Ottawa rules guide for the need of X-rays
The X-rays help to rule out fractures
The CT, MRI and bone scanning help detect subtle soft tissue and bone injuries
            │
            ▼
Proceed to management
PRICES and pain management
Expert opinion
Conservative management and rarely surgery
Adequate rehabilitation, physiotherapy and preventative measures
```

CHAPTER 7

Ascites

Jesus Daniel López Tapia, Mariana Patricia Valdez Rodríguez

INTRODUCTION

Ascites is the excess accumulation of fluid in the peritoneal cavity, inside the space between the visceral peritoneum and parietal peritoneum.

Ascites is the most common complication in cirrhosis and portal hypertension, in patients with advanced cirrhosis, the regulation of extracellular volume is frequently abnormal, and it may result in the accumulation of fluid ascites, peripheral edema, and pleural effusion.

Liver cirrhosis is responsible for 75% of cases of ascites, being this the most common complication, before hepatic encephalopathy and variceal hemorrhage.

Spontaneous bacterial peritonitis is considered the most serious complication of ascites, with a mortality between 30% and 90% in the 1st year of diagnosis.

It is important to understand the pathophysiology of ascites to give adequate treatment and decrease the mortality of these patients.

ETIOLOGY/CAUSES (TABLE 1)

- *Portal hypertension*: In patients with an advanced liver disease, portal hypertension is the main cause of ascites. There is a systemic vasodilatation and reduction of vascular resistance, mainly in the splanchnic circulation; this vasodilation in the portal circulation is due to the release of local vasodilators such as nitric oxide, vasoactive intestinal peptide, glucagon, and prostacyclins.
- *Lymphatic flow*: The lymphatic vascular system removes the interstitial fluid from the tissues of the body and returns it to the bloodstream, we call this interstitial fluid, lymph, when it enters the lymphatic capillaries. Failure of normal lymphatic function results in interstitial fluid accumulation and can lead to clinical manifestations such as lymphedema and ascites.
- *Cardiac ascites*: It is generally classified as a "postsinusoidal" cause of ascites. Dysfunction and regurgitation of the tricuspid valve, produces severe hepatic congestion because right ventricular pressures are transmitted directly to the draining vessels of the liver. Right upper pressures directly affect the hepatic veins and the small venules that drain the hepatic acini.
- *Ovarian cancer*: Ovarian cancer is responsible for 38% of malignant ascites cases in female patients in USA. There are other conditions in which malignant ascites can develop secondary to extra-abdominal tumors such as lung cancer, breast cancer, or lymphomas.

Table 1: Etiology/causes of ascites.

Etiology	Pathophysiology	Characteristics
Portal hypertension	• Systemic vasodilatation and reduction of vascular resistance, mainly in the splanchnic circulation, this vasodilation in the portal circulation is due to the release of local vasodilators such as nitric oxide, vasoactive intestinal peptide, glucagon, and prostacyclins 12. • The increase in the activity of the neurohormonal system (renin-angiotensin-aldosterone, endothelin, atrial natriuretic peptide, and sympathetic nervous system), is due to a compensatory response to maintain homeostasis, however, these compensation mechanisms may contribute to the progression of liver disease by provoking renal vasoconstriction and sodium and water retention, favoring the accumulation of ascitic fluid in the peritoneum.	• Serum-ascites albumin gradient > 1.1 g/dL • Radiologic finding of portal hypertension
Lymphatic flow (overload)	• Increased extravasation of fluid from the splanchnic microcirculation. In the initial phases of the disease, this process is compensated by an increase in the lymphatic return. • The lymphatic flow of the thoracic duct, which under normal conditions is less than 1 L/day, can increase up to 20 L in patients with advanced portal hypertension, therefore, when the production of lymph exceeds the drainage, lymphatic ascites occurs.	Serum-ascites albumin gradient > 1.1 g/dL and increase in the abdominal perimeter
Heart failure	Dysfunction and regurgitation of the tricuspid valve produces severe hepatic congestion because right ventricular pressures are transmitted directly to the draining vessels of the liver. Right upper pressures directly affect the hepatic veins and the small venules that drain the hepatic acini.	• Serum-ascites albumin gradient > 1.1 g/dL • B-type natriuretic peptide (BNP) > 364
Ovarian cancer	There is a transition from ovarian epithelial cells to mesenchymal cells, as part of the normal physiological process, allowing repair of the superficial epithelium when an oocyte is released. The peritoneal cavity is covered by mesothelial cells, which in the presence of an ovarian tumor allow an easy adhesion of mesothelin and hyaluronic acid through the CD44, CA125, and integrins cells, which finally manage to invade the mesothelium.	• Anorexia (36%), nausea (37%), and early satiety (6%). Ascites fluid with presence of malignant cells • CA125 > 35 IU/mL

- *Malignant ascites*: There are three main forms of dissemination of malignant cells to distal organs: (1) hematogenous pathway, (2) lymphatic vessels, and (3) transcoelomic spread (direct seeding in the body cavity), which is the most common way of metastasis in gastric cancer cases. Malignant ascites accompanied by peritoneal carcinomatosis is one of the most important causes of advanced stage gastric cancer morbidity and mortality.

PATHOPHYSIOLOGY OF ASCITES

In the initial phase of portal hypertension and splanchnic vasodilation, ascites may not be present, so homeostasis is maintained by the development of a hyperdynamic circulation that results in high cardiac output, heart rate, and elevated plasma volume. As this portal hypertension progresses and vasodilation is accentuated, this mechanism is insufficient to maintain homeostasis in the circulatory blood, leading to activation of compensatory mechanisms such as lowering of blood pressure, stimulation of baroreceptors, and increasing the activity of the renin system. Angiotensin-aldosterone and antidiuretic hormone causes water and sodium retention through vasoconstriction in the renal capillaries.

Other mechanisms responsible for ascites formation include alterations in the splanchnic circulation and damage in renal function that favor sodium (Na) and water retention. Circulatory dysfunctions caused by arterial vasodilatation within the splanchnic circulation are considered a primary factor in the pathophysiology of ascites formation. Inflammatory cytokines and chemokines, as well as reduced lymphatic flow, contribute to alterations of the peritoneal membrane. These changes decrease the difference in the plasma peritoneal oncotic pressure so that the direction of flow of fluid is directed to the peritoneal cavity. This leads to the accumulation of pathological volumes of fluid in the peritoneal cavity.

CLINICAL PRESENTATION

The increase in the abdominal perimeter is the most common sign within its primary presentation, and new onset ascites, as well as gain in weight, difficulty in inspiration due to diaphragmatic compression, superficial and short breaths, as well as a feeling of early satiety.

RED FLAGS

There are parameters of poor prognosis identified globally:
- Urinary sodium less than 10 mEq/L
- Serum sodium less than 130 mEq/L
- Renal insufficiency with a creatinine value more than 1.2 mg/dL or more
- Spontaneous bacterial peritonitis
- Mean arterial pressure less than 80 mm Hg.

EVALUATION

History

A clinical history should be performed evaluating risk factors such as a family history of cancer or some other cause that is related to ascites such as nephrotic syndrome or congestive heart failure, a history of hypercoagulability with a predisposition to a portal vein thrombosis, or Budd-Chiari syndrome.

Physical Examination

On physical examination, one of the most characteristic clinical signs is dullness to peritoneal percussion in the flanks, which usually occurs when the patient accumulates more than

1,500 mL in the peritoneal cavity, a change of position is made in these patients, from their position initial supine decubitus to lateral decubitus to perform percussion again, this maneuver has a sensitivity of 83% and a specificity of 56% for the diagnosis of ascites if flank halves are presented.

The physical examination may be more difficult to perform in patients with obesity. It is important to be aware of the time of evolution of ascites in all patients since it can develop as fast as a couple of days or as late as 2 weeks. However, patients with obesity may present clinical signs and symptoms months or years later.

INTERPRETATION OF FINDING

Initial laboratory tests should include a cell count of ascites fluid, total proteins, liquid albumin, and serum. If ascites of cardiovascular origin is suspected, it is recommended to request the brain natriuretic peptide or B-type natriuretic peptide (BNP) and if this is greater than 364 pg/mL, the diagnosis of heart failure can be made in 99.1% accuracy.

Imaging

The first-choice imaging study for patients with suspicion signs and symptoms of ascites is an ultrasound of the upper abdomen. Doppler ultrasound may be useful in the evaluation if portal or hepatic venous thrombosis is suspected.

Once the diagnosis is established, paracentesis should be performed to evaluate the ascites fluid.

Ascites Fluid Analysis

It is recommended to use serum-ascites albumin gradient (SAAG). It is obtained by measuring the serum albumin level and albumin level in the ascetic fluid. A gradient greater than 1.1 g/dL is categorized as elevated and has a sensitivity of 97% as an indicator of portal hypertension. A protein value in ascites fluid above 2.5 g/dL in most cases indicates obstruction of the hepatic venous circulation due to heart failure or Budd-Chiari syndrome. The measurement of a blood concentration of BNP can help distinguish ascites due to heart failure from ascites due to cirrhosis (**Table 2**).

TREATMENT

All patients with new onset or clinically detectable ascites are recommended to undergo paracentesis for initial diagnosis. Paracentesis should be performed in all patients with ascites on admission to the hospital since from 10% to 27% of patients develop spontaneous bacterial peritonitis. There are no absolute contraindications for a paracentesis. In fact, the majority of patients who undergo paracentesis have a prolonged prothrombin time with or without thrombocytopenia, thrombocytopenia figures can reach up to 19,000 cells/mm^3, platelet transfusion or fresh plasma is not indicated in these patients.

Table 2: Differential diagnosis of serum-ascites albumin gradient (SAAG).

SAAG > 1.1 g/dL	SAAG < 1.1 g/dL
• Cirrhosis	• Peritoneal carcinomatosis
• Heart failure	• Peritoneal tuberculosis (TB)
• Alcoholic hepatitis	• Pancreatitis
• Hepatic metastasis	• Nephrotic syndrome
• Myxedema	• Bowel obstruction/perforation

There are two primary interventions for the management and approach of ascites, the first is to reduce sodium intake and initiate diuretic therapy. A sodium intake of 88 mEq or 2,000 mg/day is usually recommended.

Within diuretic therapy, initial management is recommended with spironolactone, an aldosterone antagonist, in combination with furosemide, which mainly acts in the ascending and distal branch of the loop of Henle. Spironolactone monotherapy has been shown to be more effective compared to furosemide in the treatment of ascites. Even so, the use of spironolactone as monotherapy is not recommended due to the association of its use and risk of hyperkalemia. The recommended initial dose of spironolactone and furosemide is 100:40, respectively, with a maximum recommended dose of 400 mg of spironolactone and 160 mg of furosemide to achieve the desired effect, as long as the patient tolerates it.

The use of beta-blockers should be avoided in patients with refractory ascites, the use of nonsteroidal anti-inflammatory drugs (NSAIDs) should also be avoided due to the risk of gastrointestinal bleeding and acute renal failure. It is called refractory ascites to ascites which does not respond to high doses of diuretic therapy, as well as to an aggressive restriction of sodium, intolerance to diuretic therapy due to renal failure, or patients that require frequently therapeutic paracentesis.

There are several therapeutic routes for the treatment of refractory ascites, among them large-volume paracentesis, as well as a transjugular intrahepatic shunt, and liver transplantation.

The volume paracentesis consists of an aspiration more than 5 L, albumin replacement therapy is recommended at a dose of 6-8 g/L. It must be considered that paracentesis is a therapy that does not modify the mechanism of action in the formation of ascites, this means that the formation of ascites can recur. It is considered good management when there is a period of 2 weeks between a session of paracentesis and the reappearance of it.

A 10 L paracentesis manages to eliminate 1,300 mmol of sodium. Most authors agree to perform a paracentesis of the large total volume at first instance. It is important to know that this is an ambulatory procedure.

Flowchart 1: Summary of evaluation of ascites.

Practice a clinical history search for:
- Chronic history of liver disease (cirrhosis, hepatitis C)
- History of heart failure
- Risk for CA
- Obesity and/or alcoholism

Physical examination:
- Gain in weight
- Flank dullness
- Difficulty in inspiration
- Superficial and short breaths
- Early satisfaction
- Positive wave test
- Confusion

Diagnosis
By serum-ascites albumin gradient (SAAG):
- SAAG: >1.1 cirrhosis, heart failure, alcoholic hepatitis, and myxedema.
- SAAG: <1.1 peritoneal carcinomatosis, peritoneal TB, pancreatitis, nephrotic syndrome, and perforation.
- B-type natriuretic peptide (BNP) and if this is > 364 pg/mL, the diagnosis of heart failure.

Radiographic findings:
- Ultrasound of the upper abdomen is the first choice for imaging, ultrasound can quantify the volume of ascites.
- Transudates typically have homogenous, anechoic fluid with deep posterior acoustic enhancement.

Practice paracentesis if:
- It is new onset presentation ascites
- Clinically detectable ascites
- Risk factor to develop spontaneous bacterial peritonitis
- Refractory ascites
- Treatment consist of a large volume paracentesis > 5 L, albumin replacement, sodium restriction, and diuretic therapy.

■ SUMMARY

As now we know ascites is the excess accumulation of fluid in the peritoneal cavity in the space between the visceral peritoneum and parietal peritoneum. There is different etiology for this disease. The main challenge for the medical practice is to differentiate between the hepatic ascites and the nonhepatic ascites and give the proper treatment to the patient at the emergency room (ER) department, as well as make a deep clinical evaluation for the new-onset ascites including the family history and recognize the patients risk factors to develop ascites.

Ascites is often the most limiting chronic complication of cirrhosis in terms of quality of life. Patients with high SAAG (portal hypertensive) ascites benefit most from sodium restriction and diuretics.

Paracentesis must be performed in the patients with new-onset ascites and must be on admission to the hospital since from a high rate of patients may develop spontaneous bacterial peritonitis (**Flowchart 1**).

CHAPTER 8

Bleeding Disorders

Ayesha Musabbah Almemari, Hanan Salah Al Hajri, Maryam Hasan Darwish Alshehhi

INTRODUCTION

While trauma is the most common cause of bleeding seen in emergency department (ED), there are patients who would present with bleeding or other hematological symptoms or signs from abnormal homeostasis. It is crucial to recognize these patients with careful history and examination as workup and management will be different.

There is no definition of bleeding disorders and in most literatures bleeding and clotting disorders are used interchangeably to describe a spectrum of hematological diseases that affect hemostasis. Through this chapter, we will use bleeding disorders instead of clotting disorders term and we will discuss hemostasis disorders that present with bleeding or bleeding and clotting at the same time.

ETIOLOGY

Etiology of bleeding disorders can be either congenital or acquired (**Table 1**). Hemophilia A and B are among the most common congenital etiologies according to the world federation of hemophilia 2010 survey. 106 countries participated in the survey about hereditary bleeding disorders, with total number of patients with diagnosed hereditary bleeding disorder being 257,182 cases and hemophilia A and B being the most prevalent disease as there are about

Table 1: Classification of bleeding disorders based on etiology.

Congenital	Acquired
Hemophilia A (Factor VIII deficiency)	Disseminated intravascular coagulopathy
Hemophilia B (Factor IX deficiency)	Liver disease
von Willebrand disease	Vitamin K deficiency
Fibrinogen disorders	Massive transfusion of stored blood
	Acquired inhibitors of coagulation
	Heparin or oral anticoagulant therapy
	Renal disease
	Hypersplenism

162,781 cases around the world, followed by hemophilia A (125,049 cases), then von Willebrand disease (VWB) (65,100 cases).

PATHOPHYSIOLOGY

Most hereditary bleeding disorders are diagnosed at young age and usually present knowing their condition and have learned along the years about clinical symptomatology and treatment required. The challenge usually is de novo presentation to ED, which is most likely for acquired conditions where the emergency physician needs to have essential knowledge of the underlying pathophysiology of hemostasis process in order to guide his differential diagnosis and management. Hemostasis is a complex physiological mechanism that is composed of major events:

- *Primary hemostasis*: Platelet aggregation at site of vessel endothelial injury
- *Secondary hemostasis*: Consolidation of platelet plug through activation of coagulation factors
- *Fibrin clot formation*: Thrombin-dependent process where it converts fibrinogen to fibrin
- *Inhibition of coagulation*: Endogenous or exogenous inhibition of thrombin, which results in clot breakdown.

In the view of the four events described above, bleeding disorders can be generally classified as either platelet disorders, coagulation factor deficiencies, or could be the result of both disorders such as in disseminated intravascular coagulation (DIC) as outlined in **Table 2** and

Table 2: Classification based on hemostasis defect mechanism.

Hemostasis event	Disorders	—
Primary hemostasis disorders	Vascular abnormalities	Hereditary hemorrhagic telangiectasia
		Disorders of the connective tissue (including Ehlers-Danlos disease and osteogenesis imperfecta)
		Small-vessel vasculitis
	von Willebrand disease	
	Thrombocytopenia	Decreased production: bone marrow dysfunction or inadequate precursors such as vitamin B_{12} and folic acid
		Destruction or consumption like in DIC, infection, drugs most commonly heparin then some antimicrobials, antiarrhythmic, anticonvulsant, and antifungal agents, and H_2 receptor antagonists, toxins, systemic illness such as liver or renal disease, immune disease such as ITP and TTP
		Sequestration: Hypersplenism

Contd...

Contd...

Hemostasis event	Disorders	—
	Platelet dysfunction	*Hereditary*: VWB, Ehler-Danlos syndrome, Bernard-Soulier syndrome, Glanzmann's thrombocytopenia, congenital fibrinogen disorders, congenital platelets disorders
		Acquired: Drug effect such as antiplatelet
		Systemic illness: Uremia, cirrhosis, SLE
		Surgery related: Cardiac surgery, liver transplant
Secondary hemostasis disorders	Hemophilia Liver disease Vitamin K deficiency Acquired inhibitors of coagulation (antibodies) Consumptive processes (e.g. disseminated intravascular coagulation)	
Fibrin clot formation	Hyperprothrombinemia Hemophilia (A and B) Hereditary afibrinogenemia Drugs Systemic illness (chronic liver disease)	
Inhibition of coagulation	Coagulation factors deficiency	Idiopathic Rheumatic diseases Postpartum period malignancy Drugs SLE Antiphospholipid Congenital Surgery Malignancy

(DIC: disseminated intravascular coagulation; ITP: immune thrombocytopenic purpura; SLE: systemic lupus erythematosus; TTP: thrombotic thrombocytopenic purpura; VWB: von Willebrand disease)

Flowchart 1. Table 3 outlined a more simplified classification as well based on underlying etiology and pathophysiology of the hemostasis.

CLINICAL PRESENTATION

The natural history of most bleeding disorders is similar based on where the defect is in the hemostasis process, hence pertinent history and thorough physical examination are essential to establish appropriate differential diagnosis, treatment, and disposition. Not all those patients who present with bleeding symptoms have bleeding disorders hence developing a

Flowchart 1: Classification of bleeding disorder based on pathophysiology.

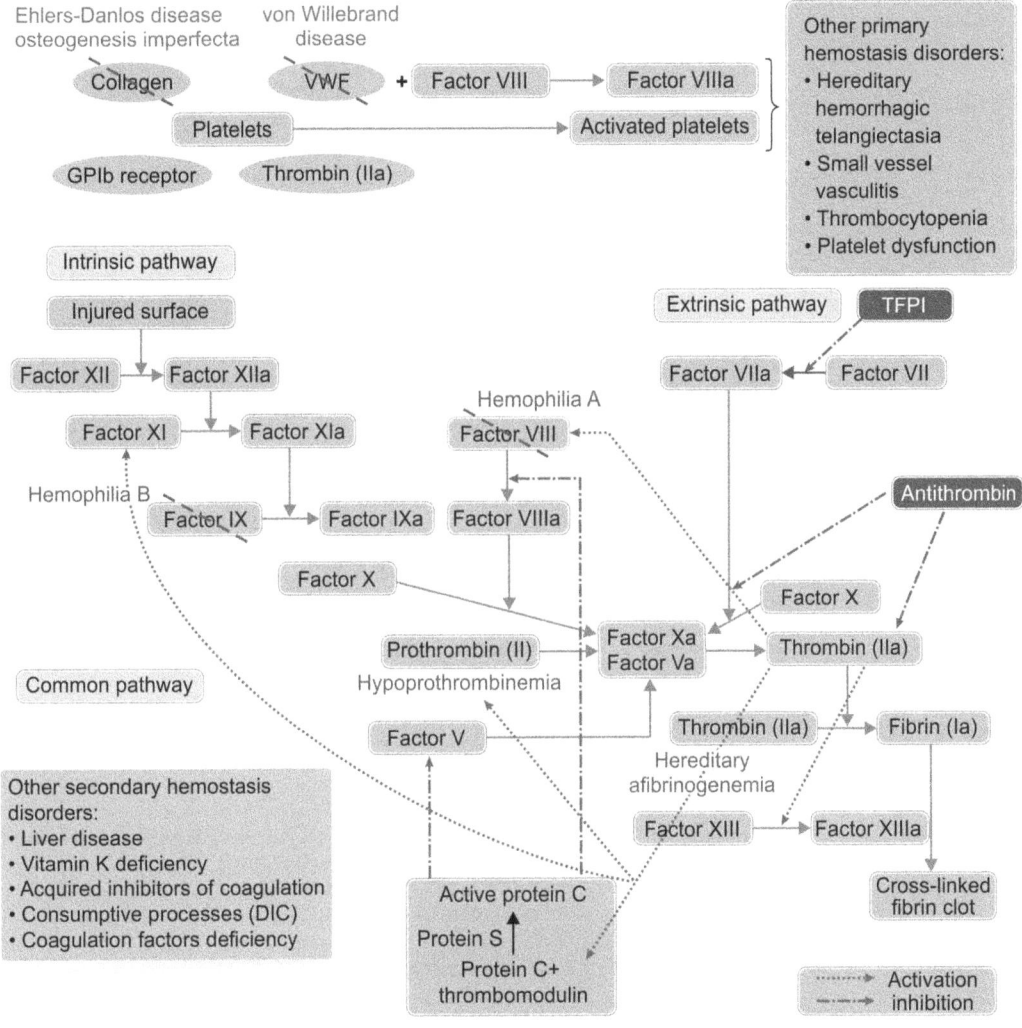

(DIC: disseminated intravascular coagulation; TFPI: tissue factor pathway inhibitor)

diagnostic approach is of paramount importance. Bleeding can be minor or life-threatening depending on the site and the underlying hemostasis defect.

History of Bleeding Patient

Patient is Underlying Diagnosed Bleeding Disorder

Those patients will likely know they have an illness and most will know or carry with them documents that will indicate their diagnosis. If they do not, physicians shall try and inquire

Table 3: Simplified bleeding disorder classification based on underlying hemostasis pathophysiology.

Platelet disorder	Low platelet number	Congenital thrombocytopenia	Wiskott-Aldrich syndrome
		Impaired bone marrow production	Impaired bone marrow production aplastic anemia, megaloblastic anemia, and bone marrow infiltration
		Increased platelet destruction/consumption	Immune-related conditions like autoimmune thrombocytopenia (ITP), systemic lupus erythematosis, drugs, and nonimmune conditions such as disseminated intravascular coagulation (DIC), thrombotic thrombocytopenic purpura (TTP)
		Splenic sequestration	Hypersplenism
	Platelet dysfunction	Inherited	Glanzmann's thrombasthenia, Bernard-Soulier syndrome and von Willebrand disease
		Acquired	Aspirin ingestion, uremia and in myeloproliferative disorders
Disorders of the coagulation cascade	Inherited bleeding disorders	Hemophilia A (Factor VIII deficiency) Hemophilia B (Factor IX deficiency) von Willebrand disease Congenital fibrinogen deficiency	
	Acquired bleeding disorders	Liver disease Renal disease Vitamin K deficiency DIC Anticoagulant therapy Massive transfusion Hyperfibrinolysis	

about guiding historical factors such as previous ED presentations, previous medications received or previous hospital admissions and procedures performed.

Patient with New Presentation of Noninjury-related Bleeding

Taking specific yet detailed history is important to exclude possibilities of underlying undiagnosed bleeding disorders. History of present illness shall focus on current presenting symptoms, onset, amount, location of bleeding, provoking factors, and any associated symptoms.

Past medical history shall inquire about previous history of prolonged or recurrent bleeding from wounds, lasting more than 15 minutes or recurring spontaneously during the 7 days after the wound, or after surgical procedures such as tonsillectomy. As well information about bruises, after minimal or no apparent trauma, spontaneous nosebleeds that lasted more than 10 minutes or required medical attention to stop and dental extractions followed by heavy, prolonged, or recurrent bleeding. In women, patient's gynecological history is important. Checking about history of heavy menses and presence of clots greater than an inch in size and/or changing a pad or tampon more than hourly, or resulting in anemia or low iron, history of postpartum hemorrhage or recurrent abortions. Additional important historical factors in patients with de novo bleeding episode are outlined in **Table 4**. Same historical factors shall be used for those known for bleeding disorders, however, when patient provide clear and concise presenting symptoms and history of bleeding disorders as much details may not be needed taking in account the goal of emergency physician when assessing any patient is to be effective and efficient.

Physical Examination of Bleeding Patient

Physical examination of a patient presenting with bleeding symptoms focuses on bleeding site assessment, control of bleeding, if actively bleeding then focus shall move to mucocutaneous manifestation of bleeding disorders such as bruises, assess if various age, size, presence of petechiae. As well assess presence of hemarthrosis; worth mentioning that bleeding disorders due to platelet pathology will manifest usually as petechiae, bruises, and mucous membrane bleeding while those due to coagulation cascade dysfunction may present with deep tissue bleeding such as hemarthrosis and deep muscle and soft tissue bleeding. Given that many systemic illnesses cause hemostasis dysfunction, hence examining for signs of chronic illness such as chronic liver disease, signs of anemia such as pale mucous membranes, and signs of end-stage renal disease.

Red Flags

The nature of the ED is that physicians see large number of patients and need to tease out those at high risk for clinical progression or deterioration in the short term hence to plan proactively management strategy to prevent further clinical worsening. Identifying red flags in various clinical presentations assist the physicians to recognize high-risk patients immediately without much thinking. There is no red flags list for bleeding disorders identified in the literature. We have looked at recognized emergency medicine textbooks as well as the hematology literature in an attempt to develop a list. There are many bleeding scores around, however, the goals of these scores are to identify the severity of bleeding disorder in primary and hematology setting and has not been validated in the ED. Most of the bleeding scores utility is in its negative predictive value though the inter-rater reliability among users vary. There some other bleeding scores that predict risk of bleeding in atrial fibrillation patients before starting them on anticoagulation. Looking at all above we developed the red flag list in **Table 5**.

Table 4: History elements in bleeding patient.

History of present presentation	Onset Location Severity Amount estimation Skin manifestation (bruises, petechiae) Systemic symptoms (dizziness, syncope, dyspnea, palpitation, abdominal or back or chest pain) Spontaneous bleeding or provoked Gum bleeding when brushing teeth
Past medical and surgical history	Prolonged or recurrent bleeding from wounds, lasting more than 15 minutes or recurring spontaneously during the 7 days after the wound, or after surgical procedures such as tonsillectomy history of blood transfusion Bruises, after minimal or no apparent trauma Spontaneous nosebleeds that lasted more than 10 minutes or required medical attention to stop
Medication history	Prescribed and over-the-counter medications including herbal medications or teas Common drugs to inquire about are the 5A's: 1. Aspirin 2. Anticoagulants 3. Antibiotics 4. Alcohol 5. Anticancer
Gynecology and obstetrics history	History of menorrhagia History of postpartum hemorrhage Recurrent abortions
Occupational history	Animal exposure (Crimean-Congo hemorrhagic fever) Working in industries that use fibrous glass material
Travel history	Ask about travel to countries at risk of hemorrhagic fever

■ INVESTIGATIONS

Obtaining a detailed patient and family history is crucial as we mentioned earlier, and once a significant bleeding history is identified, an initial laboratory evaluation is generally undertaken to determine the underlying cause. The laboratory evaluation for bleeding includes performance of initial screening tests. The most common screening tests that can be done in the emergency room are platelet counts, prothrombin time (PT), and activated partial thromboplastin time (aPTT).

For an individual with known hemophilia, routine laboratory studies (PT, PTT, and factor levels) are not indicated for a routine bleeding episode unless requested by the patient's hematologist. The clinical severity of a patient's hemophilia is gauged by his or her baseline clotting factor level, a value that remains constant throughout that person's life.

Alternatively, an individual with an undiagnosed bleeding disorder may present with abnormal hematologic laboratory studies obtained as part of routine evaluation or an

Table 5: Red flags that suggest bleeding disorders.

Bleeding from several sites	
Delayed bleeding after trauma or surgery	
Specific bleeding sites	• Bleeding into joints or deep tissue (hematoma, ecchymosis) • Spontaneous posterior epistaxis
Comorbidities	• Liver disease • Renal disease • Menorrhagia
Special population	• Pregnancy • Elderly > 65 • Pediatrics
Prior major bleeding	• Fatal bleeding, and/or • Symptomatic bleeding in a critical area or organ, such as intracranial, intraspinal, intraocular, retroperitoneal, intra-articular or pericardial, or intramuscular with compartment syndrome, and/or • Bleeding causing a fall in hemoglobin level of 20 g/L (1.24 mmol L/L 1) or more, or leading to transfusion of two or more units of whole blood or red cells
Medication usage (5A's)	1. Aspirin 2. Anticoagulants 3. Antibiotics 4. Alcohol 5. Anticancer

evaluation for surgery or for some other reason. A prolongation of the aPTT or PT of patients is not on any prescribed anticoagulant may indicate an acquired or congenital clotting factor deficiency or an inhibitor of one or more coagulation factors (**Flowcharts 2A to C**).

A mixing study should be the next step to differentiate factor deficiency from an inhibitor. In a mixing study, equal volumes of normal and patient plasma are mixed together, and the coagulation study is repeated. If the test normalized that, indicate coagulation factor deficiency, as the presence of normal plasma replaces the missing factor(s). If the PTT did not normalize after the patient, plasma is mixed with pooled plasma and this suggests presence of inhibitors interfering with one or more coagulation factors. The inhibitors are antibodies directed against specific coagulation factors hence called specific inhibitor and there are other nonspecific inhibitors (e.g. lupus anticoagulants). It is very important in mixing study to incubate the blood sample at 37°C for 1 hour minimum for accurate interpretation of the results. Technical errors can give false mixing study results.

Specific coagulation factors testing shall be done after the mixing study to identify the factor deficiency. Such testing shall be guided by hematologist instructions and guidance. Screening tests are not sensitive and do not evaluate all the abnormalities associated with bleeding including von Willebrand factor (VWF), factor XIII (FXIII), plasminogen activator inhibitor-1 (PAI-1) and others and may be insensitive to mild FVIII and FIX deficiencies,

Flowcharts 2A to C: Illustration to laboratory investigation of bleeding disorders.

Flowchart 2A

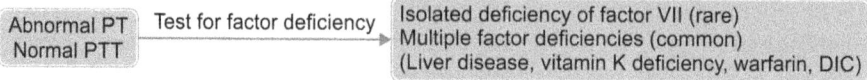

Flowchart 2B

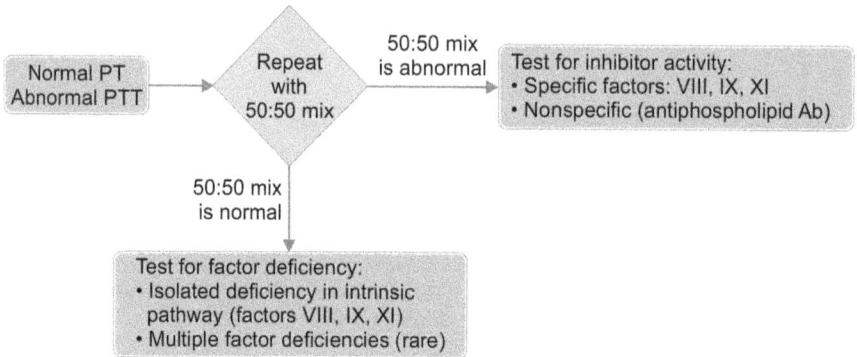

Flowchart 2C

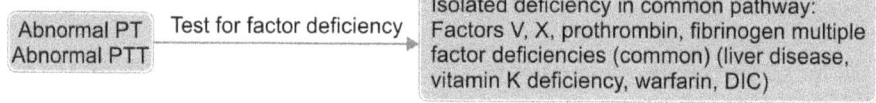

Box 1: Bleeding disorders screening and specialized workup.

- CBC and blood film
- PT and PTT, if abnormal, investigate for factor deficiencies
- If hemophilia or other factor deficiencies strongly suspected, do factor VIII, IX, XI assays
- Thrombin clotting time and clottable fibrinogen if abnormal, evaluate reptilase time and measure fibrinogen antigen
- von Willebrand disease screen, factor VIII, von Willebrand factor antigen and ristocetin cofactor levels multimers, if screen is abnormal
- Platelet aggregation with the full panel of agonists

(CBC: complete blood count; PT: prothrombin time; PTT: partial thromboplastin time)

therefore, a patients history strongly suggestive of a bleeding disorder, may warrant testing such deficiencies by referring to the hematology department for detailed investigations as in **Box 1**.

Thrombin time (TT) is of new interest to emergency physicians, as it helps them to assess bleeding tendency on patients using the new anticoagulants. The TT is the time required to convert fibrinogen to a fibrin clot, bypassing the intrinsic, extrinsic, and common pathways. Dabigatran (Pradaxa) was licensed for the treatment of nonvalvular atrial fibrillation. Routine monitoring of dabigatran is not required, testing for drug clearance may be needed in select circumstances like emergencies. The TT is very sensitive to the presence of any thrombin inhibitors in the plasma. This includes oral thrombin inhibitors such as dabigatran, as well as parenteral thrombin inhibitors such as heparin [both unfractionated and low molecular weight heparin (LMWH)], argatroban, lepirudin, and bivalirudin. TT has minimal value in the context of overdose assessment where aPTT and PT-INR (international normalized ratio) may be of more use. Another cause for a prolonged TT that may be encountered is a low fibrinogen level; which can occur with massive hemorrhage, DIC, or post-thrombolytic therapy. In this context; measurement of a fibrinogen level would be particularly useful. Uncommon causes of TT prolongation include dysfibrinogenemia, some par proteins, and high levels of fibrinogen degradation products (FDPs).

APPROACH TO PATIENT WITH POSSIBLE BLEEDING DISORDER IN ED

Considering the described pathophysiology, the clinical presentation and investigation discussed above, we recommend to follow 5-step approach in evaluating patients presenting to ED with nontraumatic bleeding who may potentially have underlying acquired or congenital bleeding disorder. The 5-step approach will help to define the type of bleeding and in providing the basis for planning management, including the initial decisions regarding administration of blood products.

Step 1

Is there a problem with the patient's platelets?
- Look for petechial hemorrhage, easy bruising, mucous membrane bleeding, epistaxis, and menometrorrhagia
- Do screening laboratory tests (platelet counts, PT, and APTT)
- Platelet aggregation will be done by the hematologist.

Step 2

Does the patient have a single factor deficiency?
- Like hemophilia A (FVIII) or B (FIX), very common or rare deficiencies like FVII, FX, FV, and FXI
- Look for purpura, hemarthrosis, muscle hematoma, and large vessels bleeding
- Screening test PT and aPTT
- Factor assays.

Step 3

Does the patient have deficiency of several vitamin k-dependent coagulation factors?
- Indicated by history of poor nutrition, vitamin K malabsorption, warfarin ingestion, symptoms, and signs of liver disease
- Warfarin and liver disease produce multiple factor deficiencies involving the extrinsic and common pathway
- Screening PT and aPTT
- Factors assays.

Step 4

Is there a circulating anticoagulant?
- Like heparin, FVIII or IX antibody, and lupus anticoagulant
- Check aPTT, 1:1 mixing, aPTT, TT, and reptilase time.

Step 5

Does the patient have consumptive coagulations?
- Like thrombotic thrombocytopenic purpura (TTP), hemolytic uremic syndrome (HUS), vasculitis, sepsis, obstetrical complication, trauma, and liver disease
- Check platelet count, PT, aPTT, TT, fibrinogen, D-dimer, and blood smear.

■ TREATMENT

Standards for emergency care of patients with known bleeding disorders have been established at national level in many countries specifically for hemophilia. Great example in UK where there are established hemophilia centers and hemophilia comprehensive care centers where registered patients have an open access during working hours. However, provision of care after hours remains ED dependent. Therefore, emergency physicians need essential knowledge of bleeding disorders and to develop an approach to assess and manage patients with established and undiagnosed bleeding disorders. It has been reported that patient always feel the care they receive at ED is poor and not up to their expectations. In a recent published report, hemophilia ED visits to ED in USA between 2006 and 2013 were about 0.016% of total ED visits. A subanalysis of 2,012 patients (4,500 patients) showed that the most common presenting complaints were cardiovascular complaints followed by injuries, hemorrhages, and sepsis. About 25% of the patients needed admission to hospital and mortality rate was quite small 0.008% and most died secondary to sepsis. Pediatric population tend to utilize ED more frequent than adults and injuries were the most frequent presenting complaint followed by joint and soft tissue disorders, fevers, and central line complications.

Prevention

This not only the responsibility of the treating physicians, emergency physicians share the responsibility of educating their patients with bleeding risk or tendency when they encounter them for any complaints. Discharge medication reconciliation is a quality metric to track.

Managing the Active Bleeding

Principle of managing patient with active bleeding in the ED is the same wither the etiology is trauma related or underlying bleeding disorder. Beginning with hemodynamic assessment is important, hemodynamically unstable patient management focus shall be controlling source of bleeding while simultaneously resuscitating with red blood cells (RBCs) transfusion initially then adding other blood products that will help to maintain hemostasis such as fresh frozen plasma (FFP), platelets, cryoprecipitate (Cryo), prothrombin complex concentrate (PCC), tranexamic acid, and calcium as well as maintaining normothermia. **Box 2** outlined the priorities of actively bleeding patient management in ED. If the patient presented with recent bleeding or nonmajor bleeding and hemodynamically stable, it is recommended to consult hematology before transfusing blood products in order to avoid harmful transfusion therapy (such as transfusing platelet to thrombocytopenic patient with possible heparin-induced thrombocytopenia or TTP may induce thrombosis); and to collect required blood samples for diagnosis as result will not be accurate once patient is transfused.

Principles of Blood Products Transfusion in ED

Red Blood Cell

Red blood cell transfusion goal is to restore oxygen-carrying capacity in bleeding patients. RBC units universally are about 220–340 mL. Rise in hemoglobin (Hb) after transfusion of 1 unit packed RBC (PRBC) is dependent on the patient weight and his blood volume, the lower the weight the higher the rise in Hb. However, in general each unit expected to raise Hb by 1 g for an average 70 kg adult patient, if no active bleeding, hemolysis, or sequestration is ongoing. Indications for PRBC transfusion in ED is mainly major hemorrhage or in cases of severe anemia where blood replacement can be started in ED and continued on the inpatient setting upon admission (**Flowchart 3**).

Box 2: Priorities of managing actively bleeding in emergency department (ED).

- Assess hemodynamic stability
- Control source of bleeding
- Activate local massive transfusion protocol, if major bleeding or hemodynamically instability believed to be due to hemorrhage
- If hemodynamically stable, replace PRBC as per estimated blood loss if needed and replace platelet, coagulation factor based on platelet, PT, PTT result and expected underlying etiology of bleeding disorder wither congenital or acquired
- Serial assessment of ongoing bleeding and response to resuscitation by repeated serum lactate, vital signs and coagulation profile (PT, PTT, INR, fibrinogen level, blood pH, and ionized Ca)
- Definitive diagnostic test to identify bleeding source based on patient presenting complaints (POCUS, CT, endoscopy, angiogram)
- Definitive bleeding site management once bleeding source or etiology is identified

(CT: computed tomography; INR: international normalized ratio; POCUS: point-of-care ultrasound; PRBC: packed red blood cell; PT: prothrombin time; PTT: partial thromboplastin time)

Flowchart 3: Blood products components derivation and average volume per unit for adult patient.

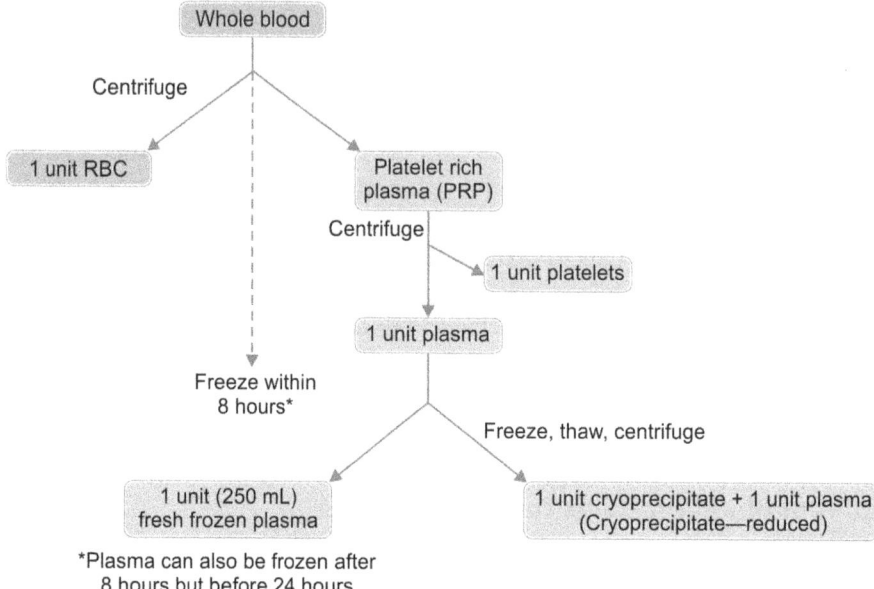

Platelet

One platelet unit is derived from a pool of 6 whole blood units and is expected to raise the platelet count by 30,000–60,000/μL in average adult patient. If patient platelet count does not increase as expected post-transfusion, the emergency physicians shall consider presence of immune or nonimmune destruction etiology such as TTP or end-stage liver disease, increase consumption such as DIC or bone marrow suppression such as in sepsis. A useful index to use to determine if lack of response to treatment is due to immune or nonimmune etiology is to calculate the corrected count increment (CCI) (**Box 3**). Indications for transfusing platelet in ED for patients with known or suspected congenital or acquired bleeding disorders are listed in **Box 4**. Platelet transfusion does not require to be ABO compatible.

Fresh Frozen Plasma

Each plasma unit is about 200–300 mL in volume and contains normal levels of plasma clotting factors with FVIII at level of 70%. Indications for plasma transfusion in ED are listed in **Box 5**. FFP shall be ABO compatible.

Cryoprecipitate

It is simply a concentrate of clotting factors that is prepared from FFP to produce a source of concentrated clotting factors including FVIII, VWF, and fibrinogen. Cryo indications are

Box 3: Calculation and interpretation of corrected count increment (CCI).

CCI = [post count (per µL) − pre count (per µL)] × BSA (m^2)/number of administered platelets (×1,011)
- A CCI > 7,500 at 1 hour and > 4,500 at 24 hours post-transfusion indicate adequate platelet responses
- A CCI < 5,000 at 1 hour indicates possible immune refractoriness
- A CCI < 4,500 at 24 hours indicates probable nonimmune refractoriness

Box 4: Indications for transfusing platelet in emergency department (ED).

- Patient with major hemorrhage and hemodynamically unstable where massive transfusion protocol is indicated
- Patient with active bleeding and platelet count is less than 50,000/µL
- Patient with thrombocytopenia due to reduce production such as in bone marrow dysfunction or inadequate precursors such as vitamin B$_{12}$ and folic acid deficiency who need urgent procedure in ED such as (LP, or central line placement) and their platelet count is less than 50,000/µL
- Patient with thrombocytopenia due to known or suspected autoimmune thrombocytopenia and life-threatening bleeding such as ICH, or major bleeding
- Patient with thrombocytopenia due to reduce production who have platelet count < 10,000/µL in attempt to prevent spontaneous ICH

(ICH: intracranial hemorrhage; LP: lumbar puncture)

Box 5: Indications for fresh frozen plasma (FFP) transfusion in emergency department (ED).

- Replacement of a single coagulation factor deficiency, where a specific or combined factor concentrate is unavailable or contraindicated
- Reversal of warfarin
- TTP
- C1 esterase inhibitor deficiency
- Massive blood transfusion
- DIC
- Acquired fibrinogen deficiency when volume resuscitation is needed as well

(DIC: disseminated intravascular coagulation; TTP: thrombotic thrombocytopenic purpura)

similar to FFP as components of clotting factors are almost the same except that Cryo is higher in fibrinogen. Transfusing 10 units of Cryo is expected to raises the plasma fibrinogen level by up to 1 g/L (60–100 mg/dL) in average adult patient. Then the main difference between Cryo and FFP in ED is that FFP has more volume than Cryo so when volume resuscitation is required, FFP is better. As well Cryo has to be ABO compatible.

Specific Coagulation Factor Therapy

Those are all blood-derived components. Most are new and has been in use over past 1 or 2 decades. **Table 6** lists their compositions and indications of use.

Table 6: Specific coagulation factors.

Product	Composition	Indications
PCCs	• Three-factor: II, IX, and X • Four factor II, VII, IX, and X	• Warfarin reversal (four factors) • Known factor II or X deficiency
Factor VIII	Factor VIII	Hemophilia A
Factor VII		• May be used in life-threatening bleeding in trauma and if in your local massive • Transfusion protocol • Consider use in ICH
Fibrinogen recombinant	Fibrinogen (derived from pooled human plasma, stored as powder in room temperature, can be prepared quite rapidly)	• Known congenital fibrinogen deficiency • Acquired fibrinogen disorder where volume resuscitation is not needed or volume can be harmful such as multiple transfusion in heart failure patient

(ICH: intracranial hemorrhage; PCC: prothrombin complex concentrates)

Nonblood Products or Transfusion Therapy

As discussed above, hemostasis process depends on many factors and not blood components only. Nontransfusion therapy includes precursors that augment hemostasis such as body temperature, calcium, and other medications such as tranexamic acid, desmopressin, and vitamin K. Maintaining patient core temperature is essential for platelet function hence to maintain hemostasis. In patients with major hemorrhage is present and patient requires massive transfusion, blood products shall be warmed if possible and patient temperature shall be monitored and maintained at normothermia. Vitamin K may be used in patients with hypoprothrombinemia due to drugs or factors limiting its absorption or synthesis such as warfarin therapy, sever liver disease, and/or biliary obstruction, pancreatic dysfunction, malabsorption, or any cause of steatorrhea or malnourished patients and chronic alcohol intake. Desmopressin may help in patients known for VWB, hemophilia A, and platelet function disorders. Calcium is essential FV and FVIII function and chelation of calcium because of the added citrate in the blood products may result in coagulopathy hence worsen the bleeding. Tranexamic acid is known as effective first-line therapy for patients with menorrhagia, and can be used with patients known for other bleeding disorders as well specifically when major hemorrhage is present and massive transfusion is required (**Table 7**).

Blood Products Transfusions Pitfalls

Technicality: Emergency physicians shall be aware that the vascular access utilized for transfusion may affect the quality of the therapy specifically with PRBC transfusion (bloody easy). Hemolysis may result, if PRBC is transfused rapidly and under pressure through a small vascular access. In adult patient, size 16–18G IV access is required when transfusion is needed

Table 7: Word Health Organization (WHO) transfusion technique recommendations for nurses.

Before transfusion	Check blood bag for: • Sign of hemolysis in the plasma, which may indicate that the blood has been contaminated, allowed to freeze or to warm • Change of color in the red cells, which often look darker/purple/black when contaminated • Clot, which may mean that the blood was not mixed properly with the anticoagulant when it was collected or might also indicate bacterial contamination due to the utilization of citrate by proliferating bacteria • Leak in the bag or that it has already been opened
	Discard blood bag, if any of the following: • It has been out of the refrigerator for longer than 30 minutes • The seal is broken • There is any sign of hemolysis, clotting, or contamination
Performing the transfusion	• Checking the patient's identity and the blood bag before transfusion. It should be done at the patient's bedside immediately before commencing the administration of the blood product. It should be undertaken by two people, at least one of whom should be a registered nurse or doctor
Time limit for transfusion	• PRBC: Within 30 minutes, if removing from refrigerator and transfusion shall be completed in less than 4 hours • Platelet, FFP, and cryoprecipitate shall be transfused immediately upon receiving it and completed within 30 minutes
Documentation required	• Time the transfusion started • Nurse shall document patient's general appearance, vital signs including (pulse, temperature, blood pressure, and respiratory rate) at beginning of transfusion, 15 minutes after starting then every hour until transfusion is completed • Time the transfusion was completed • Volume and type of blood products, blood group of each unit transfused time at which the transfusion of each unit commenced • Unique donation number of all products transfused • Any adverse effect • Signature of the individual responsible for administration of the blood

(FFP: fresh frozen plasma; PRBC: packed red blood cell)

to be given rapid and under pressure in hemodynamically unstable patient. For pediatric patient's size 22-25G is adequate with bigger size to be used for resuscitation. All other blood products can be given through any line size. On the other hand, emergency physicians and nurses shall be aware that dextrose and calcium containing IV solutions shall not be used in the same access or IV set along with blood as the former may result in hemolysis and the calcium in ringer lactate for example will antagonize the citrate in the PRBC, which may result in clotting. The clinical significance of these two reactions is undetermined. The standard is not to infuse anything along blood products except for normal saline, on the other hand, some analgesia was found not to interfere with the blood, if infused in the same line though as well the standard is to avoid infusing anything along blood products. ED nurse shall always flush the IV set with normal saline before starting transfusion. If patient condition requires the administration of steroid or antihistamine or if he had taken them shortly prior to the ED presentation emergency physicians shall be aware that transfusion reaction symptoms might appear later than usual.

Complications of Blood Products Transfusion

Transfusion reaction is considered one of the main acute complications of transfusion therapy. By definition, acute reaction occurs in less than 24 hours of transfusion and can result from ABO incompatibility, wrong blood unit administration, or poor quality product. Considering pathophysiology, acute transfusion reaction can be either of immunological etiology or of nonimmunological etiology. Causes of immunological etiology are hemolytic reaction, febrile nonhemolytic, allergic reaction, or transfusion-related acute lung injury. Nonimmunologic can result in bacterial contamination, circulatory overload, or physical and chemical hemolysis.

■ PITFALLS ABOUT SPECIFIC BLEEDING DISORDERS IN ED

Idiopathic Thrombocytopenic Purpura

- Autoimmune disease
- It is a clinical diagnosis and diagnosis of exclusion
- Can be either acute or chronic
- Acute idiopathic thrombocytopenic purpura (ITP) is a disease of children between age of 2-year and 6-year old:
  - Usually preceded by viral illness
  - Platelet count usually to less than 20,000/mm^3
  - Self-limited in most patients
  - If actively bleeding then steroids and intravenous immunoglobulin (IVIg) can be considered.
- Chronic ITP is a disease of adult age:
  - Women affected more than men
  - Not associated with viral illness
  - Presents as easy bruising, prolonged menses, and mucosal bleeding, petechiae, or purpura
  - Platelet counts between 30,000/mm^3 and 100,000/mm^3 are common
  - Treatment, if actively bleeding, is—corticosteroids, anti-D antibody (immunoglobulin) and splenectomy, if platelet count does not respond to steroids and IVIg.

Thrombotic Thrombocytopenic Purpura

- Life-threatening
- Rare

- Nonimmune disease
- Results from lack of activity in the ADAMTS13 enzyme
- Triggered by physiological stress to the body such as (e.g. surgery, pancreatitis, sepsis, and pregnancy)
- Microthrombosis in small vessels affects various systems
- Classic pentad:
  - Fever
  - Anemia (microangiopathic hemolytic anemia)
  - Thrombocytopenia
  - Acute kidney injury
  - Central nervous system (CNS) involvement (headaches, confusion, seizures, intracranial hemorrhage, and focal deficits)
- *Diagnosis*: Low ADAMTS13 protease or organ involved biopsy shows typical microaneurysms and fibrin.
- *Treatment*:
  - *Plasmapheresis*: Decreases mortality to less than 10%, needs to be started as soon as possible
  - Corticosteroids
  - Rituximab
- Do not transfuse platelet unless life-threatening hemorrhage.

Disseminated Intravascular Coagulation

- Acquired syndrome
- *Pathophysiology*:
  - Multisystem microvasculature intravascular activation of coagulation
  - Microvascular thrombi result in multisystem organ dysfunction
  - Consumptive intravascular coagulopathy and thrombocytopenia result in hemorrhage.
- *Diagnosis*:
  - Clinical suspicion
  - Calculate DIC score (**Table 8**)
  - *Treatment*:
    - Treat underlying cause
    - Correct coagulopathy, especially if active bleeding.

Hemophilia A

- Deficiency in FVIII
- 1 in 5,000 male births

Table 8: Disseminated intravascular coagulation (DIC) score.

Platelet	• >100,000/μL (0 points) • 50,000–100,000/μL (1 point) • <50,000/μL (2 points)
Increase in fibrin markers (e.g. D-Dimer)	• No change (0 points) • Moderate rise (2 points) • Strong rise (3 points)
Prothrombin time prolongation	• 3 seconds or less (0 points) • >3 seconds but <6 seconds (1 point) • Greater than 6 seconds (2 points)
Fibrinogen level	• Greater than 1 g/L (0 points) • Less than 1 g/L (1 point)
Score interpretation: • *0–4 points*: DIC is not overt, repeat score in 1–2 days • *5–8 point*: DIC probable, repeat score daily	

- *Treatment in ED*:
    - Consider factor replacement procedures such as lumbar puncture (LP), incision, and drainage
    - Replace, if actively bleeding
    - In major bleeding, always assume factor level is 0%
    - *Mild-to-moderate bleeding*: (Soft tissue, muscle, hemarthrosis, epistaxis) replace factor up to 50% (50 U/kg will likely result in 50%)
    - *Severe life-threatening bleeds*: [CNS, gastrointestinal (GI), neck/throat, major trauma] replace factor up to 100%
    - *Calculating FVIII dose:* Units of FVIII required = Patients weight (kg) × 0.5 × (% activity desired − (%) intrinsic activity.

■ PREPARING YOUR ED FOR THE BLEEDING DISORDERS PATIENT

Emergency department needs to cater for most commonly congenital bleeding disorders such as hemophilia A and B before they even approach the ED. Having ED protocol that addresses standards for triage, appropriate time to be seen by physicians (door to doctor time), diagnostic workup and factor replacement indications for various bleeding site, doses and duration of treatment will certainly improve both physicians and patient's experience. On the other hand, having pre-prepared discharge instruction sheet that can be developed with the assistance of the hematologist to guide patients on symptoms they need to watch for and when to return to ED and important phone number to call is part of the patient management process and once established, it will serve many patients for years.

SUMMARY

Bleeding disorders are common specially the acquired one. Having understanding of etiology, clinical presentation, and management is essential for safe emergency medicine practice. The 5-step approach described above will help the emergency physician to assess patients presenting with nontraumatic bleeding in order to detect possible acquired or inherited bleeding disorders. Preparing our EDs to patient with bleeding disorders will facilitate their management and enhance safety of therapy provided in ED.

Bell's Palsy

Ali Abdolrazaghnejad, Mohsen Banaie

INTRODUCTION

Facial nerve palsy is classified according to the location of the conflict (central and peripheral), the duration of paralysis (acute, subacute, and chronic), and the cause of paralysis (specific or idiopathic). Bell's paralysis is the most common idiopathic syndrome due to peripheral paralysis of the facial nerve, which is acute onset and monosymptomatic; and since Sir Charles Bell was able to describe this nerve for the first time in the early 19th century, it was called by this name for his appreciation. Although the two terms "Bell's palsy" and "idiopathic facial paralysis" are not scientifically exactly equivalent, nevertheless, in this chapter, these two terms are considered to be the same. Bell's paralysis is responsible for three-fourths of the acute facial paralysis and the most common cause of facial nerve palsy. However, due to the progress of science and diagnostic methods, it is expected that the prevalence of idiopathic facial nerve palsies will decrease over time, because finding the causes of the pathogenesis of these diseases are increasing day-by-day.

ETIOLOGY

The cranial nerve VII, or the facial nerve, is located inside a narrow canal in the temporal bone and has the longest intracranial pathway in the cranial nerves. As a result, any damage to this physical structure can disrupt the function of the nerve. For example, edema or any agent that causes edema (such as trauma, burn, infection, bacteria, viruses such as herpes zoster and herpes simplex 1, irradiation, fractures) can be a predisposing factor in the presence of peripheral facial paralysis. Bell's paralysis, or the idiopathic paralysis of the facial nerve, is a diagnosis of exclusion and occurs when there is no specific cause for the pathophysiology of facial nerve palsy.

PATHOPHYSIOLOGY

As previously mentioned, Bell's paralysis is a clinical complication of an uncertain cause. As a result, exact pathophysiology cannot be determined. However, with the advancement of technology and the ability to detect the genome of viruses using polymerase chain reaction (PCR), many gains have been made in the finding of the cause of Bell's paralysis. The findings of different studies suggest that the most important causes of this clinical syndrome can be a viral infection, in particular, herpes, vascular ischemia, and autoimmune diseases. Among the viruses responsible for the pathogenesis of Bell's paralysis, the two herpes simplex and herpes zoster viruses have the highest share. These two viruses in the infected individuals are in the geniculate ganglion of the facial nerve as a silent. After activation, these viruses cause inflammation, edema, and reversible neuropraxia in the facial nerve, which ultimately can lead to Wallerian degeneration. In a study, the disease was associated with arterial hypertension, diabetes, pregnancy, and puerperium. However, the simultaneous onset of Bell's paralysis with a disease does not necessarily suggest a relationship between them.

The natural course of the disease is benign, in most cases, and almost 70% of the patients recover without any adverse effects. However, about 10% of patients eventually lose their full function of the facial nerve and about 5% of the patients will have side effects after healing (such as spasticity, synkinesis).

CLINICAL MANIFESTATION

This idiopathic illness develops in the form of acute paralysis (usually within a few hours) of the peripheral cranial nerve VII (facial nerve), which causes one-sided facial involvement. Since this nerve, in addition to motor fibers (such as stapedius muscle fibers), has the responsibility for innervating lacrimal and submandibular glands autonomic system and also the sense of ear and the taste sensation of the two-thirds of the anterior part of the tongue through chorda tympani. Signs of damage to it can vary depending on the location of the conflict. However, common clinical manifestations in people generally include dry eye and decreased tears, pain, and anesthesia around the ear, tamper, or mandibular angle, inability to close the eyes or blink, fade nasolabial fold, and disturb the taste sensation.

RED FLAGS

As previously mentioned, Bell's palsy is benign, and almost 70% of cases are recovered without any adverse effects. But since a wide range of diseases can be manifested as peripheral paralysis of the facial nerve, attention to the differential diagnosis of this disease is of great importance. In fact, Bell's paralysis is a diagnosis of exclusion. **Box 1** lists the differential diagnosis and the underlying causes of the disease, which is based on the Finsterer study table and completed with the help of other studies.

EVALUATION

Due to the wide range of differential diagnosis for Bell's paralysis, each patient with sudden one-sided facial paralysis should be examined completely in terms of history and physical examination. When taking a history, checkpoints such as the onset of the disease, the history of any trauma, especially recent head and face trauma, high-risk behavior, recent infectious disease, history of underlying illness such as diabetes and hypertension, drug use, and history of malignant diseases in the patient and immediate family are very important. In addition,

Box 1: Differential diagnosis and predisposing factors for Bell's palsy.

Causes and predisposing factors
Infections:
- Herpes zoster
- Herpes simplex
- Influenza
- Hansen's disease (leprosy)
- Otitis media
- Mastoiditis
- Ramsey-Hunt syndrome
- Borreliosis
- Cryptococcosis
- Neurocysticercosis
- Toxocarosis
- Tuberculous meningitis
- Parotitis, parotid abscess
- Malignant external otitis
- Syphillis
- Lyme
- Guillain-Barré syndrome
- HIV Infection

Metabolic disease:
- Diabetes
- Pre-eclampsia

Stroke:
- Ipsilateral pontine infarction
- Pontine tegmental hemorrhage

Surgery:
- Removal of cerebellopontine angle tumors

Trauma:
- Head trauma (crush injury)
- Birth injury

Tumor:
- Facial nerve neurinoma
- Cerebellopontine angle tumors (neurinoma)
- Pons tumor
- Tumors of the petrosal bone
- Tumors of the middle ear
- Leukemia
- Tumors of the parotid gland
- Lymphoma

Immune system disorder:
- Guillain-Barre syndrome
- Miller-Fisher syndrome
- Systemic lupus erythematous
- Myasthenia gravis
- Sjögren syndrome

Drugs:
- Interferon
- Linezolid

Contd...

Contd...

Others:
- Moebius syndrome
- Melkersson-Rosenthal syndrome
- Sarcoidosis
- Histiocytosis X
- Autism
- Asperger's syndrome
- Parkinson syndrome

during the physical examination of the patient, in addition to examining the functioning of the cranial nerves, especially the cranial VI nerve, it should be paid attention to the parotid mass, vesicles or scabbing on the face and especially the external ear (for the rule out of herpes zoster).

INTERPRETATION OF FINDING

Since Bell's palsy diagnosis is caused by the rejection of other diagnoses, after receiving the initial history and complete physical examination, it can be diagnosed in the absence of diagnostic criteria for other differential diagnosis and based on clinical findings. Also, if you have certain clinical symptoms or a red flag during your examination, according to the results of the preliminary interpretation of the findings, it is necessary to identify the next diagnostic-therapeutic step.

INVESTIGATIONS

If there is a suspicion of a differential diagnosis for Bell's palsy during a patient's examination, we should select appropriate paraclinical method according to the type of finding. Given the wide range of these diagnoses, these actions can include blood workup, PCR, chest X-ray (CXR), computed tomography (CT) scan, magnetic resonance imaging (MRI), and so on.

TREATMENT

Treatment for Bell's paralysis generally involves the use of oral corticosteroids. Antiviral drugs can also be used in cases where there is suspicion of viral causes in the disease. However, in meta-analyses, there was no evidence of a clinically effective combination of this therapeutic regimen. In the treatment of patients with this disease, the main goals of the health team in order to expedite recovery should be psychological support and inhibition of viral replication, prevent ocular complications and side effects. The proposed diet regimens have been described as prednisolone (60–80 mg/day for 1 week), which should start within 3 days of onset of clinical symptoms.

■ SUMMARY

When dealing with a patient with acute one-sided facial paralysis and a clinical suspicion of Bell's disease, it is necessary to consider the differential diagnosis of this disease; and after ruling out other diagnosis and the confirmation of Bell's palsy diagnosis, the doctor should begin to treat the patient as soon as possible and reduce the complications and future adverse effects. Also, follow-up of patients after their treatment period is essential in order to consider the recovery process and the long-term complications of the disease on the eye, the patient's psychologic state, and probable side effects. Studies have suggested the use of botulinum toxin to improve facial muscle expression in people with muscle spasm.

CHAPTER 10

Breast Problems

Rajeev Agarwal

INTRODUCTION

Breast disease in a woman is a spectrum of benign and malignant disorders. The frequency of breast cancer varies with the age of the women and presenting symptoms. Though the vast majority of breast lesions are benign, any symptom of breast at any age should not be ignored as breast cancer though uncommon can occur as young as in twenties or thirties.

In India, women with breast disorders often present to either female physicians or gynecologists. A systemic approach and prompt evaluation is most important as any delay in the diagnosis of breast cancer may lead to worsening of prognosis. The most common breast symptoms that a woman presents to a doctor are breast pain, nipple discharge, and a palpable lump.

The uncommon presentation may be eczematous changes on the nipple, nipple retraction, thickening and redness of breast skin, isolated axillary lymphadenopathy, etc.

BREAST PAIN (MASTALGIA)

It is the most common breast symptoms in clinical practice. It may be:
- Cyclical (in relation to menstrual cycle) or noncyclical
- Unilateral or bilateral
- Continuous or intermittent
- Localized or diffuse, or
- A chest wall pain presenting as breast pain.

The *etiology* of mastalgia is unknown. Its common occurrence in premenopausal women has been suggested to be hormonal in origin but no definite correlation to hormone levels has been established. Certain nonhormonal factors, i.e. excessive intake of caffeine, physical and emotional stress have also been attributed to it.

The classification is important as the response to treatment varies in various types of pain. Overall 92% of cyclical mastalgia, 64% of noncyclical mastalgia, and 97% of those with chest wall pain will respond to medical management.

Evaluation of Breast Pain

Breast pain is often associated with benign breast conditions but presence of pain does not completely rule out a diagnosis of cancer.

A detailed history and duration of pain, its relation to menstrual cycle, trauma, drug intake, emotional stress, and lactational status are important.

A thorough physical examination should be done to exclude any localized tenderness, lump or any other physical abnormality. In the absence of a palpable mass, young woman of less than 35–40 years should undergo an ultrasonography breast and older one should undergo mammography and if needed to be supplemented by an ultrasound breast as certain benign tumor, cyst and occasionally malignant tumors may also cause pain. Any further investigations are needed if there is some abnormality detected on these investigations.

Management

In the absence of any physical or imaging findings, it is best to reassure the patient that this pain is physiological, self-limiting and may get a significant remission in 60–80% cases.

In moderate to severe pain, causing interference with day-to-day activities of patient, the one drug approval by the United States Food and Drug Administration (USFDA) is danazol in 100–400 mg/day with a response rate of 50–75% with some side effects.

Evening primrose oil has also shown to be effective in 58% of cyclical, 36% of noncyclical mastalgia with very little or no side effects.

Tamoxifen is a drug used for treatment of hormone receptor positive breast cancer in the dose of 20 mg/day. In refractory cases of mastalgia, this drug can be given in a dose of 10–20 mg/day from 10 days to 20 days of menstrual cycle has shown benefit in 90% of cyclical and 56% of noncyclical mastalgia.

Vitamin E supplements, avoidance of caffeine has not been successful in randomized trials.

Surgery has no role in the management of mastalgia without a dominant mass.

For chest wall pain presenting as breast pain, specific treatment related to the cases should be taken care off.

NIPPLE DISCHARGE

Majority of women presenting with nipple discharge have benign etiology but may happen in cancer breast also. It can be physiological or pathological.

Physiological discharge (secretion) may be bilateral, from multiple ducts and more often nonspontaneous and may be collected by aspiration, massage, and expression from ducts.

Pathological discharges are spontaneous, may or may not be associated with a mass, usually unilateral and confined to one or two ducts.

The causes of pathological discharge are:
- Duct ectasia
- Inflammatory lesion of duct
- Intraductal papillomas or papillomatosis
- Carcinoma
- Hormonal disorder—hypothyroidism, prolactinemia, pituitary adenoma

- Drugs—oral contraceptive pills, large dose of tragulizers, metachlorpromide.
It can be serous, milky, dark greenish or blood stained.

Evaluation
Careful history between physiological and pathological discharge is important.

If discharge is physiological, a thorough physical examination is usually sufficient. An ultrasound breast in young patient (35–40 years or young) and a mammography above 40 years is recommended. Nipple discharge cytology is usually not contributory.

Squeezing of nipple should be avoided for physiological discharge. Most of them resolve spontaneously and reassurance is usually adequate.

Pathological Discharge
- Localization of affected duct.
- Examination of discharge for occult blood (a dark green discharge may look blood stained by naked eye but on microscopic examination or laboratory testing, no traces of blood will be there).
- Cytology of discharge though often done has a limited value as a negative result does not exclude cancer and on the basis of positive result of malignant cytology one should not do definite treatment as it cannot differentiate between ductal carcinoma in situ (DCIS) and invasive ductal carcinoma (IDC).
- Mammography, ultrasound breast, contrast-enhanced magnetic resonance imaging (MRI) and if needed relevant image-guided biopsy is indicated.
- Excision of terminal duct may be diagnostic as well as therapeutic in benign case.
- When blood stained discharge is associated with a mass or a diagnosis of cancer is suspected on imaging, all efforts should be made to establish diagnosis by image-guided biopsy [core needle/vacuum-assisted biopsy (VAB)] and treatment as per the standard treatment of cancer breast.

BREAST MASS (LUMP)
The feeling of a breast lump or lumpiness is the second most common presenting complaints after mastalgia. Almost 90% of breast lumps are benign, but a detail workup is necessary to rule out cancer as it can occur as young as twenties and thirties.

Breast masses may be:
- Single or multiple
- Unilateral or bilateral
- Solid or cystic
- Painful or painless.

Malignant masses may be associated with other symptoms, i.e. nipple retraction, skin thickening, blood stained discharge, palpable axillary or neck lymphadenopathy.

Breast masses may be:
- Physiological nodularity in young women
- Cysts (single or complex)
- Fibroadenoma
- Prominent areas of fibrocystic changes
- Phyllodes tumor
- Chronic abscess and antibiomas
- Lactation abscess
- Traumatic fat necrosis
- Cancer.

Physiological nodularity usually occurs in young age group, in upper outer quadrant or inframammary crease and waxing and waning during menstrual cycle, usually not associated with any pathology and need only reassurance.

Dominant masses are definite lump persisting throughout the menstrual cycle and needed proper evaluation.

Cystic masses: They are common particularly in premenopausal women of 35–40 years onward and are uncommon in younger women or postmenopausal women.

Cysts are usually well defined, firm, mobile, and may be tender. Physical examination and mammography may not be helpful in differentiating solid/cystic masses. Ultrasound with or without aspiration is the best modality to establish the diagnosis. Cysts usually do not need surgery unless associated with a solid component. Then cysts should be aspirated, image-guided core needle biopsy of solid component should be done to establish the pathology and treated accordingly.

Solid masses: Palpable solid masses are always pathological (benign or malignant) and all attempts must be made by appropriate investigations to establish the diagnosis. The extent of evaluation of a solid mass depends upon the age of patient, risk status, and degree of clinical suspicion. Imaging studies define the extent of primary lump or any other nonpalpable lesion which may influence the choice of locoregional treatment.

Evaluation of Breast Mass

History includes duration, change in the size over a period of time, relationship with menstrual cycle, pain, lactational status, associated change in overlying skin or nipple, discharge from nipple, age at menarche, age at first full term pregnancy, dose of oral contraceptive or hormone replacement therapy, family history of breast and ovarian cancer in first- or second-degree relatives, any previous breast biopsy and if yes, the histology, i.e. atypical ductal or lobular hyperplasia, ductal cancer in situ, lobular cancer in situ, sclerosing adenosis, etc.

Clinical examination includes inspection of breast in supine and upright position; see any difference in the size of breast, nipple or skin changes.

Palpation includes estimate of location, size, fixity of lump to overlying skin or underlying muscle or chest wall, axillary or supraclavicular nodes, and contralateral breast.

Imaging: In younger patients up to 35 years, an ultrasound is preferred to differentiate between solid and cystic masses. In older patients, bilateral mammogram is a must in a symptomatic patient followed by an ultrasound in selected cases.

Mammography may show an area of asymmetrical density, mass, calcification (benign or malignant looking), skin changes and any other nonpalpable lesion on the same side or contralateral breast.

The MRI of breast is done in selected cases where mammography and ultrasound are inconclusive, in a diagnosed case of cancer to redefine extent of local lesion particularly in younger patients where the breasts are dense on mammography. Breast MRI should always be done contrast enhanced.

Tissue Diagnosis

Breast biopsy: Not all palpable lesions need tissue diagnosis. Cystic lesions without a solid component need not a biopsy.

Core needle biopsy is a gold standard and may be done in outpatient department (OPD) setting for large palpable lesions or image guided (mammographic, ultrasound or MRI guided) in different situations. In selected cases, an advanced form of core biopsy called as VAB is done where there is no definite mass lesion but abnormality in the form of microcalcification, or nonmass enhancement. These forms of biopsy have become method of choice and have negligible false-positive or false-negative rate. They not only give a definite diagnosis, in malignant cases, tumor markers can be done on biopsy tissue to plan the initial treatment.

Fine-needle aspiration cytology: Though commonly done in India, is not the preferred method of diagnosis due to:
- Significant risk of false-negative and occasionally false-positive rates.
- Tumor markers and other immunohistochemistry (IHC) tests cannot be performed on fine-needle aspiration cytology (FNAC) tissue.

Therefore, even if a FNAC has been negative, further evaluation must be done in the presence of a clinical or radiological suspicion.

Incisional or excisional biopsy: They are rarely done in a specialized center except wire localization excision of suspected microcalcification where stereotactic biopsy facility is not feasible or available.

Management of Breast Masses

Significant number of biopsy proven benign lesion may not need surgical excision and may be closely observed. Decision for excision may be taken on case to case basis—if the lesion is very large, suspected phyllodes tumor even if biopsy showing benign epithelial tumors, patients anxiety.

All proven phyllodes tumors and cancers must be managed as per standard guidelines.

GYNECOMASTIA

It is the most common condition of male breast. It can be unilateral or bilateral, painless or painful and occasionally tender in the retroareolar area.

Gynecomastia usually occurs in neonatal period, during puberty or in adult population beyond 50 years of age up to 7th or 8th decades of life. In majority, it is idiopathic. Other causes include certain drugs (anabolic steroids) cirrhosis, primary and secondary hypogonadism, testicular tumors hypothyroidism and renal disease.

Gynecomastia should be differentiated from pseudogynecomastia (fatty enlargement of breast without glandular proliferation). In gynecomastia, there is a firm or rubbery, mobile, disk-like mound of tissue shall be felt beneath the nipple areola complex. No such tissue is present in pseudogynecomastia.

The patient usually presents with enlargement of breast and is concerned either due to pain or cosmetic reason.

On examination, there may be a concentric firm area in retroareolar reason along with enlargement of overall breast size.

It usually does not need any major investigation and diagnosis is usually clinical. An ultrasound in younger patients and a mammogram in older patient are sufficient to reassure and exclude any underlying pathology.

Treatment

Medical therapy: Danazol, tamoxifen, and clomiphene have been tried with varying success. The best results are obtained with clomiphene in the doses of 50–100 mg/day causing reduction in breast size in almost two-thirds cases. Tamoxifen in 10 mg twice a day for 3 months has also shown good results. Similarly danazol in the doses of 50–100 mg/day is also effective in certain case but has a limited use due to side effects.

Surgical therapy: Surgery is usually reserved for cosmetic reason on patient's choice. Subcutaneous mastectomy is the standard approach.

Bowel Obstruction

Jesus Daniel López Tapia, Aldo Emigdio Bartolini Salinas

INTRODUCTION

Bowel obstruction is defined as the impairment of passage of intestinal content. It is classified according to a couple of characteristics that are the site of obstruction, the degree of obstruction, and the presence of irrigation impairment (ischemia). The sites of obstruction in general terms are the small bowel and the large bowel, which have an additional subclassification, which can be extrinsic or intrinsic (intraluminal and intramural). The degree of obstruction can be either partial or complete. In a partial obstruction, there is still some passage of intestinal content and gas which could result in constipation; in a complete obstruction, there is no passage of intestinal content and the patient might present with obstipation (incapability of passing gas or stool).

We can further classify bowel obstruction on its peristaltic characteristics (dynamic or adynamic). When the obstruction is nonmechanical or adynamic, there is an impairment in the transmission of neuromuscular innervation to the myenteric plexus, which results in paralytic ileus (aperistalsis) and colonic pseudo-obstruction. Dynamic obstruction occurs when there is a mechanical obstruction of the bowel lumen, which impairs peristalsis functionality. These obstructions can be extrinsic, intrinsic (intraluminal, intramural) as determined earlier.

It can be challenging to establish a diagnosis due to unspecified symptomatology, radiological and laboratory results. Learning these classifications can help identify these differences which have an important outcome in decision making regarding treatment choices. Mechanical obstruction will be widely discussed in this chapter.

ETIOLOGY/CAUSES

Bowel obstruction can be classified according to their etiology as being intrinsic (intraluminal, intramural) and extrinsic. The location and onset of obstruction guides us toward a specific etiology; it is important to determine if the obstruction is in the small or large bowel to be able to establish a precise diagnosis.

Postoperative adhesions are the most common etiology of small bowel obstruction (SBO) 60–85% of cases approximately, followed by hernias 30% which result in surgery due to incarceration and obstructive malignancy.

The large bowel is most frequently obstructed by a malignant etiology, rectosigmoid tumors are the most common manifestation of these; the benign etiology that obstructs the large bowel more frequently is the presence of sigmoid volvulus, followed by a stricture because of diverticulitis. Other causes of bowel obstruction are presented in **Boxes 1** and **2**.

Box 1: Causes of small bowel obstruction.

Intraluminal lesions:
- Intussusception
- Gallstones
- Congenital atresia, duplication and congenital bands
- Neoplasm
- Parasites
- Bezoars
- Foreign body
- Strictures due to nonsteroidal anti-inflammatory drug (NSAID) enteropathy
- Feces
- Meconium
- Food bolus

Intramural lesions:
- Neoplasm
- Hematoma
- Crohn's disease
- Postoperative stricture ring
- Radiation enteritis

Extrinsic lesions:
- Adhesions (congenital and acquired)
- Hernia (congenital and acquired)
- Volvulus
- Endometriosis
- Carcinomatosis
- Superior mesenteric artery syndrome
- Abscess

Box 2: Causes of large bowel obstruction.

- Neoplasm (colorectal cancer)
- Adhesions
- Strictures (diverticular disease, ischemic colitis, Crohn's disease)
- Volvulus (sigmoid volvulus)
- Hernia
- Fecal impaction
- Inflammatory bowel disease
- Bezoars
- Intussusception
- Gallstone ileus
- Endometriosis

PATHOPHYSIOLOGY

Small bowel obstruction occurs when there is a blockage of its lumen, preventing the normal passage of intestinal content through the bowel, impairing its normal functionality. When this happens, the small bowel starts to dilate proximal to the site of obstruction provoking bacterial accumulation and fermentation. Swallowed air, gas, and bacterial fermentation lead to intestinal distention, bowel wall edema and loss of absorptive function; translocation of bacterial fermentation may lead to sepsis. As this process continues, there is loss of electrolyte-rich fluid by emesis and transudation, this may result in metabolic alkalosis and hypovolemia. Continued bowel distention leads to vascular compromise, loss of perfusion, ischemia and eventually necrosis and perforation.

Large bowel obstruction (LBO) occurs in 60% of cases because of a neoplasm. Tumors that tend to cause obstruction with greater frequency are those located at the splenic flexure. Ischemia, necrosis and perforation in LBO occur due to an inflammatory reaction provoked by tumor invasion. The ileocecal valve plays an important role in the physiopathology of LBO, when the ileocecal valve is competent, a closed loop obstruction (presence of two obstruction sites) occurs due to the incapability of decompression of the bowel, resulting in ischemia or necrosis.

CLINICAL PRESENTATION

The clinical presentation of SBO and LBO differs slightly from one and other, and its symptomatology varies depending on the onset of instauration. These differences will be explained in **Table 1**.

Table 1: Clinical presentation of small bowel and large bowel obstruction.

Small bowel obstruction (SBO)	Large bowel obstruction (LBO)
Acute onset:	Acute onset:
• Periumbilical pain (colicky, cramping) • Nausea • Vomiting • Abdominal distention • Obstipation	• Hypogastric pain • Abdominal distention • Obstipation • Diarrhea • Rectal tenesmus • Rectal obstruction • Nausea and vomiting (may or may not be present)
Chronic onset:	Chronic onset:
• Develop same symptomatology of acute onset SBO, but with varying severity	• Weight loss • Weakness • Anorexia • Rectal bleeding • Develop same symptomatology of acute onset LBO, but with varying severity

Careful evaluation of symptomatology progress must be done, abdominal pain can evolve from being an intermittent cramping pain to a constant and more severe pain, which might indicate clinical complications such as ischemia and perforation. Nausea and vomiting might be more severe in patients with a proximal SBO and abdominal distention might be minimal. In distal SBO, vomiting might be infrequent and abdominal distention important.

RED FLAGS

Red flags of small bowel and large bowel obstruction have been shown in **Box 3**.

EVALUATION

History

Performing a complete medical history is a crucial step to meet to obtain sufficient information that leads us to an accurate diagnosis. Even though a thorough medical history is necessary, if a patient arrives in the emergency room, there are five main clinical features we should always have in mind. These are the presence of abdominal pain, constipation/obstipation, abdominal distention, and vomiting. Acknowledging if the patient has had a previous surgical procedure is of equal importance.

Abdominal Pain

When carrying out a physical examination in a patient with abdominal pain, careful attention must be paid to the location and onset of pain. Abdominal pain is the most common complaint.

Box 3: Red flags of small bowel and large bowel obstruction.

Small bowel obstruction:
- Prior abdominal surgery
- Inflammatory bowel disease
- Presence or history of cancer
- Hernias
- Radiotherapy

Large bowel obstruction:
- Presence or history of cancer
- Prior abdominal surgery
- Prior colorectal resection
- Inflammatory bowel disease
- Hernias
- Physiological or anatomical malformations
- Volvulus
- Radiotherapy
- Diverticulitis
- Endometriosis
- Tuberculosis
- Suppository use
- Fecal impaction

SBO pain usually is in the periumbilical area and is described as a colicky or cramping pain which is generally of severe and acute instauration. In LBO, hypogastric pain is frequently present, and generally described as a cramping pain which recurs every 20 minutes approximately. When there is a closed loop obstruction in LBO, pain can be constantly increasing. In any of these cases, if pain becomes constant and fixed in a specific area the possibility of ischemia or perforation is greater.

Constipation/Obstipation

These clinical manifestations might be present in SBO and LBO, although they are generally indicative of a LBO. Incapability to pass gas or stool might be present in an acute onset of LBO and usually occurs in a distal obstruction. Past surgical history should be acquired, as well as changes in intestinal functioning or unprogrammed weigh changes in the last few months.

Abdominal Distension

Once the obstruction develops, peristaltic activity increases in an effort to release the blockage, this process continues until intestinal motility starts to decrease due to relaxation of the bowel wall and dilation. This should be considered, since changes in peristaltic motility might be indicative of ischemia, necrosis, and perforation. In both SBO and LBO, abdominal distention is present, although usually greater in LBO, since vomiting helps alleviate this manifestation in SBO.

Vomiting

Vomiting might appear in both SBO and LBO, even though it is more frequently present in SBO as an early onset manifestation. The characteristics of the vomit are an important clue toward finding out the site of obstruction. Since unprocessed food usually indicates a proximal SBO and feculent vomit is generally indicative of a distal obstruction.

Physical Examination

A thorough physical examination should always be performed. In bowel obstruction, even though there are similar physical manifestations between SBO and LBO, paying close attention to these and other systemic features are imperative for an optimal diagnosis and treatment choice. Vital signs should be monitored. The presence of fever might be indicative of infection or other systemic complication. Heart rate monitoring is important since vomiting in SBO is usually present and this could lead to dehydration, tachycardia, hypotension, and oliguria.

Abdominal inspection is a key step, since in its fulfillment we might be able to find some previous surgery marks that could guide us toward the diagnosis. Abdominal auscultation should also be considered, in an acute onset bowel obstruction, as previously mentioned, peristalsis might be increased and accompanied by a hyper-resonant percussion differing from a chronic process in which peristalsis and percussion might be absent or hypoactive.

During abdominal palpation, we can be able to identify abdominal masses such as tumors or hernias that could be provoking the symptomatology. A rectal examination should be performed to evaluate rectal obstruction that might be caused by fecal impaction.

INTERPRETATION OF FINDING

- Persistent and increasing abdominal pain—might be indicative of a closed loop obstruction or/and ischemia, necrosis or perforation.
- Increased peristalsis—may indicate an early or recent obstruction.
- Decreased or absence of peristalsis—may indicate ischemia, necrosis or perforation.
- Persistent and increasing abdominal distention—the presence of LBO must be evaluated.
- Active vomiting—could be a sign of early proximal SBO.
- Bilious vomiting—main manifestation of intestinal malrotation and duodenal duplication cyst.
- Feculent vomiting—might be indicative of a distal obstruction.
- Presence of fever—systemic complication, bacteremia, sepsis.
- Oliguria, hypotension and tachycardia—may be found in dehydrated patients due to constant vomiting in SBO.
- Rectal obstruction—might be due to fecal impaction.

INVESTIGATIONS

After a general examination has been achieved, special attention should be paid to the abdominal (inspection, auscultation, percussion, and palpation) and digital rectal examination. A full cardiovascular evaluation is recommended, blood pressure, pulse, and capillary refill time should be considered. To detect or prevent the presence of systemic inflammatory response syndrome (SIRS), body temperature and respiratory rate must also be monitored.

Laboratory Studies

- Complete blood count with differential
- Electrolytes
- Blood urea nitrogen (BUN)
- Creatinine
- Amylase
- Arterial blood gas, serum lactate, and blood cultures (in patients with systemic signs).

Imaging Studies

- *Plain radiography (X-ray)*: It is preferred as first diagnostic tool because of its practical use. It can help determine whether an emergent procedure should be performed or not, and it can also help evaluating location and type of obstruction (partial or complete)

A plain supine abdominal radiography and an upright chest film should be done.
- Findings include:
  - Small dilated bowel loops that can be indicative of a LBO with an ileocecal valve that is incompetent in about 30% of cases. A dilated colonic diameter above 8 cm or a 10 cm or more dilation of the cecum is considered pathological.
  - If there is a dilation of the proximal bowel (>2.5 cm) with collapse of the distal bowel, it might be indicative of SBO.
  - An abdominal radiograph that shows a gasless abdomen might be indicative of a small bowel that is fluid-full. The sign of "string of pearls" might be present.
  - If volvulus is present, pneumoperitoneum, "northern exposure and coffee bean signs" might be present in LBO.
  - In an upright chest film, hydroaerial levels are found in the same levels in adynamic obstruction (paralytic ileus) while in mechanical obstruction these appear at different intestinal levels.
- *Multidetector computed tomography (MDCT) scan*: It can find the cause of obstruction in approximately 70–95% of cases and determine the specific location of the obstruction and evaluate any other masses that might be present.

  Performing computed tomography (CT) scan using contrast might be useful, but not essential, since retained fluid in the bowel can help function as contrast. Contrast imaging might be done by administering oral or rectal contrast, nasogastric tube can also be used. Intravenous contrast is another possibility although renal pathology patients are not candidates. Some findings obtained can be the presence of submucosal hemorrhage and/or edema, thickening of the abdominal wall and ascites. CT scan can also contribute in finding specific signs related with the diagnosis. For example, in volvulus a "whirlpool sign" might be found in SBO, while in LBO there might be a separation of the sigmoid wall which is described as a "split-wall" sign and "X marks the spot" which is found when there are two transition points present, in intussusception there is a "target sign" and the "cut-off sign" which is found in thrombosis.
- *Ultrasonography and magnetic resonance imaging*: These diagnostic imaging approaches are not the best tools for diagnosis of bowel obstruction. These imaging options are used in pregnant women and children.

In a study made in 62 patients with bowel obstruction, it was found that the use of CT scan for determining the site of obstruction was accurate in 91.9% of cases, while an abdominal ultrasound predicted it accurately in 82% of cases and a plain abdominal radiograph in 90.3%. To summarize, abdominal CT scan is the most effective tool for bowel obstruction location.

TREATMENT
Small Bowel Obstruction
- Fluid restoration should be done using isotonic fluid.
- A Foley catheter must be applied to assure adequate renal function and fluid restoration.

- Electrolyte imbalance should be corrected as soon as possible.
- Nasogastric tube placement is ideal for decompression.

In SBO, a prompt diagnosis and initial treatment can lead to a nonsurgical management in approximately 73% of cases. This consists of fluid restoration and stomach decompression that must be done within the 48 hours of diagnosis. If there is evidence of strangulation, ischemia, perforation or a decline in clinical symptomatology, a surgical management is the treatment of choice.

In the case of intussusception in kids, the use of contrast enemas guided by X-rays and hydrostatic pressure is the treatment of choice. When intussusception occurs in adults, surgical resection is the treatment of choice due to its high probability of being caused by a malignant process.

Surgical approach for SBO involves a laparotomy or laparoscopic management. Laparotomy is usually preferred because of the possibility of a thorough abdominal examination and is the treatment of choice when there are previous abdominal injuries, dense adhesions or complicated symptomatology. A laparoscopic approach, even though it has been increasing in popularity is reserved for well-trained doctors, due to challenging abdominal exploration. Hospital stay, morbidity and mortality are lower in the laparoscopic approach.

Large Bowel Obstruction

Large bowel obstruction treatment varies depending on the cause of the obstruction, evolution, and clinical condition of the patient. First of all, as in SBO, the patients' fluid and electrolyte imbalance should be managed, this is crucial as a beginning step in treatment. Stomach decompression can also be performed. Around 75% of LBO will require a surgical intervention eventually, but there are a series of treatment alternatives that help "make a bridge" between having to perform and emergency surgery and an elective one. These will be discussed here.

In case the patient presents a sigmoid volvulus in the emergency room, a flexible sigmoidoscopy for colonic decompression can be performed initially in order to have a programmed surgery, this procedure is successful in about 90% of the cases, even though the recurrence rates are about 50%. If the patient is in an adequate clinical condition, the first treatment should be elective resection.

Colonic stenting might be done for the same two reasons, decompression and having additional time for an elective procedure. When it is used to evade an emergency procedure, colonic stenting which is done laparoscopically, can allow resection and anastomosis to be done rather than having an ostomy done. This procedure may also be used as palliation, even though it is not a resolutive treatment, it is successful for deobstruction in the short term. Complications of this procedure might be reobstruction, perforation, and migration of the stent.

Surgical resolutions for LBO might be done at different times (one-stage, two-stage, and three-stage) and with different purposes (curative and palliative).

A one-stage procedure should always be preferred, when it is used as a curative solution, the bowel where the obstruction and dilated wall are localized is resected and reanastomosed. This procedure usually has an anastomotic leak of about 2.2–6.9%. When the one-stage procedure is

Chapter 11: Bowel Obstruction

Flowchart 1: Summary of bowel obstruction.

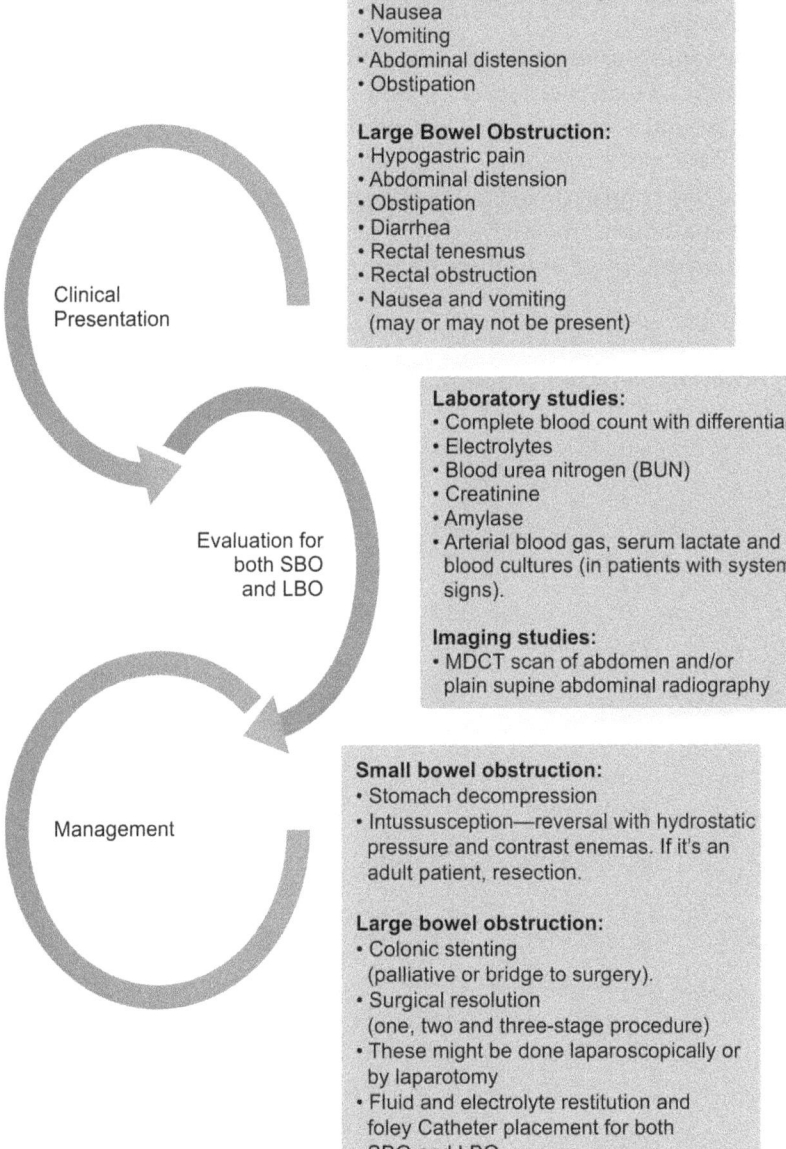

used for palliation, bowel decompression and stenting are the best options. Stenting is usually done endoscopically, and decompression is done by performing a transverse loop colostomy. Cecostomy done with local anesthetics and fluoroscopic guidance might be performed in short life expectancy patients.

Two-stage procedure involves the resection of the obstructed and dilated bowel followed by doing a colostomy or reanastomosing the bowel with a diverting loop ostomy, which is then reversed in a second step to re-establish continuity. A three-stage procedure starts with a Hartmann's procedure in which colon decompression is done by proximal diversion. After this is done, the second step consists on removal of the obstructed colon. Anastomosis can be done with an end colostomy or by a proximal diverting ostomy. To finish the three-staged surgeries, reversal of the ostomy and re-establishment of gastrointestinal continuity is done.

SUMMARY

The summary of bowel obstruction has been shown in **Flowchart 1**.

CHAPTER 12

Cervical Sprain (Whiplash Injury)

Chintan Thanki, Sanjay Shah

INTRODUCTION

The whiplash injury is a term used to describe damage to the cervical spine due to sudden acceleration-deceleration force that leads to a quick forward-backward movement of the head and neck. This is also called cervical sprain or whiplash-associated disorder (WAD). This type of injury is common after road traffic accidents especially when there is a collision from behind; and has been associated with train-related accidents in the past. It is not uncommon to ignore this type of injury due to the false belief of it being relieved spontaneously.

ETIOLOGY

Whiplash-associated disorder is more common in females and in the elderly. The classic mechanism of injury is when a patient's vehicle is collided from behind; however, any kind of road traffic accident that leads to a collision of vehicles may cause a whiplash injury. Whiplash injury has also been reported in train and roller-coaster related injuries, fall from height, assaults, child abuse, and sport-related injuries. The risk of injury is even more in patients at the extremes of age and when they are unprepared for the sudden acceleration-deceleration. When a stationary or slow moving vehicle gets collided from behind, the head and neck of the passenger and/or the driver gets suddenly hyperextended to the back followed by hyperflexion to the front. This is so because the head is usually unrestrained and the patient's torso is pushed forward by the impact. Studies have also shown that there is a simultaneous hyperextension of the lower cervical spine along with hyperflexion of the upper cervical spine leading to the whiplash injury. This leads to injury to the surrounding soft tissue, ligaments, and muscles; and an S shape of the cervical spine which is abnormal. This is due to the straightened lordotic lateral cervical curves.

PATHOPHYSIOLOGY

Due to the impact of the collision, there is a sudden acceleration of the vehicle as well as of the passengers and/or driver; followed by sudden deceleration. This leads to the patient's torso being pushed forward while the patient's head being unrestrained stays in place due to inertia. This leads to a transient extension of the head followed by the forward acceleration of the head. Flexion of the upper and middle cervical spine along with extension of the lower cervical spine can cause injury to C2–C5 and C6–T1, respectively.

The degree and direction of head rotation also has an influence on the severity and type of injury. Commonly involved and injured structures include the intervertebral disks, joint capsules and ligaments, the sternocleidomastoids and the splenius capitis. Furthermore, the cervical neural structures are at risk of stress, injury or compromise resulting in neuropathic pain. Studies have shown that females are more susceptible to whiplash injury than males due to possible genetic, anatomical, and hormonal influences. The muscular structures around the neck play important role in minimizing the damage during high acceleration but they may be slower to response during slow acceleration injuries.

An overload injury to the tendons and ligaments around the cervical spine produces cervical strain because of excessive forces on the cervical spine beyond their tensile strength. This leads to stretching or tearing of muscles and/or ligaments, edema, hemorrhage, and inflammation. The area of soft tissue around the cervical spine is particularly vulnerable to cervical strain since most cervical muscles attach directly to bone periosteum, and as a response to injury the muscles would contract. The facet joint is well innervated with C fibers and A-delta fibers with free and encapsulated nerve endings. The nociceptive nerve endings of the cervical facet capsular ligaments seem to be the source of pain in WAD as a result of the complex of stretching, bending and compressive forces during the "whiplash" movement that distends the ligaments. The pain is usually dull and aching in nature and modulated by several inflammatory factors. The C2-C3 joint is the most common source of pain referred to the head while the C5-C6 region leads to referred pain to the arms.

Whiplash injury can be further classified according to duration.
- In acute whiplash injury, symptoms are up to 4 weeks.
- In subacute whiplash injury, symptoms persist more than 4 weeks up to 12 weeks.
- In chronic whiplash injury, symptoms are present for more than 12 weeks.

CLINICAL PRESENTATION AND RED FLAGS

The common symptoms of whiplash injury include neck pain and stiffness, headache, jaw pain, and generalized tiredness. Occasionally there may be pain in the back, shoulder, and both arms. Symptoms may be delayed by several hours following the injury. Chronic disease may show symptoms of anxiety, insomnia, depression, and irritability. Some patients may also have paresthesias, weakness, numbness, vertigo, tinnitus, blurring of vision, and giddiness.

Certain red flags should be explained to the patients for prompt return to the emergency department (ED) for review and early management.
- Unsettling pain over neck, jaw, shoulder, back, and/or arms
- Excessive pain and/or severe swelling
- Unexplained anxiety, insomnia, and irritability
- Paresthesias, weakness, and numbness
- Vertigo, tinnitus, blurring of vision, and giddiness.

Whiplash injury may acutely worsen with severe neck pain/stiffness and neurological deficit requiring urgent admission and expert opinion. On the other hand, WAD may progress to a chronic condition in up to half of the patients. Pre-existing neck injury or condition, stress, anxiety, and depression are found to be associated with chronic WAD. Some studies suggest that patients having chronic WAD probably experience hyperalgesia due to alternate efferent nociceptive signals and an imbalanced descending pain modulation system.

EVALUATION: HISTORY, PHYSICAL EXAMINATION AND DIAGNOSIS

The typical history for cervical sprain or whiplash injury is twisting of the neck especially in the backward-forward motion followed by pain. Patient should be asked about past injuries, mechanism of the injury, rapidly worsening pain, paresthesias, swelling, and bruising. As for any trauma, a targeted history should rule out any evidence of head injury, headache, loss of consciousness, seizure, vomiting, ear-nose-throat (ENT) bleed, amnesia, and any injury elsewhere in the body. History should be taken regarding any comorbidities, ongoing medications, any significant illnesses in the past and related complicating conditions such as ankylosing spondylitis or any joint-related conditions. Pre-existing cervical spine degenerative condition such a spondylosis is a frequent finding in patients having the symptoms of whiplash injury. Psychological aspects such as stress, depression, anxiety, hypochondriasis, somatization disorder, malingering, etc. have to be carefully evaluated and ruled out.

Physical examination can help in ruling out fracture; and the classic look-feel-move approach can be applied. Physical examination is also aimed at identifying point tenderness and neurological deficits. Further, the range of motion (ROM) should be assessed but not before ruling out cervical spine injury through imaging. Until then a cervical collar must be applied to immobilize the cervical spine.

On inspection the person's overall posture, neck stiffness, asymmetry, rotation and any visible injury, swelling or deformity is noted. This is followed by palpation which aims to appreciate any muscle spasm, crepitus, swelling, rigidity, tenderness, and trigger points. Painful zygapophyseal joints would suggest osteoarthritis or post-traumatic irritation, whereas painful cervical facet joint would suggest whiplash injury. Furthermore, the range of movements is assessed which is significantly reduced after an acute whiplash injury.

This is followed by the patient's overall neurology examination which includes patient's affect and mental status, reflexes, sensation, coordination, and gait. In both radiculopathy or myelopathy, the coordination may be decreased. However, in radiculopathy, the muscle stretch reflexes would decrease in a myotomal pattern in the affected upper limb with normal lower limbs, whereas in myelopathy, the muscles stretch reflexes of the affected upper limb would decrease as well, but with increased muscle stretch reflexes in the lower limbs with or without spasticity.

Whiplash injury is a clinical diagnosis. Targeted history and careful physical examination remain pivotal for early diagnosis. The most common differential diagnoses include cervical radiculopathy, myelopathy, disk herniation, polymyalgia rheumatica, osteoarthritis, infections, torticollis, tumor or malignancy, malingering, and psychogenic pain.

INVESTIGATIONS AND INTERPRETATION

X-rays of the cervical spine (anteroposterior, lateral, and open-mouthed odontoid views) are useful to rule out fractures. Specialists may advice for X-rays of the neck during flexion and extension in order to appreciate lordosis and kyphosis and in cases of instability. Basic blood workup should include complete blood count (CBC), urea, creatinine, electrolytes, and erythrocyte sedimentation rate (ESR) at the least.

Computed tomography (CT) scan and magnetic resonance imaging (MRI) of the cervical spine will further identify any fractures, disk protrusion and cord compression. While CT scan is a routine imaging, MRI is indicated mostly in patients with persistent arm pain, neurologic deficits and/or clinical signs of nerve root compression. CT myelography may be indicated when CT and MRI remain inconclusive, but it is an invasive study. Bone scanning may be indicated in suspected spinal tumor, infection or occult fracture. Electromyography may be useful in diagnosing radiculopathy.

NEXUS Criteria

The criteria developed by the National Emergency X-radiography Utilization Study (NEXUS) serve as useful guidelines for sending the patient for immediate cervical spine imaging before any further manipulation. According to the NEXUS criteria, imaging is indicated in presence of any one of the following:
1. Tenderness in the midline of the back of the neck
2. Any motor or sensory focal neurologic deficit
3. Altered level of consciousness or alertness
4. Evidence of intoxication with alcohol or drugs
5. Presence of a distracting painful injury elsewhere on the body.

These criteria were studied to have 99% sensitivity and a 99.9% negative predictive value in detecting clinically significant cervical spine fractures.

Canadian C-Spine Rule

A Canadian study has shown that the Canadian C-spine Rule (CCR) is more sensitive that NEXUS rule for identifying cervical spine injuries in stable alert patients. The following algorithm is developed as the CCR:
- Are any of the following present? → "yes" indicates for cervical spine imaging
  - Patient more than 65 years old or
  - Dangerous mechanism or
  - Paresthesias in extremities.
- Are any low risk factors present allowing rotation? → "no" indicates for imaging
  - Simple rear-end motor vehicle collision (MVC) or
  - Sitting position in ED or walking after accident or
  - Delayed onset of pain or
  - Absence of midline cervical spine tenderness.
- Is the patient able to actively rotate neck bothways 45°? → "no" indicates for imaging.
- Otherwise no cervical spine radiography is required

Either of the NEXUS criteria or the CCR may be applied to patients presenting with neck pain, before proceeding to any further manipulation for physical examination.

Based on the severity of the symptoms, WAD is classified into five grades as shown in **Table 1**.

Table 1: Whiplash-associated disorder (WAD) severity grades.

Grade	Clinical findings	Imaging
0	Asymptomatic	Not required
I	Neck pain, tenderness or stiffness No other complaint; no physical signs	Not required
II	Neck pain, tenderness or stiffness plus musculoskeletal signs, e.g. decreased range of movement	Plain X-ray of cervical spine is not required unless there is suspected bone injury high-impact collision
III	Neck pain, tenderness or stiffness plus neurological involvement, e.g. sensory deficits, motor weakness, and/or decreased or absent deep tendon reflexes	Baseline X-ray of cervical spine AP, lateral and odontoid view required
IV	Neck pain, tenderness or stiffness plus dislocation/fracture with/without spinal cord injury	Same as above plus specialized imaging, e.g. CT scan, MRI, myelography

TREATMENT

Early mobilization and physiotherapy remain the cornerstones of management along with reassurance and counseling. The treatment of whiplash injury is not simple since there is no radiological evidence to support the clinical diagnosis. This is especially so when any psychological issues are associated. Moreover, there is no objective marker for improvement or response of therapy apart from patients' subjective relief of pain and/or symptoms.

In whiplash injury, early mobilization and physiotherapy within the first 4 days of injury has shown good outcome. Further, the use of nonsteroidal anti-inflammatory drugs (NSAIDs) such as cyclooxygenase (COX)-2 inhibitors has shown significant improvement in the range of movements. The use of steroids such as high-dose methylprednisolone within the first 8 hours of injury has also shown good long-term results. Medical management of whiplash injury also includes antidepressants, anxiolytics, muscle relaxants, epidural local anesthetics, and epidural corticosteroids. NSAIDs and steroids have to be avoided on empty stomach and are not recommended for long term. Opioids such as hydrocodone are advised for use in acute severe WAD grade III and in all cases of WAD grade IV.

In acute and subacute whiplash injury, several other modes of treatment have been used with variable results. These include hot and cold packs, hydrotherapy, massage, acupuncture, electrical nerve stimulation, posture training, cervical radiofrequency neurotomy, traction methods, cognitive behavioral therapy and other psychological counseling methods and chiropractic methods among others. Further, in chronic whiplash injury, other practices include cervical facet joint injections, intra-articular corticosteroids, botulinum toxin injections, etc. None of such methods is considered as single best; however, studies have shown that a multidisciplinary rehabilitation program has benefits over simple medical management in pain relief.

Surgical treatment is rarely advised. Urgent surgical opinion is recommended for any WAD grade IV, and is most likely required in presence of neurologic deficit, nerve impingement, myeloradiculopathy or instability. Subacromial decompression or cervical fusion procedures may help.

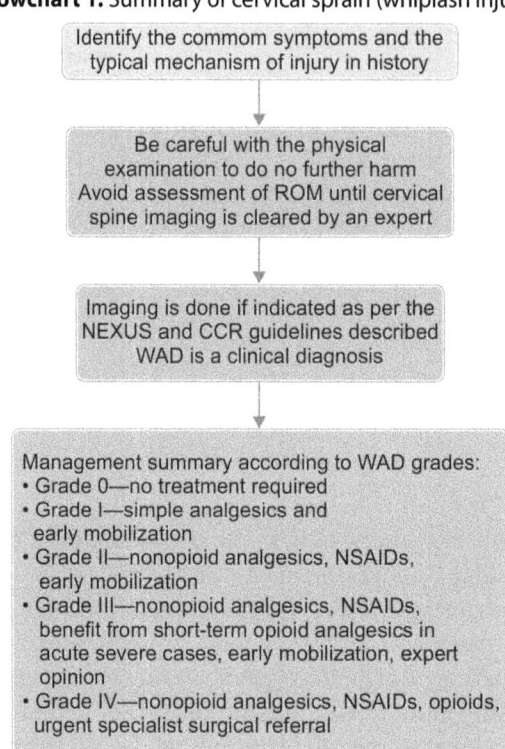

Flowchart 1: Summary of cervical sprain (whiplash injury).

SUMMARY

Whiplash-associated disorder is a frequently encountered clinical condition. Targeted history and appropriate physical examination are important since WAD is a clinical diagnosis. Imaging is indicated as per the established guidelines. Early mobilization, analgesics and psychological support remain the first line of management in WAD grades I to III. Patients having WAD grade III with excruciating symptoms and all patients with WAD grade IV require urgent specialist opinion.

Flow diagram of summary of cervical sprain (whiplash injury) has been shown in **Flowchart 1**.

CHAPTER 13

Chest Pain

Rahul Mehrotra, Shubham Chelawat

INTRODUCTION

Chest pain is one of the most common symptoms with which the patients present to the emergency department. However, chest pain can be seen in a very wide spectrum of scenarios and disease states, varying from life-threatening states requiring immediate intervention [acute myocardial infarction (AMI)] to completely benign causes (dyspepsia). As such, it is important as emergency physicians to have a sound understanding of this symptom so that they are able to recognize life-threatening conditions and initiate appropriate treatment (**Fig. 1**) while at the same time are able to identify nonemergent conditions thereby avoiding unnecessary expenditure and inconvenience to the patient. However, this is easier said than done. This is because chest pain is a very nonspecific symptom, the description by the patient may often be very unreliable, often the intensity of pain (which bothers the patient most) has no relation to the severity of the underlying disease process and there are no specific biomarkers to separate one entity from another. In view of the great importance of this symptom in every emergency department, we present here a systematic approach to evaluation of a patient presenting with chest pain.

CAUSES OF CHEST PAIN

Chest pain can have several different reasons but the general recommended approach is to differentiate cardiovascular from noncardiac causes of chest pain as a first step and then systematically rule out other possible conditions (**Flowchart 1**).

- Acute coronary syndrome
  - STEMI/NSTEMI/Unstable angina
- Aortic dissection
- Cardiac tamponade
- Myocarditis
- Pulmonary embolism
- Tension pneumothorax
- Acute chest syndrome (sickle cell disease)
- Boerhaave's syndrome (perforated esophagus)

Fig. 1: Life-threatning causes of chest pain.

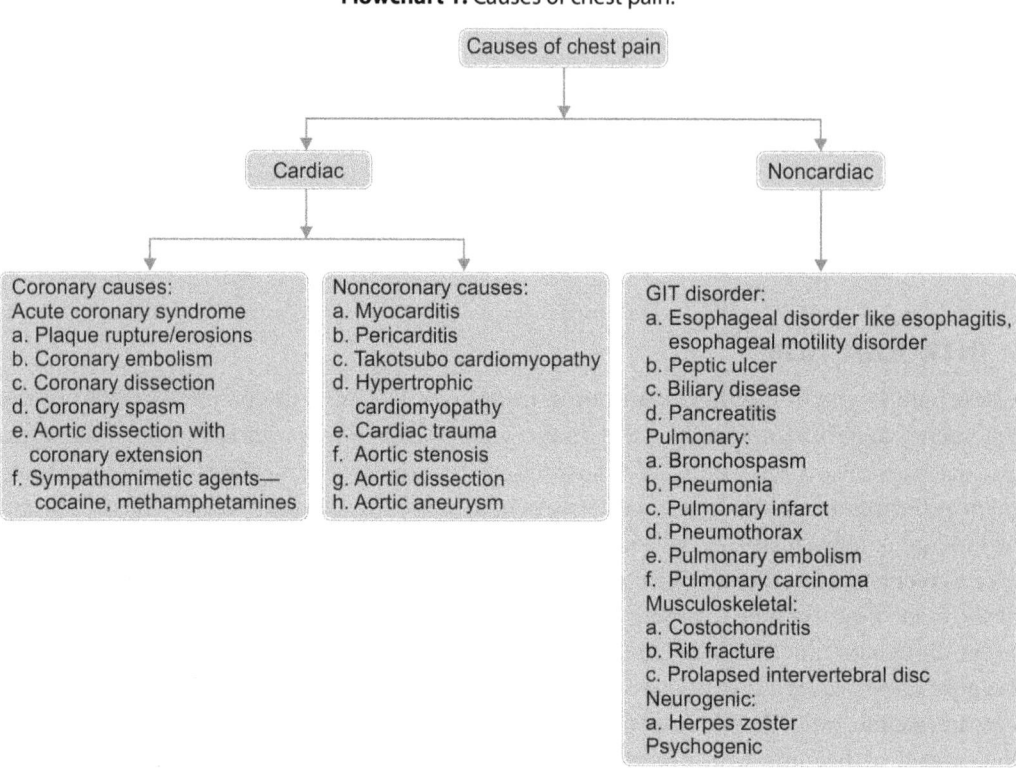

Flowchart 1: Causes of chest pain.

Cardiovascular

Angina is chest pain or discomfort that occurs when there is a mismatch between demand and supply of oxygen and blood to the heart. It is a symptom representing heart problem, most commonly coronary heart disease (CHD).

Angina is usually described as squeezing, tightness, pressure, constriction, strangling, burning, heartburn, fullness in the chest, band-like sensation, knot in the center of the chest, ache, heavy weight on chest or like a bra that is too tight.

The pain may begin with exercise or psychological stress, typically increases in intensity with time and usually radiates to the jaw, left shoulder, neck or arm.

Types of angina include stable angina, unstable angina, Prinzmetal angina, and microvascular angina depending on the underlying pathophysiology of disease and time course.

The pain of pericarditis can be severe and needs to be differentiated from other causes. The visceral surface and most of parietal surface of pericardium is insensitive to pain. Therefore, noninfectious causes of pericarditis, e.g. uremia usually cause little or no pain. In contrast, infectious pericarditis typically experience pleuritic pain with breathing, coughing, and changes in position because of involvement of surrounding pleura.

Acute aortic dissection usually causes the sudden onset of severe pain often described as ripping, tearing or shearing pain, radiating to neck or back. Pain is very severe and often not relieved even by opioids. Symptom presentation also depends on the site of origin of dissection and whether it continues to dissect. Pain in the midline of the anterior chest occurs in ascending aortic dissections, and pain in the back of the chest occurs in posterior descending aortic dissections. Dissection may occlude the large arteries supplying cerebral, abdominal, and peripheral circulations and produce related symptoms and signs.

Risk factors for aortic dissection include hypertension, Marfan and Ehlers-Danlos syndromes, bicuspid aortic valve, and pregnancy (for proximal dissections).

Pulmonary emboli often cause sudden onset of dyspnea and pleuritic chest pain, although they may be asymptomatic. Massive pulmonary emboli can cause hypotension, syncope, and signs of right heart failure. Pulmonary infarction due to smaller emboli can cause lateral pleuritic chest pain.

Pulmonary hypertension causes chest pain because of right heart hypertrophy and ischemia.

Pulmonary Conditions

Pulmonary conditions causing chest pain are usually associated with dyspnea and pleuritic symptoms. Tracheobronchitis usually causes burning midline pain, while pneumonia is associated with pain over the involved lung. Pain of a pneumothorax is usually sudden in onset and asthma exacerbations can present with chest discomfort, typically characterized as tightness.

Gastrointestinal Conditions

Acid reflux is a common cause of chest pain presenting as a burning discomfort and is exacerbated by alcohol, aspirin, and by recumbent position and relieved by antacids. It may sometimes be severe and mimic anginal pain.

Esophageal spasm leads to squeezing chest discomfort like angina.

Mallory-Weiss tears of the esophagus can occur in patients who have had prolonged vomiting episodes. Severe vomiting can also cause esophageal rupture (Boerhaave syndrome) with mediastinitis.

Peptic ulcer disease-related chest pain is usually epigastric in location and nonradiating, occurs 30–40 minutes after meals and is typically relieved by acid-reducing therapies.

Other rare gastrointestinal causes of chest pain include cholecystitis and pancreatitis.

Musculoskeletal and Other Causes

This category includes costochondritis, cervical disk disease, herpes zoster, or following heavy exercise.

Musculoskeletal syndromes causing chest pain can commonly be elicited by direct pressure over the affected area. The pain can be described as dull ache or fleeting that lasts for hours.

Panic syndrome is a fairly common cause of chest discomfort in the patients coming to the emergency department. The symptoms typically include chest tightness, often accompanied by shortness of breath and a sense of anxiety, and generally last longer.

The various causes of chest pain along with the key distinguishing features are tabulated in **Table 1**.

Table 1: Common causes of chest pain.

System	Syndrome	Clinical description	Key distinguishing features
Cardiac	Angina	Retrosternal chest heaviness/pressure; occasionally radiating to neck, jaw, shoulders, left arm or epigastrium	Exercise, emotional stress or cold weather are precipitating factors; duration 2–10 minutes
	Rest or unstable angina	Same as angina, but may be more severe	Exercise, emotional stress or cold weather are precipitating factors; duration 2–10 minutes
	Acute myocardial infarction	Same as angina, but may be more severe	Sudden onset, usually lasting ≥30 minutes; often associated with shortness of breath, diaphoresis, nausea
	Pericarditis	Sharp, pleuritic pain aggravated by changes in position; highly variable duration	Pericardial friction rub
Vascular	Aortic dissection	Sudden onset severe, ripping pain in anterior of chest, often radiating to back	Very severe pain; usually occurs in setting of hypertension or underlying connective tissue disorder such as Marfan syndrome
	Pulmonary embolism	Sudden onset of dyspnea and pain, usually pleuritic with pulmonary infarction	Dyspnea, tachypnea, tachycardia, ± signs of right heart failure
	Pulmonary hypertension	Retrosternal chest heaviness associated with dyspnea, fatigue	Pain associated with dyspnea and signs of pulmonary hypertension

Contd...

Contd...

System	Syndrome	Clinical description	Key distinguishing features
Pulmonary	Pleuritis and/or pneumonia	Sharp, usually brief, over involved area	Pain pleuritic and lateral to midline, associated with dyspnea
	Spontaneous pneumothorax	Sudden onset of unilateral pleuritic pain, with dyspnea	Abrupt onset of dyspnea and pain
Gastrointestinal	Esophageal reflux	Burning substernal and epigastric discomfort, 10–60 minutes in duration	Aggravated by large meal and postprandial recumbency; relieved by antacid
	Peptic ulcer	Prolonged epigastric or substernal burning	Relieved by antacid or food
Musculoskeletal	Costochondritis	Sudden onset of intense fleeting pain	May be reproduced by pressure over a affected joint; swelling and inflammation over costochondral joint
	Cervical disk disease	Sudden onset of fleeting pain	May be reproduced with movement of neck
Infectious	Herpes zoster	Prolonged burning pain in dermatomal distribution	Vesicular rash, dermatomal distribution
Psychological	Panic disorder	Chest pain or tightness, associated with dyspnea; lasting 30 minutes or more, not related to exertion	Patient may have other evidence of emotional disorder

EVALUATION OF CHEST PAIN: HISTORY AND PHYSICAL EXAMINATION

History

The assessment of chest pain should always begin with a clinical history that includes the characteristics of the patient's pain, including its onset (abrupt/gradual), quality, location, and radiation, the time, progression, the duration of symptoms, aggravating or relieving factors, and associated symptoms. One should try to differentiate between the various causes of chest pain on the basis of history and following points should be noted (**Fig. 2**). The history can be brief or detailed depending on the clinical stability of the patient.

- *Character of the pain*: Angina is often described as squeezing, tightness, pressure, constriction, strangling, burning, heartburn, fullness in the chest, band-like sensation, knot in the center of the chest, ache, heavy weight on chest or like a bra that is too tight. The patient may describe the pain by placing a fist in the center of the chest, known as the

- Character
- Location
- Onset
- Pattern
- Radiation
- Past medical history
- Severity
- Timing
- Aggravating factors
- Relieving factors
- Associated symptoms
- Addiction history

Fig. 2: Point to be noted during history taking.

"*Levine's sign.*" Pleuritic pain is sharp or knifelike brought on by respiratory movements or cough. Aortic dissection is often described as ripping, tearing or shearing pain of severe intensity.

- *Location of the pain*: Ischemic chest pain is usually nonlocalized and is present throughout the chest. The patient may find difficult to describe the exact location of the pain. If the patient is able to point with a finger to one area of pain, it is unlikely to be caused by cardiac ischemia.
- *Radiation of pain*: Pain of aortic dissection often radiates to neck or back. Cardiac ischemia-related chest pain often spreads to the neck, throat, lower jaw, or the shoulders and arms. Sometimes, pain is felt in the wrists, fingers, or back (between the shoulder blades).
- *Timing of the pain*: Ischemic pain tends to come on gradually and get worse over time; it generally relieves 2–5 minutes after resting if it is related to exertion. In contrast, noncardiac pain can begin suddenly, feel worst in the beginning, may last only a few seconds or may persist for hours, often unrelated to exertion. Pain that has been unchanged in severity and constant over days or weeks is not likely to be angina or myocardial infarction (MI).
- *Aggravating factors/relieving factors*: If the pain begins during an activity that increases physical exertion, emotional stress or exposure to cold, and is relieved within minutes of resting, it could be angina. The reason for this is that exercise increases the heart's need for oxygen-rich blood, and the need decreases as the person rests.
Cardiac ischemia, muscular spasms or esophageal spasm pain is relieved with nitroglycerin. If eating a meal or taking antacids relieves the pain, it could be caused by a problem with the esophagus or stomach. The pain of pericarditis often aggravates with deep breaths and relieved with sitting leaning forward position.
- *Associated symptoms*: Associated symptoms often give a clue to the system involved in causing pain. They may be systemic and nonspecific like fever, chills, sweats, fatigue, and weight loss or may be specific to a system. For example, cardiac and pulmonary system involvement is usually associated with dyspnea or palpitations, while heartburn is typically associated with gastrointestinal system.
- *Past medical history and addiction history*: History of major medical problems, especially diabetes, hypertension, dyslipidemia, coronary artery disease, bronchial asthma, chronic obstructive pulmonary disease (COPD), gastric ulcer, and addiction history including alcohol, tobacco, or illicit drug use (i.e. cocaine) should also be noted.

Physical Examination

General examination should include general appearance of the patient (distressed or with Levine's sign), pallor (exacerbate angina, heart failure), icterus, xanthoma, arcus senilis, jugular venous pressure, lymphadenopathy, cyanosis, clubbing, and lower limb pedal edema (deep vein thrombosis, heart failure).

Vitals should be noted which include pulse (rate, rhythm, regularity, volume, character, and peripheral pulses), blood pressure in the upper limbs, respiratory rate, temperature, and oxygen saturation. Aortic dissection is suggested by blood pressure or pulse disparities in between limbs depending on the location of dissection.

On inspection of chest, signs of trauma, swelling, rash of shingles, movement of chest wall, precordial pulsations, and any other visible pulsations should be looked for. On palpation, local tenderness, crepitus (rib fracture), apex beat, thrill, position of trachea, chest expansion, and vocal fremitus should be noted. Percussion is very helpful in diagnosing pneumothorax (hyper-resonant note) and pneumonia (dull note). Cardiovascular and respiratory system auscultation should be done to look for any abnormal sounds like murmur, crackles, pleural/pericardial rub, and bronchial breath sounds.

INVESTIGATIONS

A series of investigations are required to be done to confirm or rule out a diagnosis related to the chest pain. Rather than ordering a battery of tests in all patients, a systematic approach based on the most likely possibility, risk involved in missing the diagnosis, and cost should be taken into consideration. A systematic approach with the most useful and common investigations is suggested here.

Electrocardiography

The electrocardiogram (ECG) should be recorded as early as possible, ideally within 10 minutes of presentation in adult patients presenting with typical ischemic chest discomfort. It is an excellent tool for identifying acute coronary syndrome (ACS) especially ST-segment elevation myocardial infarction (STEMI). As such, the emergency physicians should be aware of the characteristic ECG changes as it has very important clinical implications on the treatment, risk, and prognosis. For example, thrombolytic therapy is only indicated in case of typical ST-segment elevation on the ECG (**Fig. 3**). However, the presence of a normal ECG does not exclude MI. Besides, ST and T wave changes may be seen in a variety of nonischemic conditions like pericarditis, myocarditis, metabolic abnormalities, pulmonary embolism, hyperventilation, ventricular hypertrophy, etc.

Electrocardiogram in pericarditis has diffuse ST-segment elevation and depression of PR-segment. ECG in pulmonary embolism can have right axis deviation, right bundle branch block, right ventricle strain—T wave inversions in leads V1 to V4, and an S wave in lead I and Q wave and T wave inversion in lead III (S1Q3T3).

> **ST elevation**
> New ST elevation at the J point in two contiguous leads with the cut points: ≥ 0.1 mV in all leads other than leads V2-V3 where the following cut points apply: ≥ 0.2 mV in men ≥ 40 years; ≥ 0.25 mV in men < 40 years, or ≥0.15 mV in women.
> **ST depression and T wave changes**
> New horizontal or down sloping ST depression ≥ 0.05 mV in two contiguous leads and/or T inversion ≥0.1 mV in two contiguous leads with prominent R waves or R/S ratio >1

Fig. 3: Electrocardiogram changes.

Posterior leads (V7, V8, and V9) can be useful for identifying ischemia in the territory supplied by the left circumflex coronary artery, which is otherwise relatively silent electrocardiographically.

Also, the availability of a prior ECG improves diagnostic accuracy and reduces the rate of admission for patients with abnormal baseline tracings. Therefore, they should be asked for whenever possible. Also, serial changes in repeated ECGs are more useful than relying on a single ECG.

Chest Radiography

Chest radiograph is useful in evaluating chest pain due to pulmonary causes. It may reveal pneumonia, pneumothorax, and pleural effusion. Hampton's hump or Westermark's sign in pulmonary embolism, mediastinal widening in acute aortic syndromes, and pericardial calcification in chronic pericarditis are some specific findings on a posteroanterior (PA) chest X-ray. Though a chest X-ray is nondiagnostic in patients with ACS, it can show pulmonary edema caused by diastolic or systolic dysfunction due to ischemia and indicate elevated left ventricular (LV) filling pressures.

Biomarkers

Cardiac biomarkers are circulating proteins released from injured myocardial cells and the rise is proportional to the degree of injury. Assessment of cardiac biomarkers is vital during the initial and subsequent evaluation of patient with chest pain suggestive of ACS.

The most sensitive and specific marker of myocardial injury/necrosis available is cardiac troponin (cTn). A second sample should be obtained after 6 hours, if the first is not elevated. Troponin level may remain elevated in the blood up to 2 weeks, hence it is not very useful in reinfarction. The diagnosis of MI should be entertained if there is a rising and/or falling pattern with at least one value exceeding 99th percentile of reference limit.

Availability of high-sensitivity troponin (hsTn) assay permits earlier detection of myocardial injury enhances overall accuracy and improved risk stratification.

Current hs-cTn assays measure cTn concentrations above the limit of detection in greater than or equal to 50% of normal individuals with less than or equal to 10% coefficient of

Cardiac causes	Noncardiac causes

• Acute coronary syndrome (STEMI/NSTEMI)
• Myocarditis
• Cardiomyopathy
  - Hypertrophic
  - Takotsubo
• Endocarditis
• Congestive cardiac failure
• Malignancy
• Chemotherapy
• Trauma
• Electric shock
• Infiltrative disease
• Post-surgery
	• Pulmonary embolism
	• Severe pulmonary hypertension
	• Renal failure
	• Sepsis
	• Stroke
	• Subarachnoid hemorrhage

Fig. 4: Causes of troponin elevation.

variation at the recommended 99th percentile, thereby increasing the ability to determine small changes in cTn.

The increased diagnostic sensitivity of hs-cTn assays comes at the expense of a lower specificity and positive predictive value to diagnose AMI.

Thus, because of a substantially lower specificity to diagnose AMI, emergency department physicians are increasingly confronted with abnormal hs-cTn values that may be related to various acute or chronic conditions other than AMI which are addressed in **Figure 4**.

Creatine kinase-muscle/brain (CK-MB) is also a cardiac biomarker which less sensitive and specific for the diagnosis of ACS but because of its short half-life it is useful in the diagnosis of periprocedural MI and reinfarction.

D-dimer assessment is useful in the evaluation of suspected pulmonary embolism. It has a very high negative predictive value. It is useful to rule out pulmonary embolism. However, patients with a higher clinical probability of embolism should undergo an imaging study.

Brain natriuretic peptide (BNP) and the N-terminal portion of proBNP (NT-proBNP) are relatively new biomarkers, very useful in diagnosis and prognostication of heart failure. Both, BNP and NT pro-BNP rise in the setting of increased ventricular wall stress. Though they are usually used in the diagnosis of heart failure, they can be elevated in the setting of transient myocardial ischemia. However, the lack of specificity of natriuretic peptide elevation for ACS limits its use as a diagnostic marker for this purpose.

NONINVASIVE IMAGING

Echocardiography and Doppler examination should be done to assess the global LV function, detect any regional wall motion abnormalities and are useful for early triage and discharge of patients with suspected MI. Echocardiography also helps in excluding other causes of chest pain like aortic dissection in appropriate clinical settings.

Manual of Signs and Symptoms

Flowchart 2: Suggestive approach to chest pain.

	Acute coronary syndrome	Pulmonary embolism	Aortic dissection	Pneumothorax
Description of chest pain	Pressure/tightness/strangling/constriction Onset over minutes Substernal/midline Radiations to arm or to jaw Exertional	Sharp Pleuritic Sudden onset over sec-mins Lateralizes to one side No specific radiation Nonexertional	Ripping, tearing or shearing pain Sudden onset over sec-mins Substernal/midline Nonpleuritic Radiation to back Nonexertional	Sharp Pleuritic Sudden onset over sec-mins Lateralizes to one side No specific radiation Nonexertional
Risk factors	DM, hypertension, dyslipidemia, smoking and other established risk factors for CAD	Immobilization Malignancy Fracture of long bones	Hypertension Smoking Marfan syndrome	COAD cystic fibrosis
Examination findings	Often normal, but may have tachycardia, tachypnea, S3, raised JVP and crackles if heart failure has developed	May have lower limb swelling Hypotension, tachycardia, tachypnea, right side S3	Tachycardia, tachypnea, BP may be unequal in arms, murmur of AR may be heard	Unilateral diminished/absent breath sounds, hyperresonance
ECG	ST-T changes; ST elevation in STEMI	Sinus tachycardia S1Q3T3 pattern	No specific findings	No specific findings
Chest X-ray	Usually normal	Usually normal, Hampton's hump or Westermark's sign	Widened mediastinum	Pneumothorax
Diagnostic next steps	• STEMI: Revascularization • Serial troponins: suspected NSTEMI/UA • Echocardiography	• Low likelihood→D dimer • High likelihood/elevated D dimer→CT angiogram	High likelihood→CT angiogram	

Chapter 13: Chest Pain

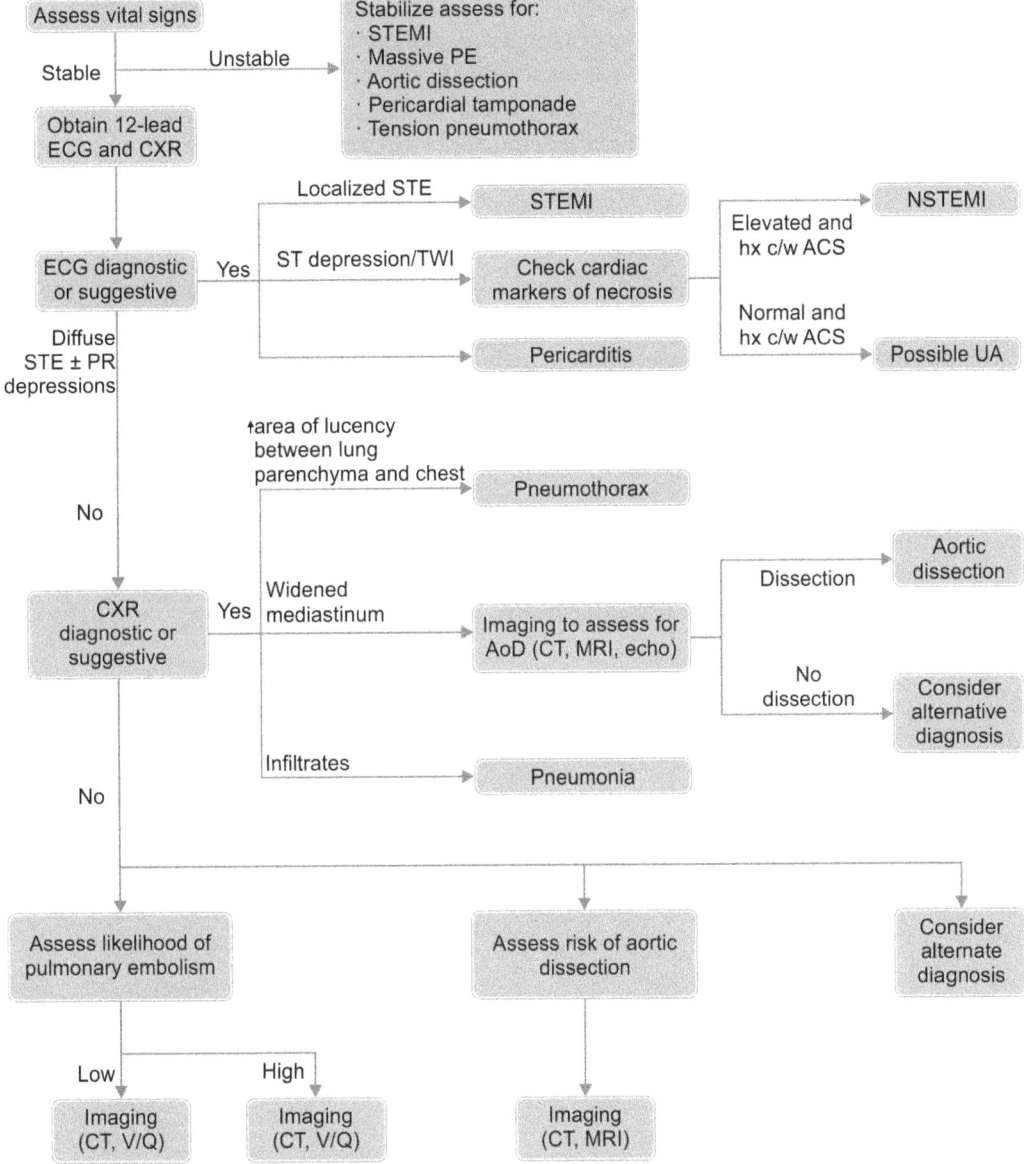

Flowchart 3: Approach to a patient presenting with chest pain.

(AoD: aortic dissection; c/w: consistent with; CXR: chest X-ray; hx: history; NSTEMI: non-ST-segment myocardial infarction; PE: pulmonary embolism; STE: ST elevation; STEMI: ST-segment elevation myocardial infarction; UA: unstable angina; V/Q scan: ventilation-perfusion scan)

Echocardiography with its modalities is very useful in the assessment of cardiac structure and function—particularly myocardial thickness and motion. Tissue Doppler and strain imaging allows quantification of global and regional ventricular function. Contrast echocardiography can be used to assess myocardial perfusion and microvascular obstruction and it also improves visualization of the endocardial border. It is extremely safe, portable, and very versatile. This makes it an indispensable tool for use in the emergency department and as such, there is more and more demand for it in every emergency department.

APPROACH TO CHEST PAIN

As discussed above, a systematic approach to a patient presenting with chest pain includes detailed history, physical examination, electrocardiography, chest X-ray, and appropriate cardiac biomarkers. Noninvasive evaluation with echocardiography can be used to reach to a diagnosis (**Flowcharts 2 and 3**).

CONCLUSION

Chest pain is an important symptom that may be indicative of a serious illness, requiring treatment in emergency (MI, pulmonary embolism, aortic dissection, and pneumothorax).

The causes of chest pain are extremely varied. A thorough history, physical examination and/or tests are required to reach to a diagnosis.

CHAPTER 14

Clubbing

Vivek Chauhan, Suman Thakur

INTRODUCTION

Examination of nails is an integral part of physical examination. While examining nails, we specifically look for presence or absence of clubbing. Diagnosis is easy when the grade of clubbing is high but clinical value lies in picking up earlier grades of clubbing. The diagnosis of digital clubbing should always be taken seriously and needs further workup. The diseases of lung, heart, gastrointestinal, and hepatobiliary system predominate the causes of clubbing. Rare presentations of clubbing include congenital clubbing and unilateral clubbing. In this chapter, we will know more about the pathophysiology and approach toward a case of clubbing.

ETIOLOGY/CAUSES

Causes of clubbing have been classified into various systems like cardiac, pulmonary, gastrointestinal, endocrinal, etc. We have classified them into common and uncommon causes for the ease of understanding (**Table 1**). With a careful history taking, examination and focused investigation, most of the common causes can be ruled out.

PATHOPHYSIOLOGY

- Historic attempts were directed at the growth hormone as the cause of clubbing but it was not found elevated in patients of lung cancer having clubbing.
- In 1987, megakaryocytes and platelet clumps were reported to be associated with clubbing. In normal patients, megakaryocytes from bone marrow get trapped in the pulmonary capillaries and are later fragmented into platelets to be released into the circulation. However, in those patients with a right-to-left blood shunt or platelet excess like cyanotic congenital heart diseases, lung cancers, subacute bacterial endocarditis, and inflammatory bowel disease, the megakaryocytes and platelet clumps get impacted in the nail capillaries.
- *Platelet-derived growth factor* (*PDGF*) released by the impacted platelets and megakaryocytes is shown to be responsible for the excessive growth of the tissue in the nail bed leading to clubbing.
- *Vascular endothelial growth factor* (*VEGF*) is another factor released by the clumped platelets which along with the PDGF was found to be significantly elevated in the patients with clubbing.

Table 1: Common and uncommon causes of clubbing.

Clubbing	Etiology
Common causes	• Lung cancer
	• Cyanotic congenital heart diseases
	• Infective endocarditis
	• Pulmonary tuberculosis
	• Interstitial lung diseases
	• Lung abscess, empyema, bronchiectasis
	• Metastatic cancers and lymphomas
	• Inflammatory bowel disease
	• Biliary cirrhosis
Uncommon causes	• Uncommon malignancies and metastatic cancers
	• Asbestosis
	• Pulmonary arteriovenous (AV) malformations
	• Celiac disease
	• Chronic active hepatitis
	• Thyroid acropathy
	• Cystic fibrosis
	• Atrial myxoma

- *Additional factors* that were studied but not found elevated in clubbing include basic fibroblast growth factor, transforming growth factor-beta 1, and carbonic anhydrase IX.
- *Hypoxia* is an important inducer of VEGF and PDGF from platelets and therefore many conditions that cause clubbing are also having hypoxemia. Octreotide is a powerful inhibitor of VEGF and hypertrophic osteoarthropathy (HOA), a form of clubbing, was shown to be responsive to treatment with octeotride. This provided strong indirect evidence of pathogenic role of VEGF in clubbing.
- *Prostaglandin E2* was demonstrated to be elevated in lung cancer patients with debilitating symptoms of HOA that reduced on taking cyclooxygenase 2 (COX-2) inhibitors and recurred on stopping them. PGE-2 can upregulate VEFG mRNA expression that is inhibited by dexamethasone. In addition, PGE-2 stimulates osteoblasts and osteoclasts and is therefore capable of inducing periostosis and acro-osteolysis, in addition to local vasodilatation, all features of HOA.
- *PDGF, VEGF, and PGE-2* are the three factors currently most strongly associated with the development of clubbing and are helped by the conditions favoring malignancy, hypoxia or right-to-left shunting of blood.

CLINICAL PRESENTATION

- Patients are mostly asymptomatic for clubbing unless it is associated with a syndrome (HOA) that involves periostosis of long bones and occasionally painful joint enlargement.

Most cases of HOA are associated with lung malignancies which gave it the name of hypertrophic pulmonary osteoarthritis (HPOA) but later it was found to be associated with nonpulmonary causes and the word "pulmonary" was thus dropped. Nonpulmonary HOA is also called pachydermoperiostosis.
- Thus, patients with clubbing can present with asymptomatic enlargement of nail folds or can be associated with painful debilitating periostosis of long bones and joints (HOA).

Various Signs of Clubbing
- *Schamroth's sign*: This sign is present in normal persons without clubbing. When the dorsal surfaces of terminal phalanges of corresponding right and left fingers are placed together, a diamond-shaped window is formed between the two fingers. This window gets obliterated in clubbing.
- *Fluctuation test*: Increased fluctuation and softening of the nail bed is the earliest sign of clubbing that can be elicited.
- *Profile sign or Lovibond's angle*: In normal people, the angle made by nail as it exists from the proximal nail fold is usually less than 180° and is called profile sign or Lovibond's angle.
- *Phalangeal depth ratio*: It is the ratio of digit's depth measured at the junction between skin and nail and at the distal interphalangeal joint. Normally, the depth at distal interphalangeal joint is more than the depth at nail bed. In clubbing fingers, connective tissue deposition expands the pulp in the terminal phalanx and the ratio becomes reversed. This ratio is also independent of age, sex, and ethnicity of population. A phalangeal depth ratio of over 1 measured by caliper or a photograph is indicative of clubbing.
- *Digital index*: It is the sum of phalangeal depth ratio of all 10 fingers. Digital index is more specific for clubbing and an index of 10.2 or higher is suggestive of clubbing.

RED FLAGS
- *HOA* is a red flag sign in a patient with clubbing as it is more often than not associated with an underlying serious disorder like malignancy. So in patients with clubbing, we must always palpate the wrists and ends of long bones for tenderness arising from periostosis.
- Presence of hoarseness, hemoptysis, engorged neck veins, generalized lymphadenopathy, pleural effusion are also red flag signs pointing toward possibility of an advanced malignancy in a patient of clubbing.
- Similarly, presence of diffuse cyanosis in a previously acyanotic congenital heart disease patient points toward Eisenmenger's syndrome that has poor prognosis for the patient.

EVALUATION
History
Careful history taking can lead us to the diagnosis of etiology for clubbing.
- *Congenital clubbing*: Long standing history since childhood points toward this etiology. Patients are mostly asymptomatic and this condition may be familial and present in

other members of the family too. Further investigation may not be needed for congenital clubbing.
- *Congenital cyanotic heart diseases*: History of cyanotic spells, differential cyanosis, repeated childhood pneumonias, palpitations, and dyspnea point toward a possibility of congenital heart diseases with right-to-left shunts. These patients will need cardiology consultation for definitive diagnosis.
- *Lung carcinoma*: Chest pain, sputum production, hemoptysis, dyspnea, hoarseness, dysphagia, swollen and engorged neck, and chest veins in a chronic smoker point toward a lung carcinoma. These patients will need a pulmonary workup to rule out lung carcinoma.
- *Biliary cirrhosis*: Prolonged Icterus, pruritus, and abdominal distention in a middle-aged female with clubbing points toward biliary cirrhosis.
- *Inflammatory bowel disease*: Chronic diarrhea with clubbing and blood in stools points toward inflammatory bowel disease.
- *Tuberculosis*: History of past or recent tuberculosis may be present in many patients with cough, dyspnea, and clubbing.
- *Pulmonary infections*: Production of excess sputum and localized chest pain point toward bronchiectasis or lung abscess and empyema, respectively.

Physical Examination

Physical examination and signs pointing toward various etiologies of clubbing:
- Engorged neck and chest veins are seen in lung cancer with mediastinal syndrome due to secondaries in lymph nodes or local spread.
- Jaundice, itch marks, and ascites are seen in biliary cirrhosis.
- In a dyspneic patient bilateral end inspiratory fine crepts, more so in the basal regions, are found in interstitial fibrosis of lungs.
- Unilateral loss of lung volume with crowding of ribs in previously treated tuberculosis is suggestive of post-tubercular lung fibrosis.
- Differential cyanosis, diffuse cyanosis, heart murmurs, parasternal heave, and precordial thrill are found in various congenital heart diseases.
- Fever with chills and rigors, heart murmurs, splenomegaly, roth spots, Janeway lesions, etc. lead toward infective endocarditis.
- Unilateral absence of breath sounds and local tenderness over the region, mostly in the basal portion of the lungs points toward empyema.

INTERPRETATION OF FINDING

- Various authors and books have divided clubbing into various grades. The earlier grades have increased fluctuation (*Grade 1*) which then leads to increase in the Lovibond's angle greater than 180° (*Grade 2*) and later increased phalangeal depth ratio (*Grade 3*). Finally, the clubbing becomes obvious due to its clubbed appearance (*Grade 4*) (**Fig. 1**).
- The clinical importance of various grades of clubbing in clinical setting is uncertain. Clubbing should be picked up early when the associated diseases are still treatable. To

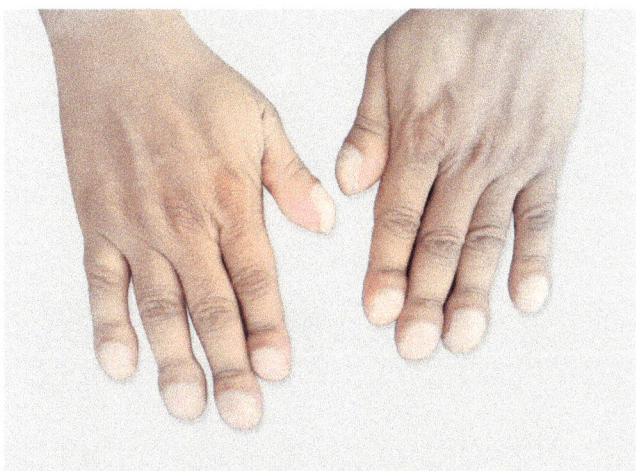

Fig. 1: Grade 4 clubbing of all nails of the hands.

be confident of early clubbing, fluctuation sign should be practiced in normal patients routinely.
- Imaging of individual fingers from a side angle using digital cameras is helpful in measurement of phalangeal depth ratio, digital index, and Lovibond's angle.
- Painful HOA must be looked for in all patients of clubbing. Its presence leads to further investigation to rule out lung cancers and other malignancies.

INVESTIGATIONS

- Investigations should be directed toward the probable etiology of the clubbing based upon history and physical examination. A chest X-ray must be done in all patients of clubbing to rule out pulmonary etiologies. Specific tests are directed toward specific etiologies, for example
    - Computed tomography (CT) chest is done for diagnosing lung cancer, idiopathic pulmonary fibrosis, lung abscess, empyema, post-tubercular fibrosis, bronchiectasis, lymphoma, etc.
    - Colonoscopy gives diagnosis of inflammatory bowel disease.
    - Ultrasound, ascitic fluid examination, and serology are needed to diagnose biliary cirrhosis.
    - Electrocardiography, echocardiography, and cardiac catheterization studies for congenital heart disease, pulmonary arteriovenous (AV) malformations, and atrial myxoma.
    - Echocardiography and paired blood cultures are done for subacute infective endocarditis.

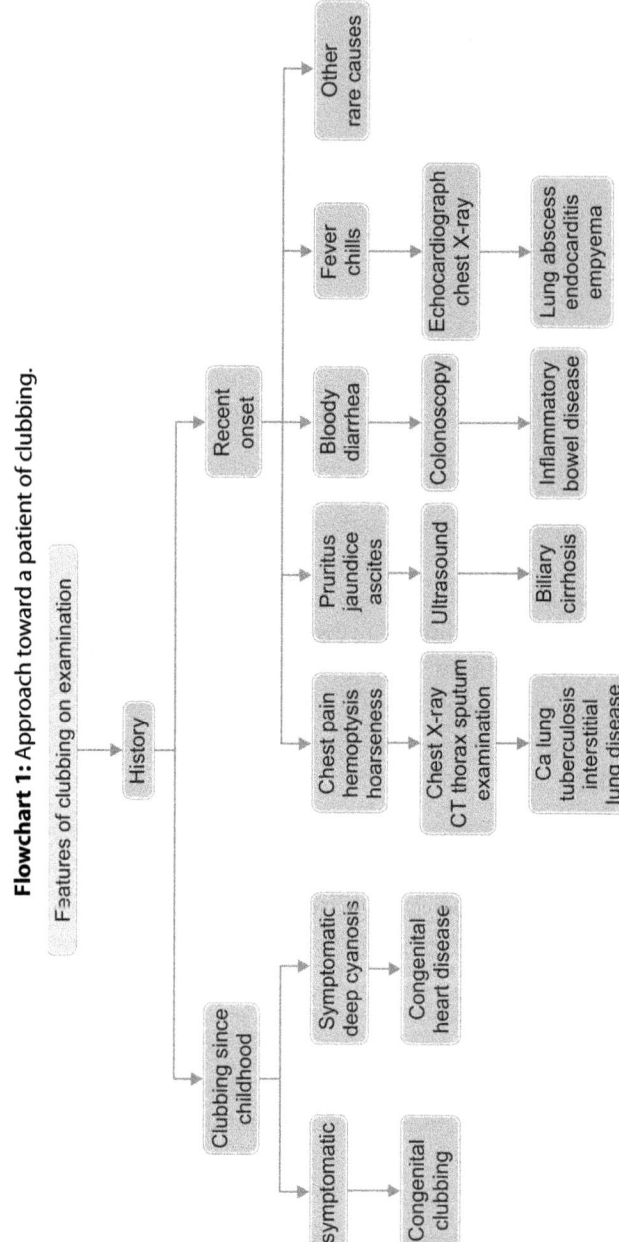

Flowchart 1: Approach toward a patient of clubbing.

- Thyroid functions must be done to rule out thyroid acropachy. It may also be associated with thyroid dermopathy and ophthalmopathy.
- Bone scan may be needed to confirm the presence and extent of HOA.

TREATMENT (FLOWCHART 1)

- In cases of clubbing, the treatment is directed toward specific etiologies. Cancers may be treatable or untreatable depending upon their stage and grade. Clubbing regresses with treatment over months.
- Many conditions associated with clubbing are treatable, e.g. lung abscess, empyema, deep abscesses, some congenital heart diseases, inflammatory bowel diseases, infective endocarditis, atrial myxoma, etc.
- The painful debilitating HOA responds to COX-2 inhibitors and corticosteroids.
- Congenital clubbing does not require any treatment and is mostly asymptomatic.

SUMMARY

To summarize, testing for presence of clubbing is an integral part of routine examination of all patients. To pick up subtle clubbing early in the disease process may be of huge clinical value as it may lead to curative treatment of cancers. Patients are usually unaware of the presence of changes in their nails and the clinical utility of various grades of clubbing beyond presence or absence of clubbing is uncertain. However, association of clubbing with HOA portends ominous value to clubbing diagnosis as it is mostly associated with malignancies. VEGF, PDGF, and PGE-2 in the setting of hypoxemia and malignancies are responsible for most proliferative changes in the clubbed nails. Careful history taking, directed physical examination and focused investigations often lead the clinicians to the etiological diagnosis of clubbing. Changes of clubbing reverse upon successful treatment of the underlying etiology but in case of malignancies and progressive disorders, it persists. Knowledge of various tests to pick up early clubbing is important for every clinician and use of digital photographs of fingers is a handy tool to diagnose and measure clubbing in fingers.

CHAPTER 15

Clavicle Fracture

Sandeep Jain

INTRODUCTION

Fractures of clavicle are one of the most common fractures owing to its superficial and subcutaneous location. It can be an isolated fracture or part of multisystem trauma with associated injuries to head, neck, and chest. Since a long time, they have been treated conservatively with either cuff and collar sling or figure-of-eight bandages. Usually they heal well with some residual deformity without any functional compromise. However, nowadays, surgery is being offered more frequently based on the location of fracture, for better cosmetic and functional results. Emergency physicians are frequently confronted with the decision for orthopedic consult and discharge from emergency department. Thus, knowledge about resuscitation and current management of these fractures is paramount.

APPLIED ANATOMY

Clavicle is the first bone in the body to ossify starting from the 5th week of gestation and one of the last to complete ossification. Its medial end fuses by 22–25 years of age. Clavicle is attached to the sternum medially and to acromion process of scapula laterally. Medially, anterior and posterior capsule of sternoclavicular joint along with interclavicular and costoclavicular ligaments provide stability. Laterally, coracoclavicular and acromioclavicular ligaments provide stability. Various muscles are attached to it—deltoid, pectoralis major, and sternohyoid originates from it while subclavius, sternocleidomastoid and trapezius have fibers of insertion on clavicle. The fracture displacement is dependent upon the site of fracture and subsequent forces imparted by these attached muscles. Behind the clavicle lie subclavian vessels and the brachial plexus, which are at risk with displaced fractures. Subclavius muscle is present between these structures and clavicle thereby providing them some protection. Apexes of the lungs are also in close proximity to clavicle.

CAUSES

- Fall on lateral shoulder causing compression is the most common mode.
- Direct trauma to the clavicle following fall or assault.
- Motor vehicle collision with high energy transfer as part of the polytrauma.
- Fall on outstretched hand is less common.

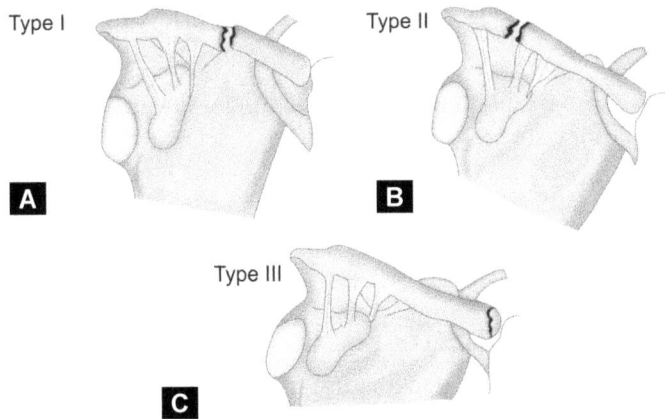

Figs. 1A to C: Allman classification of the fractures.

PATHOPHYSIOLOGY

Allman classification of the fractures is most commonly used (**Figs. 1A to C**):
- *Type I (fracture of middle third)*: The most common fractures involving junction of middle and lateral third of the clavicle. These are commonly caused due to direct force applied to the lateral shoulder as a result of fall, assault, or motor vehicle accidents. Fracture line is medial to coracoclavicular ligament with medial part of clavicle displaced superiorly by the pull of sternocleidomastoid muscle. Lateral segment is displaced inferiorly by the weight of shoulder girdle.
- *Type II (fracture of distal third)*: Caused due to direct injury to the top of the shoulder.
- *Type III (fracture of medial third)*: Caused by direct blow to the anterior chest.

CLINICAL PRESENTATION

Following trauma patient may present with:
- Pain and swelling over shoulder region
- Inability to move shoulder
- Contusion, abrasion or deformity over the affected shoulder
- Palpable bony crepitus over fracture site
- Supporting the affected shoulder with another limb
- Apparent shortening of the affected shoulder
- Breathing difficulty in case of associated pulmonary injuries—pneumothorax, hemothorax, scapular or rib fractures
- Swelling and discoloration of distal upper limb indicate associated subclavian venous injury
- Pain, pallor, paresthesia, coolness or diminished distal pulses indicate arterial injury
- Paresthesia or diminished sensations in distal limb indicate brachial plexus injury.

RED FLAG (NEED URGENT SURGICAL OR ORTHOPEDIC CONSULTATION)

- Distal vascular compromise—diminished or weak pulse, pallor, swelling, discoloration
- Neurological or motor weakness
- Open fractures
- Associated breathing difficulty or shock
- Significant displacement or shortening
- Skin tenting with impending gangrene.

EVALUATION OF THE PATIENT

All patients of trauma, including isolated fracture should be evaluated initially as per primary survey [airway, breathing, circulation, disability, and exposure/environment (ABCDE)] of Advanced Trauma Life Support (ATLS). Immediate concern of patient is pain due to fracture. All efforts should be made to alleviate pain at arrival to emergency department, enabling comprehensive evaluation. This is accomplished by supporting the limb in shoulder sling and providing analgesia. First line of drugs is nonsteroidal inflammatory drugs such as intravenous paracetamol or diclofenac. If pain persists, opioids can be added.

Examine distal pulsations, movements, and sensations. Look for associated ribs or scapular fractures and any hemothorax, pneumothorax or pulmonary contusion.

INVESTIGATIONS

- Radiographs of the clavicle and shoulder—anteroposterior (AP) view (including head of humerus and sternoclavicular joint) will detect fracture in most of the cases. An oblique view (45° cephalad) helps to define degree of displacement.
- Computed tomography (CT) scan with three-dimensional (3D) reconstruction is useful for planning of surgical fixation. It is of great value in cases of medial end fractures to detect displacement and injury to underlying structures.
- Chest X-ray—if suspected associated hemothorax/pneumothorax or rib fractures.
- Arteriography—if suspected vascular injury.
- Complete blood count (CBC), coagulation profile is done with suspected associated hemothorax or vascular injury.
- Arterial blood gas (ABG) is done if suspicion of associated pulmonary contusions.
- Bedside point-of-care ultrasonography can be used in detecting fracture lines, especially pediatric population.

MANAGEMENT

As a general guideline, most of the middle third and medial end fractures of the clavicle can be managed nonoperatively with shoulder sling or figure-of-eight bandage. Advantage of figure-of-eight bandage is that it allows patient to use both upper limbs but functional outcome is same as shoulder sling. Choice of treatment depends on patients' comfort and functional demand. Lateral third fractures have high chances of nonunion and hence need surgical fixation.

Indications for surgical management of clavicle fractures are:
- Significant displacement
- Shortening more than 2 cm
- Comminuted fractures
- Associated neurovascular compromise
- Open fracture.

COMPLICATIONS

Majority of the fractures heal spontaneously with conservative management in about 4–8 weeks, although there may be some residual cosmetic deformity. Possible complications include:
- *Nonunion*: Failure of clinical or radiographic healing in 4–6 months. Possible reasons are smoking, comminution, displacement greater than 2 cm, advanced age and osteoporosis. The nonunion rate for all mid-clavicle fractures treated nonoperatively is 6%; the rate is 15% if significantly displaced.
- *Malunion*: Majority heal spontaneously with some esthetic deformity but with minimal or no functional deformity.
- *Neurovascular injuries*: These are usually associated with middle third fractures with significant displacement or excessive callus formation.

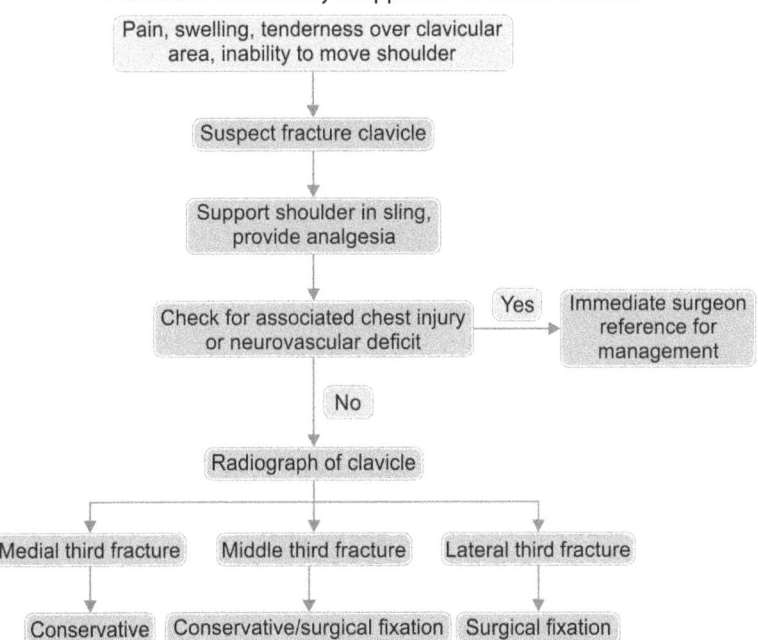

Flowchart 1: Summary of approach to clavicle fracture.

- *Intrathoracic injuries*: Hemothorax, pneumothorax, and lung contusions associated with clavicle fracture signify significant transmission of energy.
- *Post-traumatic arthritis*: Early osteoarthritis can set in case of intra-articular extension of the fracture line.
- Injury to great vessel, trachea or esophagus can be seen with displaced medial one-third fractures.

SUMMARY

Summary of approach to clavicle fracture has been shown in **Flowchart 1**.

CHAPTER 16

Concussion

Mustafa Sabak, Behcet Al

INTRODUCTION

Traumatic brain injury (TBI) is an important cause of trauma-related death and disability across the world. Emergency physicians frequently encounter patients with altered mental status following head trauma. The severity of TBI is generally classified according to Glasgow Coma Scale (GCS) and the deterioration of brain function without gross pathology in the imaging of patients with GCS 13-15 is termed *mild TBI (mTBI), or* in other words, a *concussion*. A concussion usually has a benign course, with loss of consciousness (seen in 1-14% of cases) not a necessary symptom. In the vast majority of cases of concussion, there is no reported loss of consciousness. Intracranial abnormalities may be demonstrated in some patients (contusion, bleeding, etc.) during follow-up, and these patients are more likely to have severe sequelae both in the short term and long term.

EPIDEMIOLOGY

The most frequent cause of TBI is *falls*, followed by being struck by an object and motor vehicle crashes. The incidence of concussion in males is 2:1 compared with females. The highest age group with TBI-related mortality rate is greater than 75 years. The age distribution of most likely cause of death was found to be assault in the 0-4-year age group, *motor-vehicle traffic* in 5-24 age group, *intentional self-harm* in 25-64 age group and *falls* in more than 65 years age group.

Concussions are most common in sports such as football, hockey, soccer which have body contact. Especially in soccer players who have a history of previous concussions, the risk of concussion is 3-6 times higher.

PATHOPHYSIOLOGY

Concussions occur when the brain strikes the inside of the skull often by external direct impact or acceleration–deceleration trauma. Concussion is a functional decline as opposed to an obvious structural injury. Cortical contusion may develop due to coup and contrecoup injuries. Secretion of substances such as acetylcholine, free radicals, glutamate, and aspartate causes a slight degree of axonal damage, contributing to the secondary injury. Some advanced imaging modalities other than enhanced computed tomography (CT) and magnetic resonance imaging

Table 1: Signs and symptoms.

Headache	Impaired balance
Nausea and vomiting	Loss of taste or smell
Loss of consciousness	Blurred or double vision
Alteration mental status	Sleep disturbances
Disorientation and confusion	Mood and cognitive disturbances
Retrograde and anterograde amnesia	Sensitivity to light and noise
Dizziness	

(MRI) may help to detect certain findings suggestive of concussion. Recurrent head trauma can cause damage to the cognitive functions and structure of the brain in the long term.

SIGN AND SYMPTOMS

Symptoms in mTBI patients are often seen immediately after trauma but can become evident after weeks or months. Emergency physicians must be cognizant of concussions and TBI, even in the absence of any gross pathology on neuroimaging after head trauma. mTBI can include any or all of the common symptoms listed in **Table 1**.

The three most prevalent features of concussion are feeling distracted, inability to think clearly, and difficulty in initiating action when desired. Patients usually have *confusion and amnesia*, but the loss of consciousness is not necessary. Amnesia may be retrograde or anterograde and cranial nerve deficits may be seen after trauma. Examination findings are not usually correlated with the concussion

Seizures can usually be seen in severe TBI, but in patients with the concussion of 5%, it may also be seen within the first 24 hours of trauma.

Severe TBI should be considered in the presence of a severe and resistant headache, impaired speech and cognitive functioning, changes in sensations (taste, sound, smell, etc.), impaired control and coordination in motor functions.

Worsening neurologic condition after concussion may be due to hematoma enlargement which is usually due to intracranial vascular injury. A progressive headache, lateralization signs, and lethargy can be seen which may ultimately result in the death of the patient.

EVALUATION AND DIAGNOSIS

Physical examination findings are usually normal in concussion cases. Evaluation of patients suspected of having a concussion should include a focused neurologic examination and assessment of consciousness, mental status, short-term memory, concentration, and attention. In the neurological evaluation of the patient, at minimum cranial nerves III and VII should be evaluated as well as motor strength.

Creating standardized checklists can help identify a concussion. Many tools such as *Standardized Assessment of Concussion, Post-concussion Symptom Scale and Graded Symptom*

Checklist and Sport Concussion Assessment Tool, Abbreviated Westmead Post-Traumatic Amnesia Scale (A-WPTAS), Immediate Post-Concussion Assessment and Cognitive Testing (ImPACT), Galveston Orientation and Amnesia Test (GOAT), Balance Error Scoring System (BESS) are used for this purpose.

One of these concussion scoring systems, the A-WPTAS, consists of simple questions which can be performed quickly and applied in emergency services. It is used for detecting the concussed patients who have GCS 13-15 and closed head trauma within the first 24 hours after trauma. In order to assess amnesia, the physician asks the patient to distinguish between some of the three simple pictures within 10 seconds and then to remember the same pictures again after 1 hour. The score is designed to help guide decisions for emergency department disposition (admission vs discharge).

Computer Tomography

Computer tomography (CT) is the most commonly used imaging modality in the emergency department to detect skull fractures, injury to brain structures, and intracranial hemorrhage in patients with head trauma, especially epidural hematoma which can be rapidly fatal but is potentially reversible if identified and evacuated quickly. Because of increased availability, less time required to perform imaging study and its ability to identify serious injuries that may require neurosurgical intervention, head CT is the best imaging method for the initial evaluation when imaging is warranted.

Magnetic Resonance Imaging

Magnetic resonance imaging is usually not preferred for concussion assessment in the acute phase except in subacute and chronic phases for those with lingering symptoms. MRI can be helpful in demonstrating occult vascular injuries, assessment of white matter structure, and especially to help predict clinical outcome.

Biomarkers

S100B (calcium-binding protein B antibody) and tau protein are not routinely used as biomarkers. Use of such serum biomarkers is purely experimental at this junction in time.

■ OBSERVATION AND TREATMENT

Most patients are usually discharged home. The patient should be observed at home or inpatient *at least 24-48 hours* for the possibility of developing worsening intracranial complications. If the patient is discharged, he/she should not drive and should rest during this initial period. It is very important to avoid strenuous activities because of an increased risk for another concussion within the first 7-10 days after injury, until the patient is fully recovered. There is no specific time to returning to the normal working life as symptoms and recovery are patient-specific, so patients should repeatedly follow-up with their primary care physician for gradual easing of restrictions based on presence of symptoms.

Use of a*nticoagulants, antiaggregants/antiplatelets, and nonsteroidal anti-inflammatory drugs (NSAIDs)* are not recommended immediately after a concussion. When patients are discharged home, concussion discharge instructions should be provided which specifically mention red flag signs and symptoms that warrant immediate re-evaluation including increased symptoms, nausea, vomiting, severe headache, fever, stiff neck, somnolence, altered mental status, incontinence, restlessness, weakness or numbness in any extremity. Patients who have hemorrhagic diathesis and GCS less than 15 should be admitted to the hospital (neurosurgical services recommended) if there are no relatives who can follow the patient at home. Those who are professionally interested in sports should resume activities gradually and the emergency physician is typically not the healthcare provider who decides when to resume sports activity.

Seizures are rarely seen in patients with concussion. When present, they may be focal or generalized seizures. The initiation of the antiepileptic drug as a prophylactic agent is not recommended.

Magnetic resonance imaging is recommended if it is necessary to demonstrate new or occult pathologies and to avoiding radiation exposure. Data is insufficient to demonstrate benefit from rescanning the brain by CT for clinically stable hospitalized patients who had gross brain pathology (shift, bleeding, mass effect, etc.) during follow-up.

The post-concussion syndrome which may increase symptoms (headache, dizziness, memory problems, sleep problem, decreased concentration, light and noise sensitivity, psychological symptoms such as anxiety, mood swings, etc.) may develop within about 7-10 days of recovery after the concussion. The severity of the trauma is not correlated with the possibility of development of the post-concussion syndrome. The likelihood of development of post-concussive syndrome is higher in women and the elderly. The underlying pathology is also thought to be due to damage at the microscopic level in histopathological examinations. Treatment should be guided by the patients' symptoms. Most patients recover within a few weeks. If the patient has not undergone brain imaging with MRI in an acute injury, MRI should be requested to exclude other causes if symptoms persist for a prolonged period of time. The patient should be warned about the higher chance of reinjury immediately after the initial concussion. If possible, the patient should be referred to the neuropsychologist after discharge.

SUMMARY

- Traumatic brain injury is a common problem, and the majority of TBI is composed of concussion which is usually a benign course.
- Physical examinations of the patients are usually normal.
- Patients with post-traumatic GCS 13-15 are characterized by histopathological damage, although CT scanning is usually normal. Loss of consciousness is not necessary.
- Failing to identify and diagnose concussion initially can cause worse sequelae later due to recurrent trauma as concussed patients are more injury prone.
- Particularly due to fall, the proportion of concussion is greater and the incidence of concussion in males is 2:1 compared with female.

- Symptoms are usually seen weeks or months later but also may come to exist immediately after the trauma.
- The A-WPTAS tool can be used from standardized examination techniques with simple and short questions to identify patients who have a concussion in the emergency service setting. In this way, the physician can decide the discharge of the patient or the need for follow-up.
- When in doubt, CT is recommended as the first-choice imaging method. Routine use of CT is not recommended in patients who are followed up in hospital conditions. It should be decided according to the clinical status of the patient. MRI is recommended to prevent radiation exposure and to detect minor pathologies in follow-up or subacute and chronic period.
- Potential complications should be monitored at the hospital for follow-up, or for 24–48 hours if there is a close relative that can be monitored based on the patient's clinical status.
- The patient should avoid risky activities at least 7–10 days until full recovery, and after the return to normality, the patient should be prompted to start working as soon as possible.
- Avoid antiaggregants, anticoagulants, and NSAIDs after trauma.
- Need to refer the patient to the primary physician who will follow-up the patient. Especially in athletes, the emergency physician should not decide the period of time for normal activities.

CHAPTER 17

Coma

Saleh Fares, Omar Ghazanfar

INTRODUCTION

Coma is defined as a state of consciousness from which a patient cannot be aroused in response to painful, light, and sound stimuli and is devoid of a normal sleep-wake pattern with no voluntary functions. There is clear distinction between a real coma and a medically induced coma. In addition, there is a complete absence of wakefulness and the ability to consciously feel, speak, hear, or move.

ETIOLOGY

Coma results from a number of pathological conditions. These include focal, diffuse, structural, and nonstructural insults. It may be as a result of intoxication, drug abuse or overdose, metabolic derangements, central nervous system (CNS) pathologies, biochemical, and traumatic. In certain conditions, it can also be induced artificially by medical agents to maintain core brain functions after major trauma and neurosurgery.

Forty percent of coma states are as a result of drug toxicity, which results in either damage or reduction in the function of the reticular activating system (RAS) in the brain. Pharmacological agents, which affect the heart rate, blood pressure, and respiration may also affect the RAS. Epileptogenic activity contributes via similar mechanisms. Hypoxia or hypoxemia is the second most common cause of a reduced level of consciousness and accounts for 25% of all patients. It is generally caused by a cardiac arrest and results in a disruption of neuron communication in the central nervous systems well as by affecting the cytochrome pathway causing a depletion of adenosine triphosphate (ATP). 20% of comatose states are as a result of cerebrovascular strokes, which may be ischemic or hemorrhagic. The remaining 15% is due to trauma, blood loss, hypo- and hyperthermia, and biochemical abnormalities (**Table 1**).

PATHOPHYSIOLOGY

Alertness is as a result of an intact function of the cerebral hemispheres with preservation of arousal mechanisms in the RAS. Any pathology, which involves these structures, affects the level of consciousness. For level of consciousness to be affected; the insult is generally bilateral, however, there are certain circumstances in which a unilateral condition may also impair the RAS.

Table 1: Etiology of coma.

Causes	Examples
Focal	
Structural	• Brain tumor • Head trauma (e.g. concussion, cerebral lacerations or contusions, epidural or subdural hematoma) • Hydrocephalus (acute) • Intraparenchymal hemorrhage • Subarachnoid hemorrhage • Upper brainstem infarct or hemorrhage
Nonstructural	• Seizures (e.g. no convulsive status epilepticus) or a postictal state caused by an epileptogenic focus
Diffuse	
Metabolic and endocrine disorders	• Hypercalcemia • Hypercapnia • Hypoxia • Hyperglycemia • Hypernatremia • Hypoglycemia • Hyponatremia • Hypernatremia • Hypoxia • Hypothyroidism • Uremia • Wernicke encephalopathy
Infections	• Encephalitis • Meningitis • Sepsis
Other disorders	• Diffuse axonal injury • Hypertensive encephalopathy • Hyperthermia or hypothermia
Drugs	• Alcohol • CNS stimulants (such as amphetamines) • Sedative (such as benzodiazepine and barbiturates) • Opiates • Speed • Ecstasy
Toxins	• Carbon monoxide • Lead • Solvents • Heavy metals • Radiation • Methanol • Ethylene glycol

(CNS: central nervous system)

Dysfunction of the RAS is generally a result of diffuse effects such as biochemical insults (e.g. hypoglycemia, hypoxia, uremia, and drug overdose). It may also be as a result of focal pathology, which includes upper brainstem infarcts, cerebral hemorrhage, or direct mechanical disruption. Raised intracranial pressure (ICP) can result in reduced cerebral perfusion pressure (CPP), which causes brain ischemia and affects the RAS; leading to an impaired level of consciousness.

When cerebral damage is extensive, herniation of the brain can occur due to both direct pressure effects on the brain tissue as well as increased ICP leading to hydrocephalus, which leads to brain tissue dysfunction. The ICP increase also leads to cell death by activating apoptosis pathways leading to cell destruction.

CLINICAL EVALUATION

Clinical presentation depends on the cause of the insult and the basic rules of assessing a patient should be followed.

History

Detailed history is essential to aid in reaching a provisional diagnosis. As part of the assessment, collateral history needs to be determined from relatives, police offices, paramedics as well any witnesses to the medical event. Specific questions to be asked include the onset and time course of the presentation, history or seizures, headache, vomiting, head trauma, drug use or misuse, recent travel and exposure to infectious agents, any unusual meals ingested, and consumption of alcohol. It is important to ascertain when the patient was in a normal conscious state and if available any existing medical records can be very useful.

General Physical Examination

Physical examination should be focused and includes examination of the head and face, skin, and extremities. Signs of head trauma include periorbital ecchymosis and ecchymosis behind the ear, hemotympanum, instability of the maxilla, and cerebrospinal fluid (CSF) rhinorrhea and otorrhea. Scalp contusions and small bullet holes should be looked for during the clinical examination. Findings will suggest the underlying pathology. Hypothermia or hyperthermia with environmental exposure, near-drowning, sedative overdose, Wernicke encephalopathy, and signs of sepsis, which include fever, petechial or purpuric rash, hypotension, CNS infection, also need to be considered. Needle marks suggest drug abuse and any evidence of tongue biting will suggest seizures. Breath odor may also be indicative of alcohol use, drug intoxication, or diabetic ketoacidosis.

The CNS examination determines whether the brainstem is intact and where the lesion is located.

This includes determining the level of consciousness using the Glasgow Coma Scale (**Table 2**), which is developed to assess patients with head trauma. For head trauma, the score assigned by the scale is valuable prognostically. For coma or impaired consciousness of any

Table 2: Glasgow Coma Scale.

Area assessed	Response	Points
Eye opening	Opens spontaneous	4
	To verbal command	3
	To painful stimuli	2
	No response	1
Verbal	Oriented	5
	Confused	4
	Inappropriate words	3
	Incomprehensible	2
	None	1
Motor Combined scores < 8 are typically regarded as coma.	Obeys command	6
	Localizes pain	5
	Withdraws to pain	4
	Abnormal flexion to pain (decorticate posturing)	3
	Abnormal extension to pain (decerebrate posturing)	2
	No response	1

cause, the scale can be used because it is a reliable and an objective measure of the severity of unresponsiveness and can be used serially for monitoring. Level of consciousness is evaluated by attempting to wake patients first with verbal commands, then with non-noxious stimuli, and finally with noxious stimuli.

Eye Abnormalities

There are many different pupillary presentations, which guide the clinician to ascertain the cause of the pathology. Pupils may be dilated, pinpoint, unequal, fixed in midposition, disconjugate, or absent. There may also be unusual presentations such as ocular bobbing, ocular dipping, opsoclonus, homonymous hemianopia, a loss of the oculocephalic reflex, the oculovestibular reflex, and corneal reflexes. Pupillary responses, extraocular movements, and examination of the fundi should be done in every patient encounter.

Pupillary responses and *extraocular movements* provide information about brainstem function. One or both pupils usually become fixed in coma due to structural lesions, but pupillary responses are generally preserved until very late, especially when the coma is due to diffuse metabolic disorders. Unilateral dilated pupil and causes include ocular trauma, certain headaches, and use of a scopolamine patch.

The *fundi* should be examined for papilledema, which indicates increased ICP but can take several hours to develop. Increased ICP can also cause changes in the fundi, such as disk hyperemia, dilated capillaries, blurring of the medial disk margins, and sometimes hemorrhages. Subhyaloid hemorrhage may indicate subarachnoid hemorrhage.

The *oculocephalic reflex* is tested by the doll's-eye maneuver in unresponsive patients: the eyes are observed while the head is passively rotated from side-to-side or flexed and extended. *This maneuver should not be attempted, if cervical spine instability is suspected.* If the reflex is present, the maneuver causes the eyes to move in the opposite direction of head rotation, flexion, or extension, indicating that the oculovestibular pathways in the brainstem are intact. Thus, in a supine patient, the eyes continue to look straight up when the head is turned side-to-side.

If the reflex is absent, the eyes do not move and thus point in whatever direction the head is turned, indicating the oculovestibular pathways are disrupted. The reflex is also absent in most patients with psychogenic unresponsiveness because visual fixation is conscious.

If the patient is unconscious and the oculocephalic reflex is absent or the neck is immobilized, oculovestibular (cold caloric) testing is done. After integrity of the tympanic membrane is confirmed, the patient's head is elevated 30°, and with a syringe connected to a flexible catheter, the examiner irrigates the external auditory canal with 50 mL of ice water over a 30-second period.

If both eyes deviate toward the irrigated ear, the brainstem is functioning normally, suggesting mildly impaired consciousness. If nystagmus away from the irrigated ear also occurs, the patient is conscious and psychogenic unresponsiveness is likely. In conscious patients, 1 mL of ice water is often enough to induce ocular deviation and nystagmus. Thus, if psychogenic unresponsiveness is suspected, a small amount of water should be used because cold caloric testing can induce severe vertigo, nausea, and vomiting in conscious patients. If the eyes do not move or movement is disconjugate after irrigation, the integrity of the brainstem is uncertain, and the coma is deeper, and prognosis may be less favorable. Certain patterns of eye abnormalities may suggest brain herniation.

Autonomic Dysfunction

Patients present with pathologic breathing patterns, an example of which is Cheyne–Stokes respirations, which may coexist with hypertension and bradycardia called the Cushing reflex, which may lead to a cardiorespiratory arrest.

Motor Dysfunction

A variety of motor dysfunctions may be present and include flaccidity, hemiparesis, asterixis, multifocal myoclonus, decorticate posturing, and decerebrate posturing. *Decorticate posturing* can occur in structural or metabolic disorders and indicates hemispheric damage. Decerebrate posturing indicates that the upper brainstem motor centers, which facilitate flexion, have been structurally damaged. Decerebrate posturing may also occur in anoxic encephalopathy. Flaccidity without movement indicates that the lower brainstem is not affecting movement, regardless of whether the spinal cord is damaged. Asterixis and multifocal myoclonus suggest metabolic disorders such as uremia, hepatic encephalopathy, hypoxic encephalopathy, and drug toxicity.

Psychogenic unresponsiveness can be differentiated because although voluntary motor response is typically absent, muscle tone and deep tendon reflexes remain normal, and all brainstem reflexes are preserved. Vital signs are usually not affected.

Respiratory Patterns

The spontaneous respiratory rate and pattern should be documented unless emergency airway intervention is required. It may suggest a cause. Cheyne–Stokes may indicate dysfunction of both hemispheres or of the diencephalon. Hyperventilation with respiratory rates of more than 40 breaths/min indicates midbrain or upper pontine dysfunction. An inspiratory gasp with respiratory pauses of about 3 seconds after full inspiration (apneustic breathing) typically indicates pontine or medullary lesions and can lead to respiratory arrest. Brainstem insults can cause nausea, vomiting, occipital headache, ataxia, and meningismus.

INVESTIGATIONS

Investigations include laboratory tests, both point of care and laboratory based (e.g. pulse oximetry, bedside glucose measurement, blood and urine tests). Neuroimaging (CT/MRI/MRA) may be required as well along with measurement of ICP in certain cases. Lumbar puncture (LP) or electroencephalography (EEG) may be required to reach a definitive diagnosis.

Diagnosis of impaired level of consciousness is based whether repeated stimuli arouse patients briefly or not. If stimulation triggers decerebrate or decorticate posturing, impaired consciousness may lead into coma. ABC (airway, breathing, and circulation) approach should occur simultaneously along with stabilization and investigations. Temperature is checked to look for hypothermia or hyperthermia. If there is a history of trauma, Advanced Trauma Life Support (ATLS) guidelines are followed.

Blood tests should include a comprehensive metabolic panel, complete blood count (CBC) with differential, liver function tests, and ammonia level. Arterial blood gasses (ABGs) are measured, and if carbon monoxide toxicity is suspected, carboxyhemoglobin level is measured. Blood and urine should be obtained for culture and routine toxicology screening; serum ethanol level is also measured. Other toxicology screening panels may be required (12-lead) should be done.

If the cause is not apparent, noncontrast head CT should be done to check for masses, hemorrhage, edema, evidence of bone trauma, and hydrocephalus. Initially, noncontrast CT rather than contrast CT is preferred to rule out brain hemorrhage. MRI can be done instead if immediately available, but it is not as quick as newer-generation CT scanners and may not be as sensitive for traumatic bone injuries (e.g. skull fractures). Contrast CT can then be done if noncontrast CT is not diagnostic. MRI or contrast CT may detect isodense subdural hematomas, multiple metastases, sagittal sinus thrombosis, herpes encephalitis, or other causes missed by noncontrast CT. A chest X-ray should also be taken.

If coma is unexplained after MRI or CT and other tests, an LP is done to check opening pressure and to exclude infection, subarachnoid hemorrhage, and other abnormalities. However, MRI or CT images should also be reviewed for intracranial masses, obstructive hydrocephalus, and other abnormalities that could obstruct CSF flow or the ventricular system and thus significantly increase ICP. Such abnormalities contraindicate LP. Suddenly lowering CSF pressure, as can occur during LP, in patients with increased ICP could trigger brain herniation; however, this outcome is rare. CSF analysis includes cell and differential counts, protein, glucose, Gram staining, cultures based on clinical suspicion.

If increased ICP is suspected, pressure is measured and hyperventilation, managed by an intensive care unit (ICU) specialist, should be considered. Hyperventilation causes hypocapnia, which in turn decreases cerebral blood flow globally through vasoconstriction. Reduction in partial pressure of carbon dioxide (PCO_2) from 40 mm Hg to 30 mm Hg can reduce ICP by about 30%. PCO_2 should be maintained at 25–30 mm Hg, but aggressive hyperventilation to less than 25 mm Hg should be avoided because this approach may reduce cerebral blood flow excessively and result in cerebral ischemia. If diagnosis remains uncertain, EEG may be done.

■ PROGNOSIS

Prognosis depends on the cause, duration, and depth of the impairment of consciousness. For example, absent brainstem reflexes indicate a poor prognosis after cardiac arrest, but not always after a sedative overdose. In general, if unresponsiveness lasts less than 6 hours, prognosis is more favorable.

After coma, the following prognostic signs are considered favorable: early return of speech, spontaneous eye movements that can track objects, normal resting muscle tone, and the ability to follow commands. If the cause is a reversible condition patient may lose all brainstem reflexes and all motor response and yet recover fully. After trauma, a Glasgow Coma Scale score of 3–5 may indicate fatal brain damage, especially if pupils are fixed or oculovestibular reflexes are absent.

Patients may also have non-neurologic complications, depending on the cause of impaired consciousness. For example, a drug or disorder causing metabolic coma may also cause hypotension, arrhythmias, myocardial infarction, or pulmonary edema. Prolonged immobilization may also result in complications.

■ TREATMENT (FLOWCHART 1)

Airway, breathing, and circulation are immediate priorities. Hypotension must be corrected. Patients are admitted to the ICU, so that respiratory and neurologic status can be monitored. Some patients in coma are undernourished and susceptible to Wernicke encephalopathy, thiamine 100 mg intravenous (IV) or intramuscular (IM) should be given routinely. If plasma glucose is low, patients should be given 50 mL of 50% dextrose IV, but only after they have been given thiamine. If opioid overdose is suspected, naloxone 2 mg IV is given. In trauma cases, the neck is immobilized until damage to the cervical spine is ruled out.

Historical evidence suggested the use of gastric lavage within about 1 hour of drug abuse, however, this is not currently recommended due to the risk of aspiration and pneumonitis. Activated charcoal can, however, be given via the orogastric tube. Coexisting disorders and abnormalities are treated as indicated. Core body temperature may need to be corrected. Patients may require intubation to prevent aspiration and ensure adequate ventilation. This is most often when the patient has infrequent or shallow respiration, low O_2 saturation,

Flowchart 1: Treatment and diagnostic algorithm for coma.

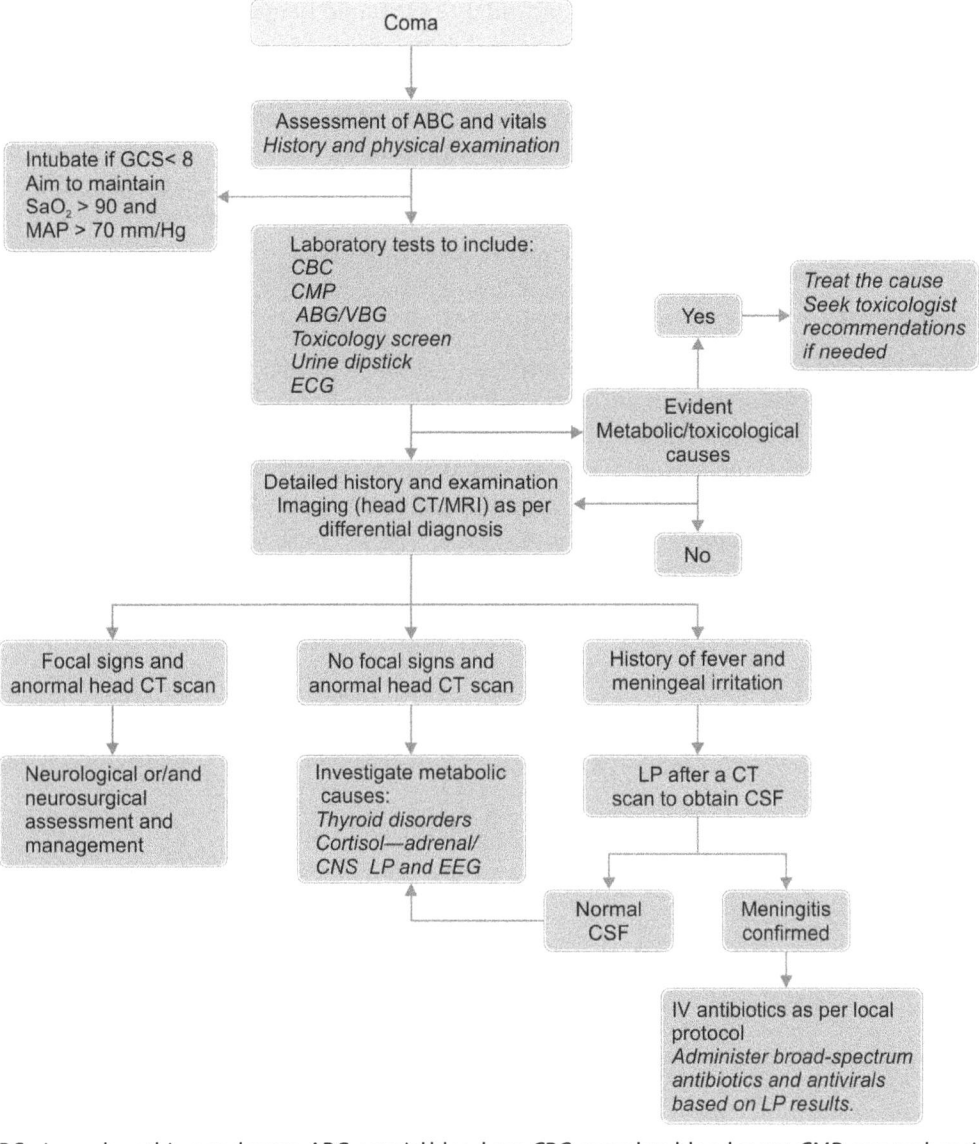

(ABC: airway, breathing, and coma; ABG: arterial blood gas; CBC: complete blood count; CMP: comprehensive metabolic panel; CNS: central nervous system; CSF: cerebrospinal fluid; CT: computed tomography; EEG: electroencephalography; GCS: Glasgow Coma Scale; IV: intravenous; LP: lumbar puncture; MAP: mean arterial pressure; VBG: venous blood gas)

impaired airway reflexes, or Glasgow Coma Scale score less than or equal to 8. If increased ICP is suspected, intubation should be done via rapid-sequence oral intubation rather than via nasotracheal intubation; nasotracheal intubation in a patient who is breathing spontaneously causes coughing and gagging, leading to an ICP and confounds the existing pathology. Pulse oximetry and ABGs (if possible, end-tidal CO_2) should be used to assess adequacy of oxygenation and ventilation. If ICP is increased, intracranial and CPP should be monitored and pressures should be controlled. The goal is to maintain ICP at less than or equal to 20 mm Hg and CPP at 50–70 mm Hg. Cerebral venous drainage can be enhanced by elevating the head of the bed to 30° and by keeping the patient's head in a midline position. Control of increased ICP involves several modalities and includes sedation, hyperventilation, hydration, diuretics, BP control, and the use of corticosteroids. Titrated hypothermia, pentobarbital coma, and decompressive craniotomy are optional treatment in some cases.

SUMMARY

Impaired level of consciousness is a as a result of multiple pathological insults, which lead to a cascade of actions within the human body leading to a state of coma. There are multiple causes as discussed and the treatment is dependent on the cause. However, there are certain basic treatment measures, which are undertaken, and ABC take priority over specific management. Immediate and long-term prognosis is largely dependent on the cause and may range from complete recovery to a long-term vegetative state.

CHAPTER 18

Constipation in Adult

Rohan N Shah

INTRODUCTION

Less than three bowel movements per week and stool dry and hard is generally considered as constipation. Stool is painful to pass. Very common complaints in outpatient about chronic constipation and few people also experience occasional constipation.

CAUSES

Primary

Most common nonlife threatening usually more than 6 months not due to any medication or medical problem. Inadequate intake of dietary fiber, fluid intake, and decreased physical activities are the common cause.

Secondary

Causes are medication such as opiates, endocrine (hypothyroidism) and metabolic disorders, and obstruction such as colorectal cancer.

Fiber in diet: Fiber promotes bowel movements and prevents constipation. Important to include good quality of fiber in diet such as fruits, vegetables, and whole grain.

Physical activity: Constipation is common in less physically active person especially in elderly group. Risk of constipation is more in bedridden patient.

Medications: Opiates, antidepressants, anticonvulsants, iron supplements, calcium channel blockers, aluminum-containing antacids, and diuretics are the drugs which frequently causes constipation.

Irritable bowel syndrome: Patient with irritable bowel syndrome (IBS) is more frequently constipated than other population.

Pregnancy: Hormonal changes in pregnancy make women more susceptible for constipation.

Problem with colon and rectum: Tumor, scar tissue, diverticulosis, and colorectal stricture prone for constipation.

Disease and conditions: Diseases of colon, rectum, or anus can cause constipation. Neurological disorders like Parkinson disease, multiple sclerosis, stroke, and spinal cord injuries can lead to constipation. Uremia, diabetes, hypocalcemia, hypothyroidism, and other systemic diseases like lupus, scleroderma, amyloidosis, and carcinoma also causes constipation.

Others: Aging, changes in routine, overuse of laxatives, not going to toilet when needed, and not drinking enough water are other causes of constipation.

■ SYMPTOMS

Hard to pass stools, infrequent, hard and dry consistency, abdominal pain, and bloating.

■ RED FLAGS

New onset without cause weight loss, blood in stool, anemia, inflammatory bowel disease, stool, and family history of malignancy.

■ DIAGNOSIS

Examination

Abdominal examination and rectal examination guide the physician to evaluate constipation further. Rectal examination will provide information about sphincter tone, presence of hemorrhoids, fecal impaction, and any other perianal irregularities. In addition to general physical examination and rectal examination, following test and procedures are required to find out the cause.

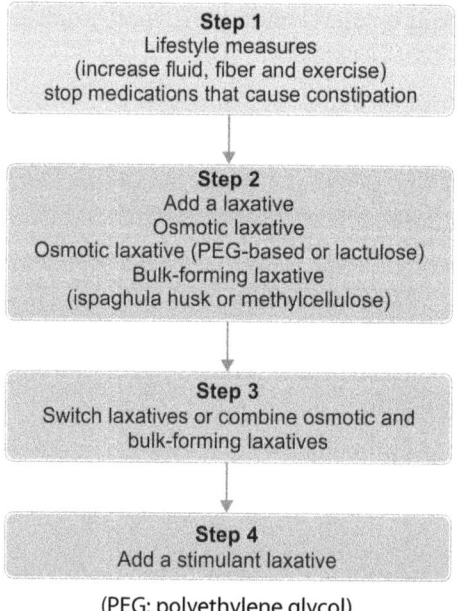

Flowchart 1: Stepwise management of constipation in adult.

(PEG: polyethylene glycol)

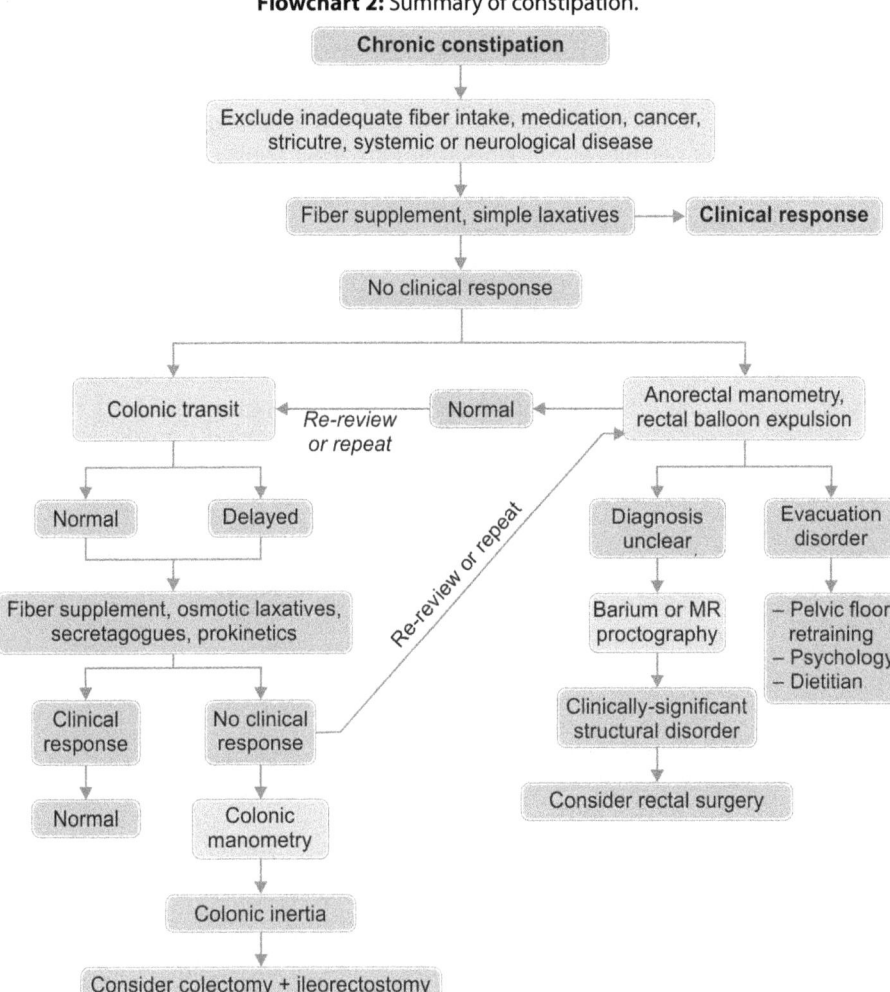

Flowchart 2: Summary of constipation.

Investigations

Blood tests, X-ray of abdomen, sigmoidoscopy (examination of rectum lower or sigmoid colon), colonoscopy (examination of rectum and entire colon), anorectal manometry (evaluation of anal rectal muscle function), and defecography (X-ray while defecation).

■ COMPLICATIONS

Hemorrhoids, rectal prolapse, anal fissure, urinary incontinence, urinary retention, and fecal impaction.

MANAGEMENT

In most of the cases, constipation resolves without any treatment. Recurrent constipation can be deal with lifestyle changes such as increase in activities, eating more fiber diet, and drinking more water, laxative can be used but carefully and only when necessary. Varieties of laxatives are available like stimulants, lubricants, stool softeners, fiber supplements, osmotic laxatives, saline laxatives, chloride channel activators, and 5-HT4 agonists. **Flowchart 1** summarizes the stepwise management of constipation.

SUMMARY

Constipation is common symptoms in general practice. For appropriate management of the constipation, it is important to know the type of constipation whether it is primary or secondary. General physical examination and rectal examination are important for further evaluation. Lifestyle changes, fiber intake, and medications are helpful in relieving the constipation. Constipation can be summarized by **Flowchart 2**.

CHAPTER 19

Convulsions in Adults

Amit Nabar

INTRODUCTION

Convulsions or seizures are common complaints in both children and adults presenting to the emergency department (ED) and account for *2% of all ED visits*.

Seizures may be ongoing upon presentation or may occur after the patient is brought to the ED or may have stopped prior to the ED physician having evaluated the patient.

It is usually the bystanders/colleagues who get the patient to the ED.

Seizures occur due to various *cerebral pathologies* similar to anemia or headache. Amongst the *various challenges posed* by a patient with seizure are:
- *Diagnosing* an event as seizure and to *differentiate* between a seizure and seizure mimic
- Effective diagnosis and *quick termination* of seizure
- Analyze the *likelihood of another episode* of seizure
- Investigate for the *possible causative factor*
- Challenge posed by *status epilepticus (SE)*.
These shall be addressed subsequently in this chapter.

What is a seizure?

A seizure is a *transient event* due to *anomalous, uncontrolled hypersynchronous discharges* from a group of *neurons in the brain*.

The sensory, motor, autonomic functions, consciousness, memory, cognitive function, or even behavior may be affected by this excessive hypersynchronous discharge, which depends on the area of origin of the discharges.

Epilepsy

Epilepsy refers to a *recurrent liability of further attacks of seizures*, which is said to be present *when two or more unprovoked seizure attacks* have occurred.

A single unprovoked seizure carries a *30–45% risk of another seizure within the first 2 years*.

CLASSIFICATION OF SEIZURE

It is essential to determine the type of seizure so as to formulate the diagnostic approach on particular etiology, to elect the appropriate therapy and to provide vital information that is of prognostic value.

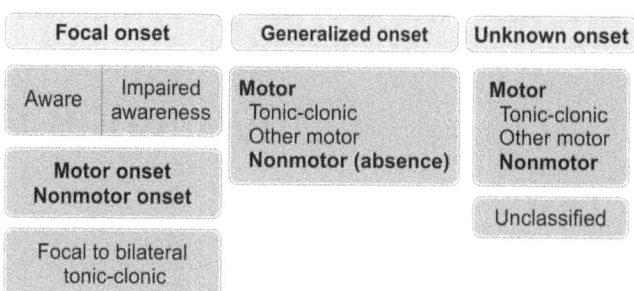

Fig. 1: International League against Epilepsy (ILAE) classification of types of seizure.

Seizure is *functionally* classified into two types, viz *focal and generalized*.
1. *Focal seizures* are focal in origin
2. *Generalized seizures* originate from bilateral networks.

The International League against Epilepsy (ILAE) has revised and classified the seizures (**Fig. 1**).

Focal Seizures

They start in the area of network of cells on one side of the brain. Here, the consciousness is preserved (earlier known as partial seizure):
- *Focal aware*: Here, the awareness is intact, (earlier known as simple partial).
- *Focal-impaired awareness*: The awareness is impaired during the seizure. The patient may have a vague recall of the event, (earlier known as complex partial seizure).

  Focal seizure may also be subclassified based on the motor involvement into:
- *Focal motor seizures*: Some movement is seen during the event, e.g. twitching, jerking, lip licking, rubbing hands, etc.
- *Focal nonmotor seizure*: This type of seizure has no motor symptoms but other symptoms like changes in sensation, strong emotions, thinking, or experiences.
- *Focal to bilateral seizure*: This seizure originates on one side of the brain and spreads to involve both sides (earlier known as secondary generalized seizure).
- *Aura*: It is a perceptual disturbance experienced by some before the beginning of a seizure. Often manifesting as the perception of a strange light, unpleasant smell, or confusing thoughts or experiences. It is usually short lived.

Generalized Seizure

It involves bilateral hemispheres (earlier known as primary generalized seizure).

They *all are presumed to affect awareness.*

They are further classified as:
- *Generalized motor seizures*: There is generalized stiffening (tonic) and jerking (clonic) seen during the seizure.

- *Generalized nonmotor seizures*: There is an abrupt loss of consciousness (absence) with cessation of all motor activity. Tone is usually preserved and the patient often appears glazed or vacant. There may be automatism like lip smacking, etc.
  - *Unknown onset*: Here, the initial onset of seizure is not known.
  - *Awareness unknown*: In certain cases, it may not be possible to ascertain the awareness. The unknown onset seizure too may have features of motor or nonmotor symptoms.

Etiology Classification
- Genetic
- Structural
- Metabolic
- Unknown.

CLINICAL PRESENTATION

The diagnostic uncertainty in cases of patients who are brought to ED after a seizure can be mitigated by *good history and a thorough clinical examination*.

It is usual for the *bystander or colleague* to get the patient to the ED.

A *detailed history* helps in accurate diagnosis of a seizure as clinical examination and the laboratory investigations may be normal in many cases.

Bystander history is the most critical tool that helps in *identifying and classifying* a seizure. History should be sought from bystander on phone if not available and should be asked for presence of awareness, motor movements, and presentation and post-event condition of the patient.

The *history from the patient* though unreliable to describe or classify the seizure can go a long way in establishing the etiological diagnosis.

The history should focus on *risk factors* and history of *seizure precipitants*.

History

Risk Factors
- History of *central nervous system (CNS) pathology (stroke, neoplasm, and recent surgery)*
- *Trauma or fall*
- History of *systemic infections, neoplasm, metabolic disorders, or toxic substance ingestion*
- *Pregnancy*
- *Family history* of seizure.

Seizures Precipitants (Provokers)
- Stress
- Fever or ill health
- Emotional disturbance
- Sleep deprivation and fatigue
- Alcohol and alcohol withdrawal

- Hypoglycemia
- Metabolic disturbance
- Noncompliance with antiepileptic drugs (AED)
- Toxins and drugs.

Physical Examination
General Examination
In *general examination*, one should search for *signs of infections or systemic illness*. It is important to observe for *tongue bite and other evidence of traumatic injuries*.

Person should be evaluated for *underlying infection* and for *organomegaly*, which may be due to *metabolic storage disease. Limb asymmetry* may suggest *brain injury early in the development*.

Cardiac Examination
It should focus on cardiac causes for loss of consciousness and can be divided into mechanical or electrical causes. Mechanical causes result in abrupt impedance the blood flow leading to systemic hypoperfusion, e.g. aortic stenosis, hypertrophic cardiomyopathy, pulmonary embolism, etc. Electrical causes manifest in the form of arrhythmias.

Skin Examination
The cutaneous signs may be subtle and can act as a window into the central nervous system. Café–au-lait spots, hypopigmentation, port-wine stain, etc. suggest an underlying neurocutaneous disorder.

Neurological Examination
A *complete neurological examination* should be performed with emphasis on eliciting signs of *focal neurological deficit or cerebral hemispheric disease*. It should include assessment of *mental status, visual fields, and fundoscopy*.

Screening test for motor functions such as *pronator drift, deep tendon reflexes, gait and coordination, and cortical sensory testing* may help in detecting the cortical lesions.

DIFFERENTIAL DIAGNOSIS (TABLE 1)
Syncope: It is a term used to describe sudden, brief, and reversible loss of consciousness usually accompanied by flaccid muscle tone and usually preceded by a presyncope.

The *diagnostic dilemma* most frequently encountered in the ED is to distinguish between a generalized seizure and syncope (**Table 2**).

Todd's paralysis: It is a reversible focal limb weakness seen after a partial seizure, which involves the motor cortex. Usually lasts for minutes to hours and generally not more than 24 hours.

Table 1: Differential diagnosis of seizures.

D/D	Key features	Tests
Syncope	Syncope is preceded by presyncope (lightheadedness, palpitations, and sweating). The syncope itself is brief (<20 seconds) without postictal confusion Convulsions may occur at the end of the syncope if hypoperfusion persists	CBC, RFT, blood glucose, ECG, Holter Check for postural hypotension; head-up tilt table test
Migraine	Symptoms gradually develop over 15–30 minutes. Hypersensitivity to light, sound, and, odors	MRI may show nonspecific white matter changes
TIA or stroke	Acute onset negative symptoms (i.e. aphasia/weakness/sensory loss) With vascular risk factors	Check HbA1c, lipid profile, carotid Dopplers, echocardiogram, and MRI brain
Transient global amnesia	Episode lasts for 4–24 hours without unconsciousness During episode, people suffer from anterograde more than retrograde amnesia with intact remote memory	MRI brain may be normal
Sleep disorders	REM sleep disorders, and hypnic jerks occur at night or just prior sleeping should be differentiated from frontal lobe seizures	Sleep study
Panic attack	Feelings of intense fear and imminent doom. Typically lasts longer than a seizure (5–30 minutes) Palpitations and sweating, with preserved consciousness	EKG and EEG should be normal
Psychogenic nonepileptic attacks	Eyes are closed during the event Movements are often bilateral with preserved awareness Pelvic thrusting is seen and episodes can be triggered by suggestion	Video EEG with capturing the event

(CBC: complete blood count; D/D: differential diagnosis ECG/EKG: electrocardiography; EEG: electroencephalography; RBD: rapid eye movement sleep behavioral disorder; RFT: renal function test)

■ PSYCHIATRIC FEATURES SEEN IN TRUE SEIZURES

Patients presenting with seizures in ED can be pseudoseizures with psychiatric manifestations but there are few true seizures, which have prominent psychiatric features which may be confused with pseudoseizures. These are:
- *Dysmnesic symptoms*: Memory disturbances such as Déjà vu, Jamais Vu, recollection of previous experiences, former life, childhood, etc.

Table 2: Diagnostic dilemma in emergency department to distinguish between a generalized seizure and syncope.

Features	Seizure	Syncope
Precipitators	Usually absent	Mental stress, pain, Valsalva, prolonged standing, pressure on the neck
Premonitory symptoms	Nil or aura	Fatigability, nausea, sweating, blackout
Duration of unconsciousness	Minutes	Few seconds
Face	Frothing at mouth, cyanosis	Pallor
Disorientation and sleepiness postevent	Many minutes to hours	Immediate recovery within few seconds of being supine
Muscles pain after episode	Likely	Unlikely
Tongue bite	Confirms seizures	Rarely
Location of tongue bite	Usually lateral tongue	If present, usually anterior tip of tongue along with lip injury
Incontinence	Common	Rare

- *Speech issues*: Patient may present with repetitive vocalization with formed words in complex partial seizures or with speech arrest.
- *Affective symptoms*: Like laughter without joy, fear, anger, etc.
- *Hallucination*: Of taste, which is usually an unpleasant sensation or hallucination of perception—vertigo differentiating feature being never severe or associated with vomiting.

DIAGNOSTIC TOOLS

History by the bystander remains the mainstay of diagnosing seizure as many patients tend to have normal laboratory and imaging findings.

There are no investigations or biomarkers, which can truly confirm the presence of seizure and so the ED assessment becomes very important.

Routine laboratory tests rarely reveal clinically important abnormalities but should include routine tests such as:
- Complete blood count (CBC)
- Serum electrolytes
- Serum calcium
- Serum magnesium
- Serum blood sugar levels
- Kidney function test
- Liver function test
- Urine analysis
- Toxicology screen
- Serum prolactin test.

Neuroimaging is essential for the first-time seizure patient and would include either a noncontrast head CT (NCCT) or noncontrast MRI of the brain.

Magnetic resonance imaging is *gold standard* (if availability and cost is not a concern) for evaluation and is highly sensitive and *identifies nearly all macroscopic lesions, e.g. tumors, vascular malformations, etc.*

Computed tomography scan is useful especially in identifying *intracranial bleeds and calcifications*. It is also used in cases where *MRI is not available or feasible* (due to the restless consciousness of the patient in the postictal phase).

The *other modalities* to evaluate the patient, though not in ED, include:
- *Electroencephalography (EEG)* is a functional test to detect epileptic activity. It should be performed before discharge since seizures are typically infrequent and unpredictable and it is often not possible to obtain the EEG during a clinical event.
- *Video-EEG recording* is needed to confirm diagnosis of pseudoseizures.

Other studies would include *ECG and 2D-echocardiography* for possible etiological diagnosis.

APPROACH TO A PATIENT WITH SEIZURE IN EMERGENCY DEPARTMENT (FLOWCHART 1)

The *goal of treatment* for a patient coming to the ED with seizures is twofold:
1. *Aborting* ongoing attack:
   - Benzodiazepine
   - Antiepileptic drug (loading dose).
2. *Preventing* further attacks:
   - This also includes efforts to address the question as to whether the patient would need long-term therapy with AED.

Earlier the treatment is instituted, *more effective* it is in halting the seizures (SE). In general, the classification of type of seizure does not help much in choosing treatment or defining prognosis (exceptions—absence seizure—sodium valproate preferred, presence of myoclonus-avoiding certain AED like phenytoin).

Three basic pitfalls during the *initial care of seizure* patient in ED include:
- *Failure to recognize seizure activity and to differentiate it from seizure mimics* (as mentioned in the Table 1 earlier):
  - It is more so in case of *generalized nonmotor seizures (absence seizures)*, which is a *rare presentation of altered mental status* and has to be considered as a differential of comatose patient. It is important to recognize a patient brought to the ED in an unconscious state, postseizures, as *SE or nonconvulsive status*.
- *Failure to control seizure activity aggressively*: There should be *low threshold for aggressive treatment* for any seizure activity, especially if it last more than 5 minutes.
  More than 20 minutes of continuous seizure activity is associated with *neurological dysfunction*.
- *Failure to consider underlying etiology*: One should evaluate and screen for *underlying infections, metabolic causes, and substance abuse. Medication noncompliance* should be ruled out.

Few things need to keep in mind while dealing with ongoing active seizure (**Table 3**)

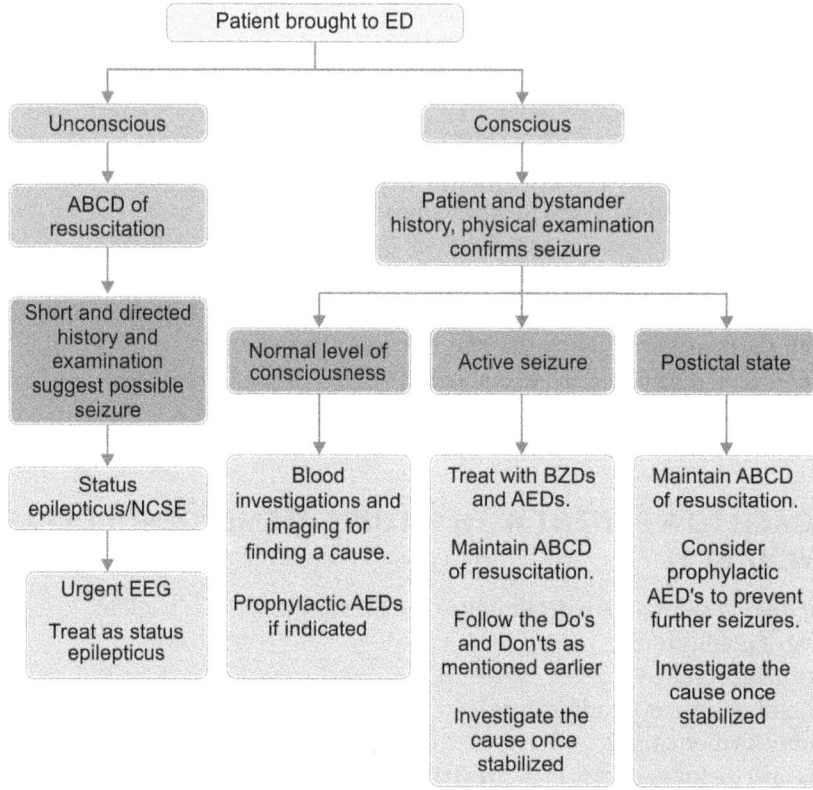

Flowchart 1: Approach to a patient with seizure in emergency department (ED).

(ABCD: airway, breathing, circulation, disability; AED: antiepileptic drug; BZDs: benzodiazepines; EEG: electroencephalography; NCSE: nonconvulsive status epilepticus)

Table 3: Do's and don'ts to deal with ongoing active seizures.

Do's	Don'ts
Patient should be made comfortable	Do not open the mouth
Made supine on the floor, *if seated and kept in lateral position*	Do not force anything between the teeth
Head should be cushioned and protected	
Tight clothing, neck wear should be released	
Efforts to prevent *injury should be made*	
Time the event and video record it, if possible	
Check vital signs, evaluate oxygen saturation and supplement with O_2 wherever indicated	

Drug Management

Benzodiazepines are the drug of choice in a seizure as they are fastest acting.
- *Lorazepam* having *longer half-life* and *less lipid soluble* is preferred.
    - Initial dose of *4 mg IV lorazepam* can be followed by a *repeat dose 5–10 minutes* after the first dose.
- *Diazepam* having *high-lipid solubility*. They carry the risk of *high first-pass concentration* and can cause *respiratory or cardiovascular collapse, if given too rapidly*. It can be given *intravenously or rectally*.
    - IV rate not exceeding 2–5 mg/min
    - Rectal dose 10–20 mg.
- *Midazolam*: Advantage is that it can be given by *buccal, rectal, or intranasal instillation or intramuscular route*.
    - Adult dose used is *10 mg instilled via catheter into the mouth or between cheeks*.

    Studies have shown that *intramuscular midazolam* is as safe and effective as intravenous lorazepam in termination of seizures.

    Parental benzodiazepines are associated with the *risk of respiratory depression, hypotension, and so monitoring the patients vitals is crucial even after the seizure has stopped* and patient is fully awake enough to protect his airway.

    Initial *failure of treatment is often due to inadequate initial dosing*.

    Although benzodiazepines offer distinct advantages due to their rapid onset of action, one should consider use of *AED* for their long-term actions.

    Antiepileptic drugs are *always loaded* to achieve the *desired therapeutic levels rapidly*.

    Antiepileptic drugs commonly used are:
- *Phenytoin/fosphenytoin*: (Fast-acting *fosphenytoin* carries advantage of being *painless* injection as against *phenytoin*, which can cause *painful thrombophlebitis*).
    - Phenytoin is the preferred medication with an IV dose 20 mg/kg at rate up to 50 mg/min, or
    - 20 mg/kg of fosphenytoin, given up to rate of 150 mg/min.

    They *act on the sodium channel* rather than gamma-aminobutyric acid (GABA) receptors, therefore present a rational alternative to patient unresponsive to benzodiazepines.

    Bradycardia and hypotension may occur from high-infusion rates with sedation, hypersensitivity amongst others being the other side effects.
- *Levetiracetam*: (It is *rapidly acting* with *lesser side effect* and *less interaction* with other drugs.)
    - Levetiracetam is often used as a *second-line agent* and can be given *1–3 g dose IV over 5 minutes or infused at 2–5 mg/kg/min*. It is generally well tolerated with mode of action not shared by other drugs.
    - *Mood and behavioral changes* are the disadvantage of long-term use.
- *Sodium valproate*: (*Broad-spectrum and rapid action*) sodium valproate has *similar efficacy when compared to phenytoin*.

- *20-40 mg/kg is given IV over 10 minutes* with *additional 20 mg/kg given over 5 minutes*, if the patient continues to have the seizures. Sodium valproate has *less cardiopulmonary side effects* than phenytoin and may be *preferred in patients with hypotension or respiratory distress*.

STATUS EPILEPTICUS

Status epilepticus refers to continuous, repetitive, discrete seizures with impaired consciousness in the interictal period.

For *epidemiological purposes*, SE is defined as *clinical or electrographic seizures lasting at least 30 minutes* or *serial seizures* in which *consciousness is not regained* between seizures.

For all *practical purposes*, seizures that *last long enough to raise concern* about an altered physiologic state (e.g. tonic–clonic seizures lasting more than 5 minutes) should be *treated as SE*.

Status epilepticus is *a medical emergency*, since prolonged seizures can lead to *irreversible neuronal injury*.

- *Generalized convulsive status epilepticus (GCSE)* is evident when patient is having visible persistent convulsions, however, if the patient stops having overt seizures and yet remains comatose, an EEG should be performed to rule out ongoing SE. Anticonvulsant treatment should be instituted without delay along with stabilizing the vitals.
- *Nonconvulsive SE* is also associated with cellular injury in the region of seizure focus and so should be treated promptly.

Protocol for Treatment of Status Epilepticus

1. *First stage of SE—early status (less than 30 min)*:
   Lorazepam 4 mg IV bolus (with maximum up to 8 mg)
   ↓   (If seizures still persists)
2. *Second stage of SE—i.e. established status (30-60 minutes)*:
   Phenobarbital IV infusion of 10 mg/kg at a rate of 100 mg/min
   Or
   Fosphenytoin* IV infusion of 15 mg PE/kg at a rate of 100 mg PE/min
   Or
   Levetiracetam IV 1-3 g over 15 minutes
   Or
   Valproate IV infusion of 25 mg/kg at a rate of 3-6 mg/kg/min
   ↓   (If seizures continue after 60 min)
3. *Third stage of SE—i.e. refractory status (>60 minutes)*:
   Use of anesthetic drugs till burst-suppression pattern on the EEG is achieved, use:
   Propofol: IV bolus 2 mg/kg, followed by a continuous infusion of 5-10 mg/kg/h
   Or
   Thiopental: IV bolus of 100-250 mg given over 20 seconds with further 50 mg boluses every 2-3 minutes until seizures are controlled, followed by a continuous IV infusion at a dose usually 3-5 mg/kg/h
   Or
   Midazolam: IV bolus of 0.1-0.3 mg/kg at a rate not exceeding 4 mg/min initially, followed by a continuous IV infusion at a dose usually 0.05-0.4 mg/kg/h.

When seizures have been controlled for 12 hours, start reducing drug dose over a further 12 hours. If repeat seizures, the general anesthetic agent should be given again for a further 12 hours and then withdrawal attempted again. This cycle may need to be repeated until seizure control is achieved.

Note: *Fosphenytoin is preferred over phenytoin as it is water soluble, so can be given faster, no phlebitis.

SPECIAL SITUATION

Seizures in following conditions need special consideration:
- *Seizures in pregnancy*: It is a complication severe untreated preeclampsia and can occur up to 4 weeks postdelivery.
  - The seizing pregnant patient should be treated similar to nonpregnant patient.
  - Magnesium sulfate is the treatment of choice.
- *Post-traumatic seizures*: They are directly related to the severity of the injury, though its occurrence is not significantly affected by early use of antiepileptics.
- *Intracranial hemorrhage*: It predisposes a patient to seizures and prophylactic antiepileptics are recommended.
- *Alcohol withdrawal seizure*: They can occur 6–48 hours after cessation of consumption of alcohol.
  - Benzodiazepines are the drug of choice to control and prevent seizures in these groups of patients.
- *Tricyclic antidepressant (TCA)* overdose and isoniazid (INH) overdose are the common causes of drug-induced seizures.
  - Apart from supportive therapy, treatment of TCA overdose is bicarbonate infusion.
  - Pyridoxine is the drug of choice for known INH ingestion.

CHAPTER 20

Convulsion in Children

Sanjukta Dutta

INTRODUCTION

Seizure is paroxysmal involuntary motor activities, changes in behavior, sensation, and/or consciousness due to abnormal electrical discharge in the brain.

Seizures are most common neurologic emergency in pediatric age group. Seizures occur in approximately 1% of children up to 14 years of age. Incidence is highest in the first year of life (120 per 100,000). Seizure may range from subtle, nonconvulsive episodes to stereotypic movements to major generalized convulsions. Severity of seizures varies widely. It may be self-limited episodes with no hemodynamic compromise like febrile convulsions to prolonged events that may ultimately be fatal in as many as 3–4% of patients. Extensive evaluation and emergency management is essential in high-risk patients as in status epilepticus, neonatal seizures.

ETIOLOGY/CAUSES

Seizures could be multifactorial. A cause is identifiable in less than 20% of children with seizures. The most common etiology of neonatal seizures is hypoxic-ischemic encephalopathy (initial 48 hours of life) and meningoencephalitis. The differences between provoked and unprovoked seizures are given in **Table 1**.

Table 1: Differences between provoked and unprovoked seizures.

Provoked seizures (seizure with an acute antecedent cause)	*Unprovoked seizures* (no immediate provoking factor)
Hypoglycemia	Cryptogenic (no known cause)
Toxic exposure	Idiopathic (genetic)
Central nervous system (CNS) infection (meningitis, encephalitis)	Remote symptomatic (preexisting brain abnormality or insult): • Hydrocephalus • Disorders of brain development • Neoplasms
Head injury	
Other precipitating factors: • Fever • Immunization	

PATHOPHYSIOLOGY

Seizures are involuntary muscle contractions with or without alteration in mental status. Generalized seizures arise from the bilateral hemispheres of the cerebral cortex. In contrast, focal seizures arise from one region or hemisphere of the brain. Aberrant electrical activity and subsequent manifestation of the seizure may range from subtle, nonconvulsive events to stereotypic movements to dramatic generalized convulsions. Neonatal seizures are typically subtler than seizures in older children and adults, given the immature nervous system of the neonate.

CLINICAL PRESENTATION

Depending upon the area in the brain where the seizure initiates and how it propagates symptoms could vary widely.
- Generalized seizures cause loss of consciousness along with purposeless full-body tonic (sustained)–clonic (interrupted) movements, atonia, and/or myoclonic jerking.
- Focal seizures can manifest as disturbances in motor/sensory/autonomic function, emotional state, cognition, behavior, or memory with or without alteration in consciousness.
- At the cessation of seizure activity, the patient will enter the postictal period, characterized by confusion, fatigue, lethargy, and/or irritability.
- Neonatal seizures may present with subtle findings, such as ocular movement or lip smacking or abnormal vitals.
- Nonconvulsive status epilepticus can present as altered mental status, mild confusion, and subtle physical movements, inexplicable sudden changes in mental status or delayed recovery after a seizure.

Febrile Convulsion

Febrile convulsion is defined as seizure in neurologically normal child of 6 months to 5 years with a temperature of greater than 38°C (100.4°F) which has no identifiable cause or previous history of afebrile seizures.

Febrile convulsion is the most common seizure disorder in childhood. It affects 2–5% of children between 6 months to 5 years age group, with peak incidence at 18 months. Around 6–15% occur after 4 years, onset after 6 years is unusual. Febrile seizures generally occur during viral or bacterial infections. They sometimes occur after vaccinations like measles, mumps, and rubella. Genetic and familial factors increase the susceptibility to febrile seizures. Febrile seizures usually take place during the initial rapid rise in body temperature, and mostly develop within 24 hours of fever onset. Typically, seizures are generalized; most are clonic, but some can manifest as periods of atonic or tonic posturing.

Febrile seizures may be simple or complex:

Simple Febrile Seizures
- Brief (<15-minute) generalized seizures
- Association with fever (temperature > 38.0°C)

- Predominantly generalized tonic–clonic seizure activity
- Only one convulsion in a 24-hour period
- Brief postictal period
- Absence of preexisting neurological abnormality (intracranial infection, metabolic disturbance, or history of afebrile seizures).

Complex Febrile Seizures
- Last greater than or equal to 15 minutes continuously or with pauses
- Have focal features
- Recur within 24 hours.

More than 90% febrile seizures are simple.

Febrile convulsion is established after exclusion of other possible causes. Fever may trigger seizures in child with previous afebrile seizures and such events are not considered febrile seizures.

Routine testing is not required for simple febrile seizures other than to evaluate the source of the fever. Complex seizures, seizures with neurologic deficits, or signs of a serious underlying disorder (e.g. meningitis, metabolic disorders), warrants appropriate investigations.

Recurrence and Subsequent Epilepsy
Recurrence rate of febrile seizures is nearly 35%. Risk of recurrence is higher if first seizure occurs in less than 1 year of age or history of febrile seizure is positive in first-degree relatives. Risk of developing an afebrile seizure disorder after having greater than or equal to 1 simple febrile seizure is slightly higher (2–5%) than the baseline risk of developing epilepsy (2%). In children who have additional risk factors (e.g. complex febrile seizures, family history of seizures, developmental delay); this risk is increased up to 10%. Prolonged febrile status epilepticus may be associated with damage to vulnerable parts of the brain such as the hippocampus.

Afebrile Seizures
A vast differential is to be considered in afebrile child with seizures. It could be a presentation of epilepsy or could be a symptom of another process, such as intracranial tumor or infection, metabolic derangement, toxic ingestion, neurocutaneous syndrome or trauma.

Status Epilepticus
Definition:
- Three or more seizures in an hour
- A single prolonged seizure lasting at least 30 minutes with a motor component
- Two or more convulsions without complete recovery of consciousness between seizures.

Approximately 10% of children presenting with active seizure to the hospital are in status epilepticus. Nearly one-third of them are related to fever, other etiologies include central nervous system (CNS) infections, ingestions, and trauma.

Nonconvulsive Status Epilepticus

No convulsive status epilepticus can present as a continuous or fluctuating "epileptic twilight" state or as a prolonged postictal state. It must be considered in any child with altered mental state where no other cause could be diagnosed.

Neonatal Seizures

The most common etiology of neonatal seizures is hypoxic-ischemic encephalopathy, usually manifesting within 48 hours of life. Still infection can be a significant trigger for seizures in neonates. So, possible meningoencephalitis is to be ruled out in this population.

RED FLAGS

- Seizure in clinically unwell child, such as, symptoms of infection, meningeal signs, dehydration
- Complex febrile seizure
- Altered level of consciousness
- Additional risks for serious bacterial infection:
  - Age less than 6 months or more than 60 months with first febrile seizure
  - Age less than 12 months with incomplete or unknown Immunization history
  - Febrile status epilepticus.
- First nonfebrile seizure.

EVALUATION

History

Most of the seizure activities stop before reaching emergency department so the detailed history usually is the guide to the diagnosis.
- Age of child
- Onset, duration, progress, and description of seizure activity
- History of trauma
- History of possible ingestion
- History of fever
- History of associated illness (vomiting or diarrhea)
- Feeding problems (especially in an infant)
- Changes in behavior
- Previous history of seizures and type of seizures
- Anticonvulsants dose and recent changes/missed doses
- Recent new medications (may alter metabolism of antiepileptic drugs)
- Allergies
- Other medical history
- Developmental history
- Family history of seizures

- Seizure specific questions can be asked:
  - Was there a warning right before the convulsion (behavioral arrest, affective change)?
  - Did the head/eyes deviate upward or to one side?
  - Did the movements start unilaterally or bilaterally?
  - What was the child like immediately after and how long to recover to baseline?

PHYSICAL EXAMINATION

In children presenting with seizure attack, a physical examination should address their cardiac, neurological, and mental status, and should include a developmental assessment where appropriate.

Some findings are important in some specific conditions:
- *CNS infection*: Fever, headache, prolonged seizure, prolonged postictal state, Stiff neck, confusion
- *Head trauma*: History, external evidence, focal deficit
- *Brain tumor*: Headache, focal seizure, focal deficits
- *Genetic syndromes and brain malformations*: Developmental delay, dysmorphism
- *Cerebral hemorrhage*: Trauma, family history of cerebral cavernous malformations, focal seizures, focal deficits
- *Neurocutaneous disorders*: Birthmarks (hypopigmented macules, café au lait spots, etc.).

INTERPRETATION OF FINDING

Seizures can be partial (simple or complex partial, or partial with secondary generalization), generalized tonic–clonic, or tonic seizures.

After stabilization of the child, it is important to determine if a seizure has occurred, and if so, if it is the child's first episode. Children can present with seizure-like symptoms that may not in fact represent actual seizures, but rather breath-holding spells, syncope, gastro-esophageal reflux, pseudoseizures (psychogenic), and other nonepileptic events. The determination that a seizure has occurred is usually based on a detailed, careful history, and neurologic examination. Tests to exclude other disorders are determined clinically.

INVESTIGATIONS

Serum Laboratory Studies

Serum glucose, sodium, calcium, magnesium, phosphorus, complete blood count, and liver and kidney function tests to rule out metabolic disorders if the history includes recent vomiting, diarrhea, or impaired fluid intake; if there are signs of dehydration or edema; or if a complex febrile seizure occurs. They are not required routinely in simple febrile seizures.

Electroencephalogram

- EEG should be performed within 24–48 hours only to support a diagnosis of epilepsy in seizures with focal features, recurrent seizures, and first afebrile unprovoked seizures.

- It is not recommended after an initial simple febrile seizure in children with a normal neurologic examination.
- When a standard EEG is not contributory, sleep EEG or long-term video or ambulatory EEG can be considered where appropriate.

Neuroimaging

Neuroimaging should be used to identify underlying structural abnormalities that cause certain epilepsies.

Magnetic Resonance Imaging Brain

Imaging investigation of choice in children with epilepsy and important in the following:
- Epilepsy before the age of 2 years, excluding those with simple febrile seizures
- Suggestion of focal onset on history, physical examination, or EEG
- Signs of increased intracranial pressure
- Failure to control seizures, worsening seizures, changes is seizure manifestations
- History of status epilepticus.

Computed Tomography Brain

- In suspected gross pathology, if MRI is unavailable or is contraindicated
- In an acute emergency, CT can be used to determine whether a seizure has been due to acute neurological lesion or illness.

Lumbar Puncture and Cerebrospinal Fluid Analysis

- Seizure in child less than 6 months
- Persistent alteration of mental status of unknown cause or failure to return to baseline
- Seizure with suspected meningitis or meningitis or intracranial infection by history or examination
- Seizures after several days of febrile illness
- Seizure with fever in those who are not fully immunized or taking antibiotics.

If increased intracranial pressure is suspected, the LP should be preceded by an imaging study of the head.

Electrocardiogram

- 12-lead ECG should be considered only in cases of diagnostic uncertainty in pediatric age group
- *Neuropsychological assessment* is suggested in selected patients.

TREATMENT

There are limited data on pediatric seizures to lead to a consensus protocol. There are varieties of guidelines and algorithms endorsed by different organizations and institutions around the globe. Though they have variations, the essential management pathways are quite similar.

For a seizing child in ED immediately:
- Secure airway
- Give high flow oxygen
- Assess breathing and circulation
- Assess vital signs
- Check blood glucose
- Secure intravenous (IV) access in a large vein
- Place patient on full monitor
- Followed by medications depending on seizure type and underlying cause.

Treatment of Febrile Seizure

- Antipyretic therapy is to be given to relive symptoms of associated febrile illness but they do not reduce seizure activity
- Supportive therapy is usually sufficient for seizures lasting less than 15 minutes as most of the seizures are brief and self-limiting
- Rectal diazepam can be used
- Seizures lasting greater than or equal to 15 minutes are treated in the line of status epilepticus
- Maintenance drug therapy is usually not indicated.

Treatment of Neonatal Seizure

Maintain airway, breathing, circulation, and temperature

↓

Collect blood for biochemistry

↓

Check blood glucose immediately

↓

Correct glucose and calcium

↓

Administer IV phenobarbitone 20 mg/kg

↓

Repeat in 5 mg/kg boluses every 15 minutes if seizure continues, upto a maximum dose of 40 mg/kg

↓

IV phenytoin 15–20 mg/kg diluted in same amount of normal saline at a maximum rate of 1 mg/kg/min over 35–40 minutes

↓

IV lorazepam (0.05–0.1 mg/kg) or diazepam (0.25 mg/kg bolus or 0.5 mg/kg rectal)

↓

Or IV midazolam as a continuous infusion (an initial IV bolus of 0.15 mg/kg, followed by continuous infusion (1 µg/kg/min) increasing by 0.5–1 µg/kg/min every 2 minutes until a favorable response or a maximum of 18 µg/kg/min

↓

100 mg pyridoxine IV or oral (if IV not available) should be given.

Treatment of Status Epilepticus

In the Community

Prolonged (lasting 5 minutes or more) or repeated (3 or more in an hour) generalized, convulsive (tonic–clonic, tonic or clonic) seizures in the community should receive immediate emergency care.

If history of previous episode of prolonged or serial convulsive seizures is present, buccal midazolam or rectal diazepam can be given. Care must be taken to secure airway and assess respiratory and cardiac function.

Patient in ED

Convulsive status epilepticus can lead to permanent neuronal injury. Majority of the seizures are brief and self-limiting. If a seizure activity lasts for more than 5 minutes, the chances are more that the seizure is likely to be prolonged. Keeping that in mind, all the status treatment protocols have used a 5-minute definition. Early treatment minimizes risk of seizures reaching 30 minutes and subsequent neuronal damage. Moreover, the adverse outcomes associated with needlessly intervening on brief, self-limited seizures are eliminated by avoiding aggressive therapy before 5 minutes.

Stabilization (0–5 minutes)

- Assess and stabilize patient's airway, breathing, and circulation
- Give high flow oxygen, if oxygenation is impaired
- Consider intubation, if assisted ventilation is required
- Take quick history
- Perform physical examination with stress on neurological examination
- Check blood glucose and correct with IV dextrose if CBG less than 60 mg%

- For children of less than or equal to 2 years: 4 mL/kg, for children more than 2 years: 25D 2 mL/kg 2 mL/h
- Secure IV or IO access immediately
- Collect blood for complete hemogram, electrolytes, toxicology screen, and antiepileptic drug levels where appropriate.

First-line Therapy (5–20 minutes)
- Benzodiazepines are the initial therapy of choice
- Any one of the following three can be used:
  - IM midazolam (10 mg for >40 kg, 5 mg for 13–40 kg, single dose)
  - IV lorazepam (0.1 mg/kg/dose, maximum: 4 mg/dose, may repeat dose once)
  - IV diazepam (0.15–0.2 mg/kg/dose, maximum: 10 mg/dose, one repeat dose can be given).
- If none of the above options are available, any one of the following can be used:
  - IV phenobarbital (15 mg/kg/dose, single dose)
  - Rectal diazepam (0.2–0.5 mg/kg, max: 20 mg/dose, single dose)
  - Intranasal/buccal midazolam.

Second-line Therapy (20–40 minutes)
- If there is a lack of response to the therapy administered in the previous phase, the following can be administered as a single dose:
  - IV fosphenytoin (20 mg PE/kg, maximum: 1,500 mg PE/dose, single dose)
  - IV valproic acid (40 mg/kg, maximum: 3,000 mg/dose, single dose)
  - IV levetiracetam (60 mg/kg, maximum: 4,500 mg/dose, single dose).
- If none of the above are available:
  - Intravenous phenobarbital (15 mg/kg, single dose, if not given already).

Third-line Therapy (40–60 minutes)
- At this juncture, no clear evidence is there to guide therapy
- If the seizure continues, second line therapy can be repeated or anesthetic doses of thiopental, midazolam, pentobarbital, or propofol can be administered. EEG monitoring is necessary at this phase.

Based on the cause and severity of the seizure, the second- or third-line therapy can be initiated at an earlier time, if necessary. If at any point, the patient responds to therapy and is at baseline, symptomatic medical care should be initiated.

Treatment of Nonconvulsive Status Epilepticus
- Less well defined
- Most forms not life-threatening
- Initial treatment: Similar to generalized convulsive status epilepticus.

DISPOSITION

Admission should be considered for:
- Infants less than 6 months
- Children with complex features
- Seizures are uncontrolled or prolonged
- Social concerns.

SUMMARY

- Airway
- Breathing
- Circulation
- Check glucose
- Stop seizures
- Prevent or correct metabolic complications
- Identify and treat underlying causes.

CHAPTER 21

Cough in Adult

Bhawana Sharma

INTRODUCTION

Cough is the most common symptom observed in pulmonary disease patients and most frequent cause of visit to clinics. The patient's anxiety associated with the serious underlying cause is significant. Troublesome-associated symptoms like—chest pain from intercostal muscle strain or even a fractured rib, cough-induced urinary or fecal incontinence may lead to fear of social isolation, besides considering cough as communicable disease symptom by peer group.

What is cough?

A forceful expiration expels mucus and foreign material from the airways protecting lung against aspiration.

Effectiveness of cough, i.e. ability to take deep breath and exhale forcefully—it depends on:
- Ability of an individual to take a deep breath
- Lung elastic recoil
- Expiratory muscle strength
- Level of airway resistance.

Cough is usually ineffective in patients with:
- Cardiopulmonary diseases
- Neurologic diseases especially involving respiratory muscles and gag reflex
- Systemic neuromuscular diseases
- Early postoperative period due to painful respiratory movements—especially after pulmonary or upper abdominal surgeries and trauma.

Often expiratory flow is limited by factors such as:
- Bronchospasm (e.g. asthma)
- Reduced lung elastic recoil (as in emphysema)
- Muscle weakness.

CONSEQUENCES OF INEFFECTIVE COUGH

- Atelectasis
- Retained secretions
- More prone to develop pneumonia and/or hypoxemia.

CHARACTERISTICS OF COUGH

- Dry
- Loose
- Productive
- Nonproductive
- Acute
- Chronic
- Relation with time (nocturnal or daytime).

Dry or nonproductive cough: Typical of restrictive lung disease such as congestive heart failure (CHF) or pulmonary fibrosis.

Loose or productive cough: More often associated with inflammatory obstructive disease such as bronchitis or asthma.

ETIOLOGY OF COUGH

Most common cause of acute, self-limiting cough is a viral infection of upper airway.

Chronic cough is one lasting 8 weeks or longer.

Chronic cough carries with it considerable frustration and anxiety for patients with decreased quality of life and depression.

When a detail history and thorough examination fail to find evidence of disease [e.g. cancer, human immunodeficiency virus (HIV) disease] and the chest radiograph is normal, more than 90% of chronic cough cases are accounted for by upper airway cough syndrome (formerly called postnasal drip), asthma, and gastrointestinal reflux.

Chronic cough has numerous common and uncommon causes that sometimes may have multiple sources (**Box 1**).

MECHANISM OF COUGH (FLOWCHART 1)

When cough receptors are stimulated by inflammation, mucus, foreign materials, or noxious gases. Receptors are located primarily in larynx, trachea, and large bronchi.

CHARACTERISTICS OF COUGH IN SPECIFIC ETIOLOGIES

The characteristics of cough in specific etiologies are described in **Table 1**.

COMPLICATIONS OF COUGH

- *Circulatory:* Decrease in cardiac output due to raised intrathoracic pressure especially in patients with cor pulmonale or right heart failure.
- *Syncope:* Posttussive—nearly always occur in man
- *Raised intra-abdominal pressure:* Hernia, collapse of rectum or vagina
- *Intraocular hemorrhage.*

Box 1: Evaluating chronic cough in adults (>8 weeks duration).

Common sources:
- Upper airway cough syndrome (formerly known as "postnasal drip")
- Pulmonary tuberculosis
- Asthma
- Gastroesophageal reflux
- Chronic bronchitis associated with cigarette smoking
- Environmental exposure
- *Angiotensin-converting enzyme (ACE)*—one cough (caused by antihypertensive drug ACE inhibitors)
- Nonasthmatic eosinophilic bronchitis.

Less common sources:
- Postinfection (e.g. pertussis, *Mycoplasma*)
- Interstitial lung disease
- Bronchiectasis
- Obstructive sleep apnea
- Primary lung cancer
- Heart failure.

Uncommon sources:
- Sarcoidosis
- Recurrent aspiration
- Chronic tonsillar enlargement
- Chronic auditory canal irritation
- Foreign body aspiration
- Endemic fungi
- Peritoneal dialysis
- Cystic fibrosis
- Tracheomalacia
- Habit or "tic cough."

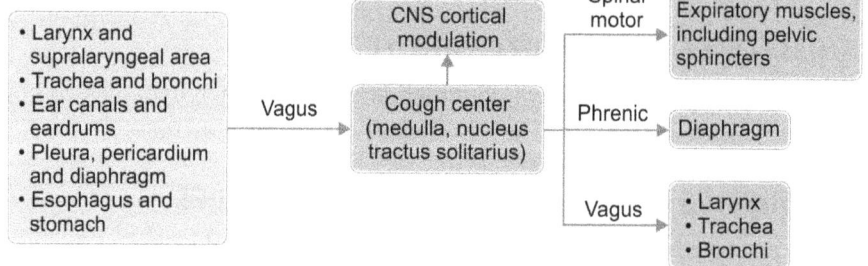

Flowchart 1: Mechanism of cough: signaling pathways in the development of cough.

(CNS: central nervous system)

ALGORITHM FOR THE EVALUATION OF CHRONIC COUGH IN ADULTS

The algorithm for the evaluation of chronic cough in adults is given in **Flowchart 2**.

Do not suppress the cough—treat the cause of cough.

Table 1: Characteristics of cough in specific etiologies.

Causes	Characteristics of cough
Sinusitis or nasopharyngitis	Cough following an upper respiratory syndrome or sinus symptoms; sensation of a need to clear the throat; postnasal drip
Acute infections of lung:	
Tracheobronchitis	Cough associated with sore throat, running nose, and eyes
Lobar pneumonia	Cough often preceded by symptoms of upper respiratory infection; dry cough—initially painful later become productive
Bronchopneumonia	Cough dry/productive, usually begins as acute bronchitis
Mycoplasma and viral pneumonia	Paroxysmal cough, productive—mucoid/blood-stained sputum associated with flu-like syndrome
Exacerbation of chronic bronchitis	Productive cough—mucoid then purulent
Chronic infections of lung:	
Bronchitis	• Productive cough on most days for more than 3 consecutive months and for more than 2 years • Mucoid sputum until acute exacerbation, when it becomes mucopurulent.
Bronchiectasis	Copious, foul smelling, purulent sputum often since childhood; forms layers on standing
Tuberculosis or fungal infection	Persistent cough for weeks to months, often with blood-tinged sputum
Parenchymal inflammatory processes:	
Interstitial fibrosis and infiltrations	Persistent, nonproductive cough—depends on origin
Smoking and inhalation of irritants	Persistent slightly productive cough, mostly in mornings, usually associated with infected pharynx, if succeeded by chronic bronchitis copious purulent sputum may be present
Tumors:	
Bronchogenic carcinoma	Nonproductive cough → productive in weeks to months, may be associated with recurrent mild hemoptysis
Adenocarcinoma in situ or minimally invasive adenocarcinoma	Same as earlier, some cases may present with copious, watery to mucoid sputum
Benign tumors in airways	Nonproductive cough, occasional hemoptysis
Mediastinal tumors	Cough with dyspnea—caused by compression of trachea and bronchi
Aortic aneurysm	Brassy cough
Gastrointestinal:	
Gastroesophageal reflux disease (GERD)	Nonproductive cough—often followed by meals or with recumbency. May or may not be associated with other symptoms of GERD (e.g. heartburn, bitter oral taste, and belching)

Contd...

Contd...

Causes	Characteristics of cough
Foreign body:	
Immediate while still in upper airway	Cough associated with progressive evidence of asphyxiation
Later, when lodged in lower airway	Persistent, nonproductive cough associated with localized wheeze
Cardiovascular:	
Left ventricular failure	Cough and dyspnea worsens when supine
Pulmonary infarction	Cough with hemoptysis, usually with pleural effusion
Drug-induced:	
Angiotensin-converting enzyme (ACE) inhibitors	More common in females, dry cough, may occur at any time (soon after starting drug or many years later)

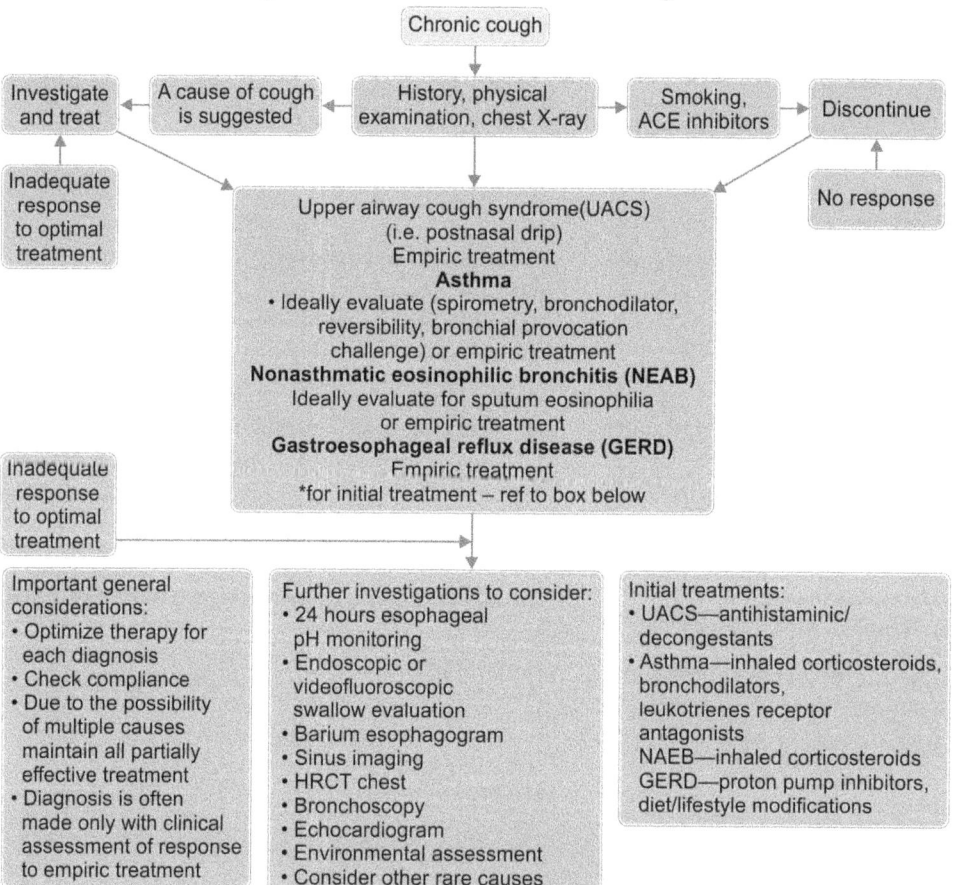

Flowchart 2: Algorithm for the evaluation of chronic cough in adults.

(ACE: angiotensin-converting enzyme; HRCT: high-resolution computed tomography)

CHAPTER 22

Cough in Children

Maninder S Dhaliwal

INTRODUCTION

Cough is a common and distressing symptom in children, which leads to frequent emergency and also outpatient visits to a pediatrician/physician. Cough is also the most common system of the respiratory system and despite it being a common symptom in all age groups, from infancy, toddler, adolescence, adult, and to old age; definite studies are lacking on same. Surprisingly, in medical literature, especially clinical and physiology textbooks contain only a small chapter on this topic. But in recent years, pediatric-specific cough guidelines have been formulated in America (US), the United Kingdom (UK), and Australia. The causes and presentation of cough in children is very different from adults; hence, the management of pediatric cough is also distinctively dissimilar. Common causes of cough in children include viral upper respiratory tract infection (URTI) or bronchitis which are generally mild illnesses with, at the most, bothersome symptoms which usually resolve spontaneously. However, occasionally cough may be the only indication of a serious underlying disorder, which can only be identified by careful evaluation. The aim of this chapter is to simplify approach to acute cough in children, with emphasis on etiology, investigations, and treatment.

ETIOLOGY/CAUSES

The following clinical details can provide clues to the etiology of cough: onset and duration, associated signs and symptoms and in particular, sound quality during coughing. The below mentioned terms and classifications, have been used in various guidelines and medical literature regarding pediatric cough.

Based on Duration

Pediatric cough can be divided into the following subtypes depending on its duration. The period of time varies among different guidelines. A brief description is mentioned here.

Acute Cough

This generally refers to cough of less than 2 weeks duration and is followed by the US and Australian guidelines. According to UK guidelines, acute cough is defined as cough lasting less than 4 weeks. As mentioned earlier, one of the most common causes of acute cough in children is viral URTI which does not require specific diagnostic evaluation. On the other hand, if cough begins abruptly and is associated with history of choking, it may raise doubt of a foreign body, in which case further evaluation including chest X-ray and diagnostic/therapeutic bronchoscopy is required. Also in cases where clinical findings suggest pneumonia or in presence of other symptoms like hemoptysis further investigation would be warranted.

Subacute Cough

This refers to cough of 4 weeks duration (US and Australian guidelines). According to UK guidelines, subacute cough is cough that lasts up to 8 weeks. The usual causes are mixed/multiple URTI's or secondary bacterial infections. Subacute cough generally requires observation and if the cough persists more than 4–8 weeks, a chest X-ray should be performed and evaluation should be done for chronic cough.

Chronic Cough

Cough continuing for more than 4 weeks, according to the US and Australian guidelines, or more than 8 weeks, according to the UK guidelines, are labeled as chronic cough and needs evaluation as per age and local infections. In India, among toddler-to-adolescent age group, cough with sputum for more than 4 weeks, tuberculosis as a possibility should be kept in mind. Chronic cough in children can be further subclassified into three etiological groups: normal/expected cough, specific cough, and nonspecific cough.

- *Normal or expected cough*: Normal children also cough. This is usually secondary to acute respiratory tract infection, bronchial hyper reactivity, and increased secretions. Young children have an average of 6–8 colds per year, associated with this type of cough.
- *Specific cough*: This type of cough is associated with clinical features suggestive of an underlying etiology. This category includes asthma, pneumonia, pulmonary tuberculosis (TB), bronchiectasis (BE), cystic fibrosis (CF), cardiac abnormalities, pulmonary interstitial disease, etc. Investigations should be carried out to find the specific etiology, so that specific treatment could be instituted.
- *Nonspecific cough*: Long standing dry cough in the absence of an identifiable respiratory etiology constitutes this division. The majority of cases are due to benign etiology (e.g. postviral cough and/or increased cough receptor sensitivity to environmental triggers) and may spontaneously resolve. Many of these cases are treated incorrectly with inhaled corticosteroids, having been wrongly labeled as "cough variant asthma."

Recurrent Cough

A recurrent cough without a cold is taken as repeated (>2/year) cough episode, that each last more than 7–14 days.

Based on Age

In children, the causes of cough vary clearly according to age, as mentioned in **Table 1**. Exposure to tobacco smoke and other environmental triggers are also a common cause of cough or are responsible for the failure of cough to resolve at all ages.

Table 1: Common age-wise etiologies of cough in children.

Causes: Age <5 years	Age >5 years
Infections	Asthma
Foreign body inhalation	Postnasal drip
Passive smoking and environmental pollution	Infection
Gastroesophageal reflux	Persistent bacterial bronchitis
Asthma	Passive smoking
Persistent bacterial bronchitis	Bronchiectasis

Table 2: Traditional recognizable cough sounds.

Cough sound	Causes
Barking/brassy	Croup, tracheomalacia
Wet	Persistent bacterial bronchitis, pneumonia, bronchiectasis, cystic fibrosis, primary ciliary dyskinesia
Dry, staccato	Chlamydia
Barking/honking	Habit/psychogenic
Paroxysmal/spasmodic/whoop	Pertussis/parapertussis

Based on Sound of Cough

Classically recognized cough sounds and the pattern of cough can help a physician point to its underlying etiology (**Table 2**).

Based on Wet or Dry Cough

"Wet" cough is a more accurate term in pediatrics and is preferred over "productive" cough. This is because young children rarely expectorate sputum; hence, cough is not actually productive; however, it is wet type due to presence of airway secretions. Wet cough usually indicates impaired mucus clearance or excessive mucus production, whereas dry cough indicates irritation/inflammation of the airway or extraneous cause. A chronic wet cough requires further investigation especially if accompanied by other symptoms like clubbing or failure to thrive. If there is presence of purulent expectoration, it can indicate presence of infection or eosinophilia. Copious purulent sputum production is classically seen in bronchiectasis. Foul-smelling expectoration usually indicates anaerobic infection of the lungs.

Pathophysiology of Cough

Cough is a protective airway reflex that helps to clear secretions and debris from the airways, enhances mucociliary function, and clears excessive secretions and airway debris from the respiratory tract. The afferent receptors for cough are distributed throughout the respiratory tract: from larynx to segmental bronchi. The usual triggers for cough reflex include mechanical

Table 3: Clinical history in children with cough and its interpretation.

History	Interpretation
Diurnal variability	Nocturnal cough: Asthma/postnasal drip Diurnal (never during sleep): Habit/psychogenic cough
With expectoration	Consider: Bronchiectasis, persistent bacterial bronchitis, cystic fibrosis, primary ciliary dyskinesia
Wheezing sounds	Asthma, pulmonary edema
Associated hoarseness	Laryngeal involvement/croup
Hemoptysis	Suppurative diseases, malformations, bronchitis
Abrupt onset	Foreign body, pulmonary embolism
Neonatal age of onset	Congenital malformations
Triggered with feeding	Aspiration/gastroesophageal reflux/tracheoesophageal fistula
Throat clearing	Post nasal drip, vocal tic
Persistent headache	Sinusitis
Dyspnea	Hypoxemia, heart failure, pneumonia, asthma
Improvement with medication	Relevant for bronchodilators/antibiotic course
Repeated infections	Underlying immunodeficiency (e.g. HIV)
Chronicity of symptoms	Athman, bronchiectasis, cystic fibrosis, etc.
Drugs	Angiotensin converting enzyme inhibitors—cough side effect

or chemical irritation. The stimulus is carried by the vagal nerve (afferent pathway) up to the brainstem and modulated by the cerebral cortex. Subsequent efferent motor response is transmitted to the respiratory muscles leading to cough production. The sensitivity of this cough is modified by disease state (e.g. upregulation in viral URTI/g gastroesophageal reflux) or medications (e.g. increased with angiotensin-converting enzyme inhibitor therapy, decreased with codeine).

Clinical Presentation and Evaluation

A good history in a child with cough should include onset and duration of cough, presence of any diurnal variation, presence of any triggering factors (exercise, allergen/tobacco exposure or temperature variation) and nature (dry or wet type) (**Table 3**). Other accompanying symptoms should also be noted. During the examination of patient, it is important to give enough time so as to observe a spontaneous cough. Failing this, the child must be asked to breathe deeply if co-operative with forceful exhalation so as to induce a cough response. Usually cough is elicitable on request in a child whose age is more than 4–5 years. This should be followed by clinical thorough examination of the patient. The examination should be divided into two parts: general and specific respiratory system. **Tables 4** (general examination) **and 5** (respiratory examination) provides a physician clinical clues to arrive at a diagnosis.

Table 4: Essential general examination findings during evaluation of pediatric cough.

Clinical signs	Interpretation
Fever	Infectious cause
Clubbing	Suppurative lung disease
Cardiac murmurs	Heart disease
Failure to thrive	Immunodeficiency, cystic fibrosis
Neurodevelopmental disorders	Aspiration syndromes due to swallowing difficulty or GERD
Skin rash	Eczema and asthma

Table 5: Essential respiratory examination findings in evaluation of pediatric cough.

Clinical signs	Interpretation
Rhinorrhea and halitosis	Posterior nasal drip
Overinflated chest	Asthma, cystic fibrosis
Deformed chest wall	Congenital malformations, severe chronic lung disease
Bilateral expiratory wheeze on forced expiration	Asthma, reactive airway disease
Unilateral wheeze with decreased air entry	Foreign body
Bilateral wheeze with fine crackle	Bronchiolitis, asthma, pneumonia
Coarse crackles	Bronchiectasis
Tracheal deviation	Foreign body, mediastinal mass
Dull note on percussion	Effusion, collapse, consolidation
Stridor	Croup, foreign body

Investigations

As discussed before, one of the most common causes of cough in children is URTI, which is a clinical diagnosis and does not need any investigations. But in some cases, depending on clinical features and signs, investigations should be carried out.

- *Blood investigations*: CBC, C-reactive protein, procalcitonin (in cases of suspected infection). Blood culture in case of suspected bacterial infections. Immunoglobulin E and eosinophil count in case of suspected allergic disorders.
- *Skin tests*: Mantoux (tuberculin sensitivity) test for suspected tuberculosis and sweat test (measurement of chloride level in sweat) for suspected cystic fibrosis.
- *Sputum*: For bacterial cultures, respiratory viruses PCR, cellularity studies. Nasopharyngeal aspirate may be used if sputum cannot be expectorated.
- *X-ray and computed tomography (CT)*: Chest radiograph should be done in case of suspected foreign body. It will also help in diagnosing effusion, consolidation, collapse, etc.

High resolution computed axial tomography chest may also be needed in selected cases.
- *Lung function test*: In cases of suspected asthma, interstitial lung disease, etc. spirometry is useful and is possible in co-operative children (usually older than 4–5 years). Improvement with bronchodilator therapy suggests asthma.
- *Flexible bronchoscopy*: The indications for flexible fiberoptic bronchoscopy include suspected foreign body, dynamic airway conditions like laryngotracheomalacia and other suspected airway abnormalities. It is also useful to perform bronchoalveolar lavage and obtain samples from within the bronchial tree for cultures, etc.
- *Esophageal pH manometry studies*: It is useful in cases of suspected gastroesophageal reflux disease.

Treatment

The objective of management of cough in children is mainly to ascertain its etiology as treatment would accordingly vary. The treatment can be divided into two parts: part 1 is treatment regarding cough with simple head colds, and part 2 covers specific cough types.

General Principles regarding Management of Cough in Children with Simple Head Cold

- In most cases of children with acute cough, the underlying cause is URTI, usually viral. Supportive management is the only treatment needed in these cases including clearing of nasal secretions, maintenance of adequate hydration, and antipyretics.
- There is no role of antitussives, decongestants, mucolytics, and antihistaminic therapy in children. They have been shown to be as effective as placebo and can lead to adverse side-effects due to which they are more harmful than beneficial. The American Academy of Pediatrics has recommended not to use dextromethorphan and codeine for cough in children.
- For children with allergic rhinitis, intranasal steroids can be prescribed as they are effective. There is no role of bronchodilators in such cases.
- Acute cough generally does not require antibiotics. The only situations where antibiotics play a role include pertussis (early macrolide therapy within 1–2 weeks of illness), streptococcal tonsillitis, and pneumonia.
- In children aged more than 2 years with cough due to URTI, honey-based products have been demonstrated to be better than placebo and may be used.
- It is important to educate both treating pediatricians and parents that acute cough in children that is caused by viral URTI and will resolve spontaneously within 2 weeks; hence, unnecessary consults and treatment should be avoided.

Other etiologies of acute cough (croup, asthma, bronchiolitis, and community-acquired pneumonia) require specific treatment and evidence-based guidelines are available for each of the same. The discussion of specific management of these etiologies is beyond the scope of this chapter.

SUMMARY

Cough in children is very common and is often the reason for emergency/outpatient consultation in pediatrics. The most common cause of acute cough in children is viral URTI which can be clinically diagnosed and needs supportive treatment only. However, certain types of acute cough and all cases of subacute/chronic cough (lasting more than 4–8 weeks) require systematic evaluation to identify etiology and treat accordingly. A wide range of etiologies exist for such types of cough and include both minor self-limiting illness and serious life-threatening conditions. Careful history, clinical examination, and appropriate investigations are essential for arriving at the correct diagnosis. Specific pediatric guidelines exist for various etiologies of cough including croup, asthma, community acquired pneumonia, etc. which differ from adult guidelines. There is no role of over-the-counter cough medications (antitussives, mucolytics and/or antihistamine) in treatment of acute cough in children.

CHAPTER 23

Crying in Infant and Children

Shweta Tyagi

INTRODUCTION

Crying is a normal response to many stimuli in nonverbal children. It gives a clue to the child's physiological state ranging from normal needs of hunger and sleep to significant pathology. Healthy children cry for about 3 hours per day on an average at 6 weeks of age with the peak occurrence between 3 pm and 11 pm. The cry is labeled as abnormal depending on the duration and its inconsolable nature. Excessive crying usually would present in concert with other manifestations of disease or distress like fever, vomiting, rash, trauma, etc. However, it can be challenging for evaluation when it is the sole presentation. A systematic and appropriate history and physical examination coupled with a suspicion for a broad range of medical possibilities need to be considered for proper evaluation. Crying is one of the most common indications for seeking medical attention by parents in the first 3 months of life. The studies have reported a range of 0.25–13.6% of all annual emergency department (ED) visits for infant crying. Although most of the times, the etiology is benign and self-limiting, excessive crying is associated with considerable parental anxiety and stress.

DEFINITION FOR EXCESSIVE CRYING

Excessive crying is difficult to define and there is little consensus available in the literature pertaining to this. It is often determined based on parental perception, which is substantiated by data indicating that parents are knowledgeable about the different cries of their infants.

The most commonly used definition is Wessel's "rule of three," which states that crying in an otherwise healthy baby aged 2 weeks to 4 months that occurs more than 3 hours per day, more than 3 days in any week for at least 3 weeks may be called excessive.

ETIOLOGY

Although the cause for excessive crying might be trivial for most of the times, yet it is pertinent for the emergency physician to integrate multiple etiologic and epidemiologic features into the evaluation of a crying infant. The evaluation in the ED should aim to identify the most common and treatable diagnosis and to avoid missing a serious life-threatening condition.

Life-threatening or serious causes of excessive crying:
- Localized infection or sepsis
- Trauma

- Dysrhythmias and congestive heart failure
- Foreign body aspiration
- Pneumothorax
- Bowel obstruction
- Intussusception
- Testicular/ovarian torsion
- Vaso-occlusive crisis (sickle cell disease)
- Insect bites
- Burns
- Pruritic eruptions
- Dehydration
- Increased intracranial pressure
- Inborn errors of metabolism
- Toxic ingestion/exposure
- Nonaccidental injuries.

Common causes of excessive crying:
- Infantile colic
- Otitis media
- Constipation
- Hunger
- Immunization reactions
- Teething
- Nasal congestion
- Gastroesophageal reflux
- Idiopathic.

PATHOPHYSIOLOGY

The first cry soon after birth of the newborn is a measure of general physiological status. Crying in infants and nonverbal children is a complex neurophysiological act, which may be a reflex activity to begin with but as the infant grows there is maturation of brain and it becomes a type of communication and form of expression.

As mentioned above, the causes for a crying infant can be varied but the following clinical pointers suggest an underlying organic cause in an excessively crying infant:
- High-pitched or abnormal sounding cry
- Any positive physical findings
- Associated symptoms like fever, vomiting, diarrhea, weight loss, or failure to thrive
- Changes in diurnal rhythm
- Maternal drug ingestion
- Excessive crying continuing past 4 months of age
- Positive family history of migraine and atopy.

PREHOSPITAL CARE

Most often, the crying infant may present to the ED with their caregivers but occasionally the ED can be called upon for dispatch of an ambulance. In the latter situation, the ED personnel should follow the standardized stabilization protocol while assessing these infants. Considering the heightened parental concern, appropriate assessment of airway, breathing, circulation, and necessary basic interventions like oxygen administration, intravenous access, fluid administration, and bedside glucose testing should be initiated. The detailed information about the presenting episode from the caregivers and vital sign assessment can be done en route. Desist from providing false reassurances to caregivers and discouraging them from ED visit as there can be a possibility of serious underlying illness in these infants.

EMERGENCY DEPARTMENT EVALUATION OF AN INFANT WITH EXCESSIVE CRYING

History

Determining the triggers for excessive crying in infants is like solving a puzzle. A comprehensive and detailed history is the key in the assessment of these patients. A good history has been reported as diagnostic in 20–86% of cases, either alone or in concurrence with examination findings.

Nevertheless all resuscitative measures must be performed prior to detailed history taking process.

Relevant history to include:
- Duration, frequency, and intensity of crying episodes with aggravating and relieving factors and details of any prior evaluations in this respect. Assess for the different crying patterns to get clinical clues:
    - High-pitched cry indicates infection of central nervous system
    - Continuous cry with grunting may indicate foreign body or respiratory infection
    - Crying with pulling of ears indicates otitis externa/media
    - Sporadic crying pattern with pallor and undrawn knees over abdomen may indicate intussusception
    - Paroxysmal crying in otherwise healthy infants of less than 4 months age usually during evening indicates infantile colic.
- Birth history, including birth weight, perinatal complications, and maternal substance use during pregnancy
- Detailed feeding history, sleep behavior, bowel and bladder patterns
- History of past illnesses, medication use, and vaccination
- Comorbid medical conditions
- Social history
- Family history of any congenital or genetic disorders.

Physical Examination

Initial physical examination should aim to assess and identify general condition of the infant to determine, if there exists a life-threatening condition associated with incessant crying.

All the vital parameters to be checked and recorded and a thorough whole body inspection should be done. Studies have proven that physical examination either alone or in addition to history can contribute to diagnosis in more than 50% cases.

A complete head-to-toe examination to be systematically done. Important considerations while examining the infant are as follows:

- *Head and neck*:
  - Examine the eye for congestion/corneal abrasion; a study by Shope et al. in 2010 found that nearly 50% of infants presenting to primary care center had corneal abrasions
  - Examine the external ear and perform otoscopic examination to rule out otitis media.
  - Oropharyngeal pathologies are not so common as a cause for crying but presence of trismus should raise a suspicion for peritonsillar abscess or deep neck space infection.
- *Nervous system*:
  - Persistent irritability and high-pitched cry points toward central nervous system cause like meningitis or encephalitis. Appropriate history, clinical examination, and requisite investigations to be considered for ruling out these serious pathologies.
  - Evaluate for occult head injury, especially in infants suspected to have nonaccidental injuries by relevant examination and imaging.
  - A bedside glucose measurement is a minimally invasive test to detect hypoglycemia as the cause for excessive crying.
- *Thorax*:
  - Clavicular fractures may occur during delivery when there is a history of difficult delivery, shoulder dystocia, or when the neonate is large for gestational age.
  - Presence of bony crepitus on palpation should raise a suspicion for rib fractures and also for nonaccidental trauma.
  - Examination of breast tissue for abscess/mastitis.
  - Examine for cardiac arrhythmias. Infants with congenital heart diseases may also present with poor feeding, fussiness, irritability, and excessive crying.
- *Abdomen*:
  - Infantile colic affects around 10–30% of infants. It has been defined as episodic paroxysmal crying for greater than 3 hours per day for greater than 3 days a week for up to 3 weeks in an otherwise healthy infant aged from 2 weeks to 4 months.
  - Many studies have proven that constipation is one of the common causes of crying infant. History and careful palpation of abdomen to be performed to rule out constipation. Rectal examination may be considered, if mandated by clinical suspicion.
  - Paroxysmal crying episodes associated with intermittent flexing of lower extremities with or without bloody stools must raise a suspicion for intussusception.
  - Palpate for an abdominal mass in the right upper quadrant in a poorly feeding infant and history of nonbilious vomiting to rule out pyloric stenosis.

- Urinary tract infection can also be the reason for excessive crying in an infant and careful evaluation regarding the same to be carried out.
- Consider evaluation for midgut abnormalities including malrotation/volvulus in an ill looking infant with nonreassuring abdominal examination.
- Examine for inguinal hernia as there is around 60% risk of hernia becoming incarcerated in the first 6 months of life.
- *Extremities*:
  - Examine for joint swelling, tenderness, erythema, and any restriction of range of movement to rule out septic arthritis.
  - In infants of less than 1 year age have high index of suspicion for nonaccidental injury in cases of suspected or detected fractures.
- *Skin*:
  - Complete exposure of the infant and evaluation for bruises and ecchymosis. The most common sites are anterior tibia, knee, or forehead. However, bruises on face and trunk are rare and their presence should raise a concern for abuse.
  - Burn injuries in the patterned shape of hot objects (like cigarettes), bilateral glove and stocking pattern (suggestive of immersion injuries) should prompt an evaluation for infant abuse. Accidental scald injuries due to spill over of hot liquids tend to usually affect the face, neck, upper limbs, anterior trunk, and are usually asymmetrical and have irregular edge and burn depth.

EVALUATION AND MANAGEMENT OF EXCESSIVE CRYING IN INFANT AND CHILDREN (FLOWCHART 1)

As the range of differential diagnosis in an excessively crying infant is extensive and there is a fear of missing a serious pathology, careful evaluation, and management become pertinent. The best approach is to individualize the workup depending on the infant's history and examination findings so as to make the evaluation high yielding, time, and cost effective.

Investigations

- The most beneficial screening laboratory test in the excessively crying infant is urine routine and urine culture to rule out urinary tract infection.
- The rest of the laboratory tests must be tailored to the individual infant for the concerns raised by the history and physical examination.
- Routine advice of imaging diagnostic tests is not helpful in screening purposes. In view of concerns of unnecessary radiation exposure and risk of associated malignancy, the risk and benefit of performing a radiological test should be weighed carefully before ordering it in the ED. When these tests are mandated by the history and physical examination, nonirradiating studies like ultrasonography (USG), magnetic resonance imaging (MRI) should be preferred.

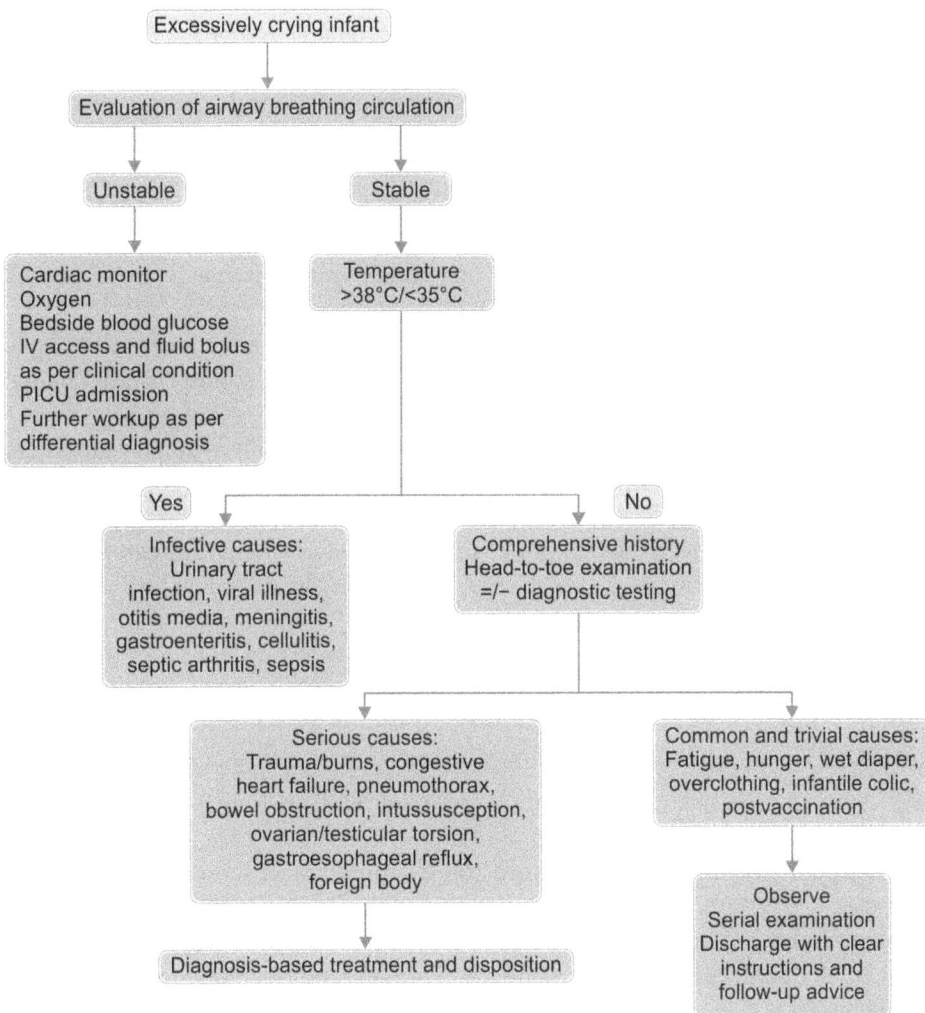

Flowchart 1: Evaluation and management of excessively crying infant.

(IV: intravenous; PICU: pediatric intensive care unit)

Serial Examinations

In cases where history, physical examination, and initial testing do not prove conclusive, a period of observation must be considered in ED and the infant should be closely monitored and re-examined for crying pattern and any new manifestations like fever, signs of acute abdominal conditions, etc. to guide additional testing and decide further disposition.

There is no consensus on duration of the observation period in ED.

TREATMENT STRATEGIES AND EMERGENCY DEPARTMENT DISPOSITION

- *Excessive crying in infants with recognizable and treatable conditions*:
  - These infants should be managed as per their diagnosed clinical condition and further disposition in terms of inpatient admission or outpatient discharge will depend on severity of clinical condition. Appropriate specialty referral should be done from ED.
- *Excessive crying in infants without clearly identifiable conditions*:
  - This is challenging and infants who appear ill looking should be considered for observation and further testing and pediatric team referral. Sick looking, hemodynamically unstable, or social concerns as poor support at home or suspicion of abuse should be admitted from the ED.
  - The infants who continue to cry but do not appear sick and have no social concerns can be considered for discharge after pediatric referral and an appropriate discharge plan and follow-up advice should be provided to the caregivers.
  - Advice for outpatient follow-up within 24 hours. Second follow-up may determine the diagnosis of these infants in almost 39% of cases.
  - Avoid prescribing medications without an unknown underlying condition.
  - Reassure the caregivers and allay their anxiety and advise them to be careful to the basic needs of infants (hunger, diaper change, fatigue, etc.), which might be the contributing cause for excessive crying.
  - Discharge advice to include clear instructions regarding red flag signs (i.e. fever, inconsolability, poor feeding, etc.), which should prompt them to return to ED.

SUMMARY

- ED visit for an excessively crying infant is common yet distressing for both caregivers and emergency physicians.
- A comprehensive history and head-to-toe examination is the key to determine the diagnosis.
- Do not be hurry in diagnosing an infantile colic, this should be a diagnosis for occlusion.
- While discharging such infants, reassure the caregivers and clear instructions for follow-up should be given.

CHAPTER 24

Cyanosis

Suman Thakur, Vivek Chauhan

■ INTRODUCTION

Cyanosis word has been derived from *cyan*, a blue-green color. Cyanosis of the skin or mucus membranes is an important finding on examination needing careful workup to find its genesis in each patient. The etiology behind cyanosis may be anything from innocuous (polycythemia of high altitude) to grave (severe interstitial lung disease). Physicians have started relying more on pulse oximeter values and oxygen saturation (SpO_2), forgetting that there are many cases where oximeters are unreliable, e.g. methemoglobinemia, sulfhemoglobinemia, carboxyhemoglobinemia. Knowledge of cyanosis, its origin, testing, and clinical implications are, thus, essential for better patient care.

■ ETIOLOGY/CAUSES

Skin and mucosae become cyanotic when concentration of any the following pigments is increased in the blood:
- Deoxyhemoglobin
- Methemoglobin (MetHb)
- Sulfhemoglobin (SulfHb)
- Methemalbumin
- Metals (silver, gold, hemosiderin)
- Miscellaneous causes (chlorpromazine, amiodarone)

The etiology for cyanosis varies with the type of pigment responsible for cyanosis (**Table 1**).

■ PATHOPHYSIOLOGY OF THE CONDITION

The normal skin color results from a combination of oxyhemoglobin, deoxyhemoglobin, melanin, carotene, and from the optical effect of scattering (Tyndall effect that gives blue color to the sky). White light that falls upon our skin has a spectrum ranging from blue at one end and red at the other. Blue skin coloration would result if the quantity of blue wavelengths reflected is disproportionately increased or if the quantity of red wavelengths reflected is disproportionately decreased. The same venous blood that gives blue color to our skin does not appear blue when taken out in a test tube. Deoxyhemoglobin is less red than oxyhemoglobin and absorbs more red spectrum, therefore, appearing bluish. By subtraction

Table 1: Various etiological causes of cyanosis in different types of pigments.

Type of pigment	Causes
Deoxyhemoglobinemia	
• Decreased arterial oxygenation	Cardiopulmonary diseases, high altitude, hypoventilation syndromes, neuromuscular and skeletal defects, vascular shunts, etc.
• Increased tissue extraction	Sluggish blood flow, heart failure, local ischemia, exercise, shock, atherosclerosis, deep venous thrombosis, Raynaud's phenomenon, hypothermia, etc.
• Abnormal hemoglobin	HbM
Methemoglobinemia	
• Genetic	Autosomal recessive
• Dietary	Fava beans, nitrate-containing foods, Ginkgo biloba
• Toxic/drug induced	Dapsone, benzocaine, nitroglycerine, nitroprusside, mothballs
• Idiopathic	
Sulfhemoglobinemia	
• Drugs	Sulfonamides, sulfasalazine, sumatriptan overdose, metoclopramide
• Industrial exposures	H_2S gas, phenazopyridine, volatile sulfur-containing compounds
Methemalbumin	Massive hemolysis
Metals	Silver, gold, hemosiderin
Miscellaneous causes	Chlorpromazine, amiodarone

of red wavelengths, the blue spectrum is allowed to predominate in the reflected light (i.e. something that is less red is more blue).

Deoxygenated hemoglobin is apparent as cyanosis on clinical examination of skin and mucosa when its amount is more than 4-6 g/dL in the capillaries. In presence of a normal cardiac output, hemoglobin, and tissue extraction of oxygen, an arterial oxygen saturation of less than 80% would be required to cause cyanosis. Cyanosis cannot be produced in severe anemia if hemoglobin concentration is below the threshold of cyanosis, i.e. 4-6 g/dL. Also anemic individuals need more profound oxygen desaturation to produce cyanosis.

MetHb is normally formed in body around 3% per day when ferrous form of iron is converted to ferric form in the hemoglobin. MetHb is not capable of binding to oxygen and thus leads to hypoxia when in excess. Cytochrome b5 reductase reduces MetHb to hemoglobin using nicotinamide adenine dinucleotide as a cofactor and keeps its levels below 1%.

SulfHb excess is relatively rare in the blood and the pigment is a greenish derivative of hemoglobin (Hb), with an absorption peak at 620 nm, but cannot be converted back to normal, functional Hb unlike deoxyhemoglobin and MetHb. In vitro, SulfHb forms when hydrogen sulfide (H_2S) is added to Hb, hence the name; in vivo, naturally occurring SulfHb is postulated to be derived from H_2S produced by intestinal bacteria, but the mode of formation has not yet clear. Cyanosis is reported to be detectable at sulfhemoglobin levels as low as 0.5 g/dL.

Gold or *silver* containing substances when ingested can produce bluish skin coloration. It is most prominent in sun-exposed portions of the body. The bluish skin color associated with *hemosiderin* deposition is more apparent in parts of the body with less melanotic pigment and a more bronze color is seen in the presence of melanin.

The oxidation products of *chlorpromazine*, when deposited in the skin and other organs, can result in a blue to purple color. A new antiarrhythmic agent, *amiodarone*, can cause lipofuscin deposition in the skin. In sun-exposed areas, a blue skin color is seen in a small percentage of patients on long-term therapy.

CLINICAL PRESENTATION

Many authors divide cyanosis into central and peripheral cyanosis:

Central cyanosis is mostly seen with systemic disorders: Some common diseases presenting with central cyanosis include chronic obstructive lung disease, pneumonia, interstitial lung disease, embolism and ventilation perfusion mismatch, acute respiratory distress syndromes, high altitude, congestive heart failure, anatomic shunts, right-to-left shunt in congenital heart disease, arteriovenous malformation, and intrapulmonary shunts.

Peripheral cyanosis: All causes of central cyanosis have peripheral cyanosis too. Isolated peripheral cyanosis; however, is seen in conditions with sluggish blood flow with increased oxygen extraction, e.g. Raynaud's phenomenon, congestive heart failure, hypovolemic shock, hypothermia, etc.

Clinical signs of dexogenation vary depending upon the etiology. A resident of high altitude can have deep cyanosis, polycythemia, and still be asymptomatic. A patient of anemia on the other hand, may be markedly desaturated with only mild or no cyanosis. Thus, knowledge of hemoglobin levels of the patient helps us understand the correlation with the severity of cyanosis and oxygen desaturation.

Cyanotic individuals are expected to have oxygen saturation levels of less than 80% and thus have worse outcomes if associated with some underlying pathological condition. Prolonged desaturation can lead to hypoxic encephalopathy, which may become irreversible.

Cyanosis occurs at MetHb levels of level of 1.5 g/dL, 15% of total hemoglobin. Anxiety, headache, and dizziness can occur at MetHb levels greater than 20%. Levels between 30% and 50% can produce fatigue, confusion, and tachypnea. At levels greater than 50%, arrhythmias, acidosis, seizures, and coma can occur.

SulfHb produces cyanosis at 0.5 g/dL levels but the patient may have normal oxygen saturation and be asymptomatic.

RED FLAGS

In the presence of cyanosis, the following additional findings may be the red flags:
- Low-blood pressure
- Altered sensorium
- Tachypnea and dyspnea.

EVALUATION

History
- History should be focused toward the presenting complaint and contributing past history of illness.
- A high proportion of cases with cyanosis have a long standing cardiopulmonary illness. The acute event like viral or bacterial infection, arrhythmia, pneumothorax, pleural effusion, myocardial infarction, pulmonary embolism, congestive heart failure, myocarditis can worsen a stable long-standing cardiopulmonary illness and produce cyanosis.
- In absence of a long-standing illness and obvious cardiopulmonary involvement, we must take history of recent drug intake or toxin exposure (both intentional and accidental) and rule out cyanosis due to rare pigments like MetHb, SulfHb, and nonheme pigments.

Physical Examination
- Since the sensitivity to detect cyanosis at the threshold levels of deoxyhemoglobin is not very high, it becomes important to know the technique and practice it routinely. Lighting is important as cyanosis is best appreciated when lighting matches the spectral composition of that of the sunlight. So, the artificial sources of light should be similar to sunlight. Tungsten filament bulbs and certain fluorescent bulbs are satisfactory for detecting cyanosis. Too intense light is also inappropriate to detect cyanosis. Some people recommend less than 20 footcandles of illumination for this purpose.
- *Sites to look for cyanosis*:
  - Parts of skin and mucosa that lack melanin pigment are appropriate to look for cyanosis. Lips, tongue, hands, and ears are the most commonly observed sites (**Fig. 1**). Trunk, nailbed, conjunctiva, and circumoral areas also have been described to look for cyanosis. The tongue is the most sensitive but lips are more specific sites for cyanosis.
- Many cases of cyanosis also have associated clubbing. These conditions mostly have some form of right-to-left shunt either within the heart, lungs, or in the periphery.

INTERPRETATION OF FINDINGS

Cyanosis as a tool for detecting arterial hypoxemia is neither sensitive nor specific. Definite cyanosis was not apparent to 25% of observers even at arterial oxygen saturations of 71–75% (PaO_2 35–40 mm Hg). In contrast, 6% and 17% of the observers believed definite cyanosis to be present when arterial oxygen saturations were 96–100% and 91–95%, respectively. The sensitivity of this sign is decreased when examining deeply pigmented individuals. In blacks, 3–6% more arterial oxygen desaturation may be required for detection of cyanosis.

Still, early detection of cyanosis may point toward an underlying serious disorder like congenital heart disease like tetralogy of fallot in children, methemoglobinemia, sulfhemoglobinemia in absence of profound symptoms of any disease.

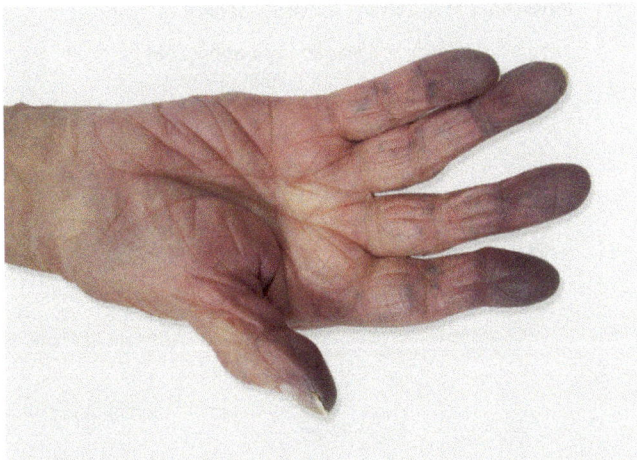

Fig. 1: Peripheral cyanosis in one of the hands of a patient.

INVESTIGATIONS

Whenever we detect cyanosis, we must confirm the arterial saturation by pulse oximetry followed by arterial blood gas (ABG) analysis. Nail polish can decrease the oximetry values by 6%; therefore the pulse oximeter should be applied sideways to the fingers.

In cases where there is a mismatch between the oximetry values and ABG, we go for co-oximetry. Pulse oximeter measures light at two wavelengths, oxyhemoglobin, and deoxyhemoglobin. Co-oximetry measures the absorption of light at four different wavelengths corresponding to oxyhemoglobin, deoxyhemoglobin, carboxyhemoglobin, and methemoglobin.

Once the diagnosis of the type of cyanotic agent is clear, we then focus our attention toward the etiological agent or disease. For deoxyhemoglobin based upon our probable diagnosis, we get further investigations done that may include chest X-ray, electrocardiogram, echocardiogram, computed tomography of chest, pulmonary and coronary angiogram, ventilation perfusion scan, sleep studies, etc. Diagnosis of the disease responsible for oxygen desaturation is often easily obtained with the above investigations.

For rarer forms of heme and nonheme pigments responsible for cyanosis, we focus our attention toward the drug, toxin, or accidental exposures. Deficiency of NADH MetHb reductase system is inherited in autosomal recessive pattern.

Abnormal hemoglobins like hemoglobin M that has decreased affinity for oxygen can be diagnosed with the help of electrophoresis.

A practical approach to the etiology of cyanosis has been described by Snider et al. (**Flowchart 1**):
- Obtain a heparinized arterial blood specimen.
- If the sample is dark red and becomes bright red on shaking in air, one should perform blood gas analysis on another specimen to confirm arterial hypoxemia.

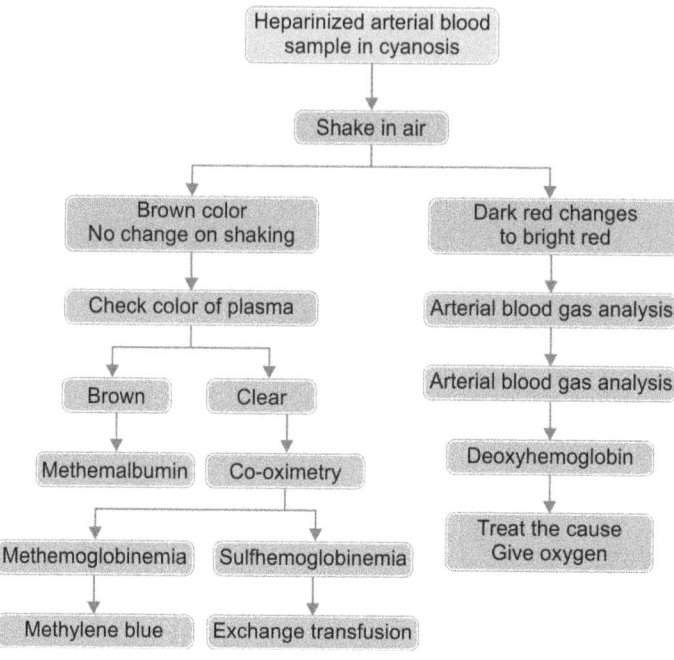

Flowchart 1: Approach toward a patient of cyanosis.

- If the specimen obtained is brown and does not change color on shaking in air, the plasma should be allowed to separate.
  - If the plasma is brown, methemalbumin is likely to be present.
  - If the plasma is clear, one should suspect the presence of methemoglobin or sulfhemoglobin.
- A bright red arterial specimen obtained in a patient with generalized blue skin color should lead one to suspect deposition of nonheme pigment in the skin.

TREATMENT

Deoxyhemoglobin: Treat the underlying cause and give supplemental oxygen to improve the hemoglobin oxygenation.

MetHb: First step in treatment of MetHb is to remove the culprit medication. This often is sufficient in mild cases. Methylene blue is the treatment of choice in severe cases of methemoglobinemia. It accelerates the reduction of MetHb via the NADPH MetHb reductase pathway and it should be given IV at a dose of 1–2 mg/kg for 5 minutes. The maximum effect of methylene blue occurs quickly, at 30 minutes. Additional doses of methylene blue may be given after 1 hour if response is inadequate. Co-oximetry is not helpful in monitoring these patients because it does not have the ability to distinguish between MetHb and methylene blue. High doses (7 mg/kg) can lead to hemolysis and a paradoxical rise in MetHb levels of up to 10%. Less responsive forms of include analine and dapsone-induced MetHb. MetHb can cause hemolysis in G6PD-deficiency too.

SulfHb: These patients can show cyanosis at 0.5 g/dL levels of SulfHb. Cyanosis is not responsive to oxygen administration. Patients may be asymptomatic at much higher levels of SulfHb and partial pressure of oxygen is usually normal. SulfHb is irreversible and stays till the life span of affected red blood cells, i.e. 120 days. Oxygen should be given to all patients and exchange transfusion has been suggested and tried as a treatment modality in cases that are symptomatic.

SUMMARY

Cyanosis is visible on specific body parts when various types of heme and nonheme pigments accumulate in our body beyond normal limits. Some of these pigments like deoxyhemoglobin and MetHb are normally produced in our body but they are regularly replaced by oxygenated hemoglobin. Many physiological and pathological states are associated with cyanosis. The clinical examination is now aided by oximetry, ABG analysis, and co-oximetry in finding the cause of cyanosis. Careful history and focused examination gives us the diagnosis in most cases. Treatment of cyanosis revolves around the inciting agent or disease. Oxygen administration helps in most cases but IV methylene blue injection in MetHb and exchange transfusion in SulfHb may be needed to remove the abnormal pigments.

CHAPTER 25

Deafness

Deepak Dalmia, Sanjaya Bahera

INTRODUCTION

Deafness is defined as a degree of loss such that a person is unable to understand speech even in the presence of amplification. Hearing loss, also known as hearing impairment, is a partial or total inability to hear. A deaf person has little to no hearing.

ETIOLOGY

Age

Advanced age leads to presbycusis (high frequency hearing loss).

Noise

Exposure to loud sound.

Genetic

- Stickler syndrome
- Waardenburg syndrome
- Pendred syndrome
- Usher syndrome
- Alport syndrome
- Neurofibromatosis type 2.

Perinatal Problems

- Birth hypoxia
- Fetal alcohol syndrome
- Neonatal hyperbilirubinemia.

Other Systemic Disorders

- Stroke
- Multiple sclerosis
- Perilymph fistula
- Measles, mumps, and rubella

- Meningitis
- Syphilis
- Otosclerosis
- Superior semicircular dehiscence syndrome
- *Demyelinating disease*: Charcot-Marie-Tooth disease.

Medications
- Nonsteroidal anti-inflammatory drugs (NSAIDs)
- Loop diuretics (furosemide, bumetanide)
- Antimalarial (quinine, chloroquine)
- Aminoglycosides (gentamicin, amikacin)
- Chemotherapeutic agents (cisplatin, carboplatin).

Chemicals
- *Asphyxiants*: Carbon monoxide (CO), hydrogen cyanide (HCN)
- *Heavy metals*: Pb, Hg, Cd, and As
- *Solvents*: Toluene, styrene, and xylene.

PATHOPHYSIOLOGY
Hearing loss can be classified as conductive, sensory neural, or mixed.

Conductive Hearing Loss
- Secondary to the disease of external auditory canal (EAC), tympanic membrane (TM), and middle ear.
- These lesions prevent sound to be effectively transferred to the inner ear.

Sensorineural Hearing Loss
Can be caused by inner ear pathology (sensory) or auditory nerve pathology (neural).

Mixed Hearing Loss
- Otosclerosis
- Otitis media superimposed in a sensorineural hearing loss (SNHL).

CLINICAL PRESENTATION
Hearing loss or hard of hearing.

Red Flags
- Unilateral SNHL
- Rapidly worsening or sudden hearing loss.

EVALUATION

History of Present Illness
- Duration
- Onset (acute, gradual)
- *Laterality*: Whether it is unilateral or bilateral
- Any history of scuba diving, barotrauma, and loud noise exposure
- Any intake of ototoxic drugs
- Ear symptoms (e.g. ear pain, tinnitus, and ear discharge)
- Vestibular symptoms and other neurologic symptoms
- In children, important-associated symptoms include presence of delays in speech or language development, visual changes, or delayed motor development.

Past Medical History
- Central nervous system (CNS) infection
- Exposure to loud noise
- Head trauma
- Family history of hearing loss
- For young children, a birth history.

PHYSICAL EXAMINATION

The external ear is inspected for obstruction, infection, congenital malformations, and other lesions.
    Otoscopic examination—The TM is examined for perforation, drainage, and otitis media.
    Neurologic examination, particular attention needs to be paid to the 2nd, 7th, and 8th cranial nerves.

TUNING FORK TEST

Rinne Test
- Positive in SNHL and normal hearing
- Negative in conductive hearing loss (CHL).

Weber Test
- Lateralized to worst ear in CHL
- Lateralized to better ear in SNHL.

Pure Tone Audiometry
Give the degree of hearing loss.

Otoacoustic Emission
To know the hearing status in neonates as a screening tool with perinatal problems.

Brainstem Evoked Response Audiometry
Ideal for small children to know the reflexes from the auditory pathway and degree of hearing loss.

INTERPRETATION OF FINDING
History and examination concludes the common problems like earwax, foreign body, and chronic suppurative otitis media (CSOM).

In case of 5th, 7th, and 8th cranial nerve palsies—vestibular schwannoma or any other cerebellopontine (CP) angle tumor.

Maxillofacial malformations may suggest a genetic or developmental abnormality.

Any child with delays in speech or language development should be evaluated for intellectual disability, aphasia, and autism.

INVESTIGATIONS
- Audiological evaluation
- *Pure tone audiometry*:
    - Measurement of pure-tone thresholds
    - Speech reception threshold
    - Speech discrimination score
    - Tympanometry
    - Acoustic reflex testing.
- *Advance testing*:
    - Otoacoustic emission (OAE)
    - Electrocochleography
    - Brainstem evoked response audiometry (BERA)
    - Auditory steady state response (ASSR).

High-resolution computed tomography (HRCT) of temporal bone/MRI of vestibulocochlear complex to know the status of vestibulocochlear nerve.

TREATMENT
- The cause of hearing loss should be evaluated and treated
- *In case of ototoxicity*: Stoppage of the offending drug
- Fluid in middle ear infusion can be drained
- *Chronic suppurative otitis media with central perforation*: Tympanoplasty
- *Otosclerosis*: Stapedotomy or reversal stapedotomy
- Hearing aid [bone conduction aid, contralateral routing of signal (CROS) aid] in case of presbycusis.

In case of prelingual deafness, diagnosed early:
- Cochlear implant
- Brainstem implant.

■ SUMMARY
- Most common causes of deafness are cerumen, genetic disorders, infections, aging, and noise exposure.
- All patients with hearing loss should be accessed with pure tone audiometry (PTA).
- Cranial nerve deficit should be searched for if present imaging should be done.

CHAPTER 26

Dental Problems

Mayank Tripathi

TOOTHACHE

The most common symptom, for a patient who comes to a dental office is toothache. Be it children or adult toothache may occur at any age and due to varying reasons. Most common finding associated with pain is dental caries, leading to inflammation of pulp causing pain. On the basis of its intensity, the time of occurrence and duration of pain, toothache may lead to diagnosis of its origin.

Here are some most common causes for which a patient visits a dental office for pain:
- Teething pain
- Pain due to caries
- Pain due to trauma
- Pain due to abscess
- Pain due to wisdom tooth eruption
- Referred pain
- Periodontal pain
- Pain in temporomandibular joint (TMJ)
- Neuralgic pain.

TEETHING PAIN

Pathophysiology

As the tooth erupts, inflammatory mediators are released at the eruption site, causing pain.

Clinical Presentation
- There is hyperemia or swelling of the mucosa overlying the erupting teeth
- Redness is visible at the mucosa
- Increased salivation and drooling.

Red Flags
- General irritability
- Loss of appetite and sleep.

History

It is a physiologic phenomenon so teething pain occurs almost in every child. Seen most commonly at the age of 4–6 months.

Physical Examination

Patches of erythema on the cheeks.

Investigations

Radiographic investigations are done.

Treatment

- Topical application of lignocaine hydrochloride over the area
- Topical application of glycerine
- Mild purgatives like castor oil, milk of magnesia are also used in treating teething.

CARIES

Caries in children as well as in adults leads to pulpitis. According to duration and severity of caries, the pulpitis is of two basic types reversible and irreversible.

Reversible Pulpitis

Pathophysiology

The pain is mainly due to rise in intrapulpal pressure due to exudative force.

Clinical Presentation

Any external stimuli like temperature change or biting force cause quick sharp pain. The response is hypersensitive or else asymptomatic.

Red Flags

- There is no spontaneous pain
- The pain subsides as the stimuli are removed.

History

There is occurrence of prolonged food lodgment because of caries exposing the pulp.

Physical Examination

- Black lesion over tooth surface
- Long-term food lodgment
- No pain on percussion.

Investigations
Intraoral periapical radiographs are preferred.

Treatment
- Treatment of choice is root canal treatment
- Nonsteroidal antiinflammatory drugs (NSAIDs) can be given to relieve pain.

Irreversible Pulpitis
Pathophysiology
With pulpal inflammation there is exudates, if the exudates come out of pulpal chamber it relieves pain, but it may cause edema. If exudates remain in pulpal chamber it causes pain.

Clinical Presentation
It may be of two types:
1. *Symptomatic:* It is associated with spontaneous pain. Pain occurs even after stimuli is removed.
2. *Asymptomatic:* No pain is felt.

Red Flags
Prolonged pain to temperature.

History
Long-term exposed pulp due to wide caries.

Physical Examination
- Caries involving very large area of tooth surface
- Tenderness on percussion is positive.

Investigations
Intraoral periapical radiographs are preferred.

Treatment
- Treatment of choice is root canal treatment
- NSAIDs can be given to relieve pain.

■ PAIN DUE TO TRAUMA
Traumatic injuries to teeth are very common and usually associated with road traffic accidents, contact sports like boxing, taekwondo, karate, etc. or fights. This is very common with children than adults while playing or falling.

Pathophysiology
Pain due to trauma can be because of exposure of pulp, avulsion, or luxation.

Clinical Presentation
Pain is severe like pulpitis but associated with bleeding.

Red Flags
Fractured crown of tooth.

History
It is very important for clinician to know cause of injury, angle of impact, and object of impact to know the extent of injury.

Physical Examination
Mobility of tooth is very common, sometimes fracture can occur at the root which is very painful but show no sign clinically. Radiographs are helpful in such cases.

Investigations
Radiographs OPG or IOPA are most commonly done.

Treatment
- If the fracture is at crown of the tooth exposing the pulp of tooth then root canal treatment is done followed by restoration of the tooth
- If there is luxation, splinting is done
- In case of avulsion, teeth can be replanted under half an hour of injury if the tooth is preserved in saliva or milk and periodontal ligament fibers are intact.

PAIN DUE TO ABSCESS
When a prolonged infection in tooth or in gingival tissue persists for a long time asymptomatically or there is sudden trauma to the tissue, there is formation of abscess.

Pathophysiology
Usually of sudden onset on marginal or interdental gingiva. Purulent exudates may be expressed.

Clinical Presentation
Localized, painful, and rapidly expands.

Red Flags
Gingiva is fluctuant.

History
Long-standing infection of tooth or gingival, forceful embedding of apple core, tooth brush into gingiva.

Physical Examination
Purulent exudate in 24–48 hr.

Investigations
Radiographs OPG or IOPA are most commonly done and FNAC.

Treatment
Removal of exudate under local anesthesia with an incision or opening the canal.

PAIN DUE TO WISDOM TOOTH ERUPTION
This pain usually occurs in the early 20s. The pain aggravates and subsides by its own periodically, but sometimes persists for a longer duration.

Pathophysiology
Infection of soft tissue surrounding the crown of partially erupted tooth.

Clinical Presentation
Spontaneous pain, operculum may get traumatized by opposing teeth.

Red Flags
Pericoronitis is seen.

History
Occurrence at the age of 21 years and onward, erupting wisdom tooth is visible.

Physical Examination
It is seen usually around mandibular 3rd molar. Edema in submandibular region and peritonsillar area.

Investigations
Circumferential bone resorption around tooth seen in radiograph.

Treatment
- Antibiotics: Metronidazole 200 mg three times for 7 days
- Drainage of abscess
- Extraction of concerned tooth
- Operculectomy can also be done.

■ REFERRED PAIN

Pain may be referred to teeth from inflamed nasal mucosa, nonspastic myofascial pain from temporalis, and masseter muscle or the pain arriving from the tooth may be referred to temporal and frontal region.

Pathophysiology
Pain occurring in the mandibular posterior tooth is referred to the area where the mandibular nerve arises.

Clinical Presentation
Pain referred to tooth is intense or sometimes mild. Pain referred from tooth is intense and involves almost half of the face including temporal and frontal bone.

Red Flags
Referring area is tender to touch.

History
Long-term inflammation of the referring area.

Physical Examination
Trismus, sinusitis.

Investigations
OPG.

Treatment
Analgesics to relieve pain.

■ PERIODONTAL PAIN

Pathophysiology
It may occur due to inflammation of periodontium directly like trauma, adjacent impacted tooth, or indirectly through pulpal infection.

Clinical Presentation
Intense pain which can be easily localized, sometimes mobility in teeth.

Red Flags
Tooth is tender to lateral percussion.

History
Inflammation of periodontium occurs due to trauma or long-term caries.

Physical Examination
Inflammation over periodontium, bleeding on probing from gingiva.

Interpretation of Findings
Acute or chronic periodontitis.

Investigations
OPG or IOPA.

Treatment
Complete oral prophylaxis has to be done.

PAIN IN TEMPOROMANDIBULAR JOINT

Pain in TMJ occurs due to trauma, infection, dislocation, or disc displacement. The pain is mild or may be sometimes severe.

Pathophysiology
Pain usually emanates from capsular ligament.

Clinical Presentation
Pain in disc occurs usually during function like opening, closing, or mastication.

Red Flags
Pain in response to pressure.

History
The pain in TMJ is usually associated with displacement of disc due to trauma, or infection in the TMJ. Patient usually gives history of sudden jerk in the associated area.

Physical Examination
Pressure bearing surface of the joint are usually painless.

Interpretation of Findings
The findings are suggestive of TMJ arthralgia.

Investigations
OPG, CBCT or computed tomography (CT) scan.

Treatment
- Occlusal disengagement of TMJ with occlusal splints
- Analgesics are prescribed to relieve pain
- Injecting local anesthesia into the joint also helps.

NEURALGIA
These are unilateral or sometimes bilateral paroxysmal pain occurring along the course of the nerve trunk.

Pathophysiology
These pains occur due to neuropathic changes occurring in the sensory fibers of the ganglion and dorsal root sometimes due to unknown causes or due to some conditions like neoplasm, trauma, aneurysm.

Clinical Presentation
Paroxysmal pain lasting for few seconds or minutes but of extreme intensity.

Red Flags
Usually unilateral pain which is aggravated by triggering factors like touch, movement of face like yawning, chewing, drinking, shaving, etc.

History
The patient gives history of sharp shooting episodes of pain occurring in response to some triggers and the pain is unresponsive to pain killers.

Physical Examination
There is no sensory loss along the nerve.

Treatment
- Drugs like dilantin, carbamazepine, baclofen, clonazepam can be given
- Injection of nerve with anesthetic solution or alcohol
- Nerve sectioning or nerve avulsion
- Electrocoagulation of ganglion.

Summary
- It is necessary to know the site of pain and the etiology associated with pain
- Pain due to pulpitis and abscess are usually same
- Abscess pain is mostly associated with swelling
- Teething pain occurs at age of 3-6 months
- Pain due to wisdom tooth eruption occurs at 20-30 years age
- Pain from teeth are referred to temporal and infraorbital region
- Neuralgias are paroxysmal of pain.

DENTAL TRAUMA
Traumatic injuries to teeth are very common and usually associated with any injury occurring in the face. Usually any person having a road traffic accident, are prone to dental trauma, also fights and contact sports like boxing and karate cause trauma over teeth.

TYPES OF DENTAL TRAUMAS
- Fracture of crown of tooth involving only enamel
- Fracture of crown of tooth involving enamel and dentin
- Fracture of crown of tooth involving pulp causing pulpal exposure
- Concussion
- Subluxation and luxation: Intrusive, extrusive, lateral luxation
- Avulsion
- Fracture of alveolar socket wall
- Injuries to gingival and oral mucosa
- Injury to facial bones.

Pathophysiology of the Condition
Trauma to tooth, if associated with the alveolar socket wall fracture, causes swelling due to release of mediators of inflammation. These mediators cause swelling and pain in the associated gingival and the face tissues.

Clinical Presentation
Fracture of tooth leading to exposed enamel does not cause any pain unless it is associated with any internal bone fracture. Pain occurs only if pulp is exposed in a fractured crown or if

there is concussion or luxation or avulsion of tooth. If the tooth fracture is associated with bone fracture like alveolar bone or maxilla or mandible then it leads to facial edema and mobility in bone fragment.

Red Flags
- If traumatized tooth is sore to percussion—concussion
- If percussion pain is associated with bleeding—luxation.

Evaluation

History
It is very important to note the: (1) object of impact; (2) angle of impact; and (3) force of impact to decide the amount of harm caused to the orofacial structures. If a soft object hits the face like tennis or rubber ball, then there are less chances of tooth fracture. If a hard object hits and the angle of impact is perpendicular to tooth, then the fracture of tooth can be at the apical, middle, or incisal. Third, if the impact is from above or the angle is from incisal to root of tooth, then it causes intrusive luxation of tooth, if impact is parallel to long axis of tooth, then there are chances of longitudinal fracture of tooth.

Physical Examination
- *Pain in percussion:* Concussion, luxation, pulp exposed due to fracture
- *Mobility of segment:* Fracture of bone.

Investigations
IOPA, OPG, PA radiographs.

Treatment
- *Concussion and luxation:* Splinting of the mobile segment is done
- *Avulsion:* Replantation of teeth, if it is preserved in saliva or cold milk within half an hour of trauma
- *Bone fracture:* Joining of bony segment with implants or mini plates.

Summary
- To know the extent of injury to teeth, it is very important to know the object, the angle, and the force of impact on the teeth
- If there is only fracture of tooth (without bone) then it is not associated with swelling
- Splinting is done in luxated tooth
- Avulsed tooth can be replanted.

DENTAL ABSCESS

Etiology/Causes
- Dental infections involving staphylococci are frequently associated with abscess
- Trauma to tooth may lead to abscess formation
- Chemical or mechanical irritation to gingival tissue.

Pathophysiology
Staphylococci produce coagulase enzyme which causes fibrin deposition and helps in walling off lesion. Small pockets of necrotic tissues are formed inside cellulitis. Then pockets join together and enlarge to form abscess.

Clinical Presentation
Severe throbbing pain, affected area is sensitive to pressure, swelling is seen in adjacent tissues. Teeth are nonsensitive to hot, cold, sweet, or sour.

Red Flags
Fluctuant swelling in the associated tissue of teeth. Swelling may extend to facial spaces.

Evaluation

History
A long-standing infection in the periodontium or trauma or wedging of food in gingiva leads to abscess formation.

Physical Examination
- Soft and fluctuant swelling in associated tooth
- The tissue of swelled surface appears taut and inflamed and becomes distended
- Patient may appear irritable, weak from pain, loss of sleep, and may have slight fever.

Interpretation of Findings
Depending upon location of abscess and the duration, it can be classified into acute periapical abscess, periodontal abscess, and acute exacerbation of chronic lesion (pericoronal abscess).

Investigations
IOPA, OPG are done.

Treatment
Drainage of the abscess either via root canal or incision.

Summary
- Soft, fluctuant swelling on tooth-associated tissues
- Rapidly expands over facial spaces
- Staphylococci-associated infection cause abscess
- Incision and drainage is the treatment of choice with antibiotics and analgesics
- It can be due to acute as well as chronic reasons.

■ BLEEDING AFTER DENTAL SURGERY

Etiology/Causes
- Single tooth extraction
- Multiple extraction
- Implant placement
- Traumatic injury.

Clinical Presentation
Bleeding after extraction can be of three types:
- *Primary:* Continuously after surgery
- *Reactionary:* After few hours of surgery
- *Secondary:* After few days.

Bleeding during surgery like implant placement is expected and usually easily controlled. However, if a large vessel is cut, then hemorrhage is uncontrolled, and it requires suturing the vessel.

Pathophysiology
After extraction of tooth, the bleeding usually occurs from small blood vessels, which stops by its own by applying pressure for few minutes. However, sometimes if there is any bleeding disorder or if a venous plexus is present at apex of root of tooth the hemorrhage can be difficult to control.

Evaluation

History
If the bleeding is persistent after surgery then past medical history is very important. Systemic bleeding disorders like hemophilia, thalassemia or von-Willebrand disease, etc. are commonly associated with uncontrolled bleeding. Other causes may include drugs like aspirin usually taken by hypertensive patients.

Physical Examination
- *Hemophilia:*
    - Most common manifestation is hemorrhage in joints, which is spontaneous and associated with warmth and muscle spasm

- Superficial trauma cause uncontrolled bleeding
- Processes like tooth eruption and exfoliation cause prolonged and severe bleeding.
- *Thalassemia:*
  - Patient appears pale, weak, with prominent cheek and other bones
  - Mongoloid appearance: Frontal head bossing with overdeveloped malar bone and short nose
  - Oral mucosa is usually pale due to chronic jaundice.
- *von-Willebrand disease*
  - Excessive bleeding even after minor trauma
  - Most common intraoral sites of bleeding are gingiva and nose
  - Menorrhagia is also very common
  - Bleeding tendencies decrease with age.

Investigations

Investigations for bleeding disorders are done before surgery based on past medical history of the patient.
- *Thalassemia:* Typical safety pin cells and nucleated red blood cells (RBCs) in circulation
- *Hemophilia:* Clotting time is prolonged but bleeding time, platelet count, and prothrombin time are all normal
- *von-Willebrand disease:* Prolonged bleeding time, normal platelet count, decreased factor VIII or factor IX.

Treatment

- Management of postsurgical bleeding:
  - As soon as continuous bleeding is detected, apply digital pressure for 2–3 minutes. If bleeding stops, close the wound by sutures to stabilize the clot.
  - If bleeding still persists, it can be due to bony vessels, apply gel foam, fibrin foam or bone wax over the area, and close with suture.
  - If bleeding still persists, then it is very important to identify the bleeding area and cauterize it with diathermy or if there is larger vessel, that can be ligated.
  - The blood sample can be sent for testing for any systemic disorder and appropriate measures should be taken like blood transfusion.
- *Bleeding after implants*: Bleeding during surgery is expected and usually easily controlled by cauterization or by ligation. Postoperatively patients are given instructions about normal expectation of bleeding and how to prevent and manage it. However, submucosal or subdermal hemorrhage into soft tissue spaces can lead to hematoma formation. Larger hematomas that occur in systemically compromised individual can cause infections. It is advisable to prescribe antibiotics in such cases.
- *Bleeding in systemic disorder patients:*
  - Hemophilia: Raise factor VIII (in hemophilia A) and factor IX (in hemophilia B) levels.

- Various replacement therapies are available like plasma, cryoprecipitate, and factor VIII concentrates.
- Thalassemia: Blood transfusion is required in severe blood loss.
  - Folic acid maybe required due to erythropoiesis.
  - Chelating agents like desferrioxamine can be given.

Summary

- Bleeding after extractions is not a major complication unless it is associated with any systemic cause or drug side effects
- Mild bleeding can be managed by patient
- Systemic diseases are associated with severe blood loss
- Apply digital pressure over the bleeding area, if it does not work, then control the bleeding by ligating the major vessels.

CHAPTER 27

Diarrhea in Adult and Travelers

Sanjay Kumar

INTRODUCTION

Diarrhea is best defined as increased fluidity of stool though increased frequency and volume is also sometimes a consideration. It is one of the most common gastrointestinal (GI) symptoms. It is the second most common cause of mortality in children and is one of the most common reason for absenteeism from job in adults globally. Most cases are self-limiting and do not require treatment but some of them could be serious due to dehydration, acute kidney injury (AKI), electrolyte imbalance, and rarely sepsis.

PATHOPHYSIOLOGY

Increased stool volume/increased fluidity or increased frequency results whenever there is excess unabsorbed fluid/stool traveling through left colon. So, this would happen either if there is excessive secretion in small bowel or defective absorption or if there is poor absorption of fluids in colon. Sometimes, there is no problem with absorption/secretion, but still there may be diarrhea like in case of increased motility, seen in functional bowel disease or hyperthyroidism.

CAUSES

Most common cause of acute diarrhea in adults is infection. Among infections, viral is most common. Causes are listed in **Boxes 1 and 2**.

APPROACH TO ACUTE DIARRHEA

Diarrhea is classified as acute or chronic, inflammatory or noninflammatory, and osmotic or secretory. But while evaluating a patient at bedside, it is more useful to ascertain whether it is small bowel diarrhea or large bowel diarrhea because that guides you to further evaluation and proper management.

Frequency and volume are most important points in history. Voluminous stool 3-6 times a day is suggestive of small bowel origin while more frequent but scanty stool is suggestive of large bowel origin.

Box 1: Causes of acute diarrhea.

- Infections: Bacterial viral, parasitic, protozoal
- Food allergies
- Food poisoning
- Medications
- Initial presentation of chronic diarrhea

Box 2: Infections that cause diarrhea.

Bacteria:
- *Aeromonas* spp.
- *Campylobacter* spp.
- *Clostridium difficile*
- *Escherichia coli* (enterotoxigenic, enteroinvasive, and enterohemorrhagic)
- *Plesiomonas* spp.
- *Salmonella* spp.
- *Shigella* spp.

Viruses:
- Adenovirus
- Norovirus
- Rotavirus

Parasites or protozoa:
- Cryptosporidium
- Cyclospora
- Entamoeba
- Giardia lamblia
- Microsporidia

Next are contents. Presence of blood/mucous suggests large bowel, i.e. colitis while profuse watery diarrhea suggests small bowel, i.e. enteritis. Crampy abdominal pain can be present in both but tenesmus points to a large bowel/rectal origin.

A detailed history will go a long way in providing clue to the cause of diarrhea and one can manage accordingly (**Table 1**).

PHYSICAL EXAMINATION

Important point to be assessed during physical examination is degree of dehydration in patient. Patient with severe dehydration generally have ill appearance, dry mucous membranes, delayed capillary refill time, increased heart rate, and abnormal orthostatic vital signs. Fever is present in inflammatory diarrhea.

Investigations

Hardly any investigations are required in routine cases. Stool routine and culture may be advised if there is suspicion of invasive diarrhea based on presence of fever and blood in stool. Hemogram and renal function tests must be done if patient is dehydrated. A film for malarial

Table 1: Clue to diagnosis based on history and examination.

History	Possible pathogen/causes
• Bloody diarrhea, abdominal pain but no fever • Eating sprouts, raw meat, and raw milk.	Shiga toxin producing *Escherichia coli*
Bloody diarrhea and fever	*Shigella, Salmonella*, and *Campylobacter*
Drinking untreated water in camping	*Giardia*
Seafood	*Vibrio* (rice-water stool)
Antibiotic use	*Clostridium difficile*
Acute onset of diarrhea in group of people after consuming same food	• Food poisoning with preformed toxins • Within 6 hours—*Staphylococcus, Bacillus cereus* • Diarrhea within 8–16 hours—*Clostridium perfringens* type

Table 2: Management of acute diarrhea.

Nontoxic patient	Symptomatic treatment, oral rehydration therapy
Toxic	• Fluid and electrolyte therapy, investigate complete blood count, electrolyte, urea creatinine, stool culture, ova parasite examination, antigen testing for *Giardia* and *Cryptosporidium*, and testing for *Clostridium difficile*. • Sigmoidoscopy or colonoscopy.

parasite may be handy if there is high fever with chills as sometimes malaria can present as diarrhea (algid malaria).

TREATMENT

Mainstay of treatment of acute diarrhea is restoring/maintaining fluid and electrolyte balance (**Table 2**).

Rehydration Therapy

Fluid deficit should be assessed by calculating difference between patient's normal weight and weight during diarrhea. Fluid deficit should be supplemented orally. Various oral rehydration formulae are available. Usually oral rehydration salt (ORS) with low osmolarity is beneficial and also recommended by the World Health Organization (WHO) in 2002. Low osmolarity ORS decreases stool frequency, vomiting, and the requirement of intravenous (IV) fluid.

If patient is having vomiting and oral rehydration is not possible, we have to give IV fluids. While giving IV fluids, best way to monitor adequacy is urine output but if patient is too sick or has comorbidities especially, chronic kidney disease (CKD)/congestive heart failure (CHF)/chronic liver disease (CLD), fluid balance should be ensured by ultrasonographic inferior vena

> **Box 3:** Points to remember in managing the acute diarrhea.
>
> *Red flags (indications for hospitalization):*
> - Severe dehydration
> - Blood in stool
> - Fever associated with diarrhea
> - Frequent episode of diarrhea and incontinence
>
> *Not recommended:*
> - Routine antibiotic use
> - Routine stool culture
> - Hospitalization if no dehydration
> - Detailed workup not indicated routinely

cava (IVC) monitoring or central venous pressure (CVP) monitoring by putting in a central venous catheter.

Antibiotic Therapy

Routine use of antibiotic is not recommended for nonsevere, watery diarrhea because acute diarrhea is mostly self-limiting and caused by viruses. Antibiotics can be used in elderly age, immunocompromised severely ill, and sepsis patient.

Zinc Supplementation

For treatment and prevention of diarrhea in children more than 2 months, zinc supplementation (20 mg/day for 10 days) may play a crucial role, particularly in developing countries.

Most cases of acute diarrhea are self-limiting and can be managed with ORS. Those who have red flags (**Box 3**) can be managed with hospitalization, IV fluids, and antibiotics. Very rare cases will develop complications like acute kidney injury or sepsis and these will require prolonged hospitalization, intensive care, and can be fatal too.

■ TRAVELER'S DIARRHEA

Traveler's diarrhea is due to eating contaminated food and drinking contaminated water. Traveler's diarrhea manifests as loose stool and abdominal cramps during a visit to a place where the climate or hygiene are different from their home. It usually begins abruptly during your trip or shortly after return from the trip. Most cases resolve within 1–2 days without treatment and completely within a week. Sudden onset diarrhea three or more stool per day, abdominal pain, nausea, vomiting are usual presentation. Fever may or may not present.

Patient should be hospitalized if severe diarrhea, continuous vomiting, fever, dehydration, and decreased urine output.

Enterotoxigenic *Escherichia coli* (ETEC) is most common causative agent for traveler's diarrhea.

Traveler's diarrhea is common in Central and South America, Mexico, Africa, the Middle East, and most of Asia including India. It is generally low in Northern and Western Europe,

Japan, Canada, Australia, New Zealand, and the United States. Greater risk of developing traveler's diarrhea is in young, immunocompromised individuals especially in diabetics, inflammatory bowel disease, and patient of chronic illnesses.

Prevention
- Do not consume raw uncooked or undercooked food
- Avoid raw milk and dairy products
- Do not eat from street vendors
- Drink boiled/bottled water while traveling
- *Follow rule of thumb*: Boil it, cook it, peel it, or forget it.

Treatment
Dehydration is the most likely complication of traveler's diarrhea, so it is important to try to stay well-hydrated. An ORSs solution is the best way to replace lost fluids. Bottled oral rehydration products are available in drug stores.

Experts generally do not recommend taking antibiotics to prevent traveler's diarrhea; some suggest taking antimotility agents like loperamide, diphenoxylate, and bismuth subsalicylate (Pepto-Bismol), which has been shown to decrease the likelihood of diarrhea. However, do not take this medication for longer than 3 weeks.

CHAPTER 28

Diarrhea in Children

Veena Raghunathan

BACKGROUND

The earliest description of diarrhea dates back to the Vedic era: it has been described in the Suktas of Atharva Veda. It was considered as a deadly disease especially in small children in the olden times. The understanding of etiopathogenesis of diarrhea and management strategies have evolved to a great deal in the modern era; however, diarrhea still continues to be one of the major causes of under-five age group mortality. In India, around 10% of infants and 14% of 0–4-year children die due to diarrhea. An average child suffers from 1.7 episodes of diarrhea per year. Diarrhea usually resolves within few days; however, the symptoms are unpleasant and the dehydration and dyselectrolytemias that accompany it can be dangerous if not properly treated. The risk of fluid and electrolyte losses is greater if the child is younger. Fluid losses can be as high as three times circulating blood volume. This accounts for the potentially life-threatening nature of this illness, especially if untreated. Acute diarrhea is usually of infective etiology in children. This chapter will focus on the definition of acute diarrhea in children, clinical assessment, and key points in management of acute diarrhea.

DEFINITION AND ETIOLOGY

There is no single universally accepted definition of diarrhea. Also, the terms acute diarrhea and acute gastroenteritis are often used interchangeably. However strictly speaking, gastroenteritis refers to underlying infectious etiology, whereas the term acute diarrhea encompasses both infective and noninfective causes like drug/systemic illness. Noninfective etiologies; however, usually lead to prolonged diarrhea. Acute diarrhea is defined as passage of loose or watery stool more than three episodes (in 24 hours) with/without vomiting. More than the frequency, it is the consistency of stool which is important. Acute diarrhea usually lasts for 3–7 days. Prolonged diarrhea (lasting >1 week) is evaluated and treated differently than an acute case of diarrhea. Globally, infective etiology predominates and viral gastroenteritis is the most common cause of acute diarrhea in children. Bacterial pathogens are less common and diarrheal presentation of protozoal infections is rare in children (**Table 1**). Acute gastroenteritis usually spreads by feco-oral route and has short incubation period (hours-days). Acute diarrhea can be secretory (producing large quantities of watery stools) or invasive (mucosal invasion leading to blood in stool and cramping).

Table 1: Etiology—acute diarrhea in children.

Infective
Viruses: • Rotaviruses • Caliciviruses • Adenoviruses
Bacterial: • E. coli • C. jejuni • V. cholerae • Salmonella • Shigella
Protozoal: • E. histolytica • G. lamblia • Cryptosporidia
Noninfective (rare) • Drug induced, e.g. antibiotic • Inflammatory bowel disease • Celiac disease • Hyperthyroidism

CLINICAL MANIFESTATIONS

On history, details about onset of diarrhea, frequency, color and consistency of stool, accompanying symptoms (fever, vomiting, etc.) must be noted. History of decreased urine frequency or concentrated appearance of urine indicates significant dehydration. Presence of any comorbidities, drug history, history of recent travel, consumption of raw/undercooked food are pertinent. Impact on usual oral food/fluid intake and activity/alertness of the child suggests greater severity of illness.

Typically infective diarrhea, especially viral presents with watery stools with no blood/mucus. Fever, vomiting, generalized malaise, and myalgias are variably present. These symptoms may precede or follow diarrhea or may not be present at all. Vomiting usually subsides by 48 hours with adequate rehydration. Choleric diarrhea has a characteristic "fishy" odor. Dysentery involves colon and rectum and presents with blood and mucus in stool, abdominal cramping, and fever and is usually due to bacterial etiology. Differentiation from abdominal conditions like intussusception and appendicitis are sometimes required; imaging studies are required in these cases. Urine tests may help to differentiate from urinary tract infections, whose initial presentation could be fever with diarrhea. Apart from dehydration, certain other complications may occasionally occur in acute diarrhea and include: seizures (due to dyselectrolytemias/hypoglycemia), encephalopathy, circulatory shock, and acute kidney injury (pre-renal). A patient with recurrent or persistent symptoms (>7 days) or malnutrition would require further evaluation by a pediatric gastroenterologist.

Table 2: Classification of degree of dehydration.

Assessment	No dehydration	Some dehydration	Severe dehydration
*General condition	Alert	Irritable, restless	Lethargic, unconscious
*Eyes	Normal	Sunken	Sunken
*Skin pinch	Goes back immediately	Goes back slowly (<2 sec)	Goes back very slowly (>2 sec)
*Thirst	Drinks normally	Thirsty, drinks eagerly	Drinks poorly
Mucous membranes	Moist	Dry	Dried out
Heart rate	Normal	Tachycardia	Marked tachycardia/bradycardia
Capillary refill	Normal	Delayed	Marked delay
Peripheries	Warm	Cool	Cold/cyanotic
Urine output	Normal/slightly decreased	Decreased	Markedly decreased
Fluid deficit as % of body weight	<5%	5–10%	>10%
Fluid deficit in mL/kg body weight	<50 mL/kg	50–100 mL/kg	>100 mL/kg

*World Health Organization (WHO) classification parameters.

It is important to correctly assess the degree of dehydration based on clinical signs and symptoms as the treatment plan would depend on it. The WHO dehydration classification system uses four items (general condition, eyes, skin pinch, and thirst) to grade patients into no, some, and severe dehydration. Decreased urine output, dryness of mucous membranes, and absence of tears are also markers of dehydration. Other signs consistent with severe dehydration/hypovolemic shock include severe tachycardia for age, delayed capillary refill time, abnormal respiration, and poor radial pulse (**Table 2**). The dehydration that ensues in acute diarrhea can be isotonic/hypotonic or hypertonic and does not depend on the causative microbe.

LABORATORY INVESTIGATIONS

Blood and stool investigations are generally not required in cases of mild/moderate illness. In cases of severe diarrhea, lab evaluation includes complete blood count, electrolytes, blood gas, renal function tests, and glucose. Elevated blood urea nitrogen has shown some correlation with degree of dehydration. Serum bicarbonate less than 17 mEq/L has been demonstrated to have 94% sensitivity for more than 10% dehydration. Inflammatory markers such as CRP and ESR cannot reliably differentiate between viral and bacterial etiologies. Blood culture is of limited utility except to detect *Salmonella*. Urine specific gravity is an indicator of degree of dehydration. Urinalysis can help to differentiate from urinary tract infection. Stool routine microscopy can reveal presence of blood, mucus, and leukocytes (in dysentery) and in rare

cases protozoal cysts/trophozoites. Stool polymerase chain reaction (PCR) tests and cultures can identify etiological agent but are not routinely required as they have little therapeutic utility. Culture reports usually take 2–3 days, by which time usually diarrhea is better. Also identification of etiological agent does not usually alter the management which is largely supportive. The few exceptions when identification of etiological agent is important include:
- Suspected hemolytic-uremic syndrome
- Hospital acquired diarrhea (diarrhea after 3 days of admission)
- Congenital/acquired immunodeficiency
- Suspected *Clostridium difficile* infection
- Infants less than 3 months, with severe course (especially preterm)
- Prolonged diarrhea more than 2 weeks: to decide on antibiotic administration

Abdominal imaging [ultrasound/computed tomography (CT)] is indicated only in cases with severe abdominal pain and tenderness or if there is strong clinical suspicion of underlying abdominal pathology, e.g. appendicitis. Endoscopy is reserved only for cases of protracted diarrhea with unclear etiology for diagnostic purpose.

TREATMENT

The mainstay of treatment is supportive care and includes rehydration, zinc supplementation, and judicious use of antibiotics. The present universally accepted management strategy is based on WHO guidelines. Mild-moderate degrees of dehydration are usually successfully treated with oral rehydration; however, severe dehydration requires IV rehydration and close monitoring, sometimes in pediatric intensive care unit (PICU) setting. The older concepts of withholding food for few hours and low-fat diet during diarrheal illness are now considered obsolete and no longer advocated. The flowchart for management of dehydration in diarrhea is described in **Flowchart 1**.

Correction of Hydration

Hydration therapy in diarrhea depends on degree of dehydration. Generally oral route of rehydration is preferred and considered better than IV, unless there is excessive vomiting or severe dehydration. Oral rehydration therapy is successful in 90% cases with mild-moderate degree of dehydration.

No Clinical Dehydration

Children with no signs of dehydration must be given extra fluid + salts to replace ongoing water and electrolyte losses in diarrhea. If such replacement is not advised, there will progression to dehydration and its deleterious effects. The child can be managed at home, provided the caregiver has been appropriately advised regarding replacement fluids and danger signs.

Type of fluid to be given: Home available fluids (salted rice water, lemon water, buttermilk, soups) or oral rehydration salts (ORS) (appropriately diluted) should be given. ORS should be prepared by adding 1 L of clean drinking water to one packet (of low-osmolarity ORS). Commercial fruit juices, carbonated beverages should not be given as they can worsen

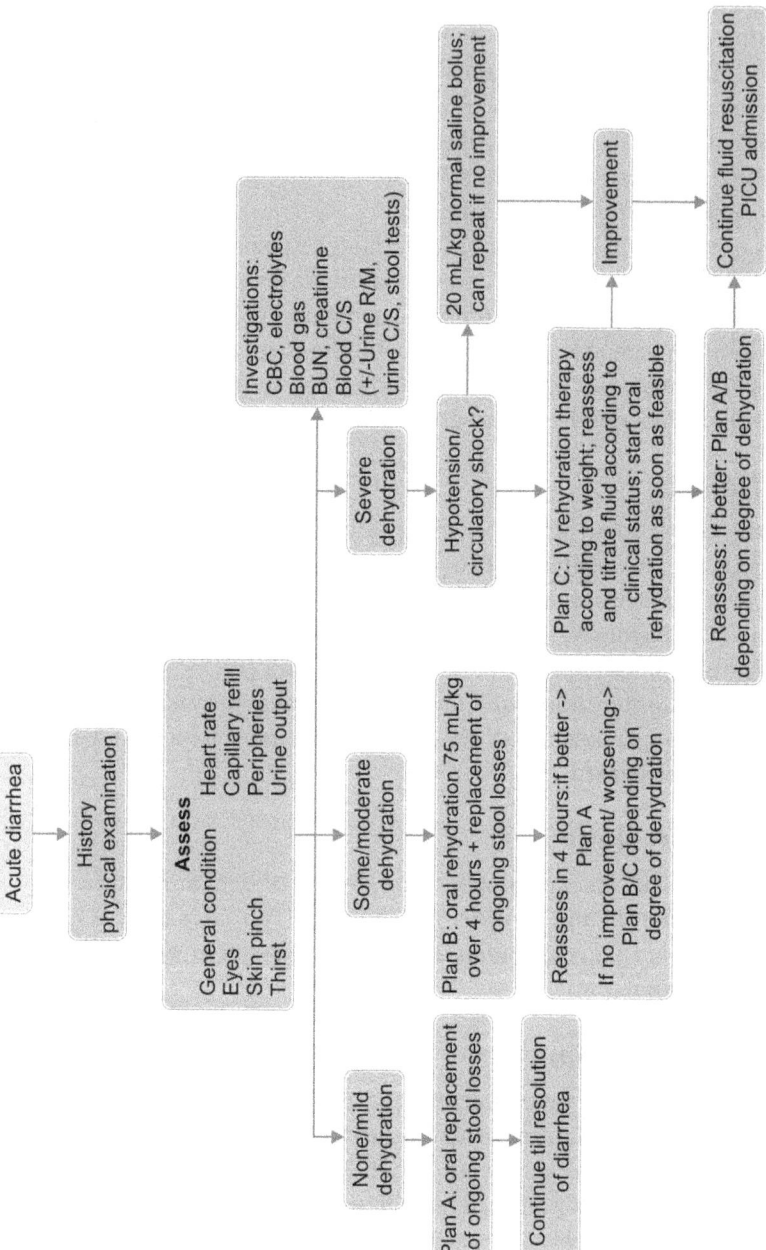

Flowchart 1: Management of dehydration in acute diarrhea.

diarrhea. The child should be fed what he/she usually eats additionally, feeding should not be withheld. There is no role of withholding milk during episode of acute diarrhea.

Amount of fluid to be given: Depends on the age. ORS and other fluids must be offered slowly by spoon/sip every 1–2 minutes. The general dictum is to give as much fluid as the child wants, till diarrhea subsides. As a general guide:
- Upto 2 months: Five spoons of ORS
- Two months to 2 years of age: 50–100 mL (a quarter-to-half a large cup) of fluid
- 2–10 years: 100–200 mL (a half-to-one large cup)

Older children: As much fluid as they want

Danger signs/when to report back to the physician

The caregiver must be explained that the child must be brought back to the physician if any of the following symptoms develop:
- High purge rate: many watery stools which cannot be adequately replaced
- Repeated vomiting/poor oral acceptance
- Lethargic/altered sensorium
- High grade fever
- Blood in the stool
- Decreased urine frequency
- No improvement in 3 days.

Some Dehydration

Children with some dehydration should receive ORS fluid according to the estimated fluid loss (*see* **Table 2**) for rehydration. Alternatively, they can receive 75 mL/kg of ORS over 4 hours. They should be continuously monitored for signs of improvement. If at any stage, there is clinical worsening of dehydration, the management to shift to plan C and IV rehydration should be carried out. At the end of 4 hours, the clinical assessment will be as follows:
- *No dehydration*: In this case, child must be advised regarding home care (as described in plan A).
- *Some dehydration*: Plan B should be repeated in this situation and close monitoring and reassessment should be carried out.
- *Severe dehydration*: IV therapy according to plan C.

Severe Dehydration

Intravenous fluids must be started immediately. Generally, Ringer lactate (RL) is used for IV rehydration; use of large amounts of normal saline can lead to hyperchloremic metabolic acidosis. If there is accompanying dyselectrolytemia (e.g. hypernatremia, hypokalemia), appropriate correction should be calculated and fluid volume and composition determined accordingly. Generally, for infants, 30 mL/kg IV RL is given over 1 hour f/b 70 mL/kg over next 5 hours. Correction in older children is done faster: initial 30 mL/kg over half-an-hour f/b

70 mL/kg over 2.5 hours. The patient should be continuously reassessed; if radial pulses are weak, fluid should be administered at a faster rate. A patient with signs of shock should be managed with fluid boluses and if required inotropic support similar to septic shock guidelines.

After stabilization with IV fluid therapy, patient can be stepped down to plan B or A depending on the amount of dehydration.

Dyselectrolytemias

Often encountered in diarrhea are hyponatremia, hypernatremia, and hypokalemia. Metabolic acidosis (normal anion gap) may also be present. All these usually will resolve with appropriate rehydration therapy. Extremely high or low sodium leads to adverse effects including seizures, cerebral edema. In hypernatremic dehydration, it is important to remember that clinical estimation of dehydration will be erroneously lower than the actual amount of dehydration. Appropriate sodium and water replacement must be administered slowly in such cases and most importantly, sodium must be closely monitored and necessary changes in fluid composition made if correction is too rapid. Oral rehydration therapy wherever feasible is helpful and safer than IV therapy as it will not lead to sudden swings in sodium. Potassium losses during diarrhea, if not replaced will lead to hypokalemia, especially in children with malnutrition. This has deleterious effects including muscle weakness, ileus, and arrhythmias (which can be life threatening). Replacement of potassium (oral or if severe IV) is essential in any acute diarrheal episode.

Zinc Supplementation

Zinc plays a crucial role in metallo-enzymes and cell membrane and function. Various studies have demonstrated that zinc supplementation reduces both duration and severity of diarrhea in children less than 5 years of age. It is recommended to give zinc supplementation to all children greater than 3 months at a dose of 20 mg elemental zinc/day during and for up to 7 days after diarrhea supplementation.

Role of Antimicrobial Therapy

There is no role for routine use of antimicrobial agents in treatment of acute diarrhea in children. Protozoal disease causing acute diarrhea is very rare in children, hence there is no role of antiprotozoal drugs (metronidazole/tinidazole, etc.) unless cysts of *E. histolytica/ Giardia* is visualized on stool microscopy. Antibiotics are indicated only in select conditions which include acute dysentery (to target *Shigella*), diarrhea due to cholera, salmonella infection, and *Clostridium difficle*. In cases of acute bloody diarrhea (dysentery), treatment with nalidixic acid/ciprofloxacin or third generation cephalosporin for 3-5 days should be given. Cholera is characterized by profuse voluminous watery diarrhea which has potential to quickly cause severe dehydration and hypovolemic shock. The episode is effectively shortened by the use of antibiotic: single dose doxycycline in an older child or 3-day course of erythromycin/azithromycin in a child less than 12 years. In cases of *Salmonella* (typhoid), prolonged antibiotic therapy usually for 10-14 days with ceftriaxone/cefixime is required. Fluoroquinolones are less effective due to increasing resistance.

Role of Probiotics

Some preliminary data suggests that probiotics are beneficial in treatment of acute gastroenteritis in children. However, most of the research on this is conducted in the West, and have included certain probiotic strains which are not available in India. Rotavirus diarrhea constituted more than 75% cases in the patients studied in the West, whereas it constitutes around 25% of diarrhea in India. So, at present, role of probiotics is still unclear.

Antiemetics

Vomiting is a very common symptom accompanying diarrhea. Antiemetic therapy should be reserved for those patients who have severe or recurrent vomiting which interferes with oral intake. Domperidone or ondansetron can be used and is generally safe in children.

Diet during Acute Diarrhea

Age appropriate feeding must be continued and not interrupted in patients with acute diarrhea; especially in cases with mild-moderate dehydration. In severe cases, or when there is excessive vomiting, feeding must be initiated as early as possible once rehydration and supportive care has been provided. Enteral nutrition is important for regeneration of enterocytes in gastrointestinal tract (GI) tract damaged by infection (breast feeding should be continued and ORS offered in between feeds in young infants). Use of special infant formulae, lactose-free milk, soy-based products is not indicated. Highly sweetened foods, carbonated beverages, and processed fruit juices should be avoided (due to high osmolar content).

There is no role of antimotility agents (e.g. loperamide), adsorbents (e.g. charcoal), bismuth, or cholestyramine in treatment of childhood diarrhea.

■ PREVENTION

After a child/infant with acute diarrhea is appropriately treated, education of care-giver about preventive steps is also vital. The importance of proper hygienic measures, including hand washing with soap and water, use of clean uncontaminated water to name a few are the best methods by which feco-oral transmission of the microbes causing infective diarrhea can be controlled.

■ CONCLUSION

Acute diarrhea is still a very commonly encountered condition in infants and young children. An accurate assessment of degree of dehydration and other coexisting problems based on history and clinical examination is essential. Once the severity of dehydration is assessed, appropriate rehydration therapy should be provided to prevent worsening dehydration and complications. The key aspects of treatment include appropriate fluids (oral preferred over IV wherever feasible) and supportive care which includes correction of dyselectrolytemias and judicious use of antibiotics. Preventive measures and family education is important to decrease overall incidence of acute diarrheal disease.

CHAPTER 29

Dysmenorrhea

Nilu Sunil

DEFINITION

Dysmenorrhea is a painful cramping sensation in the lower abdomen occurring shortly before or during menstruation. It is often accompanied by fatigue, dizziness, sweating, backache, nausea, vomiting, and diarrhea.

It is the most common gynecological problem in women of all ages and one of the most common causes of pelvic pain. Prevalence rates vary from 25% to 90% among women and adolescents. Even though dysmenorrhea is not a real threat to life but it can affect the quality of life leading to disability, inefficiency, school and work absenteeism, and reduced participation in social activities. Moderate to severe pain requires professional attention and diagnosis of underlying pathology.

ETIOLOGY

Dysmenorrhea can be categorized into two types (**Table 1**)—(1) primary and (2) secondary.

Types

1. Primary dysmenorrhea is defined as painful menstrual cycles not associated with any pelvic pathology. It begins frequently during adolescence. It is associated with ovulatory cycles.
   It is quite common in young women and is associated with a good prognosis, but interferes with quality of life. It is most intense on the 1st day of menstrual cycle and gradually lessens with menstrual flow. It usually lessens after child birth. Pelvic findings are normal
   According to epidemiologic review published in 2014 by Hong Ju, Mark Jones, and Gita Mishra regarding the prevalence and risk factors of dysmenorrhea, women's age, parity, and use of oral contraceptives were inversely associated with dysmenorrhea and there is an association with family history.
   Moderate to severe pain requires professional attention and diagnosis of underlying etiology.
2. Secondary dysmenorrhea is caused by underlying pelvic pathology, e.g. fibroids, adenomyosis, pelvic inflammatory disease (PID), and endometriosis. Endometriosis is the most common cause of secondary dysmenorrhea. The incidence is highest among 25–29

Table 1: Differences between primary and secondary dysmenorrhea.

	Primary	Secondary
Age (years)	16–25 years	30–45 years
Onset of pain	Just prior to menstruation (spasmodic)	Pain often progresses through late (congestive) phase
Pathophysiology	Prostaglandins, vasopressin, and leukotrienes	Underlying disorder
Symptoms	Usually lasts 1–3 days prior or during menstruation. Responds to OCPs and NSAIDs. Periods are normal or light	Associated with other features related to underlying diseases resistant to OCPs and NSAIDs. Periods are heavy
Signs	Not conclusive or significant	Usually depends on the underlying cause but may have a tender, fixed, enlarged, and retroverted uterus with adnexal tenderness

(NSAIDs: nonsteroidal anti-inflammatory drugs; OCPs: oral contraceptive pills)

years of age and lowest among women older than 44 years. Black women have a 40% lower incidence of endometriosis as compared to white women.

VARIETIES

- *Spasmodic dysmenorrhea:* Most common presents as cramping pain usually on the 1st and 2nd days of menstrual cycles.
- Congestive dysmenorrhea usually presents with increasing pelvic discomfort and pelvic pain a few days before the cycles begin. The patient feels better on the onset of her menstrual cycles. This is usually seen in PID, endometriosis, and fibroids.
- Membranous dysmenorrhea presents with painful cramps due to the endometrium being shed at the time of menstruation.

PATHOPHYSIOLOGY

Hyperactivity of the myometrium with uterine ischemia is the main contributory factor in the causation of pain.
- Psychosomatic due to stress and anxiety which lowers the pain threshold.
- Abnormal development of uterus such as:
  - Stenosis at the internal os or narrowing of the cervical canal which makes it difficult for the menstrual blood to escape leading to painful strong uterine contractions.
  - Septate or bicornuate uterus causing pain due to unequal muscular contractions.
  - Uterine hypoplasia leading to inadequate force to expel the blood.
  - Imbalance in the autonomic nervous control of the uterine musculature.
- *Prostaglandins:* Prostaglandins seem to be involved to a large extent in myometrial hyperactivity.
- Under the influence of progesterone prostaglandins like PGF2 alpha, prostaglandin E2 (PGE2) are synthesized from the secretory endometrium maximally during shedding

of the endometrium. PGF2 alpha being a strong vasoconstrictor causes ischemia of the myometrium, causing contractions.
- Vasopressin increases prostaglandin synthesis and is also a direct uterine stimulant.
- The more severe pain in primary dysmenorrhea could be the combined result of vasopressin and PGF2 alpha.
- Endothelins, leukotrienes, and platelet activating factor have also been associated with dysmenorrhea.

CLINICAL FEATURES

In primary dysmenorrhea, the pain is most intense on the 1st day of menstrual cycle and gradually lessens with menstrual flow. The pain could radiate to the back and the medial aspect of the thighs. It is usually associated with systemic symptoms like diarrhea, nausea, vomiting, or headache. It could also be accompanied by sweating, fainting, syncope, and rarely collapse. Abdominal and pelvic examination findings are normal. It usually lessens after child birth. Differentiating features of primary dysmenorrhea to secondary dysmenorrhea (endometriosis and adenomyosis) is described in **Table 2**.

In secondary dysmenorrhea, it is a dull pain localized to the back and front without any radiation. It usually appears 3–5 days before the menstrual cycles and decreases in intensity with the start of the menstrual cycles. The frequency and duration of the pain depends on the underlying pathology. It is usually unaccompanied by systemic symptoms. Abdominal and pelvic examination might reveal the underlying pathology or an ultrasound would help in diagnosing the pelvic cause for the pain.

In secondary dysmenorrhea, treatment aims at the underlying cause. In endometriosis, initial treatment is with nonsteroidal anti-inflammatory drugs (NSAIDs), progestin synthetase inhibitors, and oral contraceptive pills.

Table 2: Characteristic features of primary dysmenorrhea, endometriosis, and adenomyosis.

Primary dysmenorrhea	Crampy pain in the lower abdomen occurring just before or during menses and lasting 2–3 days; pain may radiate into the lower back and thighs, and may be associated with fatigue, dizziness nausea, bloating, and general malaise; pelvic examination findings are normal	It is a clinical diagnosis. Pregnancy test should be done in women of reproductive age group
Endometriosis	Cyclical or noncyclic pelvic pain occurring with menstruation; associated with dyspareunia, dysuria, constipation, and subfertility; pelvic examination findings include fixed or retroverted uterus or reduced uterine mobility, uterosacral nodularity, and adnexal masses	Transvaginal and pelvic ultrasound is highly accurate in detecting endometriosis. A magnetic resonance imaging may be indicated for deeply infiltrating endometriosis; laparoscopy with biopsy and histology is the preferred diagnostic test
Adenomyosis	Causes menorrhagia; intermenstrual bleeding; pelvic examination findings include enlarged, tender, and boggy uterus	Transvaginal sonography and if necessary, magnetic resonance imaging will usually detect endometrial tissues within the myometrium

INVESTIGATIONS

In women suffering from secondary dysmenorrhea, tests need to be conducted to confirm the underlying pathology:
- Pelvic ultrasound
- Complete blood count to rule out anemia
- Urine analysis to rule out a urinary tract infection
- Erythrocyte sedimentation rate (ESR) to rule out any inflammatory cause
- Pregnancy test
- Cervical culture for any underlying sexually transmitted infections
- Computed tomography (CT) scan/MRI pelvis, if indicated
- Diagnostic hysterosalpingogram
- Diagnostic hysteroscopy

TREATMENT

- Psychotherapy and counseling. Advised to continue routine activities and sports
- Analgesics and antispasmodics
- Advised to keep the bowels empty.

The earlier measures are relieving pain in most women.
In very severe cases, medical therapy or surgery is considered.

Medical Therapy

- Analgesics like paracetamol 500 mg thrice a day; piroxicam 20 mg twice daily
- Analgesics like hyoscine (Buscopan) thrice daily
- *Prostaglandin synthetase inhibitors (PSIs):* They are cyclooxygenase inhibitors and hence reduce the prostaglandin synthesis. They also have an analgesic effect.
  - Mefenamic acid, belonging to the fenamate group, 250–500 mg 8 hourly
  - Ibuprofen 400 mg 8 hourly or naproxen 250 mg 6 hourly (propionic acid derivatives)
  - Indomethacin 25 mg 8 hourly.
- Glyceryl trinitrate (nitroglycerine), nitric oxide donor helps to relieve the muscle spasm, also available as transdermal patches.
- Oral contraceptive pills for 3–6 cycles (for patients who desire contraception).

Surgery

- *Dilatation of the cervical canal:* Relieves pain by stretching of the fibromuscular tissues at the internal os which leads to loss of tone and there is also an injury to the sensory nerve endings blocking the pain pathway.
- Bilateral block of the sacral plexus.
- *Presacral neurectomy:* In rare cases, where all other measures fail.
- In secondary dysmenorrhea, treatment aims at the underlying cause. In endometriosis, treatment is usually initiated with contraceptive pills. Several trials have confirmed the

effectiveness of oral and depot medroxyprogesterone, levonorgestrel-releasing intrauterine system, and the etonogestrel implant. Treatment with gonadotropin-releasing hormone agonists can also be initiated. Hysterectomy is generally the last resort. In fibroids, uterine artery embolization can help relieve the symptoms.

There is limited and inconsistent evidence on the pharmacologic therapy for primary dysmenorrhea. Topical heat may be effective as NSAIDs. There is insufficient evidence for acupuncture, yoga, massages, and nutritional supplements like vitamin B, omega-3 fatty acids (**Flowchart 1**). Dysmenorrhea is summarized in **Flowchart 1**.

Flowchart 1: Evaluation and management of dysmenorrhea.

```
History consistent with primary dysmenorrhea,
          normal pelvic examination
                    ↓
   Treatment with NSAIDs, PSI, or oral
     contraceptives/psychotherapy
                    ↓
                                  Yes
     Pain/symptomatic relief  ───────→  Continue same treatment
                                         and reassess in 6 months
          No ↓
   Laboratory testing (for gonorrhea,
   chlamydia; urine analysis, ESR, and CBC)
                    ↓
                                       Treat for pelvic
     If tests are positive  ──────→   inflammatory disease
     If negative ↓
          Pelvic ultrasound
                    ↓
                              Yes
     Any pelvic pathology?  ──────→  Treat accordingly
          No ↓
          Reassess history
                    ↓
     CT scan/MRI pelvis, hysteroscopy,
        or laparoscopy, if indicated
                    ↓
   Clinical and diagnostic tests positive  ──────→  Treat pathology
          No ↓
   Chronic pelvic pain and multidisciplinary approach
```

(CBC: complete blood count; CT: computed tomography; ESR: erythrocyte sedimentation rate; MRI: magnetic resonance imaging; NSAIDs: nonsteroidal anti-inflammatory drugs)

CHAPTER 30

Dyspepsia

Ravindra Kale

INTRODUCTION

Dyspepsia is feeling of upper abdominal pain or vague discomfort which encompasses postprandial fullness, early satiety, burning, nausea, and bloating in upper abdomen, i.e. symptoms that presumably arise from stomach and duodenum. Heart burn is usually associated with these symptoms but it is considered to be a symptom of gastroesophageal reflux disease and not of dyspepsia.

ETIOLOGY

Dyspepsia most commonly results from peptic ulcer disease, gastritis, and reflux disease; but there are myriads of other causes which may lead to dyspeptic symptoms. Cardiac and pancreatobiliary conditions are particularly important to be differentiated for emergency management.

Peptic ulcer is responsible for 5–10% cases of dyspepsia. Risk factors are *Helicobacter pylori* infection and frequent use of analgesics [nonsteroidal anti-inflammatory drug (NSAID)] particularly in elderly. Complications can occur specially with concomitant aspirin use in cardiac patients as they may bleed. Reflux esophagitis is another important cause in 20% of patients and equal number of patients with reflux symptoms may not have endoscopic signs of reflux disease (nonerosive reflux disease). Gastric malignancy also causes dyspeptic symptoms. Risk increased with long-standing *Helicobacter pylori* infection. Gastroparesis usually due to diabetes is associated with postprandial fullness, nausea, and vomiting.

Medications are another important cause of dyspepsia. NSAID, theophylline, oral iron, potassium chloride, and antimalarials (chloroquine and quinine) frequently cause dyspepsia through direct mucosal injury, reflux, or idiosyncratic mechanisms.

Chronic pancreatitis and pancreatic malignancy may mimic symptoms of dyspepsia but usually have more severe pain, characteristic radiation, and weight loss. Presence of gallstones alone does not cause dyspepsia and other causes should be evaluated. Patients with hyperthyroidism, acute coronary syndrome, renal failure, and chronic obstructive pulmonary disease (COPD) can also have dyspepsia-like symptoms.

Functional dyspepsia is absence of any obvious cause for dyspepsia. Rome criteria for functional gastrointestinal (GI) disorders (Rome IV) defines functional dyspepsia as one or more of the following symptoms in last 3 months—bothersome symptoms of: (a) postprandial fullness, (b) epigastric pain, (c) early satiety, and (d) epigastric burning, with onset at least 6 months prior to diagnosis. These symptoms should be present in absence of significant structural disease (including normal endoscopy) that can explain symptoms. Functional dyspepsia can be further classified as postprandial distress syndrome (PDS) which include fullness and early satiety and epigastric pain syndrome (EPS) which include epigastric pain and burning.

PATHOPHYSIOLOGY

There are several proposed mechanisms for dyspepsia. Abnormally enhanced perception of visceral stimuli (visceral hypersensitivity), impaired gastric relaxation to meals, and delayed gastric emptying can be responsible. *Helicobacter pylori* infection can be a cause of functional dyspepsia and eradication may improve symptoms. First-degree relatives of patients have increased frequency of dyspepsia suggestive of genetic predisposition.

CLINICAL PRESENTATION

Usual presentation is of chronic upper abdominal discomfort with epigastric pain or burning, fullness after meals, nausea, and vomiting. Most of the patient are well nourished and may be obese. Some patients are on prolong NSAID therapy. Presence of anemia and/or weight loss indicates serious disorder like gastroesophageal or pancreatic malignancy or complicated peptic ulcer with bleeding or stricture. Patients with acute onset epigastric pain and dyspnea, especially on exertion and improvement after rest, should be evaluated for cardiac disease.

RED FLAGS

- Old age
- Significant weight loss
- Long-term aspirin and NSAID use
- Gastrointestinal bleeding
- Anemia
- Persistent vomiting
- Dysphagia.

EVALUATION

- *History*: All patients should be evaluated with detailed history of dietary habits and medications including complementary and alternative medicines. History of dyspnea on exertion and fatigue may suggest cardiac disease or anemia due to blood loss. History of melena, hematemesis points toward peptic ulcer disease. Dysphagia may be due to peptic stricture or malignancy. History of psychiatric disorders and past physical or sexual abuse may be relevant in those with refractory symptoms. History of diabetes and other endocrine disorders in patient/family should be enquired for. Diabetic patients can have gastroparesis and drug- (metformin, acarbose) induced dyspepsia. Improper use of abdominal exercise

techniques like *kapalbhati* (a yogic breathing exercise) may be responsible for aggravation of dyspepsia in some (personal experience).
- *Physical examination*: A detailed physical examination to be done. Presence of anemia, lymphadenopathy, abdominal lump, or ascites requires further evaluation. Succussion splash in epigastrium in a fasting patient may suggest gastric outlet obstruction or gastroparesis. Per rectal examination may show presence of blood in stools and rectal shelf deposits.

INTERPRETATION OF FINDINGS

Investigations

Young, otherwise normal patient on examination, need not to undergo any further evaluation. Age more than 50 years old; family history of malignancy; history of NSAID use; and presence of alarm features like GI bleed, anemia, dysphagia, and weight loss warrants further workup.

Initial workup consists of complete blood counts, creatinine, thyroid-stimulating hormone (TSH), blood sugar, electrolytes, calcium, liver function tests, and ultrasound of abdomen. Upper GI endoscopy is very useful and needs to be done to look for mucosal lesions. Gastric biopsy from antral region and rapid urease test for *Helicobacter pylori* can be done. At the same time, bleeding lesions can be endoscopically treated and stricture dilatation can be done. Barium examination and serology for *Helicobacter pylori* can be done wherever access to endoscopy is not available. Endoscopy is superior to barium studies in detecting mucosal lesions.

Stool test for ova, parasites, and occult blood to be done. Contrast-enhanced computed tomography (CECT) of abdomen, and manometry (esophageal and antroduodenal) are required in specific circumstances.

TREATMENT

Clinical decision to initial treatment depends on age and presence of risk factors. Young patients without any alarm features can be directly given empirical therapy with acid antisecretory medication: histamine 2-receptor antagonists (H2RAs) and proton pump inhibitors (PPIs). Both are efficient in relieving symptoms in 33–50% patients of dyspepsia, particularly in those with predominant reflux-like symptoms. Usual doses are ranitidine 150 mg BD, omeprazole 10–20 mg/day, rabeprazole 20–40 mg/day, and lansoprazole 15–30 mg/day, etc. Lafutidine is a second-generation H2RA with additional gastroprotective ability independent of antisecretory action. It activates capsaicin sensitive afferent neurons and stimulates calcitonin gene-related peptide (CGRP) which inhibits acid secretion and stimulate mucosal blood flow. Therapeutic benefits of H2RA and PPI in FD seems independent of antisecretory action.

Dietary modification and lifestyle changes should be advised in every patient. It includes eating small meals and avoiding high-fat diet. Patient should be told to avoid tea, coffee, NSAID, alcohol, and tobacco use.

Helicobacter pylori eradication can improve dyspepsia in few patients. Test and treat infection can be a strategy in those not responding to PPI. Those responding will have long-term sustained remission.

Prokinetic agents stimulate GI motility and hence may be helpful in functional dyspepsia. Metoclopramide, levosulpiride, and domperidone are dopamine receptor antagonists. Domperidone does not cross blood–brain barrier and is devoid of serious side effects. Levosulpiride additionally acts as 5-HT4 receptor agonist and is superior to other two in improving gastric emptying and alleviate dyspepsia. However, these drugs have lot of adverse effects including extrapyramidal symptoms, galactorrhea. Mosapride is a 5-HT4 agonist and 5-HT3 receptor antagonist and itopride is dopamine D2 antagonist and acetylcholinesterase inhibitor. Acotiamide is a new prokinetic and fundus relaxing drug with muscarinic antagonist and cholinesterase inhibitor action and improves gastric emptying. In doses of 100 mg thrice daily, it improves postprandial fullness, bloating, and early satiety. It is now approved for managing functional dyspepsia. It is not effective in EPS. Drugs like erythromycin which have pure prokinetic effect without antiemetic effect are not found useful.

Antidepressants especially tricyclic antidepressants have some beneficial effects in functional dyspepsia (EPS) even in absence of depression and can be added to PPI in nonresponders. Anxiolytic agent buspirone, a 5-HT1A agonist, was superior to placebo in improving dyspeptic symptoms. It enhances gastric accommodation by fundic relaxation.

Psychological interventions like cognitive therapy, hypnotherapy, and relaxation techniques may be useful in refractory patients. Meditation and yoga can also help. Referral to psychiatrist can be considered in those with associated severe psychiatric symptoms.

Rikkunshito, a Japanese herbal medicine has shown better response than placebo for treatment of FD. Another herbal preparation Iberogast (STW5), extract from *Iberis amara* plant, has fundus relaxing properties and has shown efficacy in FD in double-blind, placebo-controlled studies.

SUMMARY

Dyspepsia is a very common condition defined as epigastric pain or discomfort. Rarely, may it be a manifestation of a serious condition like malignancy. Identification of red flag signs can help in planning further management. Those with no red flags can be treated with empirical PPI initially and investigate further if no response. Management of refractory dyspepsia requires multidisciplinary approach.

CHAPTER 31

Dysphagia

Amit Mittal, Anukalp Prakash

DEFINITION

Dysphagia is an alarm symptom that requires identification of its cause and initiation of the treatment. Dysphagia, from the Greek word *dys* (difficulty, disordered) and *phagia* (to eat), refers to the sensation that food is "hindered" in passage from the mouth to the stomach. Most patients complain that food sticks, hangs up, or stops, or they feel that the food "just would not go down right." Odynophagia is painful swallowing. Globus sensation (e.g. sensation of retained food bolus, lump, etc.) is functional disorder seen commonly in women.

Food impaction (most commonly beef, chicken) is the usual etiology of acute onset dysphagia, more seen in males with increasing age especially in 7th decade of life. Management is done by upper endoscopy guided removal of food bolus by grasping devices. Nonacute dysphagia includes oropharyngeal and esophageal dysphagia.

PATHOPHYSIOLOGY

The swallowing difficulty can be caused by a problem with the strength or coordination of the muscles required to move food bolus from the mouth to the stomach or by a fixed obstruction anywhere between the mouth and the stomach. The food bolus is transported from mouth to stomach within 10 seconds with the help of the primary and secondary peristalsis of esophagus and the oropharyngeal swallowing mechanism. Dysphagia is caused by failure of development and progression of orderly oropharyngeal and/or esophageal muscular contractions. Dysphagia may occur due to low amplitude esophageal contractions causing inadequate clearance of esophagus, especially in elderly.

Mechanical obstruction of the esophageal lumen may hinder the orderly passage of a food bolus despite good peristaltic contractions. Symptoms differ with the degree of luminal narrowing, associated esophagitis and type of food ingested. Minimally obstructing lesions cause dysphagia only to large, poorly chewed boluses of food whereas the lesions which obstruct the lumen completely lead to symptoms with solids and liquids.

CATEGORIES

Anatomic versus Motility

Anatomic causes of dysphagia are usually those that cause esophageal luminal narrowing, e.g. benign or malignant, oropharyngeal or distal esophageal, mucosal, intramural or extrinsic to the esophagus. Common mechanical causes of dysphagia include esophageal stricture, head and neck or esophageal malignancies, and extrinsic compression secondary to mediastinal lymph nodes. Patients with mechanical dysphagia will have symptoms primarily with ingestion of solid, large food bolus with dense consistency.

In contrast, patients with motility-associated dysphagia are more likely to have symptoms with both solids and liquids as the propulsion of both solids and liquids is affected by altered neuromuscular forces. Motility disorders requiring greater esophageal contractile amplitude may start with solids but eventually involve liquids with disease progression. In oropharyngeal disorders, liquids may be more problematic than solids because of easier entry to the airway causing severe cough during swallowing and recurrent chest infections due to aspiration. Typical disorders of motility are achalasia or oropharyngeal dysfunction secondary to a cerebrovascular accident.

Upper Esophageal versus Mid and Lower Esophageal

The location of the patient's symptoms does not correlate well with the location of esophageal dysfunction. This has been found both clinically and through balloon distention experimentations and by radiographic impaction of a marshmallow in the distal esophagus leads to a highly variable symptom location among individuals. The factors that help determine the location are associated symptoms apart from dysphagia due to oropharyngeal dysfunctions. For example, in patients with dysphagia due to lower cranial nerves palsy will also give history of associated change in voice, nasal regurgitation, and coughing after swallowing due to aspiration.

Organ-specific versus Involvement by Another Disease

It is important to differentiate that symptoms are due to esophagus-specific disease or a systemic disease affecting the esophagus. For example, systemic neuromuscular diseases, such as scleroderma, may cause dysphagia of the lower esophagus, whereas amyotrophic lateral sclerosis or myasthenia gravis may affect oropharyngeal function. Lichen planus or Crohn's disease may lead to narrowing of esophageal lumen causing mechanical dysphagia whereas others may cause luminal narrowing due to extrinsic compression. As a result, detection of an esophageal disorder leading to dysphagia may not just stop at the esophagus.

DIAGNOSTIC APPROACH

History

Oropharyngeal or transfer dysphagia: Within 1 second of swallowing associated with cough, drooling of saliva, nasal regurgitation, choking.

Esophageal dysphagia: More than 1 second after swallowing:
- Onset (sudden, e.g. foreign body ingestion, acute esophagitis or gradual)
- Types of food, e.g. solids, liquids or both
- Progression (progressive, e.g. neoplasm, peptic stricture or intermittent, e.g. mucosal ring, web)

- Other symptoms such as loss of appetite, weight loss, fresh or old blood in vomitus, chest pain
- Medical problems like diabetes, scleroderma, overlap syndrome, acquired immunodeficiency syndrome (AIDS), stroke, myasthenia gravis, multiple sclerosis
- Frequency and severity (symptoms daily or not)
- Aggravating factors (hot or cold liquids, e.g. spastic esophageal disease)
- Relieving factors (repeated swallowing, raising arms over head, Valsalva maneuver, e.g. motility disorder)
- Ingestion of corrosives, pills, e.g. antibiotics like doxycycline, tetracycline, clindamycin, potassium chloride, alendronate, ascorbic acid, nonsteroidal anti-inflammatory drugs (NSAIDs), ferrous sulfate, quinidine (pill esophagitis)
- Treatment history in the past, e.g. surgery on larynx, esophagus, spine or radiation therapy
- Symptoms now (better or worse).

It is important to emphasize that patient with chronic diseases commonly learn techniques to adapt to their symptoms and thus ease the difficulty that attends this problem. As a result, it is important in collecting further history to inquire about compensatory mechanisms that reduce the frequency and severity of dysphagia. Such patients start eating slowly, and usually are last to finish their meals and avoid problematic food.

Patients also adapt to facilitate bolus passage. For example, patient with solid food dysphagia may give history of drinking water with every bite to facilitate bolus passage. Patients also learn techniques to clear impacted bolus. History of dysphagia must also include any family history of similar symptoms. Psychogenic dysphagia is characterized by oral apraxia, intact speech and pharyngoesophageal and neurological function.

Algorithm for evaluation of dysphagia symptoms has been shown in **Flowchart 1** and disorders causing oropharyngeal dysphagia have been depicted in **Table 1**.

Physical Examination

- Examine cranial nerves
- Look for proximal or asymmetric extremity weakness, dysarthria, tremor, fasciculation, and cognitive dysfunction
- Oral examination (thrush, e.g. candidal infection) is also necessary. Clues to the cause of dysphagia might include poor dentition, buccal lesions such as lichen planus, tongue fasciculations, asymmetrical palate elevation, and labial drop
- Suspect malignancy in patients over 40 years of age with thin built, anemia, mass or Virchow's node
- Koilonychia suggests postcricoid web (Plummer-Vinson syndrome)
- Hepatomegaly in case of suspected esophageal cancer suggests liver metastasis
- Chest examination to look for aspiration pneumonia in case of oropharyngeal dysphagia and suspected tracheoesophageal fistula secondary to esophageal cancer.

Bedside Testing

Watch the patient swallowing in the office. Observation of deglutination of a simple glass of water or bite of a solid food can give a lot of information on the patient's dysphagia. Patients

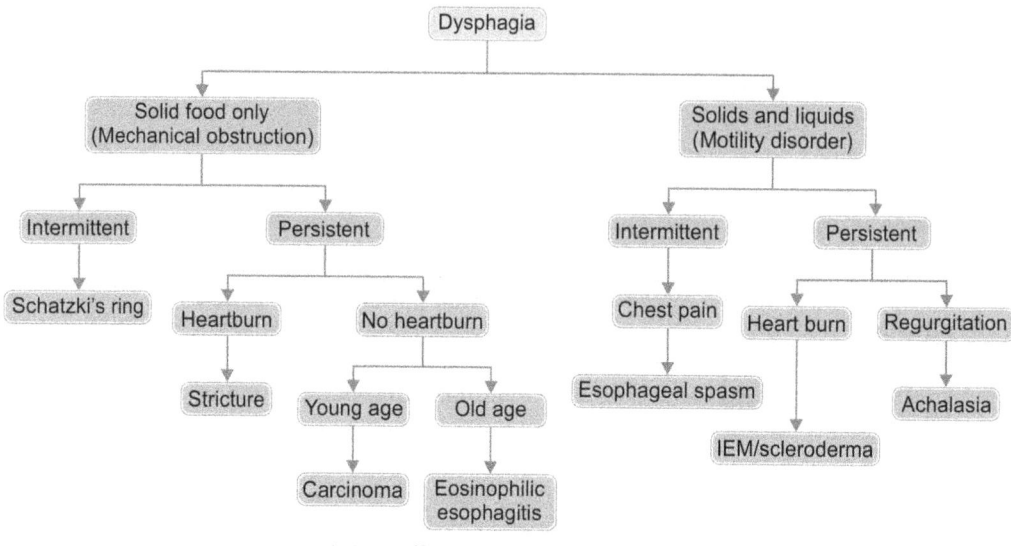

Flowchart 1: Algorithm for evaluation of dysphagia symptoms.

(IEM: ineffective esophageal motility)

Table 1: Disorders causing oropharyngeal dysphagia.

Anatomic	Neurological	Muscular
Zenker's diverticulum	Cerebrovascular accident	Polymyositis
Tumor	Post-polio syndrome	Myasthenia gravis
Enlarged thyroid	Radiation injury	Muscular dystrophy
Web	Parkinsonism	Radiation injury
Osteophytes	Head/Neck surgery	Head/Neck surgery
Abscess	Multiple sclerosis	Thyroid disease
Head/Neck surgery	Botulism	
	Supranuclear palsy	
	Amyotrophic lateral sclerosis	

commonly underestimate their degree of difficulty, but it may be revealed by observations such as multiple swallows required for a single bolus, the use of small sips of fluid or small bites of a solid, post-deglutitive throat clearing, and a general fear of swallowing.

INVESTIGATIONS

Barium Swallow versus Endoscopy

These investigations are complementary to each rather than being duplicative. Pre-endoscopy barium esophagogram is the initial test in patients with dysphagia with history of previous surgery for laryngeal/esophageal cancer, Zenker's diverticulum because blind intubation of proximal esophagus during upper endoscopy carries a risk of perforation. For distal esophageal motility disorders such as achalasia or scleroderma involving the esophagus, barium evaluation is superior to endoscopy. Barium swallow is also superior for detection of esophageal strictures. Prior esophagogram also helps to plan an endoscopic procedure, e.g. in a case of tight esophageal stricture it helps determine the need of fluoroscopy and type of dilation required.

The upper gastrointestinal (GI) endoscopy is required for diagnosing underlying cause of dysphagia, take biopsy from growth or stricture and to perform a therapeutic procedure, e.g. dilatation of stricture, stent placement. Patient with normal upper endoscopy should be evaluated with barium esophagogram to look for missed lesions, e.g. lower esophageal rings or extrinsic compression of esophagus.

High-resolution Impedance Manometry

It shall be done in case of normal upper endoscopy or on suspicion of esophageal motility disorders, e.g. achalasia cardia. This procedure (36 transducers spaced at 1 cm distributed longitudinally in esophagus) is more accurate than conventional esophageal manometry (only few transducers spaced at 3–5 cm) as it provides panesophageal pressure tracing described through a colorimetric graphic presentation (the Clouse plot). It provides assessment of sphincters and body with a single series of swallows. The final interpretation of this procedure helps in differentiating various esophageal motility disorders and determining subtypes of a particular motility disorder, e.g. achalasia cardia and plan for best treatment option (type II achalasia responds best to pneumatic dilatation) available. Ordering the appropriate diagnostic test by the referring physician helps in eliciting the next step in management of the patient's dysphagia.

SPECIFIC DISORDERS CAUSING DYSPHAGIA

Neuromuscular Diseases

The swallowing is a complex phenomenon which involves a coordinated function of brain, cranial nerve, and muscle. Any disturbance causing neural or muscular dysfunction can cause oropharyngeal dysphagia, e.g. Cerebrovascular accidents, Parkinson's disease, and progressive supranuclear palsy. Examples of primary striated muscle disease are inclusion body myositis, myasthenia gravis, and polymyositis. Management is based on treating the cause, e.g. cricopharyngeal myotomy in primary cricopharyngeal dysfunction and botulinum toxin injection in achalasia cardia.

Stricturing Diseases

Luminal narrowing of esophagus due to causes like caustic ingestion, peptic stricture causes dysphagia. Approximately 15% patients are found to have eosinophilic esophagitis. It typically affects children, adolescents, and young adults. Endoscopic findings include stacked circular rings, stricture, linear furrows, white papules, small caliber esophagus.

Esophageal Cancer

Adenocarcinoma is one of the most rapidly increasing cancers in Western society, now far outnumbering previously common squamous cell carcinoma. Barrett's esophagus is the most dominant precursor to adenocarcinoma. Dysphagia symptoms may be insidious and progressive. Other alarm symptoms that may accompany dysphagia include weight loss, anorexia, and hematemesis.

Cardiovascular Abnormalities

Vascular abnormalities compressing the esophagus are rare, e.g. double aortic arch, right aortic arch with retroesophageal left subclavian artery, large aneurysm of thoracic aorta impinging esophagus. Symptoms usually develop during childhood but they may also develop in adults.

Achalasia

Primary achalasia is disease of unknown cause characterized by loss of normal peristalsis in distal esophagus and a failure of lower esophageal sphincter relaxation with swallowing. It can occur at any age but usually diagnosed between 25 years and 60 years of age. On radiography, patients have a dilated esophagus with an incompletely opening lower esophageal sphincter, i.e. bird beak appearance. Upper endoscopy is done to exclude pseudoachalasia. Diagnosis is confirmed by esophageal manometry.

CHAPTER 32

Dyspnea

Chitra Mehta, Srinivas Monanga

INTRODUCTION

Dyspnea or shortness of breath is one of the most common presenting symptoms to the emergency department (ED). It has been observed to be reported in 50% of patients admitted in tertiary, acute care hospitals. It is one of the most dreaded symptoms to evaluate in ED. It needs to be worked up in matter of minutes as it may depict a potentially life-threatening event.

It has been defined by American Thoracic Society as "a subjective experience of breathing discomfort that consists of qualitatively distinct sensation that varies in intensity."

It has a lot of subjective overlay. So it becomes really challenging to make a rapid and accurate diagnosis, and differentiate it from the objective component.

Assessment of severity of dyspnea is very crucial as it shows the acuteness of situation, and also aids in triaging of patients to appropriate destination.

Various validated dyspnea scales available which are easy to use in, and are general or disease specific. Most popular is the New York Heart Association (NYHA) classification which is specific for chronic congestive heart failure. Another clinical scale "modified Medical Research Council" scale is also commonly used for the assessment of dyspnea in patients with chronic lung disease. Other scales are descriptions of intensity based such as visual analog scale and Borg scale. There is another multidimensional questionnaire-based scale, i.e. "Multidimensional Dyspnea Profile" scale. These scales aid physicians in understanding life-threatening or benign nature of the presenting dyspnea.

PATHOPHYSIOLOGY

Dyspnea is usually the end result if a stimulus activates the respiratory center beyond a certain threshold. Hypoxemia stimulates the carotid receptors, hypercapnia stimulates the medullary chemoreceptors, decreased compliance results in stimulating the mechanoreceptors in diaphragm, chest wall and airway, and airway resistance stimulates the airway receptors.

ETIOLOGY

The first step while evaluating dyspnea is to understand whether it is a new problem or pre-existent problem, or it is an exacerbation of a chronic lung disease, or may be a combination

Box 1: Common causes of acute onset dyspnea in emergency department.

Upper airway
- Foreign body
- Laryngeal edema
- Laryngospasm
- Anaphylaxis
- Epiglottitis.

Lower respiratory tract
- Acute asthma
- Acute exacerbation of chronic obstructive pulmonary disease (COPD)
- Pulmonary embolism
- Pneumonia
- Pneumothorax
- Massive pleural effusion
- Interstitial lung disease especially acute interstitial pneumonia
- Acute hypersensitivity pneumonitis
- Drug-induced lung disease
- Acute aspiration
- Acute respiratory distress syndrome (ARDS).

Cardiac
- Acute coronary syndrome
- Cardiac tamponade
- Arrhythmias
- Valvular heart disease
- Heart failure with reduced ejection fraction.

Others
- Metabolic acidosis
- Severe pain
- Myasthenic crisis
- Neuromuscular disorders like Guillain-Barré syndrome
- Amniotic fluid embolism
- Fat embolism
- Chest trauma
- Drug reaction
- Carbon monoxide poisoning
- Anxiety and panic attacks.

of both. Urgent decisions are needed in presence of acute dyspnea especially if severe. **Box 1** enlists the most common causes of acute dyspnea in ED.

These acute causes may be complicating a chronic lung disease state. Causes of chronic dyspnea are listed in **Box 2**.

EVALUATION OF DYSPNEA

After ensuring airway, breathing, and circulation of the patient, one proceeds to evaluation of dyspnea by taking a good history. Unfortunately, it is found to be accurate in about 56% for all causes (47% for pulmonary causes and 67% for cardiac causes). Combining physical

Box 2: Common causes of chronic dyspnea.

Pulmonary
- Chronic obstructive pulmonary disease
- Bronchial asthma
- Interstitial lung disease
- Chronic pulmonary thromboembolism
- Occupational lung disease
- Obstructive sleep apnea (OSA).

Cardiac
- Congestive heart failure
- Coronary artery disease
- Valvular heart disease.

Others
- Anemia
- Gastroesophageal reflux disease
- Thyroid disorders
- Chronic renal failure
- Neuromuscular causes.

examination and chest X-ray with history has been found to increase the accuracy to about 66% for all causes, and in 27% of cases the chest X-ray reveals a serious finding. Of all, it is the acute dyspnea in ED which is most worrisome and needs a quick workup (**Table 1**).

There are some less common causes of acute dyspnea which should be kept in mind like:
- Anemia
- Aortic dissection
- Pulmonary tumors
- Vocal cord dysfunction
- Hepatopulmonary syndrome
- Pulmonary arteriovenous malformations
- Pleuritis
- Arrhythmias
- Acquired valvular heart disease
- Methemoglobinemia and carbon monoxide poisoning
- Tetanus
- Thrombotic thrombocytopenic purpura
- Pericardial disease
- Myasthenia gravis
- Guillain-Barré syndrome
- Kyphoscoliosis and pectus excavatum
- Pheochromocytoma.

The key to diagnosis lies at the corroboration of findings on history, physical examination, and chest X-ray. After drawing a differential diagnosis, various diagnostic tests can be performed in order to establish the definite cause.

Table 1: History, clinical examination, and X-ray findings of most common etiologies of acute dyspnea.

Disease	History	Clinical examination	Chest X-ray
Chronic obstructive pulmonary disease	Chronic productive cough, chronic dyspnea, exposure to smoke, occupational exposure to fumes and chemicals, recent history of fever, sore throat, increase in sputum, and change in color of sputum	Facial plethora, pursed lip breathing, tripod position, diffuse wheezing, pulsus paradoxus, altered mentation, cyanosis, barrel-shaped chest, silent chest, and tachypnea	Hyperinflated chest, flattened diaphragms in emphysema
Asthma	Episodic seasonal wheezing, family history may be positive, history of recent viral infection, fever, sore throat, and exposure to allergens	Diffuse wheezing, silent chest, tachycardia, tachypnea, and cyanosis	Hyperinflated chest
Pneumonia	Fever, chills, cough with sputum, pleuritic chest pain, may be of 2–3 weeks duration especially in tuberculosis or fungal pneumonia, and hemoptysis	Bronchial breathing, inspiratory crepitations, cyanosis, and altered mentation	Lobar consolidation with air bronchogram, or bilateral diffuse infiltrates
Pulmonary embolism	Sudden onset dyspnea, chest pain, hemoptysis, prolonged immobilization, neoplastic disease, injury to leg, pregnancy, or child birth	Hypotension, tachycardia, neck vein engorgement, lower extremity edema, and calf tenderness	Normal or Hampton's hump, Westermark sign, and prominent pulmonary arteries
Acute coronary syndrome	Pericardial chest pain, palpitations, feeling of impending doom, radiation of pain to left arm, diabetes, and history of stroke	Cold clammy extremities, hypotension, S3 or S4 gallop rhythm, bilateral crepitations, and ejection systolic murmur	Bilateral diffuse infiltrates, batwing appearance
Pulmonary edema	Orthopnea, paroxysmal nocturnal dyspnea, chest pain, ankle swelling, end-stage renal, and liver disease	Bilateral fine rales, distended neck veins, S3 gallop rhythm, cyanosis, and altered mentation	Bilateral diffuse infiltrates, batwing appearance
Acute respiratory distress syndrome	Acute onset dyspnea, history of febrile illness, trauma, near drowning, aspiration, smoke inhalation from house fire, burns, blood transfusions medication reactions, and radiotherapy	Tachycardia, tachypnea, cyanosis, bilateral crepitations, and hypotension	Bilateral diffuse lung infiltrates
Pneumothorax	Sudden onset dyspnea with unilateral chest pain, retroviral positive, and history of cocaine use	Unilateral absence of breath sounds, tympanic note on percussion, and distended neck veins	Collapsed lung and unilateral lucidity ± mediastinal shift to contralateral side
Anxiety and panic attacks	Most common seen in young females, both sexes can be involved, previous history of anxiety or antidepressants or phobias, and discomfort in various locations	Tachycardia, tachypnea, normal oxygen saturation, sweating, frequent sighs, Chvostek sign, and Trousseau sign may be present	Normal

Contd...

Contd...

Disease	History	Clinical examination	Chest X-ray
Pulmonary contusion	History of blunt or penetrating trauma, hemoptysis	Focal decreased breath sounds, chest tenderness, and paradoxical breathing	Focal inhomogeneous opacity, with or without hemothorax
Alveolar hemorrhage	History of cough, fever, hemoptysis, anemia, and history of mitral valve disease	Tachypnea, tachycardia, ± diastolic murmur of mitral stenosis, and bilateral crepitations	Bilateral alveolar infiltrates

DIAGNOSTIC WORKUP

There are some basic investigations which are suggested for all dyspneic patients in ED. They are hemogram, D-dimer, pulse oximetry, renal function test, liver function test, electrolytes, chest X-ray, arterial blood gas (ABG) analysis, electrocardiogram (ECG), and echocardiography. These help in narrowing down the diagnosis and focus on only some specific differential causes. Some people like to measure biomarkers right at the admission like procalcitonin, B-type natriuretic peptide (BNP). Need of various investigations is dictated by the clinical context.

Pulse Oximetry

This allows detection of hypoxemia and presence of respiratory failure. Oxygen saturation may be normal in patients with anxiety, pulmonary embolism among the acute causes.

Arterial Blood Gas Analysis

This is another important investigation for dyspnea which serves various purposes. Firstly it aids in defining the type of respiratory failure, secondly it gives an idea about the severity, thirdly it defines presence of acidemia or alkalemia assisting in narrowing the differential list, and last but not the least, it sometimes may clinch the diagnosis of methemoglobinemia by either depicting mismatch between the partial pressure of oxygen in the blood and oxygen saturation by pulse oximetry, or by directly measuring the methemoglobin levels. Hypercapnia may point toward diseases like chronic obstructive pulmonary disease (COPD), asthma, obstructive sleep apnea, upper airway obstruction, or neuromuscular disease. Hypocapnia is present in acute respiratory distress syndrome (ARDS), pulmonary embolism, interstitial lung disease, pneumonia, and asthma. It basically indicates hyperventilation. Metabolic acidosis may point toward renal failure, sepsis, poisoning, and cyanide toxicity to name a few.

Arterial blood gas proves sometimes invaluable for suspecting pulmonary embolism in a patient with near normal oxygen saturation by pulse oximetry. In presence of near normal oxygen saturation, elevated alveolar-arterial oxygen gradient (A-aDO$_2$) may be the first clue pointing toward pulmonary embolism.

Other Investigations

Leukocytosis points toward an underlying infection most of the times. Eosinophilia may be observed in asthmatics, parasitic infections, and certain vasculitides. Anemia may be suspected as the primary cause. Thrombocytopenia generally indicates viral infections, thrombotic thrombocytopenic purpura, and adverse drug reaction. Deranged liver function tests may be seen in congestive heart failure, dengue, liver failure, atypical pneumonia (especially legionella pneumonia), acute myocardial infarction, viral infection, etc.

Deranged kidney function test may be the end result of primary pathology, or renal failure may be the primary cause of dyspnea.

Elevated troponin I/T, creatine kinase muscle-brain (CK-MB) may be present in myocarditis, takotsubo cardiomyopathy apart from acute myocardial infarction. Generally, in these conditions, elevated BNP levels are also seen. Elevated serum procalcitonin levels in presence of leukocytosis increase the confidence in sepsis as the primary etiology.

After the trimming of the differential list is done with the help of history, examination, chest X-ray and basic investigations, definitive tests are ordered. The list is long and may include high-resolution computed tomography (HRCT) of the chest, CT pulmonary angiography, venous Doppler of the limbs, ventilation perfusion scan, Holter monitoring, bronchoalveolar lavage, lung biopsy, chest fluoroscopy to demonstrate diaphragmatic paralysis, and sleep study to name a few.

ROLE OF ULTRASOUND IN DYSPNEIC PATIENTS

Recent times have seen a prominent role of ultrasound in evaluation of dyspnea in ED. Presence of B lines, lung sliding, pleural effusion, lung point, and inferior vena cava (IVC) diameter help in establishing the definitive diagnosis. Coupled with echocardiography, it may help physicians to arrive at primary cause in most of the cases.

MANAGEMENT

Treatment is directed toward the underlying cause. Adequate oxygenation should be ensured, and noninvasive or invasive ventilatory support should be started in presence of excessive work of breathing when appropriate. Bronchodilators and steroids with or without antibiotics are indicated in presence of acute asthma or acute exacerbation of COPD. Diuretics and antihypertensives should be started in presence of pulmonary edema. Antibiotics should be prescribed in case pneumonia or any other infection is suspected. Patients with pneumothorax or pleural effusion would need a tube thoracotomy. Anticoagulants should be started in case of pulmonary embolism.

Flowchart 1: Approach to patient with acute dyspnea in emergency department.

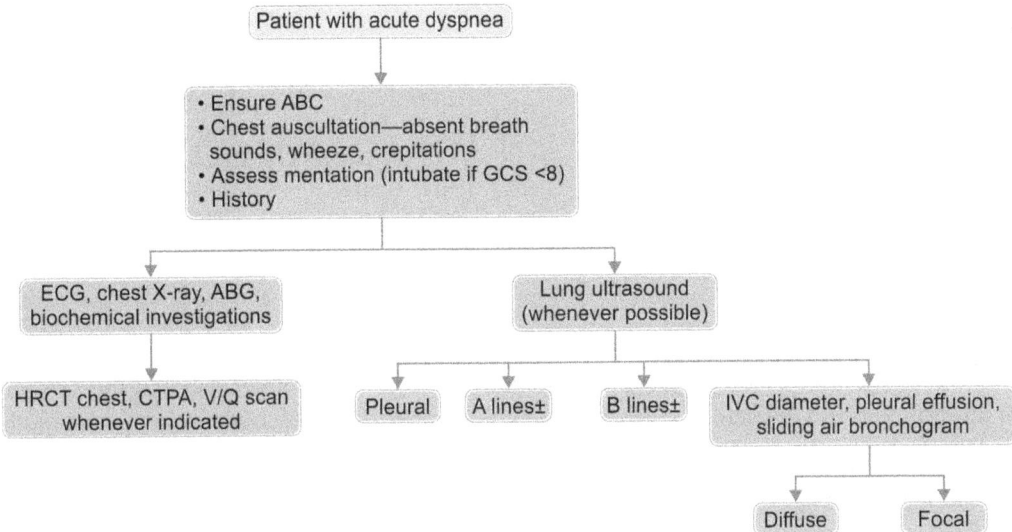

(ABC: airway, breathing, and circulation; ABG: arterial blood gas; CTPA: computed tomographic pulmonary angiography; ECG: electrocardiogram; GCS: Glasgow Coma Score; HRCT: high-resolution computed tomography; IVC: inferior vena cava; V/Q scan: ventilation-perfusion scan)

SUMMARY

Acute dyspnea is one of the most challenging conditions in ED. A thorough history, good clinical examination, appropriate laboratory investigations, and proper triaging are essential for its prudent evaluation and management. An approach to a patient with acute onset dyspnea is suggested in **Flowchart 1**.

CHAPTER 33

Earache

Deepak Dalmia, Sanjaya Bahera

■ INTRODUCTION

Earache is otherwise called otalgia. An earache may affect one or both ears. It may be constant or intermittent, and the pain may be dull or sharp. Earache can affect both children and adults and can be due to the disease related to the ear or referred from the other parts of the head and neck region.

■ ETIOLOGY

Disease-related Primary to the Ear
- Ear wax (impacted)
- External ear infection (otitis externa)
- Middle ear infection (otitis media)
- Foreign body in the ear
- Barotrauma
- Tympanic membrane rupture
- Inner ear disease: acoustic neuroma, Meniere's disease.

Disease in Head and Neck Causing Referred Pain in Ear
- Sinusitis
- Pharyngitis
- Laryngitis
- Tonsillitis
- Supraglottic growth
- Thyroiditis
- Temporomandibular (TMJ) arthralgia
- Trigeminal neuralgia
- Impacted tooth.

■ PATHOPHYSIOLOGY

Earache can occur because of the disease process within the ear itself or referred pain from any other head and neck pathology.

Pain from ear results due to a pressure gradient between middle ear and external ear because of Eustachian tube dysfunction (ETD). ETD leads to disequilibrium in middle ear pressure and atmospheric pressure and allows accumulation of fluid in middle ear. This results in inflammation and bulging of tympanic membrane (TM) causing pain.

Referred pain in ear occurs due to pathologies of nose and paranasal sinuses, teeth, tonsil, pharynx, larynx, mandible, trachea, esophagus, 5th, 9th, and 10th cranial nerves which also supplies the ear.

CLINICAL PRESENTATION
Symptoms
- Ear pain
- Fullness of ear
- Discharge from the ear
- Nose blockage or discharge from nose (sinusitis)
- Throat pain (tonsillitis, pharyngitis, laryngitis)
- Pain on TMJ joint (TMJ arthralgia)
- Pain on front of neck (thyroiditis)
- Dental pain (caries tooth).

Signs
- Fever
- Otoscopic examination (wax or otomycosis)
- Perforated tympanic membrane (traumatic)
- Fluid behind the ear with impending rupture of tympanic membrane [acute suppurative otitis media (ASOM)]
- Throat examination:
  - Inflamed tonsils, pharynx, and larynx
  - Neck examination: For thyroiditis and lymphadenopathy.

RED FLAGS
- Diabetes and other immunocompromised disease
- Mastoiditis with protrusion of auricle
- Edema of external auditory canal (EAC)
- Pain associated with other head and neck pathology.

EVALUATION
- History
- Location
- Duration
- Severity

- Intermittent or constant
- Associated with jaw movements or pain throat
- Any history of repeated ear cleaning
- History of foreign body impaction
- Recent scuba diving or swimming
- Past medical history as diabetes or another immunocompromised
- Physical examination:
  - Vital signs
  - Fever
  - Complete examination of ear, nose, and throat
  - Mastoid tenderness and forward displacement of pinna
  - Otoscopic examination
  - TM joint examination
  - Complete head and neck examination.

INTERPRETATION OF FINDINGS

If otoscopic examination shows disease in external auditory canal or tympanic membrane or accumulation of fluid behind the tympanic membrane then the cause is related to the ear.

Patient with normal ear examination may suffer from tonsillitis or pharyngitis or laryngitis.

Patient with severe sharp pain of ear for few minutes may be due to neuralgic pain.

Each patient should be examined for head and neck cancers if tympanic membrane is normal.

INVESTIGATIONS

- History
- ENT examination
- Physical examination
- In case of diabetes with otitis externa, magnetic resonance imaging (MRI) may be needed.
- In case of otitis media, a high resolution computed tomography (HRCT) of temporal bone may be needed.

TREATMENT

Oral analgesics, usually a nonsteroidal anti-inflammatory drug (NSAID) or acetaminophen, to reduce the pain. In cases of severe otitis externa, opioids may be used.

In otitis externa, treatment requires suction of debris from the ear canal and insertion of a medicated wick to allow for delivery of antibiotic ear drops to the infected tissue along with oral antibiotics.

Patients should be instructed to avoid digging in their objects. Also, patients should not irrigate their ears unless instructed by a physician to do so, and as instructed by physician.

Underlying immunocompromised status and systemic diseases should be dealt with care.

SUMMARY
- History and physical examination is paramount for diagnosis of etiology.
- Otologic causes mostly due to infection of external ear and middle ear.
- When otoscopic examination is normal, one should search for nonotological causes.

OTITIS EXTERNA (SWIMMER'S EAR)

Introduction
Otitis externa is an acute infection of the ear canal skin typically caused by bacteria. External otitis may manifest as a localized furuncle or as a diffuse infection of the entire canal (swimmer's ear).

Etiology
- Moisture (swimming, perspiration, high humidity)
- Allergies
- Psoriasis
- Eczema
- Seborrheic dermatitis
- Irritants
- Inadvertent injury to the canal caused by cleaning with cotton swabs or other objects (finger nails, hearing aid, ear plugs).

Pathophysiology
- External otitis is usually caused by bacteria, such as *Pseudomonas aeruginosa*, *Proteus vulgaris*, *Staphylococcus aureus*, or *Escherichia coli*.
- Fungal external otitis (otomycosis), typically caused by *Aspergillus niger*.
- Furuncles usually are caused by *Staphylococcus aureus*.

Clinical Presentation

Symptoms
- Ear pain and discharge
- Hearing loss if the canal becomes swollen or filled with purulent debris
- Itching (lobomycosis).

Signs
- Tragal tenderness
- Otoscopic examination is painful and difficult to conduct and shows the ear canal to be red, swollen, and littered with moist, purulent debris and desquamated epithelium.
- Furuncles cause severe pain and may drain sanguineous, purulent material. They appear as a focal, erythematous swelling (pimple).

Red Flags
- Diabetes
- Immunocompromised state
- Associated other cranial nerve palsy.

Evaluation
Otoscopic Examination
- The canal appears red and swollen.
- The ear canal shows scaly shedding of skin.
- Tragal tenderness (touching or moving the outer ear increases the pain).
- It may be difficult to see the tympanic membrane with an otoscope at the initial examination because of narrowing of the ear canal.
- The culture of the discharge may identify the bacteria or fungus causing infection.
- In severe cases of external otitis, there may be enlargement of preauricular and postauricular lymph nodes.

Investigation
- Otoscopic examination
- MRI skull base and HRCT temporal bone if associated with lower cranial nerve palsy.

Treatment
- *Cleaning of ear:* For direct contact of medication with the EAC.
- *Mild external otitis:* 2% acetic acid and by relieving inflammation with topical hydrocortisone.
- Moderate external otitis requires the addition of an antibacterial solution or suspension, such as ciprofloxacin, ofloxacin, or neomycin/polymyxin.
- Medicated ear wick should be placed into the ear canal and wetted with Burow solution (5% aluminum acetate) or a topical antibiotic 4 times/day. The wick is left in place for 48 hours.
- Severe otitis externa associated with the presence of cellulitis extending beyond the ear canal may require systemic antibiotics (fluoroquinolones and third generation cephalosporins).
- Fungal external otitis requires thorough cleaning of the ear canal and application of an antimycotic solution (e.g. gentian violet, cresylate acetate, nystatin, clotrimazole), dry ear.
- A furuncle should be drained and a medicated wick pack is to be applied.

Summary
- Acute external otitis is usually bacterial.
- Tragal tenderness is an important sign for diagnosis of external otitis.
- Gentle removal of the debris (desquamated epithelial cells or fungal debris) is required before application of wick pack.

For severe external otitis, look for the immunocompromised status and treatment of choice is debridement along with the IV broad spectrum antibiotic.

OTITIS MEDIA

Introduction

Acute otitis media (AOM) is a bacterial or viral infection of the middle ear, usually accompanying an upper respiratory infection. Otitis media is among the most common issues faced by physicians caring for children. Approximately 80% of children will have at least one episode of acute otitis media.

Chronic otitis media (COM) is a chronic inflammation of the middle ear and mastoid cavity that is characterized by discharge from the middle ear through a perforation of tympanic membrane for at least 6 weeks to 3 months despite of conservative management.

Etiology

Viral or bacterial infection
- Viral infections are often complicated by secondary bacterial infection.
    - In neonates: *Escherichia coli*, and *Staphylococcus aureus* cause AOM.
    - In older infants and children less than 14 years: *Streptococcus pneumoniae*, *Moraxella catarrhalis*, and *Haemophilus influenzae*; Group A β-haemolytic streptococci.

Pathophysiology

- AOM is a complication of ETD that occurs during an acute viral upper respiratory tract infection that creates a negative middle ear pressure leading to accumulation of middle ear fluid.
- Sterile middle ear fluid often get infected with bacteria (in 90% cases) causing pain and ear discharge.

Clinical Presentation

- Initial symptom is otalgia
- Hearing loss
- Infants may get up at night and cry.
- Fever, nausea, and vomiting often occur in young children.
- Otoscopic examination can show a budged and erythematous tympanic membrane.
- Pneumatic otoscopy shows poor mobility of the TM.
- Spontaneous perforation of the TM causes serosanguinous or purulent discharge.

Red Flags

- Age (mostly children)
- Allergies

- Exposure to other respiratory irritants
- Immunodeficiency
- Craniofacial anomaly
- Upper respiratory infection.

Evaluation
- Acute otitis media is diagnosed in patients with acute onset, presence of middle ear effusion, physical evidence of middle ear inflammation, and symptoms such as pain, irritability, or fever.
- Acute otitis media is usually a complication of ETD that occurs during a viral upper respiratory tract infection.
- *Otoscopic examination:* Tympanic membrane is budged or retracted, congested, light reflex is absent in AOM.
- In COM, there is perforation of tympanic membrane (central perforation) or pars flaccida retraction or a posterior superior retraction pocket with cholesteatoma.

Interpretation of Finding
- Presence of acute onset of pain, bulging of the TM and, particularly in children, the presence of signs of middle ear effusion on pneumatic otoscopy—acute otitis media.
- History of otorrhea more than 6 weeks with presence of a central perforation or retraction pocket—chronic otitis media.

Investigation
- History
- *Clinical examination:* Fever
- Otoscopic examination
- Aural swab culture and sensitivity
- *X-ray mastoid (oblique lateral view):* To view mastoid status
- HRCT of temporal bone.

Treatment
Acute Otitis Media
- *Analgesia to reduce pain:* Oral analgesics, such as acetaminophen or ibuprofen.
- *Nasal vasoconstrictors and oral antihistaminics:* For ET patency.
- Antibiotics relieve symptoms quicker and may reduce the chance of residual hearing loss and labyrinthine or intracranial sequelae (amoxicillin or third generation cephalosporins).
- If there is good follow-up, can safely be observed for 48–72 hours and given antibiotics only if no improvement is seen.
- *Myringotomy:* If pain not relieved by vasoconstrictors or analgesics.

Chronic Otitis Media
- Make the ear dry and safe is the first goal to treat COM.
- Adequate suction cleaning of the ear.
- Mixed ear drops and oral antibiotics depending on the aural discharge culture and sensitivity.
- Once ear is dry, plan for tympanoplasty in case of central perforation of tympanic membrane.
- *In case of pars flaccida retraction:* Modified radical mastoidectomy with ossiculoplasty.

Summary
- Give analgesics to reduce pain.
- Antibiotics should be used selectively on the patients based on the age of the patients, severity of symptoms and availability of follow-up.

PERFORATED TYMPANIC MEMBRANE

Introduction
A tympanic membrane perforation is usually a hole in the tympanic membrane which occur because of ear injury, infection, or previous surgery.

Etiology
- Otitis media
- Exposure to loud noise
- Traumatic
- Surgery (myringotomy)
- Barotrauma (sudden change in air pressure).

Pathophysiology
- In otitis media, because of fluid in middle ear, pressure builds up in middle ear which ruptures the tympanic membrane to drain in the stage of resolution.
- Poking the ear canal with a sharp subject can lead to the perforation because of trauma.
- In case of scuba divers and airplane passengers, because of the pressure changes in middle ear and the atmospheric pressure, the thin tympanic membrane ruptures.

Clinical Presentation
- Hearing loss
- Pain
- Discharge from the ear
- Nausea
- Blood from the ear
- Tinnitus (ringing sensation in the ear).

Red Flags
- Associated with vertigo and tinnitus (suggestive of associated inner ear trauma)
- Facial weakness.

Evaluation
- History:
  - Previous history of ear discharge
  - Head trauma
  - Use of foreign body in ear
  - Sudden onset pain and mild bleeding from the ear following trauma
  - Associated tinnitus
- *Otoscopic examination:* Confirms the tympanic membrane perforation with the size of perforation.
- *Tuning fork test:* Tells about the degree of hearing loss.

Interpretation of Findings
- Previous history of ear discharge with a perforation of tympanic membrane in otoscopic examination—CSOM.
- Sudden onset pain, tinnitus with fullness in ear following trauma with otoscopic examination showing perforated drum with irregular margins—traumatic rupture of tympanic membrane.

Investigations
- *Otoscopic examination:* Proper visualization of tympanic membrane
- *Pure tone audiometry:* To know the degree of hearing loss.

Treatment
- Traumatic perforation:
  - Keep ear dry
  - Oral broad-spectrum antibiotics if injury is dirty
  - If not resolved spontaneously then paper patch or surgical repair.
  - Perforation associated with otitis media tympanoplasty.

Summary
- Small perforations heal spontaneously.
- Ear should be dry during the phage of healing.
- Surgery is done for nonhealing perforations with hearing loss.

WAX IMPACTION

Introduction
Ear wax is produced by the glands (sebaceous and sweat glands) of the external auditory canal for cleaning, protection as well as lubrication of the canal.

Etiology
Excessive production of wax lead to ear wax impaction.

Pathophysiology
- *Wax is a mixture of secretions:* The glands of the EAC and sloughed epithelial cells.
- Wax impaction is accumulation of the wax in the ear.

Clinical Presentation
Patients may develop symptoms of ear fullness, blocked ear, hearing loss, and pain (because of pressure on EAC).

Evaluation
- History: the symptoms of ear fullness, blocking of ears, mild hearing loss and brownish discharge from ear.
- Physical examination:
  - *Otoscopic examination:* Visualization of cerumen
  - Associated with tragal tenderness suggestive of external otitis
  - One must see for associated stenotic ear canal.

Interpretation of Finding
- Visualization of wax

Investigations
- Otoscopic examination
- *Audiogram:* To know the degree of hearing loss if the patient complains of hearing loss.

Treatment
- Topical application of cerumenolytics (paradichlorobenzene + lignocaine)
- When wax softens, then syringing or manual removal by hook or scoop.

Summary
Ear wax is one of most common problem of hearing loss need to be diagnosed and treated in stepwise manner. Proper ENT check-up essential to exclude the cause of hearing loss.

CHAPTER 34

Ear Discharge

Sanjaya Bahera, Deepak Dalmia

INTRODUCTION

Ear discharge is also known as otorrhea. It may be mucoid, serous, or purulent in character. May be continuous or intermittent discharge and associated with ear pain, pruritus, tinnitus, hearing loss.

ETIOLOGY (TABLE 1)

Causes in the External Ear
- Foreign body in ear
- Otomycosis
- Otitis externa
- Wax
- Carcinoma of external auditory canal (EAC).

Causes in the Middle Ear
- Acute suppurative otitis media (ASOM)
- Chronic suppurative otitis media (CSOM)
- Carcinoma of the middle ear
- Following insertion of ventilation tube in serous otitis media.

Traumatic
- Cerebrospinal fluid (CSF) otorrhea.

PATHOPHYSIOLOGY

Wax is the normal secretion of the glands of the external ear canal, and most patients complain of wax discharge from the ear. A purulent discharge indicates the presence of infection may be external ear or middle ear. Recurrent episodes of purulent otorrhea suggest CSOM (may be because of a central perforation of tympanic membrane or a cholesteatoma sac or retraction pocket) while purulent otorrhea of acute onset suggests ASOM with perforation of the tympanic membrane. Bloody discharge may follow trauma or occur with granulation tissue associated with chronic infection.

Table 1: Causes of ear discharge.

Acute onset ear discharge	Findings	Diagnosis
Otitis externa	External auditory canal (EAC): inflamed, edematous with normal tympanic membrane (TM) May be infective or allergic	Otoscopic examination
Postmyringotomy tube	Grommet on TM	Otoscopic examination
Acute suppurative otitis media (ASOM)	Severe pain with relieve after ear discharge	Clinical evaluation
Cerebrospinal fluid (CSF) otorrhea following head trauma	History of head trauma and ear surgery Clear watery or blood mixed fluid	High-resolution computed tomography (HRCT) of temporal bone Biochemical examination
Chronic ear discharge		
Foreign body	Usually in children Foul-smelling discharge	Clinical evaluation
Malignant otitis externa	Immunodeficiency Severe pain Facial nerve paralysis	HRCT of temporal bone Magnetic resonance imaging (MRI) of skull base.
Chronic suppurative otitis media (CSOM) with central perforation	Long history Intermittent discharge Macerated EAC Central perforation	Otoscopic examination HRCT of temporal bone
Unsafe CSOM	Long history Persistent discharge Scanty secretion Foul-smelling discharge Cholesteatoma/retraction pocket	HRCT of temporal bone Culture
EAC carcinoma	Bloody ear discharge Pain Mass in the EAC	HRCT of temporal bone Culture
Mastoiditis	History of untreated otorrhea Redness over mastoid area with postauricular fullness	HRCT temporal bone

Most cases of CSF otorrhea have a traumatic etiology, following a head injury or surgery to the skull base.

CLINICAL PRESENTATION
- Fever
- Ear discharge
- Tenderness and fullness in the postauricular region
- Tragal tenderness
- Hearing loss
- Itching of the ear
- Tinnitus.

RED FLAGS
- Recent major head trauma
- Any cranial nerve dysfunction
- Fever
- Erythema of ear
- Swelling in postauricular region
- Diabetes or immunodeficiency.

EVALUATION

History

History of Present Illness
- Duration of symptoms and whether symptoms have been recurrent
- Associated with upper respiratory tract infection
- Associated symptoms include pain, itching, decreased hearing, vertigo, and tinnitus
- Habits, e.g. swimming, insertion of objects including cotton swabs, use of ear drops
- Major head trauma
- Whether associated with any cranial nerve deficit
- Past medical history of ear surgery (grommet insertion), and diabetes or immunodeficiency.

Physical Examination
Systemic examination for fever.

Ear Nose Throat (ENT) Examination
- Both preauriclar and postauricular region inspected for any swelling, erythema
- Tragal tenderness is examined
- Otoscopic examination of ear
- Discharge: character (mucoid, serous, serosanguinous)

- Presence of canal lesions, granulation tissue or foreign body are noted
- Examination of tympanic membrane for inflammation, perforation, and signs of cholesteatoma, polypoid mass from TM
- In case of otitis externa or when there is copious drainage, careful suctioning can permit an adequate examination and also allow treatment
- All the cranial nerves are tested.

INTERPRETATION OF FINDINGS

- *Otoscopic examination:* For perforation of TM, foreign bodies or external otitis, granulation
- Other findings are less specific but indicate a more serious problem:
    - Vertigo and tinnitus (disorder of the inner ear)
    - Cranial nerve deficits (disorder involving the skull base)
    - Erythema and tenderness of ear, surrounding tissues, or both (significant infection).

INVESTIGATION

- Otoscopic examination of ear.
- Pure tone audiogram and high-resolution computed tomography (HRCT) of the temporal bone or gadolinium-enhanced magnetic resonance imaging (MRI).
- Biopsy should be considered when auditory canal granulation tissue is present.
- *In case of clear otorrhea:* CSF should be suspected and sample should be sent for β2 transferrin, and biochemical examination.

TREATMENT

Treatment is directed toward the cause:
- *If foreign body:* It should be removed.
- *External otitis:* Broad spectrum antibiotics with medicated wick pack.
- *ASOM:* Antibiotics, nasal decongestant, ear drop.
- *CSOM:* First medical management to dry the ear followed by tympanoplasty and mastoidectomy if requires.
- *CSF otorrhea:* First conservative treatment, if the leak is large then closure of the leak by tensor fascia lata after doing mastoidectomy.
- *Tumor:* Biopsy of the sample to be done. If carcinoma detected then temporal bone resection.

SUMMARY

- Ear discharge without any immunodeficiency because of otitis externa or ASOM or CSOM.
- Patients with persistent otorrhea with cranial nerve dysfunction and systemic symptoms should be searched for skull base lesion because of malignant otitis externa and EAC carcinoma.

CHAPTER 35

Epistaxis

Sandeep B Gore

INTRODUCTION

Epistaxis is one of the common presentations to emergency department (ED). Mild episodes are either self-limiting or can be managed successfully by the emergency physician (EP). About 60% of people would experience epistaxis once in their lifespan and only 6-10% of them would require medical help. There is bimodal pattern in the incidence of epistaxis according to the age distribution, the two peaks being in children and older adults (45-65 years).

APPLIED ANATOMY

The most commonly (almost 80-90%) implicated area for epistaxis is the anteroinferior part of the nose called as Little's area. This area is richly supplied by blood and is responsible for warming and humidifying the inhaled air. The blood supply to Little's area is by following four arteries, which anastomose to form a vascular plexus called Kiesselbach's plexus.
- Anterior ethmoidal artery (branch of ophthalmic artery)
- Greater palatine artery (branch of maxillary artery)
- Septal branch of superior labial artery (branch of facial artery)
- Sphenopalatine artery (branch of maxillary artery).

ETIOLOGY

The causal factors for epistaxis are manifold ranging from local to systemic causes. By far the most frequent cause is nose picking.

Local Causes
- Local inflammation due to atopy and allergy
- Infection like rhinitis and sinusitis
- Foreign body
- Anatomic abnormalities like septal defects
- Trauma like nasal contusion or fracture
- Medications like topical decongestants or inhaled corticosteroids
- Iatrogenic, e.g. due to nasogastric tube insertion or any surgical interventions
- Malignancy like tumors of nasal cavity or paranasal sinuses
- Environmental causes such as hot or cold and dry air leading to crusting and bleeding.

Systemic Causes

- Medications like anticoagulants and antiplatelets
- Hematological causes like thrombocytopenia and hemophilia
- Systemic illnesses, which can affect coagulation like liver failure
- Uncontrolled hypertension.

■ EMERGENCY DEPARTMENT EVALUATION

The patients with epistaxis can have a wide range of presentation from light nosebleed responding to simple therapeutic methods to life-threatening hemorrhage, which would mandate admission and surgical interventions.

History

Most bleeding is from anterior part of the nose. Posterior bleeding is caused by more serious problems and must be managed with caution. The patients with posterior bleeding may present with hematemesis resulting from swallowed blood.

A careful history suggestive of intensity, duration, recurrence, and laterality of bleeding can allow a judgment to be made about the severity and urgency of treatment. Try to exclude the local and systemic causes that predispose a patient to nose bleed. Equally important is the accurate medication history, any recent surgical procedures and the details of comorbid illnesses like coagulopathy.

Physical Examination

It is pertinent for the examining physician to use personal protective equipment like face mask, protective eye gear, apron, and gloves to prevent contamination and accidental exposure to blood.

Initial assessment in ED should begin with a rapid primary survey to assess for potential airway or hemodynamic compromise.

Bleeding from nose can be frightening to patients and the fear and anxiety can lead to elevations in blood pressure. Reassurance and reassessment after hemorrhage control is generally sufficient. A modest reduction in blood pressure may be required in patients with persistent epistaxis who require packing or surgical interventions to control bleeding.

Red Flags

- Hemodynamically unstable patient
- Patient with low-blood oxygen levels and low-blood pressure
- Patients with low hemoglobin level
- Patients with coagulopathy or on anticoagulants/antiplatelets.

MANAGEMENT OF EPISTAXIS (FLOWCHART 1)

Initial Resuscitation

In extreme cases, patients can present with uncontrolled hemorrhage, standard resuscitation principles should be applied.

Airway

- Risk of airway obstruction from blood in the posterior pharynx, or decreased level of consciousness from hypovolemia.
- Place patient in position to assist in managing the blood loss, and may require frequent suctioning.
- Be prepared to secure and place a definitive airway by endotracheal intubation in case a need arises.

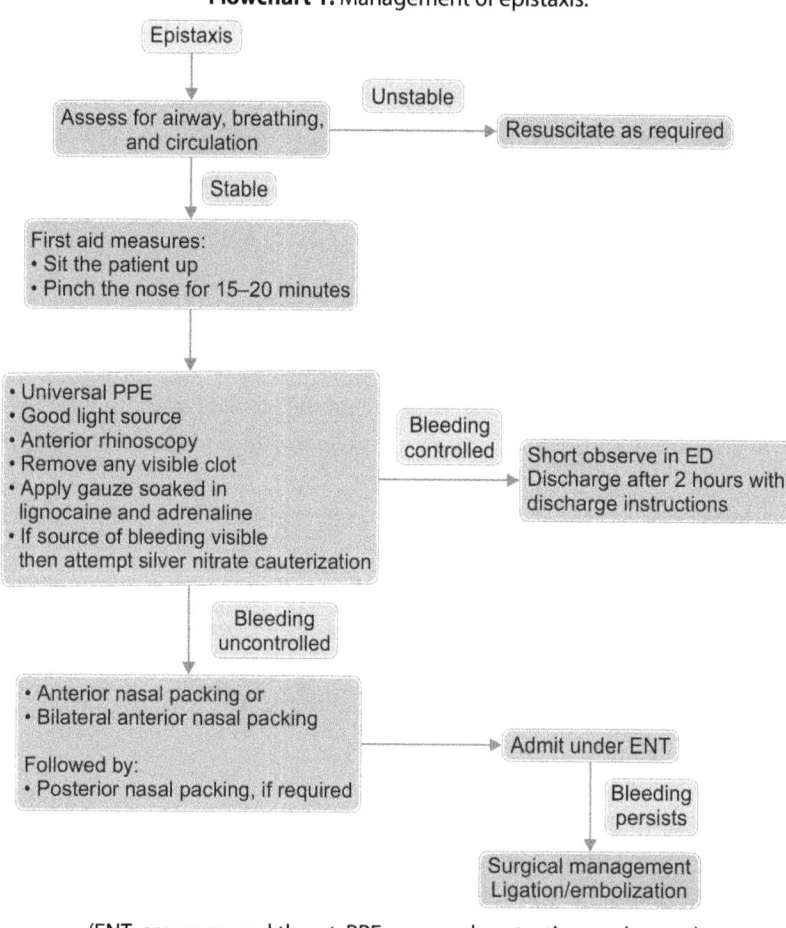

Flowchart 1: Management of epistaxis.

(ENT: ear, nose, and throat; PPE: personal protective equipment)

Breathing
- Assess respiratory rate
- Remember a noisy airway is an occluded airway
- Provide high-flow oxygen.

Circulation
- Assess heart rate, blood pressure, and capillary refill
- Patient at risk for severe hemorrhage place × two large-bore IV, check complete blood count, cross-match blood, and start fluid resuscitation.

Disability
Monitor patient's level of consciousness.

Exposure
- Keep patient warm to prevent coagulopathy
- If epistaxis is caused by major trauma, always examine for other injuries.

Specific Measures
The first step in the management of epistaxis is pinching of the anterior nares and compressing for 15-20 minutes using two fingers. The patient should be positioned in a sitting posture with leaning in forward direction to prevent the blood trickling down the pharynx.

Local application of ice with intend of vasoconstriction can be done but its value is not proven in literature.

It is important to differentiate anterior and posterior epistaxis. Generally, the diagnosis of posterior bleeding in ED is made when measures to control anterior bleeding have failed. Posterior source of bleeding should be suspected in bleeding from bilateral nares, elderly patient, or patients with coagulopathy.

Therapeutic Measures
Anterior Rhinoscopy
To locate the source of bleeding, clean clots from little's area and apply topical vasoconstrictors and anesthetics such as adrenaline (1:1,000), 0.5% phenylephrine, or 0.05% oxymetazoline solution-soaked gauze strips can be used. Due to the local vasoconstrictor effects, this step can be both diagnostic and therapeutic.

Cauterization
When bleeding persists further to two attempts at direct pressure, this is the next appropriate step. Chemical cauterization with silver nitrate is done. Preanesthetize the nasal mucosa with cotton soaked in 0.05% oxymetazoline and 4% lidocaine solution in equal concentration.

Visualize the bleeding site after anterior rhinoscopy and the silver nitrate stick can be placed proximal to the bleeding source. Once a bloodless field is obtained, apply silver nitrate directly to the bleeding site briefly. This should not be attempted on both sides of the septum, as it can increase the chances of perforation. Silver nitrate is a strong oxidizing agent and on interaction with liquids, it precipitates and leads to release of free radicals. This process oxidizes mucosa and destroys mucosal structures, which later heal with scar tissue with decreased vascularity. Following cauterization local ointment application with saline gel is recommended to avoid crusting and rebleeding. Complete recovery can take 2–3-week period. Silver nitrate cauterization has a success rate of 75–85%.

Thrombogenic Foams and Gels

These are a good alternative before considering nasal packing by nonabsorbable material when attempts at cautery have failed. They are effective hemostatic agents and by being bioabsorbable, they do not require to be removed.

Anterior Nasal Packing

As an addition to cautery local insertion of gauze can be done for physiological hemostasis, especially in cases of diffuse mucosal bleeding. If bleeding persists, anterior nasal packing is the next step. It can be used if hemostatic foams and gels are not available. Nasal tampons (e.g. Merocel—a compressed dehydrated polyvinyl acetate sponge), epistaxis balloons or ribbon gauze packing can be used. Lubricate them with local anesthetic and water-soluble antibiotic ointment prior to insertion. The drawstrings should be taped to the anterior face to facilitate easy removal and avoid posterior dislocation. Once inserted, it is kept in place for 48 hours and antibiotic and analgesic treatment is to be used during this period.

Posterior Nasal Packing

Anterior packing acts as a good tamponade at the nasal septum when done bilaterally. If bleeding persists after this then ENT (ear, nose, and throat) consult is imperative and posterior nasal packing may be required. The complications associated with posterior packing are pressure necrosis, higher rates of infection, and increased patient discomfort. Rapid Rhino pack has both anterior and posterior balloons and can be used. Foley's catheter of 12 Fr or 14 Fr with 30 mL of balloon inflation can also be used for posterior packing. All posterior packing should have an anterior nasal packs. Once done, these balloons should be partially deflated and checked after 24 hours. If bleeding persists then surgical treatment may be necessary.

Surgical Treatment

If clinically significant bleeding starts after pack removal then there is a need for surgical treatment. The bleeding will need evaluation in operating room under general anesthesia and possible bleeding vessel will need ligation or cauterization. Endoscopic clipping or coagulation of sphenopalatine artery may be necessary. The ligation of ethmoidal artery, facial artery, sphenopalatine artery, or internal maxillary artery as required may be done by endoscopic method. Interventional radiologist doing an angiography and selected arterial embolization may be necessary in intractable epistaxis. The complications involved in these procedures can include stroke and blindness, which should be discussed with the patient and informed consent must be obtained before proceeding with it.

Management of Epistaxis in Patients on Anticoagulants

Anticoagulation can be continued in minor epistaxis episodes, which can be controlled by minor interventions. Only in episodes of massive uncontrollable bleeding, adjustment of doses should be considered in consultation with hematologist and cardiologist. When anticoagulant overdose is suspected then reversal of anticoagulation is deemed necessary.

- *Antiplatelet therapy*: Normal hemostasis will be restored after a week of discontinuing antiplatelet therapy. Platelet transfusion can be considered.
- *Unfractionated heparin*: Administer protamine sulfate with a dose guided by activated partial thromboplastin time (aPTT).
- *Vitamin K antagonists*: Administer vitamin K and fresh frozen plasma, if overdose is suspected.
- *Direct oral anticoagulation*: Adjustment of doses with expert consultation. Antidote for use is available only in the case of dabigatran.

EMERGENCY DEPARTMENT DISPOSITION

- Mild episode of epistaxis, which is self-limiting and no accompanying coagulopathy can be discharged from ED after a brief period of observation. They should be provided with discharge instructions to review if recurrence of bleeding is noted. Inhaled vasoconstrictors like oxymetazoline can be prescribed.
- Patients who have anterior packs should be given oral analgesics and antibiotic cover with anti-staphylococcal cover like amoxicillin and clavulanic acid combination. ENT follow-up should be arranged in 2–3-day period.
- Patients with persistent bleeding and coagulopathy who require posterior packing preferably need ENT consult and inpatient observation.

SUMMARY

- Epistaxis is the most common ENT emergency and most of the cases are self-limiting and can be successfully treated by emergency room physicians.
- For continuing bleeding specialist ENT referral should be obtained as available.
- When the source of bleeding can be visualized cauterization can be successfully attempted.
- When diffuse bleeding is suspected hemostatic sponges and gels are a good treatment options for anterior packing.
- Epistaxis persisting these attempts will require posterior packing, immediate ENT consult, and consideration of surgical interventions.

Eye Problems

Carreen Pakrasi, Sudipto Pakrasi

INTRODUCTION

The eye is a small but essential part of the body. It is the one thing that adds quality to life. Hence, care of the eyes is as important as of any other part of the human body.

Most often, the emergencies related to the eye will be obvious, with the cause related to either injuries such as trauma and chemicals and presenting with suggestive history and complaints of severe pain and visual loss of varying degrees from 6/6 to no perception of light.

Sometimes, pain is the only presenting complaint in potentially debilitating conditions that must be detected early so as to prevent late visual complications, such as optic neuritis, temporal arteritis, and sometimes herpes zoster. A high index of suspicion and an acute clinical sense are important in early diagnosis.

Ocular emergencies are those conditions that may or may not present with ocular pain and redness and are potentially blinding. These have to be recognized and treated swiftly so as to preserve the visual functions of the eye.

The World Health Organization (WHO) studies quote the incidence of ocular injuries causing loss of work hours as 55 million. Epidemiological studies by Vats et al. have found the mean age of ocular trauma to be 24.2 years. The prevalence of ocular trauma is reported to 2.4% of the population in an urban setting in India.

We are going to try to present the various scenarios in a logical progression so that they are easily identifiable by first responders in an emergency setting. The Ocular Trauma Score has been presented according to various standard systems, of which the Birmingham Eye Trauma Terminology (BETT) is one of the most widely accepted. The terminology and classification are mostly to differentiate between penetrating and nonpenetrating ocular trauma due to mechanical cause.

CAUSES OF OCULAR EMERGENCIES

Of the patients presenting in the emergency, the cause of symptoms can be any of the following. Most classifications of ocular emergencies will focus on ocular trauma. However, in a multispecialty hospital, patients walk in with any of the following presentations:
- *Infections*:
  - *Viral conjunctivitis*: Herpes simplex conjunctivitis or epidemic keratoconjunctivitis
  - Mucopurulent conjunctivitis
  - Ocular involvement due to herpes zoster.

- *Trauma*:
- *Ocular presentations of systemic diseases*:
  - Diplopia
  - Sudden loss of vision due to vascular or neurological causes.

Culturally, in India, there are a few festivities that have a high incidence of ocular emergencies. These may be infective or there may be chemical injuries to the cornea or emergency as a result from ocular trauma. All emergencies are usually on high alert around these festivities.

Holi

Injury during the festival of Holi can be any of the following:
- Infections due to contaminated color or water going into the eye.
- Chemical injuries due to reactions to adulterated and artificial colors.
- Closed or open globe injuries due to blunt trauma with balloons filled with water hitting the eye at high velocity.

Dussehra
- Bow and arrow injuries.

OCULAR TRAUMA SCORE (KUHN ET AL., 1996)

Anatomy

The eye has a unique function, which requires clarity of its surface. It is soft, therefore susceptible to traumatic injuries. However, it also has a unique setting. It is placed inside a bony socket, which is designed to protect the eye, which by its nature of being closed on all sides except the front, serves as a buffer against direct impact. The front of the eye is protected by the eyelids, which are very sensitive to light, wind and are served by a highly reactive nervous system, which closes the lids whenever there is a threat to them. Any loss of function of the lids will therefore increase the risk of injury to the eye itself.

The entire body is protected by skin, which is tough and capable of protecting the underlying tissue from direct injury. The eye, however, has skin that is soft, transparent, and susceptible to injury. This is because of its function of gathering light rays and transmitting them to the retina, so that an image can be generated. The cornea, the most anterior part of the eye, has to be as clear as any clear glass. Disturbance in this clarity will result in an alteration in the visual acuity.

In the same way, the arrangement of cells in the minutest way is very crucial to the proper functioning of the central part of the eye in the visual axis, which is responsible for good vision. The cornea, lens, the chambers of the eye, the retinal layers, and the optic nerve are all part of this visual pathway which culminate in the visual cortex, in the brain which is, ultimately the seat of vision perception. There are conditions, which present as ocular emergencies with loss of vision, or doubling of vision, which have nothing to do with the eye, but instead have diseases of the brain and the nerves that originate there, the cranial nerves.

With this minimalistic overview of the relevant anatomy, we will approach the various cause of ocular anatomy by first dividing them into following major categories:
- Traumatic ocular emergencies: those related to injury.
  – Penetrating injuries
  – Nonpenetrating, blunt injuries.
- Nontraumatic ocular emergencies: causes not arising from injury.
  – Infections
  – Inflammations
  – Vascular
  – Neurological.
- Chemical injuries.

Penetrating Ocular Injuries

History: The maintenance of the integrity of the globe is the most natural instinct served by vision to protect the eye and it has an inbuilt protective mechanism in the following ways:
- The orbit serves to protect the globe from injuries by serving as a physical block against any oncoming projectiles unless they are directly approaching it from the front.
- The eyelids also protect the globe with their ability to respond to sudden external insult by shutting the lids to cover the cornea. The lids themselves are soft so it is common for penetrating injuries of severe nature to go through the lid into the globe.

In penetrating injuries, there will be a history of any of the following projectiles entering the eye:
- Stone
- Bullet
- Sharp object
- Finger with great force
- Pencil
- Crackers.

The scenarios in which these injuries happen are:
- School—in the classroom as well as in the playgrounds and laboratories
- Road traffic injuries
- Factories
- Construction sites
- Diwali and Dussehra celebrations because of the crackers swords used for play
- Sports, especially those that involve sharp implements and speed
- Any situation can result in eye injuries of varying levels if they involve implements that are sharp or pointed, hence, preventive measures are always to be followed as per protocols.

Signs/symptoms: The signs/symptoms that indicate an ocular emergency can be any of the following:
- Sudden, acute pain
- Sudden drop in vision
- Bleeding from the eye or around it
- Swelling
- Doubling of vision
- Flashes/floaters
- History of injury/intraocular foreign body.

Examination: The clinical signs will vary according to the severity of the injury.
- *Associated injuries*:
  – Head and neck injuries
  – Facial injuries
  – Orbital fractures
  – Neurological damage
  – Multiple injuries.

The BETT is the most widely accepted classification of ocular trauma as shown in **Box 1**.

The BETT provides a logical key to understanding of all injuries to allow better understanding of the extent and prognosis. It is desirable that it becomes the language for everyday clinical practice. We are further simplifying the signs and symptoms so that all physicians may be able to grade and treat presenting ocular emergencies more efficiently.

A sharp object will easily penetrate the eye and may not have expensive associated ocular trauma. On the other hand, blunt objects need higher kinetic energy to cause rupture of the globe. They can cause extensive damage to the intraocular structure without globe rupture.

The injuries are the following depending on which part of the eye is involved.
- *Lid lacerations*: There can be tears of the eyelids and the skin around the eye. Often, in the presence of a penetrating injury, it would be wise to look for a track, which may point to the site of penetration of the eyeball.
- *Conjunctival tears*: These can be accompanied by hemorrhage in the affected area. If any hemorrhage is seen, it is wise to look for an injury in the sclera under the hemorrhage.

Box 1: The Birmingham Eye Trauma Terminology (BETT) classification of ocular trauma (Kuhn et al., 1996).

The BETT classification of eye trauma:
- Closed globe
  – Contusion
  – Lamellar laceration
- Open globe
  – Laceration: Penetrating
  – Intraocular foreign bodies (IOFBs)
  – Perforating

Table 1: New classification for ocular trauma (Shukla et al.).

Local	Associated injuries	Cause of injury

• Mechanical:
  – Globe
  – Destructive
  – Adnexal:
    ♦ Orbital
    ♦ Palpebral
    ♦ Conjunctival
    ♦ Lacrimal
	• Head injury
	• Facial injuries
	• Multiple injuries
		• Industrial
		• Sports related
		• Road traffic
		• Assault
		• Agricultural
		• Daily activities

• Nonmechanical:
  – Chemical
  – Thermal
  – Radiation
  – Electrical		

New classification for ocular trauma (Shukla et al.): New classification for ocular trauma (Shukla et al.) has been shown in **Table 1**.
- *Penetrating scleral injury* will often be found if there is a local contusion in the conjunctiva.
- *Penetrating corneal injuries:* The extent of the corneal tear will determine the extent of the injury.

Closed Penetrating Corneal Injury

- If the injury is small, it may be self sealed or partial and the integrity of the globe will be maintained, this may be still a closed globe injury because the injury is partial thickness or sealed.
- The iris may seal the wound.
- If there is a knuckle of the iris in the wound, it is imperative for the iris to be repositioned in order to avoid the dreaded complication of sympathetic ophthalmia in the other eye.
- There may be blood in the anterior chamber of the eye known a hyphema. In the process of the blood been mobilized out of the anterior chamber, there may be blood cells which block the anterior chamber angle from where drainage from the anterior chamber takes place. This will lead to a rise in the intraocular pressure.
- It is imperative to look for a retained intraocular foreign body, which may be imbedded in any of the intraocular structures, that is, the cornea, the iris, the lens or the retina.
- There can also be blood in the vitreous cavity of the back of the eye, which makes it difficult to see the retina. In these cases, if an iron foreign body causes the penetrating injury, a simple X-ray of the orbit will reveal the embedded foreign body. It is important to remove these foreign bodies because these are toxic to the eye.
- If there is an accompanying retina injury, the retina may be detached or may have a hemorrhage.

- Direct optic nerve injuries are rare but penetrating injuries have been known to sever the optic nerve completely causing optic avulsion.

Open Globe Injury
- When there is full thickness corneal wound and open globe.

Closed Globe Injury
- Nonpenetrating or blunt ocular injuries.

The eye is a finely balanced instrument of vision and in order to achieve its perfect functionality, all the anatomical arrangements in the path of the light have to be in perfect alignment. Any injury, which leads to misalignment or alteration of the normal anatomy of these anatomical structures, will cause an aberration in its function, which results in loss of vision to varying extents.

Symptomatic presentation: The patient may have any of the complaints following blunt trauma to the eye.
- Watering
- Foreign body sensation
- Inability to keep the eye open
- Photophobia
- Loss of vision
- Pain
- Doubling of vision.

Clinical findings: Again, the approach to localizing the diagnosis must be logical and methodical, examining the eyeball and noting the findings from the outer part of the eye and progressing inward.

Contusions (Nonpenetrating Injury): In contusion injuries, there may injury to the eye wall, i.e. the sclera and the cornea.

Look for any swelling in the supraorbital margins, the eyebrows or the eyelids. The discoloration of the lids will be evident if there is a localized hemorrhage anywhere on the forehead or eyebrows. Pooling of fluid will follow the gravitational pull and swelling will usually extend downward toward the cheekbones presenting as a *black eye*.

Supraorbital Injuries

Injuries in the area of the eyebrow line with a swelling over the lateral one-third of the eyebrow must be looked at carefully. Very often there will be an indirect optic nerve compression injury. In such cases, the pupillary reaction must be closely evaluated to indicate any afferent pupillary defect. These are often overlooked in the face of other seemingly more serious injuries and can result in permanent loos of function of the optic nerve and visual loss. The only indicator will be an afferent pupillary defect in the presence of the supraorbital injury because the optic atrophy will not be apparent in the initial stages. A timely course of systemic steroids can save the optic nerve from damage due to local inflammation and edema and need to be given immediately, on detection.

Subconjunctival Hemorrhage (Fig. 1)

These are alarming to look at but will be harmless and easily treated by local cold compresses alone with lubricating eye drops to ease any foreign body sensation.

The important possible underlying injury to look for is that of a scleral rupture which can be hidden by the hemorrhage.

There may also be an involvement of the ocular muscles with accompanying diplopia.

Corneal Abrasions (Fig. 2)

- These are the most common injuries after any impact. The cornea is intact but the continuity of the surface is compromised.
- The presence of corneal injury will typically give rise to acute and copious watering accompanied by unbearable foreign body sensation. This is a protective response, which helps to protect the cornea from drying and infection when the surface is abraded.

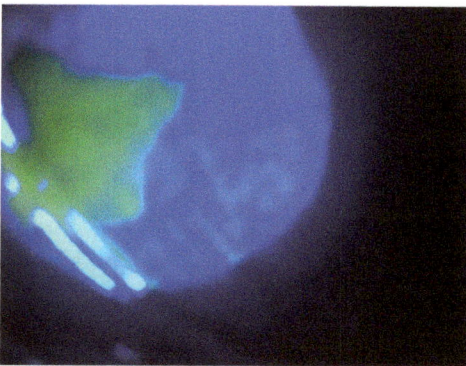

Fig. 1: Subconjunctival hemorrhage.

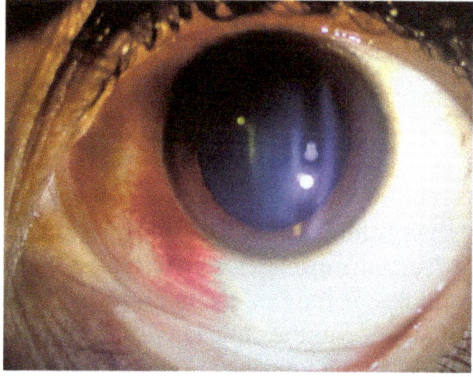

Fig. 2: Corneal abrasion.

- The eye remains closed and the pain is acute.
- On staining the cornea with fluorescein dye, a tell-tale fluorescence will be clearly detected indicating a breach in the corneal epithelium.
- These require pad and bandage with an antibiotic ointment to assist resurfacing for as long as the corneal epithelium takes to heal completely. Examination must be done every 24 hours with a repeat pad and bandage everyday until the epithelium is resurfaced and the cornea no longer registers staining.
- Healing can sometimes result in various levels of scarring.
- Depending on the site of the initial injury, the vision can be variously affected with central scars obviously causing the maximum loss.

Hyphema: Blood in the Anterior Chamber
- The presence of blood in the anterior chamber of the eye can follow open (penetrating) as well as closed (nonpenetrating) injuries of the eye.
- Whenever there is a history of significantly severe force, any blunt injury of the eye can cause blood to collect in the anterior chamber. This occurs due to direct force on the iris causing it to bleed.

Associated Injuries
There can be various nonobvious effects that can accompany a bleed into the anterior chamber. These have to be detected early to prevent future vision loss.
- Angle recession must be ruled out with a good gonioscopic examination of the anterior chamber angle.
- The incidence of angle recession can be anywhere between 20% and 90% of all ocular traumas and of these 5–20% will develop angle recession glaucoma.
- Angle recession of the angle of more than 180° has a high risk of raised intraocular pressure.
- Raised intraocular pressure will also result due to the hyphema itself, concomitant uveitis or anterior dislocation of the lens. All or any of these can cause blockage of the trabecular meshwork.
- The patient must be given a pad and bandage to rest the eye and speed the mobilization of heme from the anterior chamber.
- The patient is also encouraged to lie in a semireclined position as the resolving hyphema can result in deposition of heme pigments on the anterior surface of the lens.
- In case the hyphema is increasing over the first few days, look for iris injury.

Iris Injuries
- Injuries to the iris will give a good indication of the presence of an angle recession. The iris sphincter damage will result in a dilated nonreacting pupil with no loss of a consensual response to light.

Vitreous Hemorrhage
- Retinal hemorrhage, retinal tears or posterior vitreous avulsion can also result in a bleed into the vitreous cavity. This will result in severe loss of vision.
- The fundus glow will be lost on distant direct.
- Ultrasound examination (preferably B-scan) will reveal the extent of the injury and can identify any retinal detachment, which significantly decreases the visual prognosis.

Retinal Injuries
Injuries to the retina may or may not result in immediate loss of vision. If the injury is sparing the macula and is not in the visual axis, the vision may not be affected on primary examination.

Floaters are a good indicator of the presence of vitreous liquefaction and may be a retinal tear. Flashes will most certainly accompany a tear in the peripheral retina. Careful history taking is a must, to determine this. In case there are any complaints of floaters or flashes, the peripheral retina must be screened repeatedly over the following weeks to make sure that small tears in the retina is not missed. These are potentially blindly and timely treatment is preventive.

Retinal hemorrhages can be present without symptoms and can be easily detected by careful examination of the retina with a 90-diopter lens as well as careful indirect ophthalmoscopy. They need no treatment except observation and follow-up.

Berlin Edema
This is caused by contrecoup injury to the macular due to impact over the anterior part of the globe. It is also called commotio retinae in keeping with the pathophysiology, where the injury is indirect, due to the transmission of the force across the tissues causing damage across the point of impact. There is retinal swelling, which can cause a significant drop in the visual acuity, which usually resolves spontaneously in a couple of weeks.

Extraocular Muscle Involvement
Any involvement of the extraocular muscles will give rise to diplopia.

Any complaint of diplopia demands a thorough evaluation of the surrounding orbital spaces and bony structures for any inflammation or fracture and trapping of any of the ocular muscles within the fracture.

The diplopia will usually resolve spontaneously with anti-inflammatory medication and requires observation till healing is complete before contemplating surgical management.

Blowout fractures involve fracture of the inferior wall and may sometimes need surgical correction without which the diplopia will not resolve.

Chemical Injuries
As far as ocular injuries go, chemical injuries are the most dreaded and difficult to contain. It is absolutely essential that they should be recognized immediately and managed efficiently

as this will determine the visual prognosis. The load of contaminant, the response time and type of contaminant determine the success of treatment. The goal is to eliminate the causative substance and restore the conjunctival spaces to the normal pH level as soon as possible so as to limit the seepage of the contaminant into the deeper layers of the ocular surface tissues.
- *Alkali burns*: In this respect, alkali burns continue to be the most challenging situations because of the nature of alkali. They can saponify the cell membrane and penetrate the cornea rapidly into the anterior chamber causing the pH of the aqueous to rise thereby damaging the iris and ciliary body. The vascular supply can be affected causing ischemic damage to the cornea leading to rapid deterioration of the integrity of the ocular surface.
- *Acid injuries*: On the contrary, the nature of acid burns is to coagulate and fix the ocular tissues so that there is limited penetration to the deeper structures. They may cause expensive immediate damage but will contain themselves after the initial insult.

Management: Immediate and copious irrigation of the affected eye should be carried out and continued until pH testing of the conjunctival sac returns to normal. This helps the offending substance to leach out gradually, thereby limiting the extent of penetration into the deeper tissues.

After sufficient irrigation has been carried out, a detailed history of the type of chemical involved in the injury. In case there is evidence of any solid particles, these must be carefully removed from the conjunctival sac so that there is no risk of continued penetration.

The presence of limbal ischemia is an indicator of the extent of injury and will determine the prognosis. Corneal epithelium integrity has to be determined by fluorescein staining of the cornea.

In the presence of alkali burns, 10% potassium ascorbate drops have been seen to be useful in limiting damage to the ocular tissue by scavenging free radicals released by degranulating polymorphs.

Further management will best be done by an ophthalmologist and will involve prevention of scarring with the use of antibiotic-steroid combinations ointment and pad and bandage. Further surgical may be required to treat any scarring that is bound to occur if the injury is extensive.

Nontraumatic Ocular Emergencies

Contact lens-related emergencies:
- *Displaced or broken contact lenses*: This is a common complaint. The patient may or may not be aware of the contact lens inside the eye.
- Presenting history of pain, foreign body sensation, and red eye.
- A careful history will determine that the patient is a contact lens user.
- Detailed examination of the eye must be done to detect the presence of a contact lens in the conjunctival sulcus.
- Removal of the lens and antibiotic along with lubricating eye drops will suffice as treatment.
- Sometimes, the patient would have tried unsuccessfully to extract the contact lens and may have abrasion on the cornea. This will require a pad and bandage with antibiotic ointment for 24 hours.

Conjunctivitis: These will sometimes report to the emergency room and working knowledge is useful even though they are rarely sight threatening and have very few complications apart from superficial corneal scarring.
- Allergic or infective inflammation of the conjunctiva can occur suddenly and without warning making it an ocular emergency.
- Allergic conjunctivitis will most often be accompanied by edema of the surrounding adnexa. The eyelids will be swollen without much inflammation and increased local temperature. The conjunctiva will reveal typical pupil response with causing acute dry eyes and foreign body sensation. The discharge will be watery if there is not accompanying infection.
- Bacterial conjunctivitis will by typically accompanied by mucopurulent discharge and matting of the lashes. A conjunctival swab from the lower fornix for Giemsa stains and culture sensitivity before treatment would be prudent to allow specific antibiotic therapy according to the sensitivity pattern.
- Viral conjunctivitis will be accompanied by decreased corneal sensations and this simple test can prevent unnecessary antibiotic exposure. The symptoms will vary little except for the lack of mucopurulent discharge.
- Epidemic keratoconjunctivitis must be treated with close follow-up and will usually not require topical antibiotic unless the picture is of a mixed infection with superadded infection. Prevention of transmission of this highly contagious disease is as important as the treatment of the disease itself in order to limit the proportion of the epidemic. Personal hygiene lessons must be given along with other management.

Corneal ulcers:
- Corneal ulcers are a dreaded condition, which unless treated immediately and well, can lead to nonhealing and chronically debilitating complications that are potentially blinding.
- They can be of bacterial or viral infective origin and can also be degenerative.
- These will all present with similar symptoms of red eye accompanied by extreme pain and photophobia.
- *Bacterial corneal ulcers*: Examination will reveal a staining ulcer on the cornea of varying depth and extent depending on the severity of the condition. If caught early, a course of broad-spectrum oral antibiotics, along with local fortified antibiotic drops will prevent further deterioration and promote restoration of the normal epithelial integrity. Mydriatic eye drops will alleviate pain and redness and relieve the photophobia.
- Viral corneal ulcers can be identified by the classical dendritic pattern on staining. Topical and systemic antiviral medication will be required to promote healing. Mydriatic eye drops will alleviate pain and redness and relieve the photophobia in these conditions as well.

Uveitis:
- This potentially debilitating condition can present as an anterior, posterior or panuveitis, involving both the anterior as well as the posterior chambers of the eye.

- The patient will present with complaints of a varying degree of pain and photophobia depending on the severity of the inflammation.
- If caught early, the treatment will prevent deterioration otherwise the inflammation progresses to create keratic precipitates (KPs) on the endothelium with outpouring of cells into the anterior chamber resulting in an increased stickiness of the iris. Unless the ciliary muscles are kept in motion by the prescription of a medium long-acting mydriatic eye drop, the sticky iris will form posterior synechiae with the anterior lens surface.
- *Management*: Immediate management aims to decrease the inflammation by the administration of topical and if severe enough, oral corticosteroids to control the inflammatory response. The prescription of mydriatic eye drops is necessary in order to prevent synechiae and also to relax the ciliary muscles thereby decreasing the pain.
- Long-term management must include all tests for the detection of an underlying cause.
- Pointers toward possible cause are the type of KPs (Fine KPs in nongranulomatous uveitis and thick mutton fat KPs in granulomatous uveitis). These are not in the purview of emergency management.

  Glaucoma emergencies: High intraocular pressure in the eye will result in the following:
- Pain due to stretching of the ocular structures
- Blurring of the vision and haloes due to corneal edema
- The pupillary reactions will be sluggish
- If the patient has angle closure glaucoma, the anterior chamber will be flat with possible iris bombe if there is a pupillary block.

Angle Closure Glaucoma

This is a very typical presentation with a patient complaining of headache accompanied by generalized congestion of the conjunctiva with blurring of vision. Bringing the intraocular pressure down is immediately rewarding with alleviation of symptoms. Further management on follow-up will require preventive neodymium:yttrium-aluminum-garnet (Nd:YAG) laser peripheral iridotomy.

Angle closure glaucoma will cause most glaucoma emergencies but the intraocular pressure can also be high in untreated open angle glaucoma, secondary glaucoma or steroid-induced glaucoma, resulting in similar symptoms without flattening of the anterior chamber.

Neuro-Ophthalmology Emergencies

Ocular emergencies of neurology origin will bring the patient into the emergency room with any of the following complaints:
- *Sudden loss of vision*: The most ominous and urgent complaint that can result from optic neuritis, temporal arteritis, intracranial lesions affecting the optic tract or papilledema.
- *Diplopia*: This is a very debilitating condition that can arise from loss of innervation to any of the muscles groups or isolated muscles.
- *Ptosis*: Usually resulting from underaction of the third nerve alone or in conjunction with other nerves.

- Proptosis or periorbital swelling in case of thyroid ophthalmopathies and orbital tumors. Management will involve investigation to isolate the cause and treatment of the cause itself if one is found.

Optic neuritis:
- Inflammation of the optic nerve will result in swelling of the optic nerve head with loss of vision to varying degrees.
- The pupil will show afferent pupillary defect in the side involved.
- Management with intravenous (IV) methylprednisolone or a short course of oral steroids is indicated and visual outcome is dependent on early initiation of treatment. If systemic steroids are not instituted early, they have questionable efficacy in the late stage.
- Central vision may be maintained, with a significant peripheral field loss so a visual field test (VFA) and an optical coherence tomography (OCT) to demonstrate optic nerve abnormality are highly indicated.

Papilledema:
- Routine evaluation of hypertensive patients may reveal the presence of papilledema, which then becomes an emergency. On evaluation, the blood pressure may be found to be dangerously high.
- Neurological emergency patients may present with papilledema, in which case, the pupils may be sluggish and the visual fields indicative of the pathology.

Vascular Emergencies

- Sudden loss of vision may be a complaint in patients with vascular abnormalities resulting in hemorrhages in the retina or the vitreous cavity.
- Dilation of the pupil will reveal the pathology.

Venous occlusion—CRVO and BRVO—semiemergencies:
- *Symptoms*: Sudden onset of floaters and varying degrees of visual loss depending on the volume of hemorrhage.
- Venous occlusions are the most common causes of visual loss in diabetic retinopathy.
- Central retinal vein occlusion (CRVO) at the optic nerve is one of the causes of sudden visual loss. About 90% of these occur in people over 80 years.
- Branch retinal vein occlusion (BRVO) will also cause visual loss but occurs in the branch veins.

Central retinal artery occlusion (CRAO)—an acute emergency:
- *Symptoms*: Sudden and complete loss of vision, which may or may not be accompanied by history of acute, transient, pain, or headache.
- This is one of the most dreaded causes of sudden loss of vision. It involves blockage of the central retinal artery resulting in acute ischemia. The treatment requires quick diagnosis and lowering of the eye pressure with ocular massage and medication. Only one out of four patients will retain good vision on recovery.

Table 2: Presentations, causes, investigations and treatment of ocular emergencies.

Presentation	Possible causes to look for	Investigations	Treatment
Acute foreign body sensation accompanied by watering and conjunctival congestion	• Corneal or conjunctival foreign body • Conjunctivitis	Fluorescein staining/evert the upper lid and check the palpebral conjunctiva/check the conjunctival fornices	• Antibiotic eye drops and ointment • Moisturizing eye drops • Removal of foreign body and pad and bandage with antibiotic ointment for 24 hours and close follow-up.
Acute foreign body sensation accompanied by watering	*History of injury:* paper edge/blunt trauma/pointed substances/finger/eye pencil	Fluorescein staining	Pad and bandage with antibiotic ointment for 24 hours and repeat if there is residual staining with fluorescein under observation in cobalt blue filter
Acute pain with circumciliary congestion of the conjunctiva	Flare and cells in the anterior chamber/presence of posterior synechiae	CBC with ESR/ACE/ANA/tubercular antibodies	
Acute pain with congestion, photophobia and haloes	Flattening/shallowing of the anterior chamber accompanied by high intraocular pressure	Check the intraocular pressure and do a gonioscopy to determine the presence and grade of angle closure	Antiglaucoma agents, specifically pilocarpine eye drops to induce miosis causing the intraocular pressure to drop. If insufficient, injection mannitol can be given in IV bolus over 20 minutes after checking the blood pressure
Sudden painless loss of vision	Optic disk edema or hyperemia/disk hemorrhages/optic disk pallor/retinal ischemia (CRAO, CRVO, BRVO)	OCT and fluorescein angiography/visual field test/check pupillary reaction	Refer to ophthalmologist for OCT/visual field test and fluorescein angiography before starting any treatment. In case of CRAO, immediate paracentesis and ocular massage is very essential
Sudden painless loss of vision/floaters and flashes	Gray fundus reflex/retinal detachment on indirect ophthalmoscopy	Screening of the peripheral retina to rule out any holes/tears or retinal detachment	Refer to ophthalmologist for treatment of retinal detachment
Sudden blurring of vision with history of mild pain or painful movements	Afferent pupillary defect/field defect and blurring of the disk margins to suggest optic neuritis	Visual field test/OCT	Systemic steroids have a role if started early otherwise their role is debatable

Contd...

Contd...

Presentation	Possible causes to look for	Investigations	Treatment
History of injury/dog bite/RTA/blunt injuries	Look for penetrating injuries or orbital fracture/history of abuse/look for supraorbital injury	X-ray orbit to rule out retained intraocular foreign body/diplopia charting/pupillary reaction	Dog bite protocol has to be followed according to guidelines. The face is a very sensitive area. May need repair/refer to ophthalmologist. Seidel sign test: Put fluorescein in the eye and check for aqueous leak on the slit lamp
History of splash or contact with chemical agents/sprays	Detailed history is required to determine the agent and classify it as an acid or alkali. The treatment is specific must be instituted immediately		Wash the eye from the medial to the lateral side for at least 30 minutes with normal saline or water if none is available. Find and remove all crystals. Irrigate till the pH reading returns to 7 to 7.3. In alkali injuries, 10% potassium ascorbate has been shown to decrease morbidity

(ACE: angiotensin-converting enzyme; ANA: antinuclear antibody; BRVO: branch retinal vein occlusion; CBC: complete blood count; CRAO: central retinal artery occlusion; CRVO: central retinal vein occlusion; ESR: erythrocyte sedimentation rate; OCT: optical coherence tomography; RTA: road traffic accident)

Vitreous Hemorrhage

Symptoms: Sudden, painless loss of vision to varying degrees depending on the extent of the hemorrhage.
- Examination in all these cases will reveal loss of vision with abnormal fundus glow.
- The eye will be quiet and there is usually no pain unless the intraocular pressure is high.
- The intraocular pressure must be checked, as it can be associated with abnormal vasculature that can be the cause of both the hemorrhage as well a rise in the intraocular pressure.

Management: Vitreous hemorrhage is not an acute emergency. The symptoms are very mild, apart form the vision loss.

The patient needs to be thoroughly examined to rule out the presence of a retinal detachment.

Manage any comorbidity like hypertension or cardiac disease, which may be the pathogenesis of the condition. Modify blood thinners if any.

The immediate management of CRAO is directed at bringing down the intraocular pressure to facilitate greater perfusion. This is done by undertaking anterior chamber paracentesis and with the help of medical management to bring down the intraocular pressure. Efforts must be then made to isolate possible causes with full blood work and cardiology workup.

■ PRESENTATIONS, CAUSES, INVESTIGATIONS AND TREATMENT

Presentations, causes, investigations and treatment of ocular emergencies have been shown in **Table 2**.

CHAPTER 37

Emergency Contraception

Goma Bali Bajaj

■ INTRODUCTION

Emergency contraception can stop pregnancy before it starts. Emergency contraception is a safe way to prevent unintentional pregnancy due to unprotected sex, contraceptives failure, rupture, slippage condom or diaphragm forgotten oral pills or following sexual assault, rape resulting in unintended pregnancies causes mental, social burden to the women and society as a whole. Emergency contraception intervenes and prevents number of unwanted pregnancies by reducing the maternal, mortality, and morbidity. Emergency contraception also known as morning after or post coital method. It is similar to oral contraceptive but hormone doses are higher. Developing embryo, established pregnancy is not affected by emergency contraceptives. Emergency contraceptive is effective only if taken first few days of unprotected sexual exposure before sperm fertilizes the ovum.

■ EMERGENCY CONTRACEPTIVE USE IN INDIA

India was the part of research trial by the World Health Organization (WHO) in 1995-1997 and 1998-2001. Report and recommendations released in 2001 and emergency contraceptive was approved by Drug Controller General of India. Nowadays emergency contraceptive is important method of contraception for unprotected sex and most effective if taken within 12 hours of unprotected sex. Awareness is required among women about timing of dose of the emergency contraception. This method is one time use only so efficacy cannot be calculated by Pearl index. In India, maternal mortality is high and mostly due unsafe abortion. Judicious use of emergency contraceptive plays an important role in reducing mortality and morbidity due to unsafe abortion.

■ EVALUATION FOR EMERGENCY CONTRACEPTIVE USE

History of last menstrual period, length of cycle, and time since last unprotected intercourse, any history of chronic illness, physical examination is not generally required but urine pregnancy test if pregnancy is suspected.

■ TYPE OF EMERGENCY CONTRACEPTIVE PILLS

- *Ulipristal*—more effective than progestin-only or combined pill in preventing the unprotected pregnancy, approved in 2010 and can be taken up to 120 hours after unprotected intercourse.

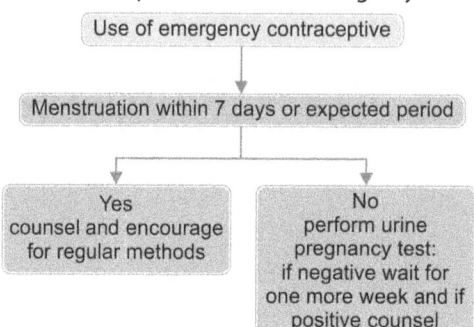

Flowchart 1: Follow-up after the use of emergency contraceptive.

- *Progestin-only pill*—progestin levonorgestrel 1.5 mg single dose or 750 µg 12 hours apart in two doses, can be taken up to 72 hours.
- *Combined pill*—contains both estrogen and progestin in higher dose. It delays the ovulation most effective within 3 days of unprotected intercourse.

Side Effects

No serious side effects, only mild, resolves within 24 hours. Mild side effects are as follows:
- Nausea
- Vomiting
- Mild headache
- Mild tenderness in breast
- Dizziness
- Fatigue
- Delay in menstruation.

FOLLOW-UP AFTER THE USE OF EMERGENCY CONTRACEPTIVE

Follow-up after the use of emergency contraceptive has been shown in **Flowchart 1**.

SUMMARY

There are high maternal mortality rates in country due to abortion resulting from unprotected and unwanted intercourse. Thus, creating social and economic burden over for society. Encouragement and awareness are required from family planning for regular use of oral contraception as well as counseling for emergency contraception, if required.

CHAPTER 38

Facial Swelling

Ashok K Taneja, Akshat Taneja

INTRODUCTION

Facial swelling is defined as the term which involves the localized or generalized swelling over the face. This may involve neck or throat region also. Facial swelling can present as a chronic case in the outpatient department (OPD) or as catastrophic event in emergency. To treat the facial swelling, one must have a deep insight into the anatomy, physiological features involving face so that the etiology can be identified promptly and clearly. This necessitates appropriate and timely treatment. As face is the mirror of body, any small or large swelling can be seen very early and hence, the treatment is never delayed.

ETIOLOGY

The facial swelling, etiologically, can be grouped into two types:
1. Localized
2. Generalized.

Let us discuss few of important causes in both categories.

Localized

- *Ocular congestion*: It causes allergic conjunctivitis, infective conjunctivitis, endophthalmitis, or orbital bone infections.
  Treatment includes antibiotics, decongestants, cold compresses, intraocular steroids (endophthalmitis).
- *Angioedema*: There is a swelling below the eyes. Normally, a drug or food-induced allergic reaction or insect bites, accompanied with urticaria and itching. Additionally, may have urticarial and itching on hands, legs, or other areas of body. Patient may have abdominal cramps also. If severe, may cause emergency situation. Diagnosis can be done on physical exam and eosinophilia, C1 esterase inhibitor test and complement components C2 and C4. Treatment includes cold compresses, antiallergic drugs (oral or injectable depending on the situation), cetirizine, avil, steroids, SC adrenaline in anaphylaxis.
- *Sinusitis*: It is the infected inflammation of facial sinuses mainly frontal and maxillary. If not treated may lead to chronic SOM or thrombosis, which may migrate to cavernous sinus in the midbrain.

Treatment is antibiotics, decongestants, and surgical drainage.
- *Abscesses like Stye*, local nasal or facial hair furunculosis or abscesses in the dental/gum areas.

  Treatment includes cold compresses, antibiotics, anti-inflammatory, and finally surgical drainage.
- *Goiter*: A goiter is a swelling caused by enlarged thyroid gland, which, is not functioning properly. Worldwide, over 90% of goiter cases are caused by iodine deficiency. It may be associated with hypothyroidism or hyperthyroidism. Goiter may be uninodular, multinodular or diffuse. These nodules may be just inactive or toxic. Causes may include iodine deficiency, autoimmune (Hashimoto's), Graves' disease, congenital, or neoplastic in origin. It may be a part of systemic disease or drug induced also. Look for the cause very carefully and order investigations according to the list of differential diagnosis made, based on clinical examination.

  Note: Do not order investigation just as a buffet spread (as it may lead to erroneous diagnosis and hence mismanagement), but rather, as a la carte to make proper diagnosis.

  Treatment depends upon hypo or hyper or euthyroid status. Broadly includes iodine solution, L-thyroxine replacements, steroids (in autoimmune diseases), radioactive iodine, surgery, etc.
- *Parotitis (mumps)*: Parotitis is an inflammation of one or both parotid glands. Parotids are the major salivary glands located on either side of the face and mostly affected by inflammation. Infectious parotitis can be acute bacterial parotitis (patient reports progressive painful swelling of the gland and fever; chewing aggravates the pain); acute viral parotitis-mumps (patient presents with pain and swelling of the gland lasting for 5–9 days, moderate malaise, anorexia, and fever. Mostly seen as bilateral involvement); human immunodeficiency viruses (HIV) parotitis (patient present with nonpainful swelling of the gland and mostly patient is asymptomatic); parotitis in tuberculosis (patient present with chronic nontender swelling of one parotid gland or a lump within the gland with clinical evidence of tuberculosis).

  Treatment includes, local heat in chronic and cold compresses in acute, gentle massage of the gland from posterior to anterior, and hydration and sialagogues. If pus is expressed from the Stensen duct, culture and sensitivity studies guide antibiotic selection. Intermittent irrigation of the ductal system with saline, steroid solution, and/or an antibiotic and mechanical removal of inspissated mucous or pus from the ducts can also be done. Treatment of the primary disease (e.g. HIV, rheumatoid arthritis) is advocated. IV antibiotics in severe acute bacterial infections (for methicillin resistant (MRSA)-vancomycin-linezolid-tigecycline-colistin) may be required.
- *Lymphadenopathy (LAP)*: Enlargement of lymph nodes, essentially is a result of infection somewhere else, the area from where the lymph is drained. LAP of face and neck is an important marker for metastasis of malignancy on any part of the body. LAP can be infective, inflammatory (secondary to chronic diseases like Koch's/HIV/sarcoidosis, etc.) or neoplastic (part of lymphoma, metastatic of nearby organs like lungs/bronchus/thyroid, etc.

or from far away primary). The LAP needs to be investigated thoroughly and treatment depends on the primary cause.

Note: Important thing is to examine and identify the small LAP in submaxillary/ submandibular or supraclavicular area which gives you a clue to the early diagnosis of systemic diseases like Koch's, lymphoma or metastasis. Early diagnosis is the key to good treatment.

- *Cushingoid*: Cushing syndrome or features like Cushing syndrome also called hypercortisolism. High production of cortisol can produce some of the hallmark signs of Cushing syndrome—a fatty hump between your shoulders, a rounded face, and pink or purple stretch marks on your skin. Cushing syndrome can also result in high blood pressure (BP), bone loss, and occasionally, type 2 diabetes. It can also cause thinning, fragile skin that bruises easily with slow healing of cuts, insect bites, and infections. May also cause acne, decreased libido, erectile dysfunction, fatigue, muscle weakness, depression, and cognitive difficulties. Causes include pituitary gland tumors (adenoma), ectopic ACTH producing tumors (carcinoma of lung, pancreas, thyroid, or thymus), primary diseases of adrenals or drug induced (steroid therapy: chronic or overdose). Patient presents with moon like face with hypertension.

Treatment depends on removal of primary cause and medications to control excessive production of cortisol at the adrenal gland like ketoconazole (Nizoral), mitotane (Lysodren), and metyrapone (Metopirone).

Generalized

- *Preeclampsia*: Preeclampsia is gestational hypertension plus proteinuria (>300 mg of protein in a 24-hour urine sample). Severe preeclampsia involves a blood pressure greater than 160/110, with additional medical signs and symptoms. HELLP syndrome is a type of preeclampsia. It is a combination of three medical conditions: hemolytic anemia, elevated liver enzymes, and low-platelet count. It is a medical emergency.
  Treatment:
  - *I/V magnesium sulfate:* Loading dose of 4–6 g in 100 mL saline to be given in 30–40 min, followed by infusion of 2 g/hr (Magpie Trial). It reduces the risk of eclampsia by 50%. In women who already have seizures, magnesium sulfate is a better choice than phenytoin.
  - *Aspirin (enteric coated):* If administered early in pregnancy, prevents development of preeclampsia in high risk patients. It showed 17% reduction. Recommended dose: 75–100 mg daily.
  - Calcium supplementation also helps.
  - *Three agents should not be used:* Progesterone, low-molecular weight heparin, and nitric oxide donors (e.g. nicorandil, glyceryl trinitrites), ACE or ARB inhibitors.
- *Anasarca*: Generally referred to as edema, which is generalized and present all over the body. As Claude Bernard said "edema is merely a result of expansion of milieu interieur—the extracellular fluid of the body." So, it is defined as abnormal accumulation of extravascular extracellular (interstitial fluid) over the body. All edema comes from the circulating blood,

hence, its composition is similar to plasma and contains electrolytes, glucose, urea amino acids, and many more crystalloids. The protein contents depend on the cause of edema. Edema of the face is a sign common to a variety of disorders and recognized very early.

Commonly the causes of anasarca includes nutritional (hypoproteinemia, anemia, cachexia, beriberi), cardiac disorders (heart failure, pericardial effusion, constrictive pericarditis); renal disorders (nephritic-nephrotic syndromes-CKDs); hepatic disorders (cirrhosis-portal hypertension); drug induced (vasodilators); blood malignancies (leukemias, etc.); infections (filaria, chronic malaria); autoimmune (Raynaud's disease, vasculitis); endocrine disorders (hypo/hyperthyroidism), and edema of pregnancy.

Management depends on the cause. Treatment of the cause in emergency room depends on the sickness of the patient.

- *Anaphylaxis*: It is usually an emergency which can be a life-threatening condition and hence, timely and adequately critical care is necessitated. It is an allergic reaction with rapid onset of sign and symptoms on exposure to allergen. The signs and symptoms usually include urticarial, rashes, itching over the body swelling over the face. If exposure to allergen is large (in case of drugs) or hypersensitivity of patient is enhanced (as in G6PD deficiency), there can be fall in blood pressure, respiratory distress, mental confusion, and shock.

Treatment includes IV fluids, antihistaminic drugs, steroids (preferably hydrocortisone or methyl prednisolone); SC adrenaline if shock is persisting. In advance cases, patient may require ventilatory support, pacemaker (to cover bradycardia); vasopressors or hemodialysis.

EVALUATION AND MANAGEMENT

In emergency department: Following evaluation of the patient is done.

History

Whether swelling is acute, chronic, or acute on chronic.
Acute:
- H/O Trauma
- H/O Fever, cough with expectoration, hemoptysis
- H/O Severe headache, tremors, slurred speech or fits
- H/O Drug intake or food ingested
- H/O generalized diseases like hepatic, cardiac, renal, thyroid disorders, etc.
- Dyspnea or orthopnea/PND/palpitations.

Examination

- Look for features of trauma on face like bruises, reddish, or bluish discoloration patches, hives, insect bites.
- If trauma: feel for features of nasal, orbital, maxillary, or mandibular fractures.

- Look for acute ocular, dental, auricular, gum, parotid infections.
- Orthopneic or normal respiration.
- Systemic exam—like pulse, BP; JVP; cardiac, hepatic respiratory or central nervous system (CNS) exam.
- Pregnancy associated with high BP. R/O preeclampsia. If present, treat as described above.

Note: Examination should be thorough. No short cuts. Normally proper history gives you a good clue to the diagnosis. Never under estimate the power of good history and physical examination. In 95% of cases, the diagnosis is accurately made with this basic and simple method.

Management

If the situation is life-threatening as in case of anaphylaxis due to insect/snake bite, food or drugs causing respiratory distress or severe trauma obstructing airways, one has to act with lightning speed.

- Take care of IV fluids, O_2 support, airways clearing, BP monitoring (vasopressors if required); fresh blood transfusion (in case of severe bleed); IV avil + hydrocortisone/methyl prednisolone (in case anaphylaxis or allergy). Patient may require SC adrenaline in case of severe anaphylaxis (of normally snake bite or food items especially mushrooms or sea food).
- Drainage of the abscess: If causing severe pain, fever, and obstructing vital organ. Be careful not to overdo. Preferably do it in operation theater (OT) not in ER. As the infection or infected thrombus may move to CNS and cause cavernous sinus thrombosis or CNS abscess.
- Ventilatory support (if patient is not able to maintain O_2 saturation).
- Pacemaker if in severe bradycardia (snake bites and mushroom poisoning).
- Hemodialysis, CytoSorb's or ECMOs, if situation warrants.
- Look for underlying cause, in case of acute on chronic swellings. Treat it accordingly.
  Caution:
  - Do not try to fix any fracture of face manually in ER, as it may cause further airway block or thromboembolism or fresh bleed.
  - Do not rush for investigations except the basics tests like electrolytes, ECG, hematocrit, blood gases, KFT, etc. first stabilize the patient and then send him for computed tomography (CT) scans or magnetic resonance imaging (MRIs), etc.
  - Never forget cold compresses for local painful swelling or bruises or hives.

■ SUMMARY

Facial swelling, localized to generalized, may be just innocuous or may be life-threatening. The dictum is to recognize the cause at the earliest and accurately. The prompt diagnosis helps in adequate and correct treatment. Stye on the eye to dental infections to parotitis, lymphadenopathy all point to the underlying sinister cause. Since face is the mirror of the body, the systemic diseases may show their signs on face as edema. Treating the underlying cause resolves facial edema.

CHAPTER 39

Fatigue

Au Kin Heng Constantine

INTRODUCTION

Fatigue or tiredness is a physiological state that presents with reduction in alertness, motivation, attention, capacity for mental performance like reasoning, and physical activity. The Allied Pilots Association found that the performance level of a person with 20 hours of continuously being awake was the same as a person with 0.05% blood alcohol content (BAC). This level of BAC is equivalent to driving drunk in many countries. Take note that a fatigued person is sleepy, but sleepiness is not equal to fatigue, although inadequate sleep or poor quality sleep is a common reason for fatigue. Many behavior and medical conditions can cause fatigue. Fatigue can be transient or chronic. Because fatigue is so common in life, only 1 in 400 may seek medical advice. The subjective characteristic of fatigue also complicates the issue. Fatigue not only affects the person (not necessarily a patient), but it can pose great danger to others. The aviation industry, the health care industry, drivers, and pedestrians have many disastrous examples of fatigue-based accidents or injuries.

ETIOLOGY

Causes of fatigue can roughly be divided into physiologic fatigue, sleep disorders, and fatigue secondary to medical conditions.

Physiologic Fatigue

Physiologic fatigue is caused by inadequate quality sleep or healthy sleep and disruption of the circadian rhythm (body clock) and occurs in the absence of any major medical conditions. The primary factors used to determine fatigue are the duration of wakefulness and activity level. After 16 hours of continuous wakefulness, performance starts to drop significantly. Poor quality sleep can be a result of inadequate sleep duration, a lack of deep sleep despite adequate total sleeping hours, and sleep disorders, such as sleep apnea. Sleep is necessary for the body and mind to restore metabolic balance. A sleep cycle is in divided into different stages. Usually, Stage 1 of sleep lasts for about 5 minutes and is light in nature. In Stage 2, sleep spans for the next 25 minutes. It is deeper than Stage 1, and the sleeper has a reduced heart rate and temperature. Stages 3 and 4 (or a combined Stage 3) are a deep form of sleep and body repair is at its peak during this stage; brain activity is the lowest at this time. The next stage is called the rapid eye movement (REM) stage, which is when dreams and rewiring of neurons occur. Usually, 25% of sleep time is allocated to REM, but this time varies with age. A usual sleep cycle consists of about 90 minutes. Deep sleep is important for the restoration of the mind and body. Any disruption to deep sleep leads to relatively strong fatigue. Long working hours lead to inadequate sleep duration. Waking up during light sleep gives rise to a relatively low-sleep inertia, and alertness can be regained shortly. On the other hand, being woken up during deep sleep leads to a relatively longer sleep inertia with impaired alertness. A high activity or exercise level leads to fatigue due to lactic acid accumulation. Vibration, such as in an aircraft, causes fatigue as well. Both too much noise and too less noise in the environment can cause fatigue or can disturb sleep, as can extreme temperatures. Sudden changes in life style, such as increasing exercise duration and changing diet, can also lead to fatigue or disturb sleep quality.

Our body follows a circadian rhythm, which lasts a little longer than 24 hours (24 hours and 12 minutes). The synchronization of the circadian rhythm and the environment may be the third most important determinant of fatigue. This circadian rhythm synchronizes with the environment via zeitgebers, which means time-giver in German, and light is the most important zeitgeber. Blue light resembles daylight and is more effective in waking people up, while red light resembles dusk and dawn and is less effective in waking. The intensity and duration of exposure to light is also a factor that must be considered. Social activities and exercise and fitness are zeitgebers and affect alertness and sleep quality.

Food is a zeitgeber. Regular meal time contributes to the body's clock. The amount of food and type of food can affect alertness. A heavy meal may cause sleepiness. Food consisting of complex carbohydrates, proteins, and fats are less tiring and can even be refreshing. Dumping syndrome and postprandial hypoglycemia lead to fatigue. Drugs, both over-the-counter (OTC) and prescription, affect the circadian rhythm. Examples of these include alcohol, caffeine, sedative antihistamines, and melatonin. A little bit of alcohol may help one fall asleep, but it may disturb the sleep quality and the diuretic effect is certainly not favorable. The hangover effect is a histotoxic hypoxia, and it may impair alertness for a long time. Caffeine keeps one alert by binding to the adenosine receptors in the brain, but over-use or withdrawal may impair alertness. Mistiming caffeine consumption can disturb sleep as well. Nicotine as in cigarettes may help alertness but it may cause harm in the long run and may disturb sleep.

Two windows of circadian low (WOCLs) exist. Usually, the primary WOCL spans from 02:00 to 06:00, and the secondary WOCL spans from 14:00 to 18:00. During WOCLs, our alertness is relatively lowered. Usually, sleeping during a WOCL is more efficient than sleeping during the other windows. A circadian challenge is when we have to work during a WOCL. Working the night shift is a typical example. Health care providers have much personal experience with this.

With the advancement of aviation technology, one can cross a few time zones within a few hours. This achievement has a short history of only about 100 years, and our bodies and minds have not yet evolved to adopt to jet lag. Jet lag happens when our body's clock and the environment's clock are unsynchronized. Usually, traveling westbound is easier for the body than traveling eastbound. The body normally takes 1 day to adjust for every 1-hour of time zone crossed. Jet lag complicated with shift-work is a perfect circadian challenge. Pilots, crews, and other personnel in the aviation industry have to face this challenge almost daily. Fatigue is a known threat in the aviation industry and is reported to be at least one of the contributing factors to many aviation disasters. Nowadays, rules and regulations govern the number of working hours and rest hours in the aviation industry, and many airline companies have imposed fatigue management programs to guide pilots and crews in rest and duty planning. Flights are cancelled if not enough fit-for-duty crew is available. It is a pity that the health care industry is slow to follow this example. Repeated days of inadequate sleep can add up to accumulated fatigue or sleep debt. Adequate quality sleep or healthy sleep may be the only way to "pay off" sleep debt.

Sleep Disorders

Sleep disorders like sleep apnea and narcolepsy often disturb sleep. A sleep apnea patient may wake up hundreds of times while sleeping, making deep sleep impossible. In narcolepsy, the brain cannot regulate the sleep-wake cycle normally. Other sleep disorders are periodic limb movement disorder (PLMD), somnambulism (sleepwalking), nocturnal enuresis, and parasomnias (night terrors).

Secondary Causes of Fatigue

These are the underlying medical conditions that may cause fatigue. Any pathology can cause fatigue and disturb sleep. It is estimated that a medical condition exist in about 20–30% of cases. This kind of fatigue usually lasts longer than 1 month, and the list is very long. One can follow a diagnosis aid, such as the surgical sieve, to help the thought process. The following discussion is a modified mnemonics of vitamin CDE. The word, "PreScribe," was added to the front so as to represent "physiologic causes" and "sleep disorders." This list, "PreScribe Vitamin AI," cannot cover all causes but serves as an aid for handling a fatigued patient.

Vascular: Ischemic heart disease, and heart failure cause pump failure occurs in the circulatory system. Cerebellar vascular diseases may lead to hypoxia and inefficient removal of metabolic waste in the brain, causing fatigue. Infectious/Inflammatory: Any acute infection in the respiratory tract, urinary tract, and the gastrointestinal tract or reproductive system, etc. cause fatigue. Arthropod transmitted diseases like Lyme disease cause fatigue. Such an infection can be subtle or subclinical, and the patient may not be aware of it at all. Any chronic infection, such as tuberculosis, human immunodeficiency viruses (HIV), brucellosis, can cause fatigue. Traumatic: Blood loss leading to anemia and pain, causing poor fatigue and sleep. Anemia/Autoimmune: Common causes of anemia include acute gastrointestinal bleeding, major trauma, thalassemia, malaria, iron-deficiency, and so on. The body's immune system malfunctions in autoimmune diseases. Lots of unnecessary cellular activities take place, and many of these activities damage the body. Repairing this damage requires energy. Rheumatoid arthritis, polymyalgia rheumatica, Crohn's disease, and systemic lupus erythematous (SLE) are some examples. Metabolic: Both catabolism and anabolism need and use energy. Any imbalance in demand and supply causes fatigue. Examples are hypoglycemia, hyperglycemia, acidosis, hyperthermia, hypothermia, hypokalemia, hypocalcemia, and dehydration. Iatrogenic: Both OTC and prescription drugs cause fatigue, even when used within the suggested dosage. Some examples include sedative antihistamines, benzodiazepine, beta-blockers, opioid (analgesics), and hypnotics. Any invasive procedure and even minor surgery can cause fatigue. Reasons can include the upset of body physiology, pain, or mental stress. Neoplastic: Cancer cells consume a lot of energy, and the immune system uses a lot of energy to defend the body against cancer cells. The absorption of nutrients, gaseous exchange, ventilation, and circulation may also become disrupted, causing fatigue. Abuse/Toxic: Abuse of alcohol, hypnotics, sedatives, and drug overdose and withdrawal can all cause fatigue. Pay special note to the possibility of withdrawal. If there is a cluster of patients, exclude the possibility of poisoning like water source, carbon monoxide (e.g. a leaking pipe). Behavior: Any behavior leading to poor sleep, such as exercising just before bedtime, using a smartphone (which has blue light) before bedtime, or drinking coffee in the late afternoon, all cause poor sleep. Chronic fatigue syndrome presents in all age groups. The major criteria include fatigue lasting for more than 6 months, fatigue not being be resolved with bed rest, and having daily activity reduced by 50%. Physical criteria include a low-grade fever, nonexudative pharyngitis, and lymphadenopathy. There is also a list of minor criteria. A diagnosis is made when all major criteria are met or when eight minor criteria or six major criteria plus two physical criteria are met. Depression or other psychiatric illnesses can be comorbid conditions or stand-alone conditions. Health care providers must bear these in mind. Endocrine: Many endocrine diseases, such as hypothyroidism, hyperthyroidism, diabetes, and Addison's disease, cause fatigue. Fibromyalgia/Failure: Fibromyalgia may present together with irritable bowel syndrome, chronic headache. Failure in any organs or systems: Examples of such failures are heart failure, respiratory failure, liver failure, and renal failure. Nutrients and oxygen cannot be absorbed or metabolized properly, and a lot of excessive energy is needed, such as in dyspnea. Gynecological/Gastrointestinal (GI). Conditions: Pregnancy, recent abortion, and pelvic inflammatory diseases cause fatigue. Occasionally, a woman may not be aware of being pregnant, especially during the early stages. As the old school adage says, any lady is pregnant is proven otherwise. GI tract upset can lead to poor nutrient and water absorption or loss, such as with diarrhea. Dumping syndrome and postprandial hypoglycemia lead to fatigue. Hypoxia: High altitude in mountaineering and even in pressurized aircraft may lead to subtle hypoxia. A working environment in which fuel is burned may cause hypoxia and carbon monoxide poisoning, and patients may not be aware of hypoxia and carbon monoxide poisoning. Idiopathic: The underlying cause may not be at all obvious. **Table 1** summarizes the common possible causes of fatigue.

PATHOPHYSIOLOGY

Sleep maintains the metabolic-caloric balance; hence, poor sleep leads to fatigue. Over-activity, infection, organ failure, malignancy, and so on all cause a metabolic-caloric imbalance. Other mechanisms, such as a decline in blood pH (e.g. lactic acidosis), a rise in body temperature, dyspnea, activation of J receptors in the lungs, and neural impulses from the muscles, cause

Table 1: Mnemonics for causes of fatigue—PreScribe vitamin AI.

Mnemonics	Category	Examples
Pre-	**P**hysiologic	Inadequate quality sleep, excessive activity, unfavorable life-style; circadian challenge, jet lag, shift work.
Scribe	**S**leep disorders	Sleep apnea, narcolepsy, periodic limb movement disorder, somnambulism (sleepwalking), nocturnal enuresis, and parasomnias (night terrors).
V	**V**ascular	Ischemic heart disease, heart failure, intracerebellar vascular diseases.
I	**I**nfectious/Inflammatory	Acute/chronic respiratory tract, urinary tract, gastrointestinal tract, and reproductive system infections. Arthropod-transmitted diseases like Lyme disease. Infection can be subtle.
T	**T**raumatic	Blood loss and pain.
A	**A**nemia/Autoimmune	Acute gastrointestinal bleeding, major trauma, thalassemia, malaria, and iron deficiency. Rheumatoid arthritis, polymyalgia rheumatica, Crohn's disease, and systemic lupus erythematous (SLE).
M	**M**etabolic	Hypoglycemia, hyperglycemia, acidosis, hyperthermia, hypothermia, hypokalemia, hypocalcemia, and dehydration.
I	**I**atrogenic	Any over-the-counter (OTC) or prescription drugs (even used within the suggested dosage). Any invasive procedures and even minor surgeries that cause fatigue.
N	**N**eoplastic	Any cancers.
A	**A**buse/Toxic	Abuse of alcohol, hypnotics, sedatives, drug overdose, and substance withdrawal.
B	**B**ehavior	Any behavior leading to poor sleep, such as exercising just before bedtime and using a smartphone (blue light) before bedtime.
C	**C**hronic fatigue syndrome	Includes major criteria, physical criteria, and minor criteria.
D	**D**epression or other psychiatric illnesses	Depression or other psychiatric illnesses can be a comorbid conditions or stand-alone conditions.
E	**E**ndocrine	Hypothyroidism, hyperthyroidism, diabetes, and Addison's disease.
F	**F**ibromyalgia/Failure in any organs or systems	Fibromyalgia may present together with irritable bowel syndrome, chronic headache. Failure in any organs or systems like the liver, kidney, the circulatory system, and the respiratory system.
G	**G**ynecological conditions **G**astrointestinal tract	Pregnancy, recent abortion, and pelvic inflammatory diseases. Poor nutrient and water absorption or loss, such as with diarrhea; dumping syndrome, postprandial hypoglycemia.
H	**H**ypoxia	High altitude, such as in mountaineering, air-travel, and work environments in which fuel is burned (may have CO poisoning as well).
I	**I**diopathic	Does not include any obvious causes.

a sensation of fatigue. Circadian challenges, such as night shift work, disrupt the body's clock and causes fatigue.

Pathological conditions can lead to the poor absorption of nutrients, an excessive use of energy, poor oxygen supply, and the accumulation of metabolic waste.

CLINICAL PRESENTATION

The presentation of fatigue can be categorized into mental, physical, and emotional groups.
- Mental presentation of fatigue includes a reduction in alertness, motivation, attention, and the capacity for mental performance, such as reasoning, loss of situational awareness, and increased reaction time and poor decision-making.
- Physical presentation of fatigue can be generalized as weakness or a lack of energy.
- Emotional presentation of fatigue includes a loss of temper, moodiness, and indifference.

RED FLAGS

- *The underlying cause:* Fatigue and poor sleep are so common that health care providers and even the patients might have ignored their significance. Causes other than poor sleep must be identified. Fatigue can be the only symptom of anemia and tuberculosis and the first sign of malignancy. Chronic fatigue may be a symptom of depression.
- *Occupation:* Fatigue can lead to disasters in certain occupations, such as with pilots, drivers, and health care providers.
- *A cluster of patients:* Exclude the possibility of toxicology. A leaking pipe may cause carbon monoxide poisoning in a household. Heavy metal poisoning of the water source is another example.
- *Other risks:* The intention of self-harm or harming others must be handled with care. It can also be a sign of substance abuse.

EVALUATION

History

Take a full history. The duration of fatigue must be noted. Recent changes in life style and milestones in life must be considered. Any symptoms, such as Type B symptoms (unexplained weight change, fever) in Hodgkin's lymphoma and melena, must be asked about. Check for drug history, including the OTC drugs, supplements, therapeutic drugs, and recreational drugs. Ask about occupation history and beware of any possible causes of and risks for fatigue. Interviewing the spouse or partner may help to identify sleep quality and the presence of heavy snoring.

Physical Examination

During the general exam, look for edema, pallor, shortness of breath, a goiter, or lymph node enlargement. Look for signs of any major organ failure, such as jaundice. Skin wound suggesting arthropod contact (bite, sting, scratch, etc.).

INTERPRETATION OF FINDINGS

Fatigue is common, and only 1 in 400 patients bother to seek medical consultation for fatigue, so take it seriously. Seek more information from the history. Pay attention to subtle signs. Think of possible medical causes and possible risks.

INVESTIGATIONS

A sleepiness scale, such as the Stanford Sleepiness Scale, and other tools may quantify the severity of fatigue and help with monitoring treatment. It was found that only 5% of persons or patients who have fatigue benefit from doing laboratory investigations or imaging. Tests must be ordered in the context of a full history and physical examination, or else the tests are useless.

Basic tests that should be considered are a complete blood count, a liver function test, a renal function test, and a glucose test. Other tests that can be considered are a thyroid function test, an erythrocyte sedimentation rate (ESR) test, a cortisol test, an immunological marker test, a drug-screening test, a chest X-ray, an electrocardiogram (ECG), an HIV test, a pregnancy test, and possibly a sleep test. Please choose tests according to the findings from the history and physical examination.

TREATMENT

General Approach

There is no magic bullet to counteract fatigue, and adequate quality sleep or healthy sleep may be the only solution. Plan for rest, diet, exercise, and other activities. Timing, duration, and the amount of each must be considered. As lifestyle is quite personal, the following serve as a guide for consideration only.

- Sleep hygiene may be improved with a sleep diary. Record factors that affect sleep quality. The spouse or partner may give valuable advice.
- Plan for sleep and rest. Pilots and crews use protocol and computer programs to plan rest and meals. Factors like duty hours, time zones, and ground hours are taken into account.
- Create a favorable sleeping environment. Take care of the temperature, background noise, and so on. **Figure 1** is a good summary of how to create a favorable sleeping environment.
- A presleep ritual may help. Avoid too much excitement like watching horror movies or reading blue light from a smart phone before sleep.
- Lifestyle modifications may work. Exercise therapy shows high evidence in counteracting fatigue. Appropriate time and plan of exercising and consuming coffee and tea is important. The effects of these factors vary from one person to another. In some cases, a change of occupation may be the only effective solution.
- Napping may help improve alertness. Napping is the most effective during the WOCLs (i.e. 02:00 to 06:00 or 14:00 to 18:00). The duration of a nap should either be less than 30 minutes or about 90 minutes. This is because one should avoid waking up during Stage 3 deep sleep (which usually happens between 30 min and 90 min after falling asleep), and if time

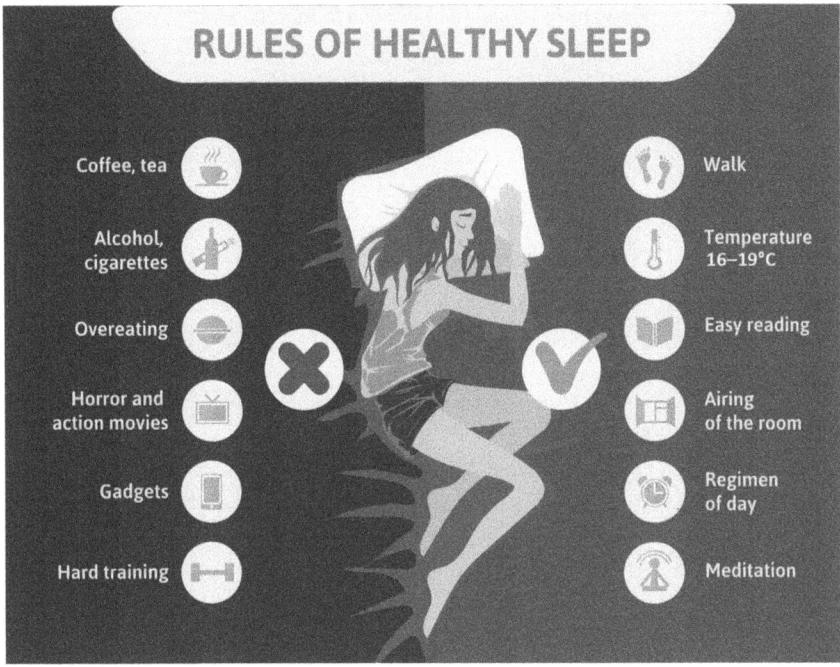

Fig. 1: Rules of quality of healthy sleep.

permits, it is better to complete one sleep cycle. Napping for about 3 hours (i.e. two sleep cycles) is usually all right, but napping for more than 4 hours in the afternoon may disrupt the circadian rhythm and disturb nighttime sleep.
- Cognitive behavior therapy is effective in adults with chronic fatigue syndrome.
- Massage, physiotherapy, meditation, and acupuncture may relieve some fatigue and facilitate sleeping. Effects may be transient though and may have to be repeated regularly.
- A sleeping aid (OTC) like vitamin B_{12} and melatonin may help. Energy drinks may contain a high volume of caffeine and sugar, so consume them with care, as they may complicate the situation.
- Prescription drugs like benzodiazepine and zolpidem are also commonly used. Doctors must be careful of patients' occupations, as pilots and drivers may face a taking-drugs-while-on-duty issue. Drug tests are used in the aviation industry and in other industries. A false negative (positive and indeterminate results) carries legal implications. In the aviation industry, clearance is assumed for five half-lives of a drug. Doctors must carefully consider the time of drug use and the dosage. Sometimes, a reduced dose may be good enough to help the patient fall asleep and may allow a shorter clearance time.
- In the past, amphetamines were prescribed to armies to keep them awake. Modafinil is now the choice for the armies or shift-duty workers. However, drugs can never replace sleep and should be used with a great deal of precaution.

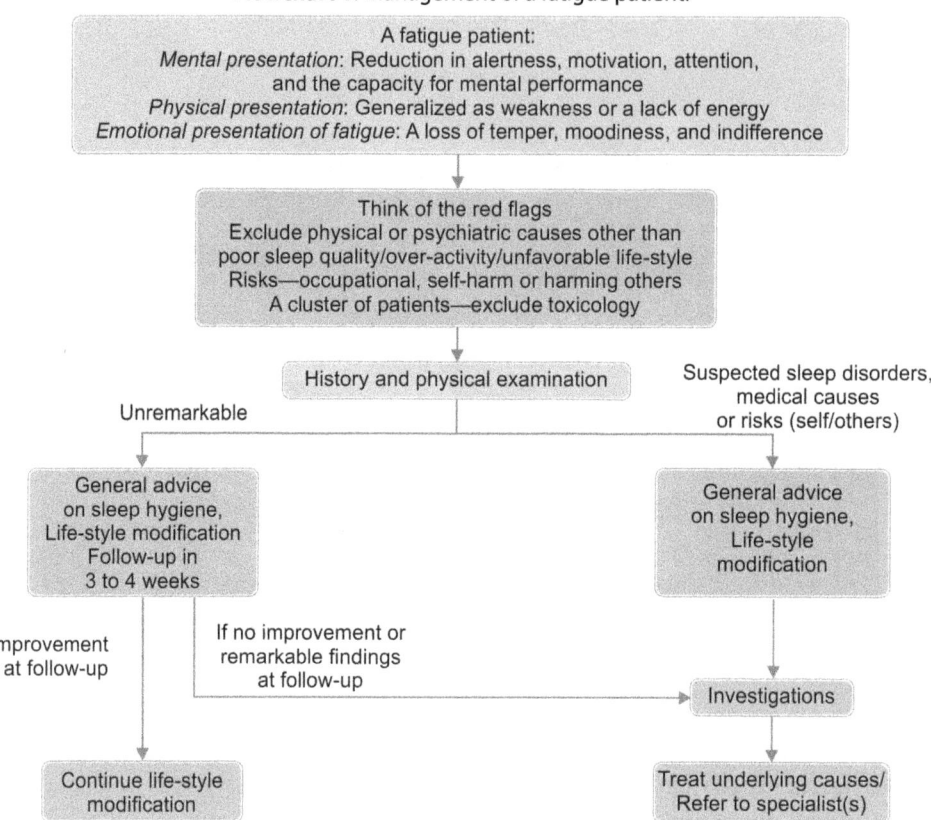

Flowchart 1: Management of a fatigue patient.

- Continuous sleep problems lasting 3 weeks or more may need assessment by a sleep specialist. Sleep apnea is often underdiagnosed.
- Offer follow-up to assess the condition.

Specific Treatment for Sleep Disorders and Medical Causes

A sleep test and consultation with respiratory physicians or neurologists may be needed. Treat the underlying medical conditions. Sometimes, a simple measure is good enough: oxygen helps with hypoxia, and descent to a lower attitude helps with mountain sickness and in aviation. Refer to relevant specialists, such as psychiatrists and rheumatologists, if needed.

SUMMARY

Fatigue is a common phenomenon. The main causes are inadequate quality sleep, over-activity, a lack of synchronization between the circadian rhythm and the environment, and sleep disorders. However, health care providers should not ignore this complaint and must check for the possibility of underlying medical conditions, psychiatric diseases, the risk of self-harm, occupational risks, and risks posed to others. Fatigue is summarized through different steps mentioned in **Flowchart 1**.

ACKNOWLEDGMENT

Thanks to Dr Quintin Kwok of the Accident and Emergency Department of Queen Elizabeth Hospital, Hong Kong for his comments on the draft of this chapter.

CHAPTER 40

Fever

Akanksha Rastogi, Amit Mittal

INTRODUCTION

It is the elevation in core body temperature exceeding the daily variation with a rise in hypothalamic set point.

Normal temperature variation: At 6 AM, maximal normal body temperature is 37.2°C (98.9°F) while at 4 PM to 6 PM, maximal normal body temperature is 37.7°C (99.9°F). Normal circadian variation is 0.5°C or 1°F.

TYPES OF FEVER

1. *Continuous*: Fever that never touches the baseline and does not fluctuate more than 1°C during 24 hours period.

   The most common causes of this fever are:
   - Enteric fever (usually in 2nd week)
   - Acute rheumatic fever
   - Pneumonia
   - Meningococcal meningitis
   - Miliary tuberculosis
   - Connective tissue disorders.

2. *Intermittent*: Always touches the baseline during 24 hours period. Further classified as:
   - *Quotidian fever*: Fever spikes occur daily. For example:
     – Urinary tract infection
     – Pent-up pus anywhere
     – Amebic liver abscess
     – Septicemia
     – *Plasmodium vivax* infection.
   - *Tertian fever*: Fever occurs on alternate days, usually seen in benign tertian malaria by *P. vivax* and malignant tertian malaria by *Plasmodium falciparum*.
   - *Quartan fever*: Fever occurring with a gap of 2 days. It is caused by *Plasmodium malariae* and is rarely seen in India.

3. *Remittent*: Fever never touches the baseline and fluctuation is more than 2°C.

Fever of unknown origin: Fever of unknown origin (FUO) has multiple origins. It was derived in 1961 by Petersdorf and Beeson as:
- Duration of fever for at least 3 weeks.
- Fever more than 38.3°C on several occasions.
- Uncertain diagnosis despite of 1 week of investigations in hospital.

Hyperpyrexia: Body temperature more than 41.5°C or 106.7°F is termed as hyperpyrexia, usually seen in central nervous system (CNS) hemorrhages, heat stroke, neuroleptic malignant syndrome, serotonin syndrome, etc.

Relative bradycardia: Normally there is increase in pulse rate by 10 beats/minute for per degree Fahrenheit rise of body temperature. Failure to rise in pulse rate by 10 beats/minute for 1 degree Fahrenheit rise in temperature results into relative bradycardia.

Causes:
- Viral fever
- First week of enteric fever
- Scrub typhus
- Brucellosis and leptospirosis.

ETIOLOGY/CAUSES

It is broadly classified as:
- *Infectious causes*: Fever with chills and rigors is most suggestive of infection. *Viral* like dengue, viral hepatitis, cytomegalovirus (CMV), Epstein-Barr virus (EBV), human immunodeficiency virus (HIV) infection, etc.; *bacterial* like typhoid fever, tuberculosis, abscesses in any organ, infective endocarditis; *parasitic* causes like malaria, amebiasis, toxoplasmosis; *unusual infections*: rickettsiosis, brucellosis, legionellosis, leptospirosis, Lyme disease; *fungal* infections.
- *Tropical fever*: Also termed as Monsoon fever. Fever which is seen in tropical and subtropical areas. Diseases to be considered are malaria, dengue, scrub typhus, rickettsiosis, leptospirosis, enteric fever. Tropical fevers have very high morbidity and mortality rate. Symptoms overlap and it is difficult to differentiate at the time of presentation. Empiric therapy needs to be initiated at the time of onset.
- *Noninfectious inflammatory causes*:
  - *Autoimmune conditions*: Mixed connective tissue disorders, systemic lupus erythematosus, rheumatoid arthritis, relapsing polychondritis, polymyositis, antiphospholipid syndrome, ankylosing spondylitis, and sarcoidosis.
  - *Vasculitis*: Churg-Strauss syndrome, Takayasu arteritis, giant cell arteritis, and allergic vasculitis.
- *Malignant conditions*: Most commonly seen with malignancies of reticuloendothelial origin like leukemia and lymphoma. Other causes like multiple myeloma, plasmacytoma, myelodysplastic syndromes, renal cell carcinoma, malignant histiocytosis, aleukemic leukemia can also present only with FUO. Solid tumors and metastasis from breast, colon, lung, and pancreas.

- *Thermoregulatory disorders*: Central (brain tumor, encephalitis, stroke) and peripheral (exercise-induced hyperthermia, hyperthyroidism).
- *Less common causes*:
  - *Factitious fever*: Artificially induced by the patient, e.g. intravenous injections by contaminated water, more common in young women working as health care professionals.
  - *Drug fever:* It is relatively a common condition but remains frequently undiagnosed. Usually associated with rash and eosinophilia (seen in 25% cases) but may not be always present. Drugs like barbiturates, antibiotics like carbapenems, cephalosporins, minocycline, nitrofurantoin, and vancomycin.

PATHOPHYSIOLOGY

Pathophysiology of fever has been shown in **Flowchart 1**.

Fever with Chills and Rigors

Rise in hypothalamic set point → neurons in vasomotor center get activated → cutaneous vessels of hands and feet vasoconstrict → shunting of blood away from periphery to the internal organs essentially decreases heat loss from the skin and the person may shiver violently.

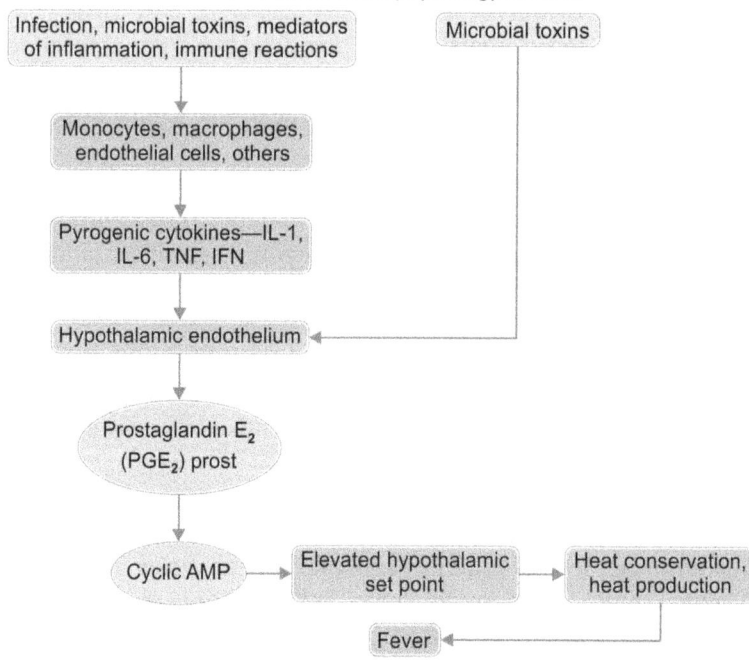

Flowchart 1: Pathophysiology of fever.

(AMP: adenosine monophosphate; IFN: interferon; IL: interleukin; TNF: tumor necrosis factor)

Once the higher temperature is reached, heat loss starts and cutaneous vessels dilate for dissipation of heat. Patient feels hot and sweating starts.

EVALUATION

Importance of a good history, physical examination and focused laboratory testing makes the diagnosis in majority of cases.

History

History should be taken from the patient or from the person most familiar with the patient. Duration of fever, onset of fever, associated localizing sign and symptoms, significant weight loss, night sweats should be asked. Pattern of fever is important. Special focus should be on history of recent travel, exposure to pets, and intake of raw milk, immunosuppression, and drugs including antimicrobials, presence of skin rash, eschar, high-risk behavior, and contact to a patient having tuberculosis.

History of presence of oral ulcers, joint pains should also be looked for:
- Past history
- Social history
- How are the symptoms now?
  - Progression or improvement with the ongoing treatment.

Physical Examination

General and systemic examination in detail is must. Special focus on musculoskeletal system if diagnosis is uncertain. Hydration and perfusion status are also assessed. Presence of hemorrhagic manifestations, erythematous mottling of skin, facial flushing, signs of circulatory failure or vascular permeability, lymphadenopathy gives an idea of the illness.

Investigations

- *Routine*: Complete hemogram with differential, erythrocyte sedimentation rate (ESR), chest X-ray, liver function test (LFT), renal function test (RFT), specific investigations pertaining to tropical fever syndrome like dengue serology, malarial antigen, Weil-Felix, *Brucella* serology, blood cultures, urine routine and microscopy, ultrasound abdomen.
- *Specific*: Sputum microscopy and culture, lactate dehydrogenase (LDH), tuberculin test, antinuclear antibody (ANA), extractable nuclear antigen (ENA) profile, triglycerides, prostate-specific antigen, ferritin levels, serum protein electrophoresis. Lumbar puncture and cerebrospinal fluid (CSF) analysis in clinically indicated cases.
- *Serological*: Epstein-Barr virus polymerase chain reaction (PCR), CMV, HIV.
- *Radiological*: Contrast-enhanced computed tomography (CECT) chest and abdomen, CECT brain/magnetic resonance imaging (MRI) brain.
- *Transesophageal echo* if indicated to look for infective endocarditis.
- Bone marrow aspiration and biopsy.

- *Positron emission tomography-CT (PET-CT) scan of whole body, biopsy* of lymph nodes or any significant soft tissue swelling if other tests are elusive.

TREATMENT
- Main objective is to reduce the elevated hypothalamic set point and facilitate the heat loss from the body.
- Majority of fever are self-limiting, e.g. viral fever.
- Antipyretics are indicated in all kind of fever for symptomatic relief.
- Cooling blankets have role in hyperpyrexia.
- Treat the underlying cause.
- Specific therapy of malaria to be started only when peripheral smear or rapid diagnostic test for malaria is positive. Empirical therapy is not indicated.
- Antibiotics in case of enteric fever (drug of choice—ceftriaxone).
- Empirical therapy for typhoid, scrub typhus, and leptospirosis is to be initiated at the earliest.
- Role of glucocorticoids, nonsteroidal anti-inflammatory drugs (NSAIDs), disease-modifying antirheumatic drugs (DMARDs), biological agents used in autoimmune conditions.

SUMMARY
- Fever of unknown origin is a great clinical challenge for the treating physician.
- Fever is a common characteristic of infectious diseases but can also be seen in noninfectious conditions as discussed above.
- The ability to develop fever in elderly is impaired and their baseline temperature is lower than younger population.
- High index of suspicion is required.
- Multiple diagnostic tests and modalities need to be used.
- An aggressive line of management is required.
- Follow guidelines of specific disease.
- Risk of opportunistic infections increases with use of biological agents in autoimmune conditions.
- Update about necessary immunizations to the patient (e.g. vaccination for typhoid, influenza, pneumococcal pneumonia, hepatitis A, varicella in specific population).

PROGNOSIS
Overall prognosis of FUO depends upon the underlying cause. Today due to the availability of extensive and panoptic investigations and treatment, FUO-related mortality rates have declined over the years. In patients where there is no diagnosis is established, prognosis is generally good and mortality is low. Up to 75% patients experience spontaneous resolution of fever, although it may take longer time. The fact is *different diseases have different outcomes.*

CHAPTER 41

Fever in Infants and Children

Sandip Kumar

INTRODUCTION

Fever is a rise in core body temperature due to specific biological response mediated by cytokines and controlled by central nervous system. Fever in infants and children is defined as temperature of more than 100.4°F (in rectum), or oral temperature of 99.5°F, and axillary temperature above 99°F.

Normal body temperature varies throughout the day from 97.8°F in morning to 100.2°F and follows circadian rhythm. Our body temperature is maintained by anterior hypothalamus thermoregulatory center, which regulating the steady state of body temperature by keeping balance between heat production by various metabolic activities in muscle mass and liver and dissipation through the skin surface and the lungs.

Esophageal and rectal temperature reflection is considered as core body temperature, and oral temperature is usually 1°F lower than rectal temperature.

Fever without localizing signs (FWLS): Children with acute onset of shorter duration of fever (<1 week), without any other complaints and signs or symptoms involving any of the organ system are categorized as FWLS. Most common age group presenting with FWLS are neonates and infants up to 36 months (3 years).

Fever of unknown origin (FUO): FUO is defined as a fever which is documented by healthcare professional, for which no cause is identified after 3 weeks of outpatient evaluation or 1 week of inpatient management with proper history taking, physical examination and laboratory assessment.

ETIOLOGY

One of the most common presenting complaints in pediatric age group is fever, which is associated with several illnesses. All types of fever can be divided into four main groups based on the etiology, i.e. infectious, inflammatory, neoplastic, and miscellaneous. Each of them shows certain characteristics, which can provide us clue about the underlying etiology. Such as fever related to viral infections is typically associated with a slow declining fever with relatively shorter duration, which may be up to 1 week. Whereas in a bacterial infection the fever gets subsided promptly after administration of proper antibiotics. Usually the pathogens are eliminated once the antimicrobial therapy is employed, but still the fever may persist for few more days as a result of tissue injury and related inflammatory changes.

Cause of very high-grade fever, i.e. higher than 105.8°F is usually associated with noninfectious cause, and most importantly due to central nervous system dysfunction.

Intermittent fever: Fever with exaggerated circadian rhythm that includes a period of normal temperature.

Septic or hectic fever: Fever with wide fluctuations throughout.

Sustained fever: There is a persistent temperature with variations not more than 0.9°F per day.

Remittent fever: Persistence of fever and variations of more than 0.9°F per day.

Relapsing fever: Febrile period is separated by interval of normal temperature.

Biphasic fever: It indicates a single illness with two distinct periods, characteristically seen in poliomyelitis, enteroviral infection, leptospirosis, dengue fever.

Causes of prolonged fever, lasting for more than 14 days, have different etiologies; however, infectious cause still remains the most common, below are the other etiologies of prolonged fever:

- Infectious—tuberculosis, human immunodeficiency virus (HIV), chronic fungal infection, liver abscess.
- Inflammatory diseases—rheumatoid arthritis, systemic lupus erythematosus (SLE), Kawasaki disease, Behçet's disease, polyarteritis nodosa.
- Malignancies—lymphomas, leukemia, neuroblastoma, Wilms tumor.
- Hematological and immune deficiency—spherocytosis, hemolytic anemia, Langerhans cell histiocytosis, disorders of phagocytosis and T or B cell.
- Other causes—drug fever, anhidrotic ectodermal dysplasia.

PATHOPHYSIOLOGY

Our body temperature is regulated by thermosensitive neurons which are located in the anterior hypothalamus, which responds to any change in temperature of blood and also through the warm and cold receptor located at skin and muscle. To maintain the temperature either the blood flow is redirected to or from the cutaneous vascular bed, regulating the extracellular fluid volume and also by increasing or decreasing the sweating.

There are three main mechanisms for producing fever:

In the first mechanism the pyrogens play a big role in inducing fever, by raising the hypothalamus temperature set point. These pyrogens may be endogenous and exogenous. Endogenous pyrogens are mainly cytokines like interleukins 1 and 6 (IL-1, IL-6), tumor necrosis factor-α (TNF-α), interferons β and γ. Other endogenous pyrogen includes leukemia inhibitory factor-M (LIF), ciliary neurotrophic factor (CNTF), and oncostatin-M.

In cases of febrile illnesses, higher levels of IL-6 have been seen, and also the IL-6 induced by IL-1 or the combination with TNF contributes in clinical pyrexia. Some prostaglandins

(PGE, PGE2) which are produced by stimulated leukocytes, and some other cells, in response to the exogenous pyrogens via activation of Toll signaling.

Exogenous pyrogens include the bacterial cell wall components like lipopolysaccharide (LPS), drugs, enterotoxins, and exotoxins.

Prostaglandin E2 is the ultimate pyrogen in the whole cascade, which in turn attaches to the prostaglandin receptor site located on the hypothalamus and produces a net temperature set point. Many exotoxins like drugs, malignancies, and inflammatory diseases can also produce fever by production of endogenous pyrogens. Among all exogenous pyrogens, endotoxin is one of the substances which can directly alter the thermoregulation center in hypothalamus, and stimulates endogenous pyrogens as well.

Another mechanism in which the heat production is in excess to the release, for example, in case of salicylate poisoning and malignant hyperthermia. The third mechanism, where the loss of heat is defective, is seen in cases of ectodermal dysplasia and victims of severe heat exposure.

In febrile illnesses, there is a raise in an iron-binding protein ferritin which is stimulated by low serum iron levels. This is one of the host defense mechanisms to devoid bacteria from utilizing free serum iron. Another protective mechanism of fever is to enhance various immunologic functions, which require moderately rise in temperature, like increased bactericidal activity of polymorphonuclear leukocytes, as well as increase in production of interferon along with increasing body temperature.

Febrile illness is associated with increase in metabolic activity, increase in consumption of oxygen and increased production of carbon dioxide which leads to the increased demand on cardiovascular and pulmonary system, and aggravates cerebral injury too.

CLINICAL PRESENTATION

Unlike in adults, adolescent and elder children, young infants and younger children have certain differences in clinical presentations, as they may become irritable and show fatigue, without any other apparent symptoms. Fever in children makes them very much uncomfortable. Fever can present in wide range of symptoms in children from no symptoms at all to extreme malaise. They may be having facial flushing appearance, experience shivering, and complain of feeling hot or even cold. Various other symptoms may be manifested like loss of appetite, and some clinical features may be typical for specific diseases and can be used to point out the etiology, for example any sick child with fever and petechial rashes, raise suspicion toward meningococcemia or acute bacterial endocarditis.

Change in the heart rate from baseline is the most prominent clinical finding, and most of the patients have fever associated with tachycardia (increase in heart rate by 10, for each raise in temperature of 1.8°F). Disproportionately, increase in the heart rate is commonly seen in noninfectious conditions, or in infections in which toxins play role in clinical manifestation, in contrast, relative bradycardia.

In children of age group 6 months to 60 months (5 years), children may present with episodes of febrile convulsions.

■ RED FLAGS

- Parent concerns or physician instincts to evaluate further
- Inconsolable cry, change in crying pattern
- Rapid breathing or shortening of breaths with any duration of onset
- Findings like decreased breath sounds, or crackles on respiratory examinations
- Poor peripheral circulation, hypotension, appearing cyanosed on examination
- Fever associated with rash
- Seizures during the febrile illness
- Fever with meningeal irritation signs, neck stiffness or photophobia
- Child presenting with cyanosis, breathlessness
- Poor hydration status, and decreased skin turgor
- Drowsiness or lethargic or in altered consciousness
- Fever with chills and rigor, or bleeding manifestations.

■ EVALUATION (FLOWCHART 1)

Majority of the febrile episodes in an otherwise normal host can be diagnosed by a thorough history taking, physical examination and a few laboratory tests. Careful and detail history taking is the key component for the correct diagnosis, and must include onset, pattern, and accompanying signs and symptoms of fever. History of previous severe or major illness, any underlying immune deficiencies or ill person at home, school or day care, recent history of traveling or medication should also be noted.

Physical examination is mandatory in all cases to reach a diagnosis. Starting from getting vital signs, along with pulse oximetry should also be checked. Followed by head to toe screening is recommended, so that not to miss any important clue, for example, eschar can be seen in rickettsial infection, palm and sole lesions give a clue for coxsackievirus infection. Detailed system examination is must to identify the focus of fever, for example, abnormal breath sounds heard during chest auscultation may tell us about lower respiratory tract infection, and on the other hand organomegaly during per abdomen examination, gives a clue about infections like malaria, enteric fever, dengue, septicemia.

There are certain findings which can lead us toward possible diagnosis, narrow down the etiology and guide us for the need of further appropriate investigations. Hence it is also helpful in minimize the number of investigations.

Fever with rash: It can be seen in infectious conditions like meningococcemia, dengue, measles, rubella, varicella, herpes simplex; certain malignancies like leukemia and histiocytosis; vasculitis like Henoch-Schönlein purpura, Kawasaki disease, juvenile idiopathic arthritis (JIA), and SLE.

Fever with lymphadenopathy: It is most commonly seen in suppurative lymphadenitis, pharyngitis, tonsillitis, dental infections, and scalp infections. Also, it is seen in conditions like histiocytosis, HIV infection, tuberculosis, and some other connective tissue disorders like JIA, sarcoidosis, Kawasaki disease.

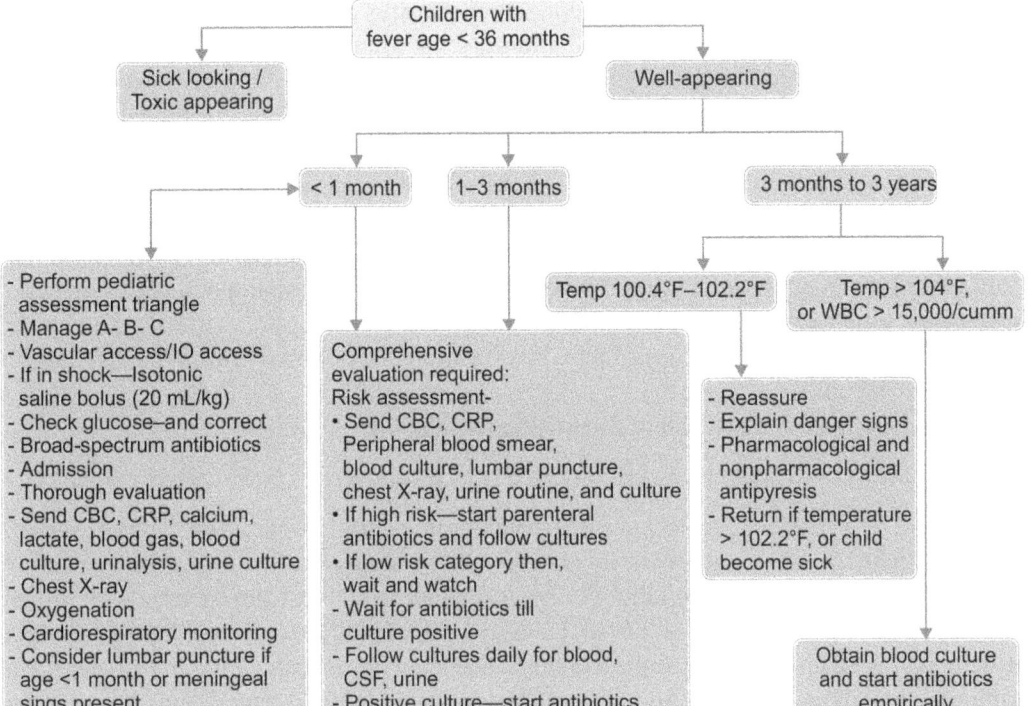

Flowchart 1: Evaluation for fever in infants and children.

Fever with hepatosplenomegaly: It is most commonly seen in infectious diseases like malaria, enteric fever, kala-azar, tuberculosis, infectious mononucleosis, brucellosis, rickettsial diseases, TORCH [toxoplasmosis, other (syphilis, varicella-zoster, parvovirus B19), rubella, cytomegalovirus (CMV), and herpes infections] group of infections, dengue and infective endocarditis.

Malignancies related to fever with hepatosplenomegaly are leukemia, lymphomas, histiocytosis, infantile hemangioendothelioma, and hepatoblastoma.

Connective tissue diseases like SLE, JIA, sarcoidosis, scleroderma, and rheumatic fever are the disorders associated with fever with hepatosplenomegaly.

INVESTIGATIONS

In case of febrile illness, once the thorough and careful history is collected, and on examination there is an obvious focus of infection, the laboratory investigations may not be required in all cases. But these days it has become very common that the cause of fever is not apparent. In these cases, laboratory investigations should be considered on case to case basis, to reach the diagnosis, and guide the initiation and follow-up of the treatment.

Also, laboratory evaluations may be required in conditions with obvious focus of fever but there is not improvement in the patient's condition after initiating appropriate treatment, or in cases where the fever is prolonged and does not follow the usual course to recovery. The history of presentation and physical examination leads us to laboratory evaluation. Any child with respiratory symptoms and hypoxia may require a chest X-ray and antigen testing for respiratory syncytial virus or influenza virus, similarly when presenting with pharyngitis, rapid antigen testing for group A streptococcus and throat culture may be helpful.

A child presenting with predominantly urinary complaints, or having a history of dysuria, pyuria, warrants a urinalysis, urine culture, and radiological evaluation. A complete blood count and blood culture are required in all sick children, and essentially before starting of antibiotics. When the primary focus of fever is known, then the laboratory evaluation for the specific etiology along with the basic blood investigations are done to confirm the diagnosis in case of any sick child.

Judicial use of laboratory testing and imaging is valuable.

Following are the important investigations need to be considered for fever workup:

Urinalysis and urine culture: Because urinary tract infection is a common cause of serious bacterial infection presenting with fever, urinalysis remains the key factor for evaluation of fever in infancy and early childhood. As it is difficult to collect urine sample with proper technique, most of the time, it is omitted. It has to be sent for all kids younger than 24 months, with unexplained fever. Urine sample should be collected by catheterization or by suprapubic aspiration technique, but also can be taken by clean catch method after cleaning around the urethra in children with voluntary control.

Blood cell counts and blood culture: White blood cells (WBCs) counts and absolute neutrophil counts are used to identify severe bacterial infections. Current guidelines recommend a complete blood count with differentials and blood culture for all infants under 3 months. Usual cutoff of WBC count in low-risk group of infants up to 3 months is 5,000–15,000/mm^3.

Stool examination: Stool WBC and culture for diarrhea with fever is not routinely recommended in children and it is most commonly seen in viral infections, but can be used in young infants as it suggests systemic illness and, in those children, presenting with dysentery.

Inflammatory markers: C-reactive protein (CRP) is one of the biomarkers which is widely used to identify serious bacterial infections. Although the use of CRP to identify bacterial infection has clear cutoff value, also it may be elevated in other inflammatory conditions, as well as viral infections.

Another biomarker procalcitonin is also used to identify serious bacterial infections and also has a high sensitivity, specificity as well as better predictive value than WBC count. Among other laboratory tests, procalcitonin is relatively costlier, poor availability and delayed results are the limitations. And, moreover, it is not very clear that whether procalcitonin test result affects clinical decision to administer antibiotics in febrile child.

Cerebrospinal fluid (CSF) analysis: After introduction of vaccination against *Streptococcus pneumoniae* and *Haemophilus influenzae* type b (Hib), the incidence of meningitis in infants has significantly reduced and so as the indications for lumbar puncture. Lumbar puncture is recommended for all the infants and the younger children with clinical signs of meningitis. For the infants younger than 3 months, WBC counts in CSF (cerebrospinal fluids) up to $5/mm^3$ and absence of bacteria on Gram Stain's are considered as cutoff point as per Pittsburg guidlines. However, few guidelines suggest that lumbar puncture can be omitted for a well appearing and previously healthy young infants without any focal signs of infection, WBC count between $5,000/mm^3$ and $15,000/mm^3$, and no pyuria or bacteriuria on urinalysis.

Imaging: Chest radiography should be taken in all neonates' unexplained fever, and in young children presenting with respiratory symptoms. Also, chest radiography is required for children with a temperature of more than 102.2°F and WBC count of more than $20,000/mm^3$.

These are the basic investigations required to find out the etiological basis of fever; however, there are other laboratory tests which are routinely used as a part of screening of organ functions in a sick child presenting with fever like liver function test, renal function other biomarkers.

Few of the tests are done as a part of fever workup in a child requiring hospitalizations in an endemic zone for an illness like dengue serology, rapid antigen testing, and smear for malaria, serology of leptospirosis and scrub typhus.

TREATMENT

Antipyresis includes use of both pharmacological and nonpharmacological approach. However, use of antipyretics may help to manage the child overall, but it does not appear to play any role in occurrence of febrile seizures.

Nonpharmacological Antipyresis

Environmental modification: Keeping the room temperature cooler (21–22°C) in order to enhance the heat loss by convection and minimal clothing can be helpful in bring the body temperature lower.

Hydration: Due to raised body temperature, there is an increase in metabolism and increase in insensible water losses, i.e. for each 1°C of increase in temperature above 37.2°C, insensible water loss increases by 7 mL/kg. Hence by increasing fluid intake is recommended in febrile patients.

Hydrotherapy or sponging: Tepid water sponging helps to lower the temperature by evaporation, conduction, and convection. It lowers the temperature gradually, but it does not lower the thermoregulatory set point, and also soon it limits the further body cooling by inducing vasoconstriction and shivering. Hence the hydrotherapy should be always accompanied by pharmacological therapy.

Pharmacological Antipyresis

Antipyretic agents act upon the arachidonic acid pathway. The main action is to competitively bind on cyclooxygenase (COX) enzymes catalytic site competing with arachidonic acid, hence inhibiting production of prostaglandin 2.

Paracetamol: It is recommended in dose of 10–15 mg/kg, at 4–6 hourly intervals (maximum 60 mg/kg/day). Antipyretic effect takes 30–60 minutes to initiate. Paracetamol helps in reduction of body temperature by 1–2°F within 2 hours of administration. Greater the initial temperature, greater the fall of temperature after the drug intake.

Ibuprofen: This drug can be used at dose of 10 mg/kg, as a first-line antipyretic. No great differences have been shown in safety and efficacy as compared to paracetamol. Although combination of these two can be more effective, but not recommended routinely in children because of associated improper drug dosages.

Mefenamic acid: This is an effective antipyretic, mainly in controlling the high-grade fever at the dose of 6–7 mg/kg/dose (20 mg/kg/day is maximum). Commonly practiced as to give one dose of mefenamic acid for high temperature and then subsequently to follow with paracetamol.

Care should be taken while prescribing antipyretics. Physician should be aware about clinical data on safety, efficacy, adverse effects and cost of the pharmacological agents. Paracetamol is safest antipyretic in children in therapeutic dosage, but also is associated with most serious cause of hepatotoxicity in children. Ibuprofen is also known for overdose and is relatively difficult to manage as compared to paracetamol. Aspirin should be avoided in children due to its adverse effects like Reye's syndrome, other side effects like blunting of immune response, increased risk of gastritis and gastrointestinal bleeding.

CHAPTER 42

Fingers and Nail Problems

Aditya Agarwal, Vimlendu Brajesh, Sukhdeep Singh, Hardeep Singh, Sanjay Mahendru, Pooja Sharma, Madhusoodan Gupta, Saurabh Garg, Deepika Gupta, Rakesh K Khazanchi

■ FINGER DISLOCATION (PROXIMAL INTERPHALANGEAL JOINT)

Introduction

Dislocation of proximal interphalangeal (PIP) joint is the most common ligament injury in the hand. PIP joint is a bicondylar hinge joint with minimal movement in more than one plane.

The PIP joint has a ligament box configuration with collateral ligament supporting on either sides and volar plate on the volar side, permitting movement full range during flexion but minimal or no degree of extension or lateral movement.

Dislocation of PIP joint requires ligament box disruption in at least two planes.

Etiology

All type of heavy ball games (basketball, football, volleyball, etc.) can lead to such types of injury.

Pathophysiology

Dorsal dislocation is a condition where the middle phalanx gets displaced out of the PIP joint due to some hyperextension force along with longitudinal compression.

Clinical Presentation

Finger appears crooked, swollen and is painful. It may be bent upward or at strange angles, may lead to vascular compromise and finger may appear pale; may be associated with numbness and tingling; associated breech in the skin may or may not be present.

Investigations

Anteroposterior (AP) and true lateral view of the involved finger to assess articular surface fracture.

Computed tomography (CT) scan may occasionally be needed to assess suspected articular depression.

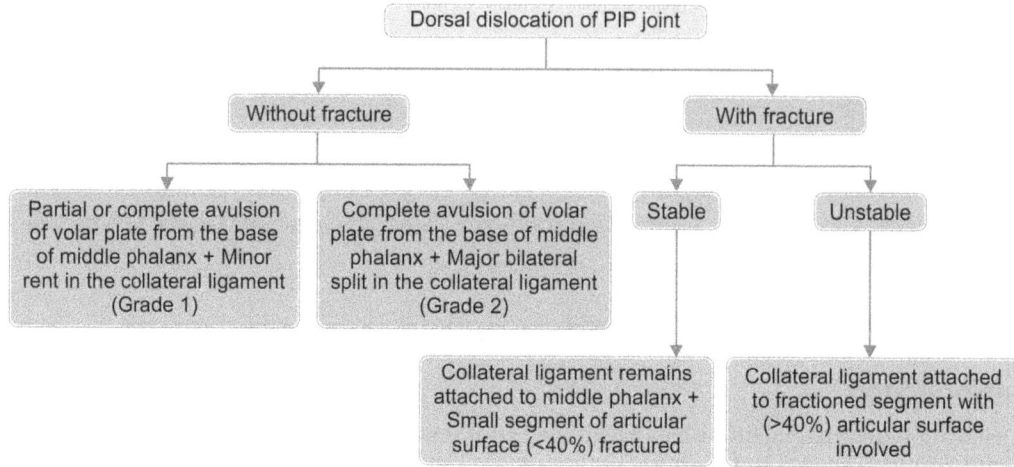

Flowchart 1: Classification of proximal interphalangeal (PIP) dorsal dislocation.

Classification

It depends on the direction of dislocation—dorsal, volar, and lateral and it refers to the position of the middle phalanx relative to proximal phalanx.

Dorsal dislocation of the PIP joint being the most common. The classification of PIP dorsal dislocation depends on degree of soft tissue injury and associated fracture of articular surface of middle phalanx (**Flowchart 1**).

Volar dislocation is less common where the proximal phalanx gets trapped between the central slip and lateral band.

Treatment (Flowcharts 2 and 3)

Dorsal dislocation is treated by applying simple traction force under digital block to reduce the dislocation, if reduction fails by this technique the injury pattern is recreated by producing hyperextension and simultaneous pressure applied to the base of the middle phalanx dorsal to volar direction to achieve reduction.

Once reduced stability revaluated by radiography and clinical test for stability.

Reduction is followed by immobilization with dorsal splintage with 20–30° flexion for 3–5 days (grade 1) and 7–14 days (grade 2). After full-time splinting, buddy taping and early active flexion is started.

Fracture dislocation if stable involving less than 40% of articular surface of middle phalanx can be treated with reduction and splintage for 4 weeks followed by active flexion.

Dynamic skeletal splint is more useful for comminuted fractures.

Volar plate arthroplasty is useful for fractures where K-wire fixation not possible.

Postoperative Management

Distal interphalangeal (DIP) joint movement started immediately.

Flowchart 2: Treatment of dorsal dislocation of proximal interphalangeal (PIP) joint.

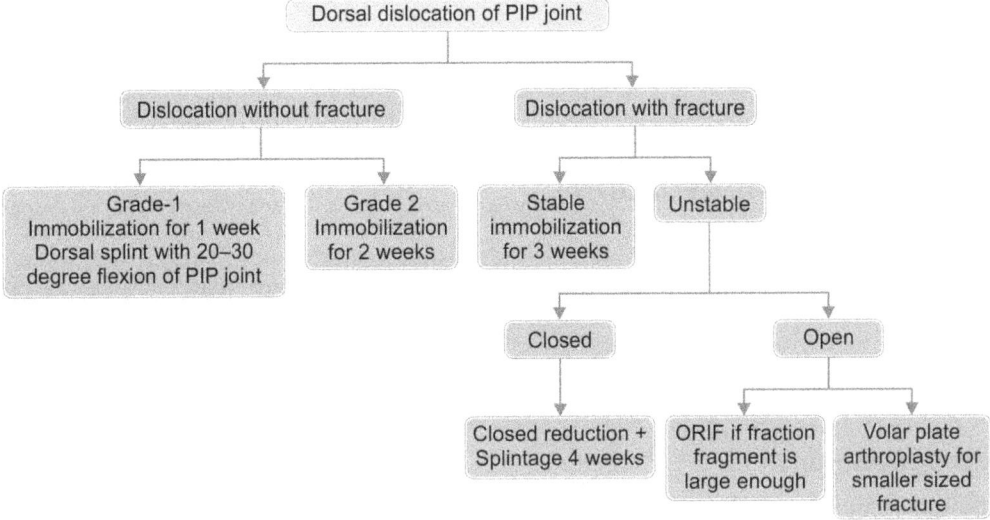

Flowchart 3: Treatment of dislocation without fracture.

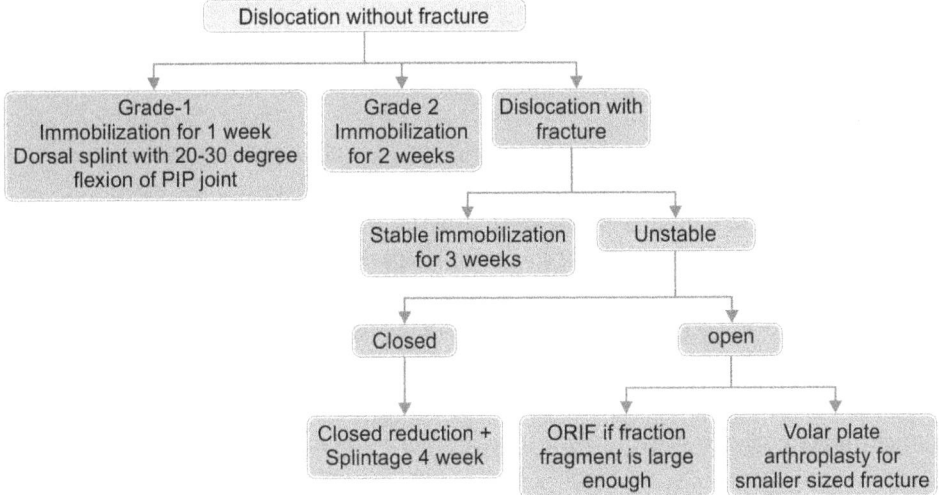

Three weeks after surgery K-wire removed and active flexion of PIP joint started using extension block splint. Unrestricted active extension started after 4 weeks.

If full active extension is not achieved after 4 weeks, dynamic extension splinting is begun. Sports activity started after 8 weeks with a buddy tape and continued for 6 months.

Red Flag

Normal PIP function unlikely despite best efforts but satisfactory functional recovery is possible.

Complications
- Redisplacement
- Angulation
- Flexion contracture
- DIP stiffness.

■ FINGER/TOE NAIL AVULSION

Introduction
The nail comes out of its attachments to the nail matrix (sterile + germinal).

Etiology
Crush injury mostly due to getting crushed by the door or smashed by heavy object.

Pathophysiology
Often the nail has attachment to the underlying sterile matrix of the nail bed which gets disrupted partially or completely, and there may be associated nail bed laceration with or without distal phalanx fracture.

History/Clinical Presentation
- Patient often gives a history of his finger being crushed by some heavy object or long nails getting suck to some object.
- Avulsion may be partial or complete. Partial nail avulsion may present with pain, discoloration of the nail, subungual hematoma leading to excruciating pain.
- Patient may present with or without the avulsed part of the nail.
- The avulsed nail may have a part of sterile nail matrix attached to its undersurface.
- Exposed distal phalanx may be seen if nail bed is avulsed along with nail.
- It may have associated pulp injury or fracture of the tuft of distal phalanx.

Investigations
Simple AP and lateral view of the involved digit to rule out associated fracture of distal phalanx.

Treatment (Flowchart 4)
Exploration of nail bed under local anesthesia (digital block) or general anesthesia (pediatric age group) with nail bed examination under magnification for any laceration. Repair of the nail bed with 6-0 Vicryl/catgut to achieve close approximation of the nail bed laceration with minimal debridement of the ragged edges is done. The nail is replaced as a splint after creating a small rent to allow for egress of blood, and if the nail is missing a silicone sheet or aluminum foil of suture is cut into shape of the nail and used as a substitute. The nail or splint is fixed to the pulp by figure of eight suture to prevent its displacement. Most of the time suturing of laceration itself serves as a splint for the underlying distal phalangeal fracture.

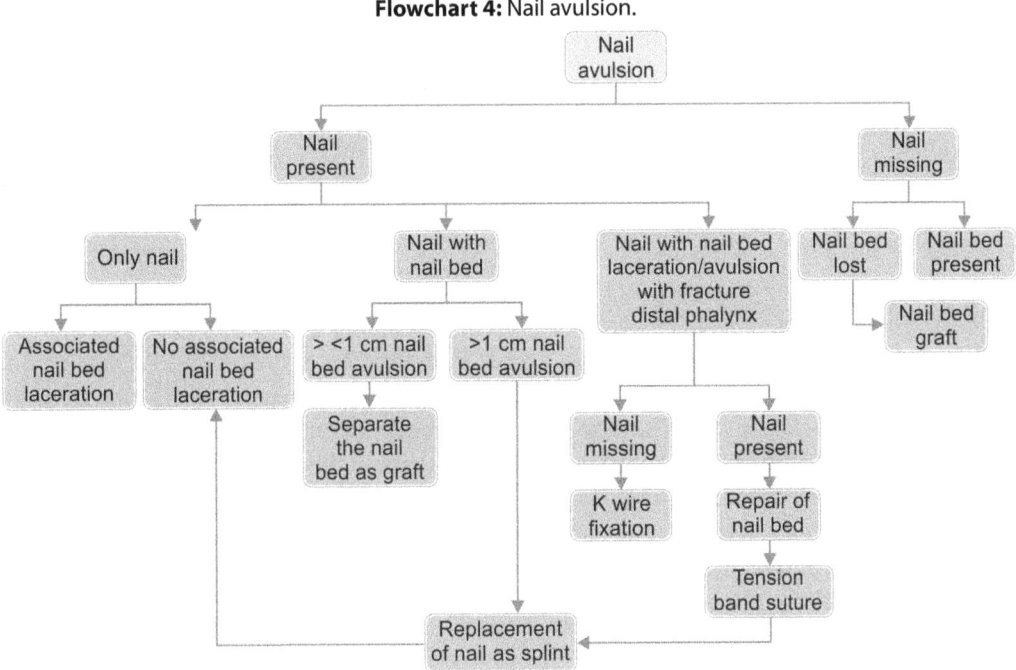

Flowchart 4: Nail avulsion.

NAIL ROOT DISLOCATION, SUBUNGUAL ECCHYMOSIS, SUBUNGUAL HEMATOMA, AND NAIL BED INJURY

Nail and fingertip injuries are commonly encountered in an emergency department and constitute the most common hand injuries seen. These are generally caused due to blunt trauma leading to crushing of the fingertip. Most common age group is between 4 years and 30 years and is seen more in males. The nail bed injuries occur in 15–24% of fingertip injuries and about half of these are associated with phalangeal fractures. The aim in the management of these injuries is to have a smooth nail bed without any scars so as to prevent secondary deformities of the nail. The final result is generally evaluated after 1 year.

The spectrum of the nail bed injuries ranges from nail root dislocation, subungual ecchymosis, subungual hematoma with or without nail bed laceration and associated phalangeal fracture. The involved finger should be examined in detail for posture, any deformity, nail avulsion, nail bed lacerations if visible, foreign bodies. X-ray (AP/lateral/oblique) should be done in patients with significant trauma.

Nail Root Dislocation

This occurs due to blunt crushing trauma and the nail root comes to lie over the eponychial fold rather than under it in its usual position. The cuticle which marks the position of attachment of the eponychial fold continues to be attached at the same position. This occurs as the nail is not strongly adherent to the nail bed in the region of the lunula. An X-ray rules out any bony injury.

Under digital nerve block and a finger tourniquet, the dislocated nail root is lifted and the nail bed inspected for any laceration. The nail bed and the germinal matrix should not be debrided and if present the laceration is repaired with absorbable 6-0 suture. The nail root is repositioned under the eponychial fold and may be secured in position with two nonabsorbable sutures on the side which are removed after 5 days. An undisplaced fracture gets splinted with the nail plate only. For a displaced fracture, it should be reduced and splinted or fixed with a K-wire.

Nail Bed Ecchymosis

This presents as light brown to light blue-brown discoloration of the nail and is caused due to minor crushing of the fingertip leading to accumulation of some amount of blood between the nail plate and the nail bed. The associated pain generally settles in about 30 minutes and slight sensitivity might remain when the patient presents to the emergency. An X-ray of the part should be considered in case of history of significant trauma. Such a discoloration without the history of trauma should raise a suspicion of a melanoma, Kaposi sarcoma, and infective endocarditis. Nail bed ecchymosis does not require any intervention other than analgesics and elevation of the affected hand and a fingertip splint in cases of persistent sensitivity (common simple emergencies).

Nail Bed Hematoma

Nail bed hematoma occurs due to more severe trauma to the nail bed. The blood collects in between the tough nail plate and the nail bed. As this is a very constricted space, it is intensely painful condition. The pain tends to settle in 48–72 hours due to stretching of the tissues. One should check for associated lacerations of the paronychium, eponychium or nail root avulsion. X-ray should be done to rule out phalangeal fracture. If the hematoma involves less than 25% of nail plate area then no treatment is needed. If the area involves is more than 50% then as per traditional teaching it require exploration and repair of the nail bed but recent studies have shown equivalent results with just trephination and drainage of hematoma even in presence of an underlying nail bed laceration or a stable fracture. If there is laceration involving the nail plate or the nail folds then patient can be taken up for removal of nail plate and repair of laceration along with the evacuation of the hematoma.

Trephination for the evacuation of the hematoma can be done without any anesthesia as the nail plate is insensitive. Children and some adults may need some forms of anesthesia for this procedure. Electrocautery, an 18-gauge hypodermic needle or a heated metal pin can all be used to make few holes in the nail plate to drain the blood and relieve the pressure. Care should be taken to avoid injury to the underlying nail bed. It results in immediate relief of pain. A simple dressing and a finger splint are then applied to the affected digit. The nail outgrows the discoloration of the hematoma in about 3–12 months.

Nail Bed Laceration

These may be transverse but are generally stellate when caused due to crushing. These are often seen along with nail fold lacerations, avulsion of the nail, pulp lacerations, and half of these are associated with phalangeal fractures for which X-ray is required.

Principles of management are use of magnification, minimal debridement, tension-free repair of the nail bed with good approximation of the edges. The procedure is generally done under digital nerve block and a finger tourniquet. Children may need general anesthesia. After removing the nail plate from the nail bed, wound lavage and minimal debridement, the repair is done with 6-0 or finer absorbable suture and the nail plate or a nail substitute is placed in its position under the eponychial fold after making a hole in it and secured with a figure of eight suture. Recently octyl cyanoacrylate glue (Dermabond) has also been advocated for the nail bed repair instead of sutures with equivalent results. A tuft fracture may not need any intervention if the nail bed has been repaired which tends to splint the fracture. In more proximal transverse or oblique fractures of the distal phalanx shaft with displacement, a K-wire or a 21-gauge needle may be used to reduce and fix the fracture along with nail bed repair. Dressing and splint are given.

If a nail splint has been used, it is removed in 3 weeks. A repositioned nail is outgrown itself by the new growing nail. It takes about 3–4 months for the new nail to grow completely but may take longer. Nail deformity, especially in severe trauma, nonadherence of the nail plate to the nail bed, infection are the likely complications.

■ FOREIGN BODY UNDERNEATH NAIL

Introduction

Subungual foreign bodies are often difficult to treat. Foreign bodies such as wood or metal splinters, pencil lead, thorns, spines, or hair may become lodged beneath the fingernail. Tradesmen such as carpenters, landscapers, auto mechanics, and individuals who work without hand protection with materials that produce small splinters are at risk for this type of injury. Subungual foreign bodies may also present less commonly under the toenails.

Foreign bodies may enter the subungual space at the distal fingertip beneath the nail, or may penetrate the nail plate directly. In either event, separation of the nail from the nail bed results in severe pain and acts as nidus for infection. Patients frequently attempt to remove the foreign body immediately because of this intense pain. Removal of foreign body offers relief from pain, reduces the risk of infection and can be performed in most outpatient settings.

Clinical Presentation

Patients generally present for medical intervention with pain after unsuccessfully attempting to remove the foreign body. Prior removal attempts often result in breakage of the foreign body or pushing it further beneath the nail, both of which complicate the next extraction attempt.

Complications
- Infection
- Abscess
- Foreign body reaction with granuloma formation
- Nail deformity
- Osteomyelitis.

Evaluation
The most common error in the management of subungual foreign bodies is the failure to detect their presence. A patient's suspicion that a foreign body may be present must be taken seriously. It is important to obtain a careful history, inquiring about the nature of the injury, the composition of the material most likely involved, and the presence of any foreign body sensation if the foreign body is not readily visible.

The timing of the injury is important in evaluating subungual foreign bodies. Older injuries may present as infection, inflammation, induration, or granuloma formation. The composition of the foreign body dictates the reaction of the tissues. Wood, thorns, spines, and other vegetative foreign bodies are considered highly inflammatory, whereas glass, metal, and plastic are relatively inert materials

An array of diagnostic tools is available for detecting splinters. Standard radiographs are the most practical means of screening for a foreign body. It can also detect the presence of fracture of phalanx.

Management
Most of the splinters are lodged in the distal portion of the nail and their removal does not result in nail dystrophy. However, for a more proximal subungual splinter, caution must be exercised not to disturb the nail matrix because this may result in failure of the nail to grow back normally.

Digit should be anesthetized by means of a digital nerve block before removing the foreign body to make the procedure pain free.

Foreign bodies' removal can be accomplished by a variety of methods depending on the location (**Flowchart 5**).

Equipment
- Syringe with 26-gauge needle/insulin syringe
- Bupivacaine (0.25%) without epinephrine
- Lignocaine (1-2%) without epinephrine
- Antiseptic preparation solution (Betadine)
- Fine forceps
- Fine scissors
- No. 11/15 scalpel blade
- Dressing.

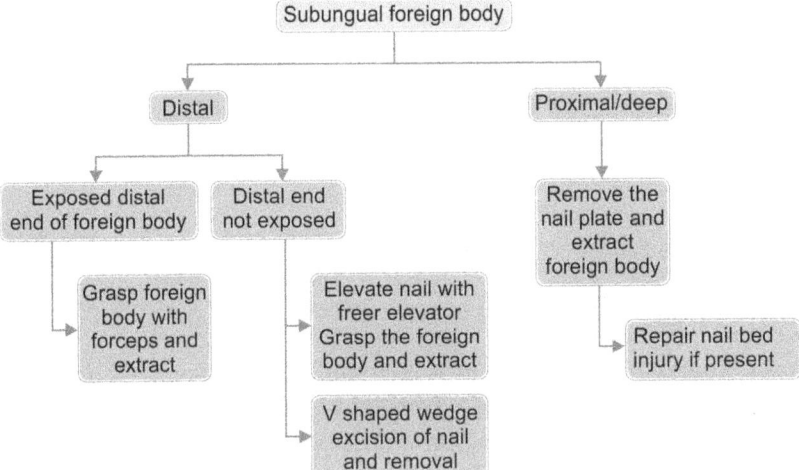

Flowchart 5: Algorithm of subungual foreign body removal.

Procedure
1. Distal subungual foreign body
   a. Grasp foreign body with forceps and extract if the distal end of foreign body is exposed
   b. Elevate nail with freer elevator (avoiding nail bed injury). Grasp the foreign body and extract
   c. V-shaped wedge excision of nail. The point of the V is at the proximal tip of the splinter. The splinter is grasped and removed, taking particular care not to push the splinter further into the nail bed.
2. Proximal and deep subungual foreign body
   a. Nail plate is removed to extract foreign body and repair nail bed laceration if present.

Summary
- Subungual foreign bodies are extremely painful and failure to remove them completely leads to infections or osteomyelitis of the distal phalanx
- Perform a radiographic evaluation as needed to confirm the presence of a foreign body
- Perform a digital nerve block if necessary
- Remove the foreign body using appropriate technique
- Clean and irrigate thoroughly
- Apply a protective dressing
- Prescribe antibiotics if there are signs of infection.

CHAPTER 43

Gait Abnormalities

Nikhil Tambe, Sandeep B Gore

INTRODUCTION

Walking is a complex daily activity. It is a complex interplay of neurological system, cardiorespiratory system and musculoskeletal system. Apart from these physiological mechanisms, age, mood, and personality also affect person's gait. Gait disturbance reduces the quality of life and independence. Prevalence of gait disorders increases with age. Gait abnormalities and loss of balance result in falls in elderly leading to debilitating injuries. Gait disorders are often underdiagnosed in emergency and receive inadequate evaluation, especially in elderly population. Gait disorders are largely due to neurological, orthopedic, and other medical problems. In elder age, gait problems are also due to poor vision, osteoarthritis of knee and hip and neuropathy. Careful history taking, observation of gait, neurological and orthopedic examination is important for evaluation and management of gait disorders.

CLASSIFICATION OF GAIT DISORDERS

The classification of gait disorders has been shown in **Table 1**.

Table 1: Classification of gait disorders.

Level	Disorder	Abnormalities
Low-level gait disorders	Disorder of proprioception or musculoskeletal system	Arthritic gait Muscle weakness Peripheral sensory problem • Sensory ataxic gait • Vestibular problems.
Mid-level gait disorders	Distortion of appropriate interaction of postural and motor processes or synergies	Hemiplegia Paraplegia Motor or cerebellar ataxia Parkinson's disease Dystonia, chorea, other movements
High-level gait disorders	Involve structures or processes that choose the appropriate responses for the support surface, body position in space, and intention of the patient	Senile gait (cautious gait) Frontal ataxic gait Apraxic gait (gait ignition failure) Frontal disequilibrium

TYPES OF GAIT ABNORMALITIES

Hemiplegic Gait

Clinical Features

Clinical features include increased tone with clasp-knife spasticity, hyper-reflexia with or without clonus, upgoing plantars (i.e. positive Babinski) reduced power, the upper limb may have flexor posturing of elbows and wrist with shoulders and fingers in adduction.

Differential Diagnosis

Unilateral upper motor neuron lesion:
- Ischemic/hemorrhagic stroke
- Brain tumor
- Trauma
- Demyelination (e.g. multiple sclerosis)
- Space-occupying lesion.

Diplegic Gait (Scissoring Gait)

Similar causes as hemiplegic gait but with complete transection of the spinal cord and/or bilateral brain involvement.

Spinal cord lesion (sensation usually affected):
- Prolapsed intervertebral disk
- Spinal spondylosis
- Spinal tumor
- Transverse myelitis
- Spinal infarct
- Syringomyelia
- Hereditary spastic paraparesis.

Bilateral brain lesion:
- Cerebral palsy
- Multiple sclerosis
- Bilateral brain infarcts
- Midline tumor (e.g. paraspinal meningioma).

Motor neuron disease:
- Associated with lower motor neuron findings.
  Quadriplegia—a term used to describe upper motor neuron weakness found in all four limbs.

Parkinsonian Gait (Festinating Gait)

Hypomimia and reduced arm swing may be early features of Parkinson's disease before the development of the characteristic short-shuffling gait. Idiopathic Parkinson's disease classically presents with a triad of tremor, rigidity, bradykinesia. There may be other associated features including cogwheel rigidity, asymmetrical tremor (typically pin-rolling), bradykinesia and difficulty getting up from a seated position.

Ataxic Gait

Ataxic gait implies cerebellar, vestibular, or sensory impairment. If cerebellar disease is the cause, other signs of cerebellar disease may be present. If the cerebellar lesion is unilateral then the signs are present on the same side of the lesion.

Cerebellar Ataxia
- Nystagmus (on the affected side of the lesion if unilateral cerebellar lesion)
- Ataxic dysarthria
- Dysmetria (i.e. past pointing or undershooting)
- Intentional tremor (on the affected side of the lesion if unilateral cerebellar lesion)
- Dysdiadokokinesia (on the affected side of the lesion if unilateral cerebellar lesion).

Sensory Ataxia

Sensory neuropathy gives the appearance of an ataxic gait due to impaired limb sensation. Signs include positive Romberg's sign, impaired proprioception (joint position sense), impaired vibration sense and the absence of other cerebellar signs (e.g. dysmetria, nystagmus, dysarthria, etc.).

Vestibular Ataxia

Vestibular disturbance can give a gait similar to an ataxic gait and associated with vertigo, nausea and vomiting.

Differential Diagnosis

Unilateral cerebellar disease (unilateral cerebellar findings):
- Ischemic (posterior circulation infarct) or hemorrhagic stroke—vascular events produce hyperacute symptoms
- Space-occupying lesion.

Bilateral cerebellar disease (giving bilateral cerebellar findings):
- Multiple sclerosis
- Alcoholism
- B_{12} deficiency
- *Drugs:* Phenytoin, carbamazepine, barbiturates, lithium
- *Genetic:* Friedreich's ataxia, spinocerebellar ataxia, ataxia telangiectasia

- Paraneoplastic disease
- Multisystem atrophy—associated with parkinsonian and autonomic features.

Neuropathic Gait (High Steppage Gait)

It is caused by a motor weakness of the nerves supplying the ankle dorsiflexor muscle (tibialis anterior).

Clinical Features

Ankle-foot orthoses: Aid to keep ankle fixed in dorsiflexion.

Unilateral foot drop with sensory impairment: Common peroneal nerve disease usually with a sensory loss on the dorsum of the foot and lateral calf. L5 nerve root disease usually with sensory loss in the distribution of the L5 dermatome.

Bilateral distal muscle weakness with foot drop: Seen in peripheral neuropathies or motor neuron disease. The appearance of pes cavus and "inverted champagne bottle calf" are features of hereditary motor and sensory neuropathies.

Reflexes: Reduced or absent in peripheral neuropathies. Brisk with upgoing plantars and fasciculations (a mixture of upper and lower motor neuron signs) in motor neuron disease.

Differential Diagnosis

Foot drop implies weakness of the muscles of ankle dorsiflexion (tibialis anterior) supplied by the common peroneal nerve (L4, L5, and S1 nerve root).

This is due to either:
- Isolated common peroneal nerve palsy
- L5 radiculopathy (weakened foot inversion) or
- Part of generalized polyneuropathy involving multiple nerves.

Unilateral foot drop with no other muscles or nerves involved suggests an isolated neuropathy—common peroneal palsy or L5 radiculopathy, and not a polyneuropathy. Common peroneal nerve palsy or L5 radiculopathy is usually unilateral, but can be bilateral.

A bilateral foot drop with other neurological features (muscle wasting, reduced reflexes, impaired sensation in a distribution outside common peroneal nerve/L5 dermatome, and weakness in muscles other than ankle dorsiflexors) is seen in more diffuse disease.

Polyneuropathies:
- Diabetic neuropathy
- Hereditary motor and sensory neuropathies (Charcot-Marie-Tooth disease is a type of hereditary motor and sensory neuropathy)
- Vasculitis
- Guillain-Barré syndrome
- Motor neuron disease—associated with upper and lower motor neuron findings.

Sensory Gait (Stomping Gait)

It is caused by sensory impairment.

Clinical Features

Romberg's test positive:
- Balance is maintained by vestibular input, visual input and proprioception (joint position sense). We need two out of three to be intact in order to maintain balance. In a healthy person when visual input stops (closed eyes), we rely on vestibular and proprioception (two inputs) to maintain balance.
- In a patient with peripheral sensory impairment (proprioception impaired), when the eyes are closed (visual input removed), they only have their vestibular input to maintain balance. One input is not enough and so the patient becomes unsteady.
- Stomping is exacerbated in the dark. Impaired sensation to the feet must be present in order to confirm the diagnosis. Usually due to diseases affecting the spinal dorsal columns (dorsal column disease causes impaired proprioception and vibration sense).

Differential Diagnosis

- Dorsal column diseases:
  - B_{12} deficiency
  - Tabes dorsalis (syphilis).
- Peripheral nerve diseases:
  - Diabetes
  - Vasculitis
  - B_{12} deficiency
  - Hereditary motor and sensory neuropathies (e.g. Charcot-Marie-Tooth disease)
  - Guillain-Barré syndrome
  - Postinfection.

Myopathic Gait (Waddling Gait or Trendelenburg Gait)

Trendelenburg's sign positive: When the patient stands on one leg, the pelvis drops toward the contralateral side.

Signs of proximal myopathy: Difficulty standing from a seated position without using arms. Difficulty standing from a squat or sitting up from a lying position.

Evidence of systemic disease or a muscular dystrophy causing proximal myopathy. Any cause of a proximal myopathy including: systemic disease, hyperthyroidism, hypothyroidism, Cushing's syndrome, acromegaly, polymyalgia rheumatic, polymyositis, dermatomyositis, muscular dystrophies, Duchenne muscular dystrophy, Becker's muscular dystrophy, myotonic dystrophy.

Choreiform Gait (Hyperkinetic Gait)

Involuntary movements are usually present at rest. However, walking can accentuate these movements.

Basal ganglia diseases:
- Huntington's disease
- Sydenham's chorea
- Cerebral palsy (choreiform type)
- Wilson's disease
- Dopaminergic medications (e.g. Parkinson's medications).

Antalgic Gait (Painful Gait)

Any cause of pain in the lower limb such as:
- Osteoarthritis
- Inflammatory joint disease
- Lower limb fracture
- Nerve entrapment (e.g. sciatica).

▮ EXAMINATION FOR GAIT ABNORMALITIES

During normal gait the body is erect, the head is straight, arms hang relaxed by the sides, each movement is rhythmic. There should be coordinated flexion of the hip and knee, dorsiflexion of the foot and the foot should just barely clear the ground. The heel normally strikes the ground first.
- Observe the patient sit upright on the stretcher.
- Have the patient rise, stand, and walk, turn around and sit back down.
- Have the patient walk heel-to-toe.

Abnormal results:
- Inability to hold themselves up in a seated position
- Wide base gait
- Truncal or ambulatory unsteadiness
- Irregularity of steps
- Lateral veering
- Inability to walk heel-to-toe
- Unsteadiness when rising from a chair, turning suddenly or when abruptly asked to stop walking.

▮ DIAGNOSIS

A patient with acute gait failure over hours to days needs thorough evaluation in the emergency department (ED), often requiring computed tomography (CT) scan and magnetic resonance imaging (MRI), or lumbar puncture if cerebrospinal fluid infection is suspected. Acute ataxia or gait disturbance may also be evaluated by consultation if available, and possible admission, in contrast to a patient with gradual loss of abilities over weeks or months where outpatient referral and evaluation may be more appropriate.

■ TREATMENT

Hemiplegic/diplegic gait: Physiotherapy is more helpful and in some cases botulinum toxin is helpful.

Parkinsonian gait: Management includes antiparkinsonian medication; modification of the antiparkinsonian medication, orthostatic hypotension, can be managed by medical and nonmedical treatment Walking aids, such as 4-wheel walkers with brakes, and physiotherapy may be helpful.

Ataxic gait: Treatment should target the underlying cause if possible. Physiotherapy including gait and balance training should be offered although the effect of this approach is often limited. Walking aids appropriate for each disease stage need to be considered.

Neuropathic gait: Peroneal splints and orthopedic footwear are usually helpful.

Sensory gait: Treatment of underlying cause—B_{12} deficiency, infection, etc.

Antalgic gait: Analgesics for pain, RICE THERAPY (rest, ice, compression, elevation) may aid in normalizing the gait.

■ SUMMARY

- Gait is an important feature that helps in diagnosing a disease.
- Thorough history and physical examination forms a key to classify gait abnormality.
- Gait abnormalities must be addressed as falls are the major reason for debility in elderly.
- Medication-induced gait disorders are preventable, measures need to implement to reduce the burden of falls in the geriatric population.
- Gait disorder of Parkinson's disease, levodopa is the drug of choice. Medication also helpful in myoclonus and orthostatic tremor.

CHAPTER 44

Goiter

Dheeraj Kapoor, Ruchi Kapoor, Ranjana Bhatt

INTRODUCTION

Goiter is defined as enlargement of thyroid gland irrespective of its pathology. Thyroid gland is a butterfly-shaped gland with two lobes connected by an isthmus located in anterior part of neck (**Fig. 1**). Normal thyroid gland weighs 12–20 grams with a highly rich network of blood supply. Thyroid gland comprises of a number of follicles which contain follicular cells in the periphery surrounding a proteinaceous fluid called colloid in center harboring thyroglobulin-precursor for thyroid hormones. Hormones secreted from thyroid are thyroxine (T4) and tri-iodothyronine (T3) after stimulation by thyroid-stimulating hormone (TSH) secreted from the anterior pituitary gland. Thyroid hormones affect basal metabolic process of almost all body tissues (b). Thyroid gland enlargement can be simple, i.e. diffuse enlargement or nodular with single or multiple nodules. This enlargement when associated with excess thyroid hormone production is termed as toxic and with normal thyroid hormone levels is termed as nontoxic goiter.

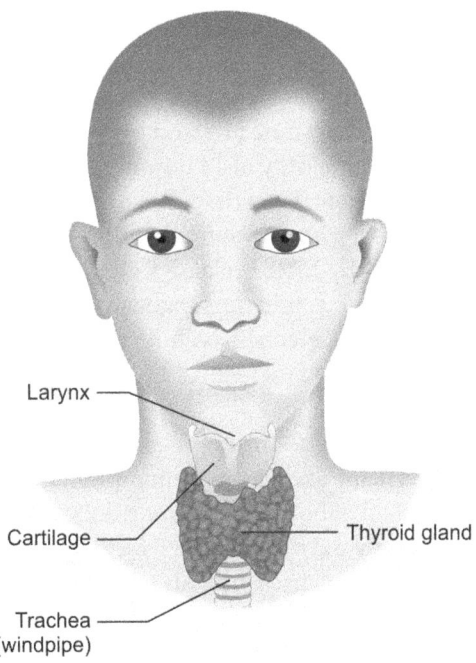

Fig. 1: Position of thyroid gland.

ETIOLOGY

- Iodine deficiency
- Autoimmune:
  - Graves disease
  - Hashimoto disease
- Inflammatory:
  - Subacute thyroiditis
  - Granulomatous thyroiditis
- Colloid cyst
- Nodular thyroid disease:
  - Solitary nodule
  - Multinodular
- Thyroid neoplasm
- Physiological:
  - Pregnancy
  - Pubertal
- Rare:
  - Drug induced: lithium, salicylates
  - Environmental goitrogens: cassava root, cruciferous vegetables
  - Biosynthetic defects: familial/sporadic.

PATHOPHYSIOLOGY

Iodine is the key element required in thyroid hormone synthesis. Epithelial cells in thyroid have Na/I symporter that aids in iodide concentration in plasma as per requirement and this iodide through oxidation (by thyroid peroxidase enzyme) is converted to iodine. The iodine thus formed gives rise to tetraiodothyronine (T_4) and tri-iodothyronine (T_3) via a number of organic reactions within the gland. Majority of T4 hormone is directly produced from thyroid but most of T_3 (80%) is converted from T4 in tissues like pituitary, liver, and kidney. Thyroid hormones thus formed are stored with the thyroglobulin moiety which is released in the circulation under the influence of TSH. TSH release from anterior pituitary is influenced by release of TRH from the hypothalamus and thus regulation of thyroid hormone synthesis is predominantly by a negative feedback mechanism from thyroid hormones wherein raised T3, T4 levels blunt TSH and TRH secretion and low T3, T4 levels stimulate TSH and TRH release (**Fig. 2**).

Increased demand of thyroid hormone during pregnancy, adolescence, or iodine deficiency states initially stimulate TSH release and cause compensatory diffuse thyroid follicular cell growth to meet the increased need of hormone. Prolong deficiency may cause few follicles to enlarge more leading to nodular thyroid disease which further increases susceptibility of gland for autonomous functioning and thus present with toxic disease. Autoimmune conditions like Graves disease cause thyroid follicular cell hyperplasia via TSH receptor antibodies, Hashimoto's thyroiditis causes infiltration of lymphocytes and mononuclear cells, sporadic

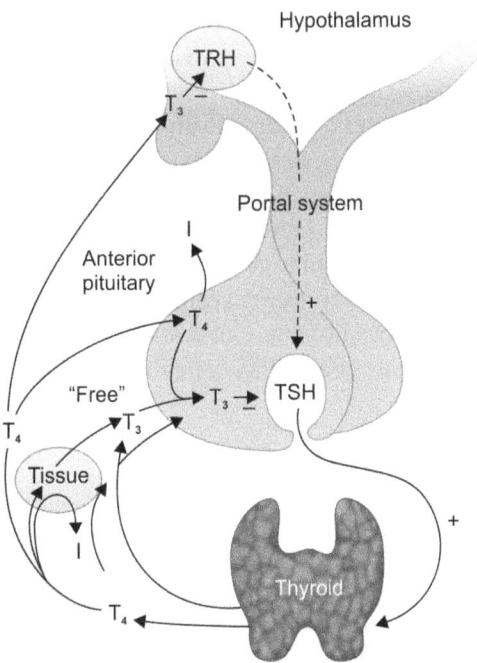

Fig. 2: The hypothalamic-pituitary-thyroid axis.

cyst or colloid deposition in gland or bleeding/calcifications in long standing cysts or cancerous growth are other such mechanisms of thyroid gland enlargement.

Thyroid hormones are required for somatic and neurological growth and development of children and adults. Thus, iodine recommendation for different age groups by World Health Organization (WHO) are mentioned here:
- 90 µg of iodine daily for infants and children up to 5 years,
- 120 µg for children 6–12 years,
- 150 µg daily for children more than or equal to 12 years and adults,
- 250 µg daily during pregnancy and lactation.

Median concentration of urinary iodine is used as a tool for epidemiological assessment of iodine sufficiency. Normal levels are described as 100–299 µg/L for children and adults (male, nonpregnant females), 150–249 µg/L in pregnancy, and below 100 µg/L is labeled epidemiologically as iodine deficiency.

CLINICAL PRESENTATION

With preserved thyroid function, most goiters are asymptomatic and frequently present with swelling in the neck. The clinical presentation of patients is variable and depends to a great extent on the size and functional status of the thyroid gland. Based on etiology, functional thyroid status of patient can vary from being hypothyroid to euthyroid to subclinical or overt thyroxicosis.

Prodrome of low-grade fever, myalgia, throat pain, or pain radiating to ear can be seen in few cases of thyroiditis. In cases of toxic goiter (Graves disease or toxic nodular goiter), patient can present with the following symptoms: palpitations, excessive sweating, diarrhea, fatigue, weight loss, loss of appetite, muscle weakness, oligomenorrhea, irritability, insomnia, tremors, gritty sensation or bulging of eyes, bone pains. In cases of suppressed hormonal profile (Hashimoto atrophic thyroiditis), patient can present with tiredness, constipation, excessive sleep, lethargy, puffiness of face, feeling of cold, dry skin, hair loss, hoarseness of voice, menorrhagia. However, if the swelling is large [large multinodular goiter (MNG)/colloid goiter/neoplasms] or has substernal extension, it can cause compressive symptoms including difficulty in swallowing, breathing, or facial congestion or choking. Cases with sudden onset pain in swelling or recurrent laryngeal nerve palsy raises possibility of hemorrhage or malignancy.

■ EVALUATION

History

- Targeted history regarding onset, duration, and progression of neck swelling
- History of prior low-grade fever, malaise, sore throat, or pain radiating to ear (s/o subacute thyroiditis)
- Associated features of over activity or under activity of thyroid gland (as described above)
- Associated features of difficulty in swallowing, breathing, repetitive coughing, or sensation of choking (compressive symptoms)
- Recent onset hoarseness of voice, facial congestion
- Abrupt onset pain in thyroid swelling (s/o hemorrhage or malignancy)
- History of any prior radiation exposure to head and neck region
- History of similar swelling or thyroid neoplasms in family.

Physical Examination

- *Vitals:* Pulse, blood pressure, temperature, respiratory rate (bradycardia in hypothyroidism, wide pulse pressure in thyrotoxicosis)
- *Neck examination:*
  - Inspection: Location, size, movement with deglutition
  - Palpation: Temperature, tenderness, extent, consistency
  - Auscultation: Bruit for increased vascularity.
- *Eye examination:* In cases of proptosis
- *Nail examination:* To look for onycholysis, thyroid acropachy
- *Skin examination:* Dry, coarse thick skin in hypothyroidism, pretibial myxedema, warm moist skin in toxicosis
- *Reflexes:* Hung-up jerk (biceps, ankle commonly seen) in uncontrolled hypothyroidism, brisk jerk commonly seen in cases of hyperthyroidism or toxicosis
- *Pemberton's sign:* To look for retrosternal extension of goiter, patient is asked to raise and hold up both extended arms above head for 3 minutes. Presence of facial congestion/breathlessness/discomfort are all suggestive as positive signs.

INVESTIGATIONS

1. *Thyroid profile—T3, T4, TSH:* Suppression of TSH with normal or raised T3, T4 is seen in an overactive thyroid gland suggestive of subclinical and overt thyrotoxicosis, respectively. High TSH with suppressed T3, T4 levels are seen in an under functioning thyroid gland.
2. *Thyroid autoantibodies—anti-TPO, anti-Tg, anti-TSHR:* Anti-TPO antibodies are found in autoimmune diseases of thyroid (Hashimoto's disease, Graves disease), postpartum thyroiditis, sporadic goiter, and nodular thyroid diseases. Antibody testing should be done in cases of suspected autoimmune thyropathy.
3. *Ultrasound thyroid:* Ultrasonography helps in assessment of size, shape, and architecture of gland and screens out potentially cancerous nodules or swelling which require further evaluation. Following features such as poorly defined or irregular margins, solid, hypoechoic nodule with microcalcifications or increased vascularity are suggestive malignancy. Computed tomography (CT) or magnetic resonance imaging (MRI) can be used for cases with retrosternal thyroid extension.
4. *Thyroid nuclear scan:* Nuclear scan detects functional autonomous activity of the gland or nodule. Gland with autonomous activity is labeled "warm or hot" and "cold" if nonfunctioning. All cold lesions on thyroid scan need further evaluation to rule out malignancy. Thyroid scan also helps to localize retrosternal thyroid tissue.
5. *Fine needle aspiration and cytology* (FNAC): It gives an accurate cytological classification of the gland and henceforth decides the line of definitive treatment. USG-guided FNAC is now routinely done on thyroid nodules which are nonautonomous/cold or show features on USG-favoring malignancy or in patients with positive family history or prior radiation exposure.

The Bethesda System revised in 2017 is a standardized and worldwide acceptable system of reporting thyroid FNA samples and is composed of six categories. Each category associated with the estimated risk of malignancy and proposed line of treatment is outlined in the **Table 1**.

Table 1: Bethesda system for reporting thyroid cytopathology.

Categories	Malignancy risk (%)	Treatment
Nondiagnostic or unsatisfactory	1–4	FNAC to be repeated
Benign	0–4	Follow-up
Atypia of undetermined significance	5–15	FNAC to be repeated or follicular lesion of undetermined significance
Follicular neoplasm or suspicious of a follicular neoplasm	15–30	Surgical lobectomy
Suspicious for malignancy	60–75	Near-total or total thyroidectomy or surgical lobectomy
Malignant	96–99	Near-total or total thyroidectomy

TREATMENT

Observation
Observation with regular follow-up should be done in cases of small, asymptomatic goiter with normal thyroid functions.

Medical Management
1. *Antiinflammatory*: In cases of subacute thyroiditis high-dose aspirin or nonsteroidal antiinflammatory drugs (NSAIDs) can be given to reduce pain and inflammation. In cases of no relief short course of glucocorticoids can also be used.
2. *Suppression of TSH, levothyroxine replacement*: Thyroxine should be given in cases of hypothyroidism in order to suppress levels of TSH which may decrease the associated symptoms and partially shrink the enlarged thyroid gland.
3. *Antithyroid drugs*: Cases who present with thyrotoxicosis should be managed with thionamides (carbimazole, methimazole, propylthiouracil), which reduce oxidation and organification of iodine.
4. *B-Blockers*: Long-acting B-blockers atenolol or propranolol are helpful to reduce adrenergic symptoms in cases of thyrotoxicosis, before the effect of antithyroid drug starts. It also inhibits the peripheral conversion of T4 to T3 and is also used in thyrotoxic crisis.

Radioactive Iodine
Radioiodine treatment is a thyroid ablation method used in cases where diffuse or nodular goiter is caused by an overactive gland. Radioiodine use for nontoxic MNG to reduce size of the enlarged gland is not a widely used and acceptable option. At present, ^{131}I is the most commonly used therapy with use of a fixed dose of isotope (e.g. 15 mCi or 550 MBq). Progressive destruction of thyroid cells occurs by radioiodine and in order to avoid thyroid crisis pretreatment with antithyroid drugs to attain euthyroid levels becomes a prerequisite. It is also used in cases of thyroid malignancy as a postsurgical radio ablation method for remnants of thyroid tissue. Radioiodine is contraindicated in pregnancy and breastfeeding. Most patients progress to hypothyroidism in follow-up years and require levothyroxine replacement.

Surgical Management
Subtotal or near total thyroidectomy is the preferable treatment for patients with large multinodular goiter, retrosternal goiter, thyroid malignancy, cases with suspicion of malignancy in due course, goiter with features suggestive of compression on trachea, esophagus, and in patients with cosmetic issues.

Regular Follow-up
Patients with goiter should be under regular follow-up with thyroid function, imaging, fine-needle biopsy (FNB) to assess the function, and progression of the disease.

Flowchart 1: Course of action for the management of thyroid nodules.

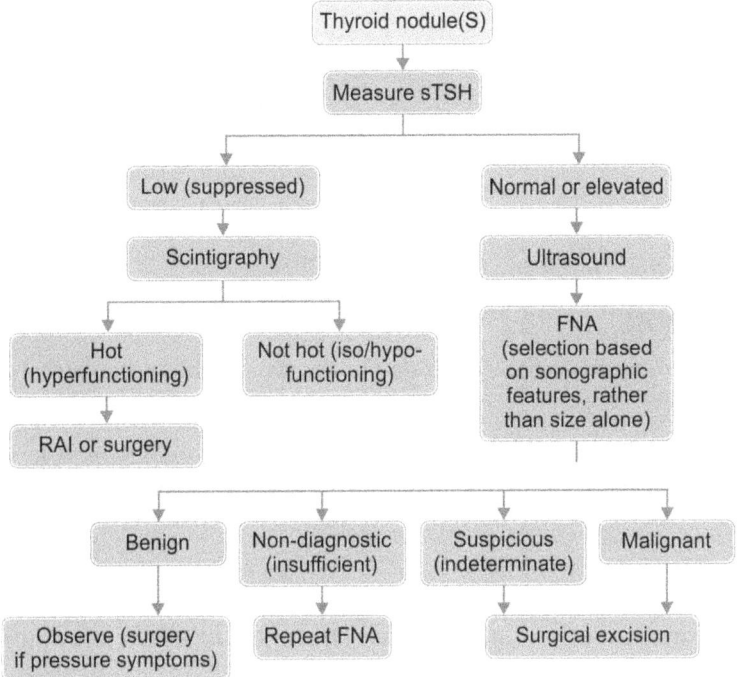

SUMMARY

Autoimmune diseases, deficiency of iodine, and nodular disease of thyroid are the commonly seen factors causing thyroid enlargement. The initial enlargement of the gland is usually diffused which subsequently becomes nodular as few of the follicles multiply, increase in size, or undergo cystic changes or calcify. Therefore, due to iodine deficiency, children and adolescents generally present with diffuse thyroid enlargement, while adults with longstanding deficiency develop nodular disease. TSH testing with assessment of functional thyroid in diffuse and nodular thyroid disease usually determines the further course of action as described in **Flowchart 1**.

In endemic or nonendemic areas neonates, children, and pregnant females should be assessed for iodine sufficiency followed by nutritional supplementation. Toxic cases should be made euthyroid with antithyroid drugs followed by radioiodine ablation or surgery depending on size and associated symptoms while observation, clinical follow-up with regular ultrasonography should be done in cases of benign or euthyroid goiter.

CHAPTER 45

Gum Disorders

Avdi Tahiri, Lumturije Njazi Asllani-Hashani

■ INTRODUCTION

Gum is part of the oral mucosa, partly fixated in the alveolar bone, cement of the root of the tooth, and partly free.

Gingivitis: It means disease that is manifested in the gum. Gingivitis is a mild form and first stage of gum disease, but without proper treatment it can lead to the more serious periodontitis.

■ ETIOLOGY/CAUSES

Plaque is the primary cause of gum disease. However, other factors can contribute to periodontal disease. These include:
- Hormonal changes
- Illnesses
- Medications
- Bad habits
- Poor oral hygiene
- Family history of gum disease.

■ PATHOPHYSIOLOGY

When gingivitis is left untreated, it can advance to periodontitis. In a person with periodontitis, the inner layer of the gum will pull away from the teeth and form pockets. These small spaces between teeth and gums collect debris and can become infected. The body's immune system fights the bacteria as the plaque spreads and grows below the gum line.

Toxins produced by the bacteria in plaque as well as the body's "good" enzymes are involved in fighting. Infections start to break down the bone and connective tissue that hold teeth in the place. As the disease progresses, the pockets deepen and more gum tissue and bone are destroyed. When bacteria build up in the mouth, it forms plaque, a condition characterized by red, inflamed sensitive gums. When this happens, teeth are no longer anchored in place, they become loose, and tooth loss occurs. Gum disease is the leading cause of tooth loss in adults.

RISK FACTORS
- Age
- Osteoporosis
- Poor hygiene
- Smoking
- Genetic.

RED FLAGS
- Bleeding gums
- Canker sores
- Receding gums
- Chronic bad breath and itchy
- Feeling around the gum line.

CLASSIFICATION
Gingivitis, based on the location in the gum, is classified as exudative, proliferative, and necrobiosis. Types of gingivitis are discussed here.

Gingivitis Catarrhalis (Gingivitis Superficialis)
These are inflamed gums with exudative reaction.
- *Epidemiology*: Gingivitis catarrhalis is a disease that happens often. It is considered that 95% of the population, who have their own teeth, have this disease.
- *Etiology*: Poor dental hygeine, dental carries, bad habits, poor nutritional staus diabetes, few physiological states like puberty menstrual periods and pregnancy responsible for the condition.
- *Symptoms*: In gingivitis catarrhalis, the color, size, form, and consistency of gingiva changes. Also, it is followed by subjective problems, bleeding and being sensitive to other things.
- *Therapy*: Therapeutic maze is getting rid of local factors, removal of dental plaque, and dental tartar. To use antiseptic preparation like H_2O_2 3%. Besides that, oral hygiene should be correct.

Gum Hyperplasia
It is manifested with exudative inflammation of gingiva.
- *Epidemiology*: It is a rare disease. It appears in children and teenagers.
- *Etiology*: Etiology factors are of the local nature like: dental plaque, poor dental hygiene, and teeth tartar. In this disease, medicine has an impact on the epilepsy disease. It is said that the gingivitis hyperplastic is a hereditary disease.

- *Symptoms*: Characterized swelling of gingiva, it is more common in the upper jaw and in the labial part. Gums are soft and red. There is no pain, but there are problems while chewing and bad breath.
- *Therapy*: The removal of teeth tartar, removing the local factors, use antiseptic preparation, treatment with sympatholytic and gingivoplastia.

Gingivitis Fibromatosa (Gingivitis Neoplastic)

Gum disease, which happens from unknown factors and these factors have an impact in the forming of connective tissue.
- *Epidemiology*: It is a rare disease. It affects mostly kids from 8 to 12 years old.
- *Etiology*: The cause is not known. It is believed that this disease is hereditary, but dental plaque does not have an impact in the forming of this gingivitis.
- *Symptoms*: This disease is characterized by hyperplasia of gum, without exudative inflammation, that is why it becomes very hard and pale. Hyperplasia is localized in the region of lateral teeth in the upper jaw, it can cover the teeth entirely. The patient can have problems during chewing and talking.
- *Therapy*: The healing process is mostly done by surgery. It can happen again.

Gingivitis Necroticans Ulcerosa

This is a gum disease which appears with alterative inflammation type. It appears in form of ulcer-necrotic changes in the gum.
- *Epidemiology*: It is a frequent disease. It affects young people from the age 20 to 30 years old. After the age of 45, the disease never appears. The illness has sessional characters and it appears during fall and winter.
- *Etiology*: It has infected etiology. Two microorganisms cause it, one is *Bacillus fusiformis* and the other is *Borrelia vincentii*. They stay in dental plaque and gingival sulcus and are apoptogenic. For the infection to happen, the dental plaque and poor oral hygiene has to be present. Some toxic materials like heavy metals (antimony, mercury, and lead) can toxically damage and favor infection. Smoking favors infection. Illnesses favor infection: diabetes, malnutrition, leukemia, agranulocytosis, and bad social and economic conditions.
- *Symptoms*: Gum is swollen and red, ulceronecrotic changes are localized in the top of interdental gum, covered with yellow or green membrane.
- *Therapy*: For the elimination of the diseases factors, antibiotics and antiseptics are used. Consequences of the illness are curable with chirurgical intervention, gum massage, and electrophoresis with vasodilatation preparations.

Gingivitis Desquamative

This is a rare disease. Because of the desquamation of gum mucosae, the gum becomes really thin.
- *Epidemiology*: It appears more on females. It affects at the ages 20–40 years old.
- *Etiology*: It is believed that it is due to hormonal imbalances.
- *Symptoms*: There are three forms of gingivitis desquamative.
- *Therapy*: Avoiding dental tartar and dental plaque, taking care of oral hygiene, usage of corticosteroids, vitamins therapy, and hormonal therapy. Even using the therapy, the illness can last months or even years.

CHAPTER 46

Heat Illness

Omar Ghazanfar, Saleh Fares

INTRODUCTION

Heat illness is a spectrum of disorders due to environmental exposure to heat. It ranges from minor conditions such as heat cramps, heat syncope, and heat exhaustion to the more severe condition known as heatstroke. A number of heat illnesses exist across a broad spectrum of presentations (**Table 1**).

SYMPTOMS OF HEAT ILLNESS

The symptoms of the different types of heat illness have been shown in **Table 2**.

Table 1: Types of heat illness.

Heat cramps	Muscular pain which happens after exercise in hot conditions
Heat edema	Cutaneous condition characterized by dependent edema from vasodilatory pooling
Heat rash	Irritation of the skin that results from excessive sweating during hot and humid weather
Heat tetany	A result of short periods of stress in intense heat. Symptoms may include hyperventilation, respiratory problems, numbness or tingling, or muscle spasms
Heat syncope	Dizziness as a result of excess heat
Heat exhaustion	A precursor of a heatstroke; which includes heavy sweating, rapid breathing and a fast, weak pulse
Heatstroke	A core body temperature of greater than 40°C (104°F) due to environmental heat exposure with either a lack or dysfunction of the central and peripheral thermoregulation center. Symptoms include dry skin, rapid, strong pulse and dizziness

Table 2: Symptoms of heat illness.

Heat illness	*Symptoms*
Dehydration	Dry mouth, headache, reduction in urine output, and dark urine
Heat rash	Red bumps in the skin on the neck, chest, and skin folds
Heat cramps	Excess sweating with muscular pain
Heat exhaustion	Excess sweating, nausea and vomiting-syncope or syncope, weakness, irritability and confusion, tachypnea and tachycardia
Heatstroke	Increased core body temperature, syncope, confusion, impaired level of consciousness, coma, and sometimes death

RISK FACTORS AND INVESTIGATIONS FOR HEAT ILLNESSES

The risk factors and investigations for heat-related illnesses have been shown in **Boxes 1 and 2**.

DIFFERENT TYPES OF HEAT ILLNESS

Heat Cramps

Heat cramps are muscular spasms which result from a loss of salt and water due to excessive exercise. Heat cramps are associated with cramping in the abdomen and calves. This is caused by inadequate intake of fluid and electrolytes. Heavy sweating can also result in heat cramps, especially when the water is replaced without electrolyte replacement.

Box 1: Risk factors for heat-related illness.

- Age >65 or <15
- Cognitive impairment
- Heart or pulmonary disease
- Poor access to ventilation
- Psychiatric illness
- Obesity
- Physical disability
- Poor fitness level
- Sickle cell trait
- Excess physical activity in high temperature
- Urban residence especially on high floors
- Heat wave
- Drugs
- Current febrile illness
- Skin disease
- Lack of acclimatization
- Previous heatstroke
- Increased heat index
- Alcohol consumption
- Lack of sleep, food, and water

Box 2: Investigations in heat-related illness.

- Monitor core body temperature regularly
- Complete blood count (CBC)
- Liver function tests (LFTs)
- Urea and electrolytes (U&E)
- Glucose
- Urate—may be a predictor of acute kidney injury
- Creatine kinase—may be a predictor of rhabdomyolysis
- Coagulation studies
- Arterial blood gases
- Urinalysis—may show myoglobinuria and impending acute kidney injury
- Electrocardiography
- Chest X-ray (CXR)—to check for aspiration/pulmonary edema

Heat cramps can be quite painful, but they do not result in permanent damage but can be an early symptom of heat exhaustion and heatstroke. Heat cramps can however indicate a more severe pathology in patients with heart disease or if it lasts for a prolonged period of time. Prevention includes oral rehydration during severe exercise or strenuous work and consumption of eat potassium-rich foods like bananas. After heat cramps occur, the affected patient should avoid strenuous work and exercise for several hours to allow adequate recovery.

Heat Edema

Heat edema is a skin condition characterized by edema in dependant body areas as a result of vasodilatory pooling. Heat causes the blood vessels to dilate, resulting in gravitation of body fluids so body fluid moves into the hands or legs by gravity. The balance of salt in the body is also a risk factor for heat edema. If salt loss is less than normal, the increased salt level draws fluid into the hands and legs. Elderly patients have an increased risk of heat edema, especially if they have other medical conditions that affect their circulation. People visiting hot climates from colder climates may also have an increased risk of heat edema.

Heat Rash

Heat rash occurs when the skin's sweat glands are blocked, and the sweat produced cannot get to the surface of the skin to evaporate. This causes inflammation that results in a rash. Common symptoms of heat rash include red bumps on the skin, and a prickly or itchy feeling to the skin (also known as prickly heat). The rash appears as reddened skin with tiny blisters and is due to inflammation. It often occurs in skin creases or areas of tight clothing where air cannot circulate. Heat rash usually fades when the skin is allowed to cool. Medical treatment is necessary only if the area becomes infected. Heat rash can be prevented by avoiding hot, humid conditions, wearing lose fitting clothes, and using air-conditioning or fans to allow air to circulate.

Heat Tetany

Heat tetany (hyperventilation and heat stress) is usually related to short periods of stress in intense heat environments. Symptoms may include hyperventilation, respiratory problems, numbness or tingling, or muscle spasms. Treatment includes removing the affected person from the heat and slowing the breathing pattern.

Heat Syncope

Heat syncope occurs in a warm environment when the blood pressure drops due to dilatation of the arterioles in the skin to radiate heat. This condition usually occurs within 5 days of heat acclimatization, before the actual blood volume expands. This subsequently leads to reduction blood to the brain, causing lightheadedness and near syncope during sudden postural movements or if the patient remains standing for a prolonged period of time. Individuals who perform strenuous work outside in warm climates are at particular risk.

Symptoms
Symptoms can include faintness, dizziness, headache, increased pulse, restlessness, nausea, vomiting, or brief loss of consciousness.

Diagnosis
The diagnosis of heat syncope is through a history and physical examination. During the physical examination, the health care provider should assess the vital signs including postural blood pressure and the pulse. If the patient experiences heat syncope, the patient is usually hypotensive and tachycardic. Excess sweating is also being a key sign. A detailed history is imperative. If the patient develops symptoms during physical activity in high temperatures, then the diagnosis of heat syncope can be made.

Treatment
The basic treatment for heat syncope is similar to other types of syncope. The patient is positioned in a seating or supine position with legs raised. If the patient can tolerate it, oral rehydration with salt or a drink containing electrolytes, can be administered slowly, and the patient is moved to a cooler area preferably under a shade. The affected person should be advised rest; as heat syncope can lead to heat exhaustion and subsequently heatstrokes.

Prevention
Physical activity in extremely hot weather should be avoided. In the event of symptoms, the patient should be moved to a shaded or cooler location. It is also recommended to avoid alcoholic beverages in hot weather as this can lead to dehydration which may exacerbate symptoms. Patients should also be encouraged to increase the intake of oral fluids during physical activity.

Heat Exhaustion
Heat exhaustion is often a precursor of heatstrokes if the patient is not treated appropriately and in a timely manner. Etiology and risk factors include hot, sunny, humid weather along with physical exertion in extremes of heat. Impaired thermoregulation in extremes of age results in geriatric and pediatric patients suffering from severe heat illness even at rest, if the weather outside is hot and humid with a lack of ventilation. Drugs including diuretics, antihistamines and beta-blockers and agents of misuse such as alcohol, ecstasy, and amphetamines can also increase the incidence of heat exhaustion. During physical exertion, risk factors for heat exhaustion include, wearing dark, padded, or insulated clothing; hats; and/or helmets in some professions, having a higher percentage of body fat, and lack of fluid intake leading to dehydration as well as pyrexia.

Symptoms

Symptoms include dizziness, nausea, headache, increased thirst, raised core body temperature, increased sweating, and reduced urine output.

Treatment

Basic management includes moving the person to a cool place with removal of extra layers of clothes. Passive cooling by fanning wet towels and increase intake of oral fluids if the patient is conscious. Specific management includes following the usual airway, breathing and circulation (ABC) approach. Supplemental oxygen may be required and if the patient is confused with impaired level of consciousness and/or vomiting, intravenous fluids and electrolyte replacement is needed.

Heatstroke

Heatstroke is a type of severe heat illness that results in a core body temperature of greater than 40.0°C and associated with confusion. Other symptoms include red, dry or damp skin, headache, and dizziness which can be sudden or gradual. Complications can include seizures, rhabdomyolysis and renal impairment.

Heatstroke results from extreme high environmental temperatures or severe physical exertion. There are certain risk factors including heat waves, humidity, and medications which include diuretics, beta-blockers, and alcohol as well as cardiac disease and skin pathology. Extremes of age and individuals with long-term chronic illness not associated with physical exertion typically occur in extremes of age or with chronic health problems. Heatstroke is a type of hyperthermia and is a pathological increase in the body's core temperature set point.

Drinking sufficient fluids and avoiding excessive heat can be an effective preventative measure. Treatment includes rapid physical cooling of the body and supportive measures. Spraying the patient with water and using a fan, or placing the patient in an ice bath, or giving cooled intravenous fluids are some of the measures which can be taken. Adding ice packs is not routinely recommended.

Heatstroke results in more than 600 deaths a year in the United States. Rates have increased in the last decade. The risk of death is over 5% in those with exercise-induced heatstroke and greater than 65% in those with nonexercise-induced cases.

Symptoms

Heatstroke presents with a hyperthermia of greater than 40.0°C in conjunction with disorientation and anhidrosis. Early signs include dizziness, mental confusion, headaches, and weakness. In exertional heatstroke, the affected person may sweat excessively. Pediatric patients may have seizures. Eventually there is impairment of consciousness, multi-organ failure, and death.

Etiology

Heatstroke occurs when the thermoregulation system is overwhelmed by a combination of excessive metabolic production of heat, excessive environmental heat, and insufficient or impaired heat loss. Alcohol, stimulants, medications as well as extremes of age can result in nonexertional heatstrokes. Exertional heatstroke can occur in young individuals without existing health problems or medications and the spectrum of patients includes athletes, outdoor workers, military personnel on outdoor maneuvers as well as emergency medical service (EMS) first responders wearing heavy personal protective equipment (PPE). In hot and humid environments, the humidity tends to reduce the degree to which the body can self-regulate the temperature by sweating and evaporation. Excessive body temperature can disrupt enzymes regulating biochemical reactions that are essential for cellular respiration and organ functions.

Young children, elderly adults, or disabled individuals left alone in a vehicle are at high risk of heat developing a stroke. In child deaths in hot cars, approximately 50% happened because parents forgot that the child was in the car, 18% happened after parents intentionally left the child in the car without understanding how hot it could get, and 30% happened after the child climbed into the car to play. This can have medical as well as legal consequences.

Prevention

The risk of heatstroke can be reduced by observing precautions to avoid overheating and dehydration. Light, loose-fitting clothes will allow perspiration to evaporate and cool the body. Wide-brimmed hats in light colors help prevent the sun from warming the head and neck. Vents on a hat will help cool the head. Strenuous exercise should be avoided during daylight hours in hot weather, as should remain in confined spaces (such as automobiles) without air-conditioning or ventilation. Adequate hydration is recommended to prevent dehydration.

Treatment

Treatment of heatstroke involves rapid mechanical cooling along with resuscitation measures. The body temperature must be lowered quickly. The patient should be moved to a cool area which is either indoor or in a shade and clothing may need to be removed to promote passive clothing. Active cooling methods include immersion in cold water, or a hyperthermia vest can be applied. Cold compresses to the torso, head, neck, and groin will help in bringing the body core temperature down. A fan or dehumidifying air-conditioning unit may be used to aid in evaporation of the water

Immersion should be avoided for an unconscious person, but if there is no alternative, the patients' head must be held above water. Dantrolene a direct-acting paralytic which abolishes shuddering and is effective in many other forms of hyperthermia has no individual or additive effects to cooling in the context of heatstroke, showing a lack of endogenous thermogenic response to cold water immersion. Aggressive ice-water immersion is the gold standard for life-threatening heatstroke.

Box 3: Drugs contributing to heat illness.

- Alcohol
- Alpha-adrenergic agonists
- Amphetamines
- Anticholinergics
- Antihistamines
- Benzodiazepines
- Beta-blockers
- Calcium channel blockers
- Cocaine
- Diuretics
- Ephedra-supplements
- Laxatives
- Neuroleptics
- Phenothiazines
- Stimulants

Adequate hydration is essential adjunct to cool the temperature. In mild cases of dehydration, it can be achieved by drinking water, or isotonic sports drinks. In exercise- or heat-induced dehydration, an imbalance of electrolytes can occur and is exacerbated by overconsumption of water. Hyponatremia can be corrected by intake of hypertonic fluids. Absorption is rapid and complete in most people but in the event of confusion, impaired conscious level or if the patient is unable to tolerate oral fluid, then an intravenous rehydration and electrolyte replacement may be required. The person's condition should be reassessed at regular intervals including the vital signs to ensure stability.

Prognosis

It was believed that heatstrokes rarely lead to permanent deficits and that the recovery is almost complete. However, research has showed that patients with heatstroke severe enough to require intensive care can leave to high percentage of morbidity and mortality. Some patients can have permanent loss of independent function or severe functional impairment at discharge which was persistent even 12 months after discharge from the health care facility.

■ DRUGS CONTRIBUTING TO HEAT ILLNESS

Medications and substances that contribute to heat-related illness have been shown in **Box 3**.

■ SUMMARY

Heat illness is a wide spectrum of different symptomatology which can range of heat cramps to heatstroke with a multitude of pathologies within the spectrum. Extreme heat can affect any individual; however, the elderly and children are more susceptible to heat stress along with people with pre-existing medical problems. Heat stress generally occurs when the body's thermoregulatory systems are unable to cope with extremes of temperatures and can lead to a wide spectrum of heat-related illnesses ranging from the simple heat cramps to the life-threatening heatstroke. Treatment revolves from instigating basic measures to remove the individual from the source as well as more advanced treatment strategies which include passive or active cooling as well as intravenous fluid and electrolyte replacement. The emphasis should however be on prevention strategies especially in extremes of ages where heat stress can be life threatening and result in significant morbidity and mortality.

CHAPTER 47

Heel Pain

Vivekanshu Verma

INTRODUCTION

Heel pain is common presentation in the foot and ankle outpatient department. Heel pain also known as various name like heel spur and plantar fasciitis. Regardless of terminology symptom is well known and diagnosis is easy. Usually patients complain of heel pain early in the morning upon arising or after rest.

CAUSES

Most common cause of plantar heel pain is mechanical overload; it may be due to biomechanical faults, overweight, working habits. Local nerve entrapment is also contributing factor for heel pain.
- Neurologic cause
- Arthritic cause
- Mechanical causes
- Traumatic causes
- Other.

Mechanical causes are responsible for most of the heel pain. In elderly population, the atrophy of heel pad is the common cause of heel pain; apophysitis of calcaneus (self-limiting condition) is cause of pediatric age group. During pregnancy, hormonal changes—weight gain may cause heel pain.

RISK FACTORS

- Obesity, standing for prolonged period, running, jumping, diabetes, thyroid dysfunction, and inflammatory spondyloarthropathy.

EVALUATION

History

Before coming to physician, patient attempts self-remedies. Patient describes heel pain as burning, aching and stabbing, worse early in morning with first step but decreases as person walks.

Flowchart 1: History taking in patient of heel pain.

- **Accessing heel pain**

Timing
- Is there any particular activity that precipitates heel pain?
- How long did heel pain last?

Severity
- How painful were the heels?
- Did anything worsen or lessen the pain?
- What impact does this have upon their activities of daily living?

Location
- Ask the patient about the which side of heel pains—medially, laterally.
- How far can they walk before the symptoms occur?

History should include duration of the heel pain, type of shoes, type of activities and any history of trauma, in case of history of radiating pain and if any sensory symptoms, neurological pathology should be ruled out. **(Flowchart 1)**.

Examination

Make observation about any swelling, range of motion of foot and ankle, dorsiflexion of ankle, palpation of heel and plantar fascia for atrophy of heel pad especially in elderly population. Gait evaluation should also be considered along with assessment of alignment of the foot. Assessment of tenderness if it is increases with the passive dorsiflexion of the toe.

After history and physical examination, appropriate radiograph especially weight-bearing radiograph may be helpful for further treatment. Heel spur can also be identified by radiological evaluation.

TREATMENT

Stepwise treatment recommended for plantar heel pain.

First Step

Padding and strapping, stretching exercise of plantar fascia, arch support, appropriate shoe, anti-inflammatory drugs, physiotherapy.

First step treatment should be continuing for at least 6 weeks.

Second Step

Continuation of initial treatment along with corticosteroid injection, night splint immobilization. This should be continuing for 6 months.

Flowchart 2: Summary of plantar heel pain.

> **Planter heel pain**
> Planter fasciitis heel spur syndrome planter fasciosis

> **Significant history**
> Isolated planter heel pain, pain on weight bearing,
> Post rest, morning pain
> Poor shoe or barefoot walking

> **Evaluation**
> Pain on palpation,
> Obesity, defective foot architecture, radiology

> **Three steps in management**
> Limitation of activities, stretching exercise, padding, strapping, anti-inflammatory, corticosteroid
> Surgery: Planter fasciotomy, heel spur resection ESWT

Third Step

Consider surgical management, plantar fasciotomy (in-step fasciotomy or endoscopic fasciotomy).

Extracorporeal shock wave therapy (ESWT) is alternative to traditional surgical approach. Nerve release and plantar fasciotomy for heel pain due to nerve entrapment. Recently radiofrequency ablation of plantar fascia and radiofrequency nerve ablation and cryoprobe methods are being used as alternative to surgical approach for chronic heel pain.

■ SUMMARY

Summary of plantar heel pain has been shown in **Flowchart 2**.

CHAPTER 48

Hematemesis

Sanjay Kumar

INTRODUCTION

Hematemesis is one of the most dreadful medical emergencies. Feeling of blood coming out of mouth is always scary for the patients and onlookers.

All patients presenting with history of hematemesis need thorough evaluation. Though some of them have a non-gastrointestinal (GI) cause which is known as spurious hematemesis like in epistaxis/dental bleed/oropharyngeal bleed, but most cases arise from an upper GI tract lesion. Common causes are summarized in **Box 1**.

APPROACH TO A PATIENT WITH HEMATEMESIS

It is of utmost importance to evaluate these patients at the earliest in terms of severity and triage them accordingly. There are various scoring systems for upper gastrointestinal (UGI) bleeding, viz. Rockall, Glasgow Blatchford, AIMS65, Baylor bleeding score (BBS), Cedars-Sinai Medical Center Predictive Index (CSMCPI), etc. Rockall score (**Box 2**) is practical to use but requires endoscopy to do complete scoring. When you have a patient with UGI bleeding, first thing is to assess vitals, ensure airway and plan for an UGI endoscopy. UGI endoscopy is not only diagnostic but therapeutic too in most cases. Best time to do UGI endoscopy depends on severity/scoring. Even in severe bleeding, UGI endoscopy is urgent but not emergent as studies have shown that most death are due to comorbidity and failure of proper resuscitation rather than failure to do an early therapeutic endoscopy.

Box 1: Sources of bleeding in patients hospitalized for upper gastrointestinal (UGI) bleeding.

- Ulcers*—gastric, duodenal or Cameron ulcer
- Varices*—esophageal, gastric or ectopic varices
- Mallory-Weiss tears
- Gastroduodenal erosions
- Erosive esophagitis
- Neoplasm—gastric cancer, lymphoma, leiomyoma, gastrointestinal stromal tumor (GIST)
- Vascular ectasias and gastric antral vascular ectasia (GAVE)
- Dieulafoy's lesion
- No source identified

*In most studies, ulcers and varices together account for 60–70% of UGI bleed cases.

Box 2: Rockall scoring.

<3 Score carries good prognosis
>8 Score carries high risk of mortality
- Age:
  - 0-<60
  - 1-60-79
  - 2->80
- Shock:
  - 0-None
  - 1-BP>100 mm Hg, HR>100/min
  - 2-BP>100 mm Hg
- Comorbidity:
  - 0-None
  - 2-Cardiac ds
  - 3-Renal/Liver failure, disseminated malignancy
- Diagnosis:
  - 0-Mallory-Weiss, no major lesion
  - 1-All other Dx
  - 2-Upper GI malignancy
- Recent hemorrhage:
  - 0-None
  - 2-Blood in upper tract, clot adherence or visible spurting

MANAGEMENT

Step I: Resuscitation and Quick Evaluation

- Maintain airway, maintain blood pressure, transfuse blood/blood products as required [in portal hypertensive bleeding, target hemoglobin (Hb) should be around 7 g% and in nonvariceal bleed around 9 g% while in coronary artery disease patients, it should be kept around 10 g% irrespective of cause].
- Assess blood loss:
  - Resting tachycardia means about 15% volume loss
  - Postural hypotension >15% volume loss
  - Supine hypotension (shock) >40% volume loss.
- Put nasogastric (NG) tube for bleed assessment and cleaning.
- Triage the patient as per your evaluation.
- Start proton pump inhibitor (PPI) infusion.
- Start somatostatin infusion if known portal hypertension and chronic liver disease.
- Start broad-spectrum antibiotics (if known portal HT/CLD).

Step II: Prepare for Endoscopy

- Inform surgeon
- Counsel family.

Step III: UGI Endoscopy (Keep All Accessories Ready for Therapeutic Interventions)

Emergency endoscopy helps in managing severe bleeding cases by providing endotherapy (as in variceal bleeding/arterial spurt from peptic ulcer/Dieulafoy's lesion). And also helps in minor bleed patients to decide about triage and early discharge.

No patients of UGI bleeding should go home without an UGI endoscopy unless clinical condition does not permit an endoscopy or patient/family fails to give an informed consent. Endoscopes should preferably be done under sedation.

- Portal HT—esophageal or gastric varices/gastropathy bleeds
  - Options:
    - Endoscopic variceal ligation/sclerotherapy for esophageal varices
    - Glue injection of fundal varices
    - APC for PHG/hemorrhagic gastritis.
- Nonportal HT bleed—ulcer/MW tear/(Dieulafoy's lesion/hemorrhagic gastritis/esophagitis)
  - Options:
    - Injection therapy/heater probe/hemoclip/APC/hemospray/or a combination.

It is recommended that for optimum result a combination of two modalities is preferred over single intervention.

For example, Injection + clip or injection + heater probe.

Step IV: Careful Monitoring of Patient for Ongoing Bleed

- Serial Hb level—every 6–8 hourly
- NG aspirate color
- Color of stool
- Blood urea nitrogen (BUN).

Step V: Relook Endoscopy

- May be required in select cases depending upon assessment of endoscopist during first endoscopy to confirm continued hemostasis or to repeat endoscopic therapy in case of failure hemostasis.

Step VI: Surgery

- In patients who continue to bleed and in whom requirement of blood is very high or rare blood group or if family prefers surgery over a repeat endoscopic treatment.

CHAPTER 49

Hematuria

Asit Misra

INTRODUCTION

The presence of blood in the urine is known as hematuria. Hematuria is divided into two major groups: gross and microscopic. Gross hematuria is any hematuria that is (visible to eyes) and microscopic hematuria that is (visible through microscope). Any hematuria with more than 3 RBC/hpf (red blood cells/high power field) is marked as significant and needs further investigation and management. Patients having gross hematuria often visit the emergency department for urgent evaluation and management. Any unexplained hematuria in adults over 50 years of age may be a result of an underlying malignancy of the urinary tract and demands thorough evaluation. Although unexplained hematuria is common in younger and older adults.

ETIOLOGY

Hematuria is a resultant of an underlying pathological condition or disease. The causes of hematuria vary depending upon: (1) age, and (2) location of the pathology in the urinary tract (**Table 1**).

Due to the broad range of etiology, the risk factors of hematuria are dependent on its etiology. It is important to note that smoking is the most significant risk factor for the development of urothelial malignancies, which leads to hematuria. The most common cause of gross hematuria in adults over 50 years is bladder cancer.

PATHOPHYSIOLOGY

In normal physiological condition, human kidneys do not excrete RBCs and the urine in normal condition should contain less than 3 RBC/hpf. Therefore, any presence of RBCs in urine over the normal limit is pathological until proven otherwise. Further, we can divide hematuria due to the pathology of kidneys (glomerular hematuria) or due to pathology of urinary tract (nonglomerular hematuria). In glomerular hematuria, blood mixes in the urine during the formation of the urine whereas; in nonglomerular hematuria, blood mixes in the excreted urine when it passes through the distal urinary tract. We can further divide nonglomerular hematuria based on medical and surgical causes. Underlying causes of medical nonglomerular

Table 1: Causes of hematuria.

1. Causes of hematuria classified by age:	
Young adults and children	Glomerulonephritis
Over 20 years	Nephrolithiasis
Over 40 years	Benign prostatic hypertrophy (in males)
Over 50 years	Malignancy
All ages	Urinary tract infections
2. Causes of hematuria classified by location in urinary tract:	
Upper collecting system	*Lower collecting system*
Papillary necrosis (sickle cell disease)	Radiation
Renal vein thrombosis	Cystitis
Renal artery embolism	Traumatic catheterization
Benign or malignant renal mass	Urethritis
Glomerular bleeding (Alport's syndrome, IgA nephropathy)	Malignancy (squamous cell carcinoma, transitional cell carcinoma)
Pyelonephritis	Urethral diverticulum
Malignant hypertension	Trauma
Hydronephrosis	Anticoagulation
Polycystic kidney disease	Transurethral resection of the prostate
Arteriovenous malformation	
Renal or ureteric calculi	
Ureteric stricture	
Postsurgical complications	
Trauma	
Anticoagulation	

hematuria can be systemic, renovascular, and tubulointerstitial disorders except renal tumors. Causes of surgical nonglomerular hematuria are stones, urologic tumors, and urinary tract infections.

Microscopic examination is warranted to distinguish the differences between glomerular and nonglomerular hematuria. In glomerular hematuria, the presence of RBC casts, dysmorphic erythrocytes, and proteinuria is detected, whereas in nonglomerular hematuria, erythrocyte casts are absent and circular erythrocytes are present. It is also important to understand that urine dipstick test used in the emergency department can result in a false positive for blood in urine in cases of myoglobinuria and hemoglobinuria. Presence of RBCs should be confirmed by a microscopic examination of the urine, which will show no RBCs in the specimen. Some other causes resulting in red or brown urine are mentioned in **Table 2**.

Table 2: Different causes of red or brown color urine.

Food	Medications	Endogenous	Other
• Berries • Beets • Rhubarb • Fava beans • Paprika • Artificial food colorings	• Phenytoin • Nonsteroidal anti-inflammatory drugs (NSAID) • Rifampin • Quinine • Phenothiazines • Nitrofurantoin • Metronidazole • Chloroquine • Levodopa • Methyldopa • Prochlorperazine • Sulfonamides	• Myoglobin • Free hemoglobin porphyrins • Bilirubin • Melanin • Amorphous urates • *Serratia marcescens* infection	• Malingering • Drug-seeking patients • Munchausen's syndrome

CLINICAL PRESENTATION AND RED FLAGS

Clinical presentation of hematuria is associated with its underlying cause. To help in the investigation, it is important to focus on the characteristics of hematuria and the clinician should consider looking for the answer to the following questions:

- **Is the hematuria microscopic or gross?**

  Identifying microscopic or gross hematuria helps the clinician to determine the degree of hematuria, and the chances of identifying any significant pathology increases. It is commonly seen that patients with gross hematuria have significant underlying pathology versus those with microscopic hematuria.

- **Any presence of pain associated with hematuria?**

  Painful hematuria is linked with upper urinary tract hematuria with obstruction of the ureters with clots. During the passage of these clots, the patient experiences colicky flank pain similar to ureteric colic. Another painful cause of hematuria is cystitis. Gross painless hematuria is seen in patients with bladder cancer.

- **When does the hematuria occur during urination? (entire stream, beginning or end of stream)**

  By knowing, the timing of hematuria during urination, one can figure out the site of the origin of hematuria. Early stream hematuria indicates the involvement of urethra (due to inflammation), end stream hematuria is linked with the pathology of the bladder neck and/or prostatic urethra, and entire stream hematuria occurs due to the pathology of the upper urinary tract and/or bladder.

- **Is there any presence of clots in urine? If yes then what is the shape of clots?**

  Presence of any blood clots in the urine sample increases the chances of identifying any significant pathology in the patient. In case of hematuria originating from the upper urinary tract, one can see the presence of vermiform (worm-shaped) blood clots. On the other hand, hematuria originating from the bladder and the prosthetic urethra will have amorphous clots.

EVALUATION

History

In the history taking of the patient with hematuria, the clinician should look for the following clues:
- Family history of renal disease, sickle cell disease, polycystic kidney disease, and diabetes.
- Recent upper respiratory tract infection (can lead to possible postinfectious glomerulonephritis, vasculitis, anti-glomerular basement membrane disease).
- Recent fever with pyuria and/or dysuria (indicates urinary tract infection).
- Any recent flank pain-radiating groin (suggestive of ureteral obstruction due to blood clot, calculus, and malignancy).
- History of hesitancy and dribbling in older men (suggestive of prostatic obstruction).
- Bleeding due to excessive anticoagulation. Studies suggest that chronic anticoagulation is not a cause of hematuria and patients on anticoagulants should be evaluated thoroughly to find the underlying cause of hematuria, as one will evaluate in other patients.
- Recent episode of strenuous exercise or trauma.
- Stay or travel history to places endemic for tuberculosis or *Schistosoma haematobium*.
- Is there a history of smoking or any drug abuse?
- Hematuria in suspected analgesic abusers, diabetics and in African-Americans is caused by papillary necrosis.

Physical Examination

In the physical examination of patient presenting with hematuria the clinician should focus on the cardiovascular system, blood pressure, and volume status (important when considering glomerulonephritis). In the examination of abdominal system, one should palpate for any mass that may be a tumor or hydronephrosis. Any positive costovertebral angle tenderness is indicative of nephrolithiasis, pyelonephritis, and/or ureteropelvic junction obstruction. In genitourinary system examination, one should feel for palpable bladder after micturition, which indicated obstruction or urinary retention. During auscultation, any bruit over renal area is suggestive of a vascular pathology. In the examination of genitals and rectum, it is vital to look for any evidence of meatal stenosis, epididymitis, prostatitis, and prostatic hypertrophy. A pelvic examination in women is necessary to rule out any vaginal or uterine bleeding.

INTERPRETATION OF FINDINGS

It is crucial for the clinicians to consider various factors when considering the causes of hematuria such as: the age of the patient, gender, habits, demographics, history of recent genitourinary procedure (instrumentation), and any other risk factors.

For obtaining an appropriate urine sample, one should ask for a midstream catch. It is suggested to collect urine sample via catheter from women having menstrual/vaginal bleeding or vaginal discharge. Foley's catheterization itself produces iatrogenic hematuria in 15% of the cases.

Glomerular versus Nonglomerular Hematuria

Red or pink urine with clots with normal RBC's morphology is suggestive of extraglomerular source whereas dark red, smoky brown, or coca cola color urine with some dysmorphic RBC's suggests the glomerular origin of hematuria. Also, hematuria of glomerular origin is differentiated from nonglomerular on the basis of related significant proteinuria and presence of cast.

INVESTIGATIONS

Urine Dipstick

This test is a common point of care test in the emergency department. It can identify the presence of blood, glucose, protein, ketones, bilirubin, and leucocytes in the urine. A positive urine dipstick test for blood is indicative of hematuria, myoglobinuria, or hemoglobinuria. This test uses a chemical reaction to detect blood in urine, which is based on peroxidase like activity of the hemoglobin. Dipstick test detects 150 mg/L of free hemoglobin which is similar to 5–20 intact RBCs/mL on microscopic analysis of the urine. Urine sample having high concentration of ascorbic acid and high specific gravity can result in false-positive dipstick test. Free myoglobin, hemoglobin, and porphyrins in urine sample also give false-positive dipstick test. Clinicians must send the sample for confirmatory microscopic examination for the cases where clinical picture and dipstick test results have a mismatch.

Microscopic Examination

Microscopy of the urine sample helps to identify white blood cells in addition to the RBCs indicating infection. It can also reveal proteinuria, dysmorphic RBC's, and cellular casts which indicates glomerular disease.

Imaging Studies

Computer tomography (CT) with or without contrast is the initial imaging study of choice in hematuria of nonglomerular origin. CT has high sensitivity for detecting stones, in identifying renal tumors and other nongenitourinary tract abdominal pathologies that lead to hematuria. The disadvantage of CT scan is the need of intravenous contrast and radiation exposure to the patient. CT is also not safe for pregnant females.

Renal ultrasound is the next best initial imaging modality in case CT is not available or contraindicated. If initial imaging modalities are inconclusive to identify the source of hematuria then cystoscopy should be planned. In case of suspicion of upper tract involvement, a retrograde pyelography is helpful to identify the source of hematuria.

Magnetic resonance urography (MRU) is another imaging modality used to identify causes of hematuria where CT is contraindicated. MRU is accurate in diagnosing renal lesions over urothelial lesions. It is also safe for patients contrast allergy and for pregnant women.

Blood Tests

Kidney function test should be performed to evaluate the status of renal function. Complete hemogram, urine culture, and coagulation study is necessary to find out any evidence of systemic infection (sepsis) and coagulopathy. Blood grouping and cross matching may be needed in cases of gross hematuria.

Flowchart 1: Approach for the evaluation of hematuria.

```
                            Hematuria
                                │
              Yes               ▼               No
         ┌──────────── Acute onset with ────────────┐
         │              flank pain?                 │
         ▼                                          ▼
   Evaluate for        Yes   Any symptoms      No
   kidney stones   ◄──────── of UTI? ────────┐
                                │            │
                              ▼              ▼
                           Treat UTI    Is hematuria visible
                                        to naked eyes?
                                        (Red, pink or brown
                                         color urine)
                                         │
                             Yes ────────┴──────── No
                              │                    │
                              ▼                    ▼
   Get a CT of abdomen and pelvis   Yes       Gross           Microscopic
   with and without contrast, and ◄────── hematuria           hematuria
   urgent referral to urology                │
                                              ▼
                                        Visible blood     No    Any evidence    Yes
                                        clots in urine? ─────► of glomerular ──────┐
                                                               bleeding?           │
         Any evidence of glomerular ◄──┐                            │              │
         bleeding?                     │                            ▼              ▼
                                       │                      Look for the following   Refer the
                                       │                      risk factors:            patient to
                                       │                      1) Age >35 years         nephrologist
   Yes ─┐              No              │                      2) Any history of smoking
        │              │               │                      3) History of analgesic abuse
        ▼              ▼               │                         or heavy use
   Refer the    In females of child bearing                   4) History of urological disease
   patient to   age rule out pregnancy                        5) History of painful, frequent
   nephrologist and get a CT of abdomen                          urination
                and pelvis with and without                   6) History of chronic UTI
                contrast, referral to                         7) History of pelvic irradiation
                urology for cystoscopy
                         │                                        Yes              No
        ▲      No        ▼
        └──────── Cause identified?
   Treat the              │
   cause    ◄──────── Yes
```

TREATMENT

Treatment of hematuria is based on the etiology. In cases presenting to the emergency department, one should assess the hemodynamic stability of the patient first. In hemodynamically stable patients, without any life-threatening cause of hematuria, it is advised to have an outpatient follow-up. As per the recommendations of American Urological Association guideline, patients with microscopic hematuria without any benign cause should be referred to urology service for assessment of urinary tract malignancy.

Patients with gross hematuria may present to the emergency department with acute urinary retention due to bladder outlet obstruction and intravesical clot formation. This condition is treated by Foley's catheterization and may be followed by a bladder wash in consultation with the urologist.

Hemodynamically unstable patients with pain, intolerance to oral medications and fluids, other comorbid conditions with bladder obstruction or with life-threatening cause of hematuria should be stabilized in the emergency department and are to be admitted under appropriate specialist.

SUMMARY

The presence of red blood cells in the urine is called hematuria. It can be gross (visible to naked eyes) or microscopic (detected by dipstick or microscopic examination). In adults, any unexplained hematuria is assumed malignant until proven otherwise. Patients with gross hematuria should undergo a mandatory evaluation of the upper and lower urinary tract whereas patients with asymptomatic microscopic hematuria should have urologic evaluation upon ruling out of the benign causes. The evaluation should include urine analysis, renal functions test, cystoscopy, renal and genitourinary ultrasonography, and computed tomography. The approach to evaluation of hematuria is summarized in **Flowchart 1**. Treatment of hematuria is based on the etiology. Hemodynamically unstable patients should be stabilized in the emergency department and are admitted for further management.

CHAPTER 50

Hemoptysis

Veerottam Tomar

INTRODUCTION

Hemoptysis is the expectoration of blood from the airways, it can originate from the alveoli to glottis. Hemoptysis is derived from Latin *haemo-* "of blood" + Greek *ptusis* "spitting". It can range from blood-tinged to severe life-threatening. For most patients, any degree of hemoptysis can be frightening and needs earliest medical evaluation. It is very scary to see patients dying from asphyxiation even in spite of intubation. It is the most challenging emergency faced by intensivist because course of bleeding is unpredictable and varies from trivial to large amount.

Hemoptysis is a manifestation of underlying disease process. Till now there is no consensus regarding the optimal management of these patients. A quick history, examination, investigations, and timely intervention play a very crucial role in the management of hemoptysis. At the same time, it is very important to differentiate hemoptysis from pseudohemoptysis, hematemesis, and epistaxis (**Table 1**).

There is no clear definition for the degree of hemoptysis, however, according to the general consensus:

Minor hemoptysis usually is less than 15–20 mL/day and is commonly seen to resolve spontaneously.

Table 1: Differentiation from hemoptysis.

Symptoms	Hemoptysis	Hematemesis	Epistaxis
Cough	Common	Uncommon	Uncommon
Dyspnea	Common	Uncommon	Uncommon
Abdominal symptoms	Uncommon	Common	Absent
Frothy secretions	May be present	Absent	Absent
Mixed with food	Absent	May be present	Absent
Mixed with sputum	Common	Uncommon	Uncommon
Color	Bright red	Coffee	Bright red
pH	Alkaline	Acidic	Alkaline
Chest symptoms	May be present	Absent	Absent
Nasal bleed	Absent	Absent	Present

Table 2: Grading of hemoptysis.

Grade	Amount/24 hours	
Mild	<50 mL	
Moderate	50–200 mL	
Severe/Major	>200 mL	150 mL/12 hours or >400 mL/24 hours
Massive	>600 mL	
Exsanguinating		1,000 mL total or 150 mL/hour
Life threatening		200 mL or 50 mL/hour in a patient with chronic respiratory failure

Massive hemoptysis ranges from greater than or equal to 100 mL in 24 hours to greater than 1 L in 24 hours. It can also be judged by its clinical consequences such as requiring hospitalization, the risk of airway occlusion, laboratory evidence of blood loss or even risk of death.

The most common causes of mild hemoptysis are bronchitis, bronchiectasis, bronchogenic carcinoma, and tuberculosis. Approximately 20-40% of cases of minor hemoptysis are due to bronchitis and bronchiectasis; while bronchogenic and metastatic carcinomas account for 20% of the cases. However, in India, tuberculosis is the most common cause of mild to massive hemoptysis, where it can be seen in active disease or as its sequelae. In western part of the world, malignancies are the main causes of massive hemoptysis.

It is important to keep in mind that the cause of death in hemoptysis is asphyxiation and not blood loss. It is also dependent on rate of blood loss and underlying lung condition. We can grade hemoptysis into the following grades (**Table 2**).

PREDICTORS OF MORTALITY

- 71% in patients who lost => 600 mL of blood in 4 hours
- 22% in patients with = 600 mL within 4–16 hours
- 5% in those with 600 mL within 16–48 hours.

BAD PROGNOSTIC FACTORS

- Bleeding rate: ~ 1,000 mL /24 hours
- Aspiration into contralateral lung
- Massive bleeding requiring single lung ventilation
- Bronchogenic carcinoma as an underlying etiology.

When considering the etiology of hemoptysis, it is important to be familiar with the pulmonary circulation. Lung has dual blood supply from pulmonary and bronchial circulations. Pulmonary circulation is mainly for gas exchange and accounts for 99% of total blood supply to the lungs. It is a low-pressure (25 mm Hg systolic—8 mm Hg diastolic, 15 mm Hg mean) high-flow system that receives the entire cardiac output and causes bleeding in less than

10% of cases. The bronchial circulation is high-pressure (systemic), low-flow system, which tends to be the major source of hemoptysis because it is more likely to be the source of the collaterals and neovascularization that characteristically occurs in the setting of chronic infection or malignancy. It supplies bronchial mucosa by formation of anastomosis in the peribronchial space and gives rise to small penetrating arteries in mucosa. It causes bleeding in 90% cases.

Nonbronchial circulation can also contribute to hemoptysis especially in lung parenchymal diseases where pleural involvement is present. The neovascularization arises from internal mammary, thyrocervical, coronary, and carotid arteries.

ETIOLOGY OF HEMOPTYSIS

- Airway diseases
  - Airway trauma
  - Bronchitis: Acute or chronic
  - Bronchiectasis
  - Bullous emphysema
  - Bronchovascular fistula (e.g. aortic aneurysm with erosion in to airway)
  - Bronchial adenoma
  - Bronchogenic carcinoma
  - Dieulafoy's disease (subepithelial bronchial artery)
  - Metastatic cancer to bronchus or trachea
  - Foreign body in airway
- Infection
  - Tuberculosis, active or cavitary
  - Invasive mycetoma
  - Bronchiectasis, cystic fibrosis
  - Pneumonia—*Staphylococcus, Klebsiella, Legionella*
  - Lung abscess
  - Hydatid cyst
  - Paragonimiasis
- Pulmonary vascular diseases
  - Congenital heart defects
  - Congestive heart failure
  - Mitral stenosis
  - Tricuspid endocarditis
  - Pulmonary arteriovenous malformation
  - Pulmonary artery pseudoaneurysm
  - Pulmonary embolism
  - Pulmonary veno-occlusive disease
  - Pulmonary hypertension

- Disorder of coagulation
  - Anticoagulant and antiplatelet medications
  - Disseminated intravascular coagulation (DIC)
  - Thrombocytopenia
  - Liver disease
  - Von Willebrand disease
- Iatrogenic
  - Bronchoscopy with endobronchial biopsy or transbronchial lung biopsy (TBLB) or transbronchial needle aspiration (TBNA)
  - Transthoracic needle aspiration
  - Pulmonary artery catheterization
  - Airway stent
- Miscellaneous
  - Drugs and toxins
    - Argemone alkaloid-contaminated cooking (epidemic dropsy)
    - Bevacizumab treatment
    - Catamenial hemoptysis
    - Cocaine use
    - Nitrogen dioxide toxicity
- Trauma
  - Blunt trauma chest
  - Penetrating lung injury
- Pulmonary-renal syndrome (Wegener's granulomatosis, Goodpasture's syndrome)
- Immunologic lung disease
- Systemic lupus erythematosus (SLE)
- Idiopathic pulmonary hemosiderosis
- Genetic defects of collagens (Ehlers Danlos syndrome)
- Bone marrow transplantation
- Idiopathic.

EVALUATION OF PATIENT WITH HEMOPTYSIS

Hemoptysis can be mild or severe requiring intensive care unit (ICU) admission, so in initial evaluation first step is a thorough history and complete physical examination to confirm that the patient truly has hemoptysis and not hematemesis or epistaxis.

Massive hemoptysis remains a challenge for critical care expert. After a quick physical examination of the patient, resuscitation should be started without delay.

The clinical manifestations of hemoptysis have been shown in **Table 3**.

The initial approach to managing life-threatening hemoptysis involves resuscitation and protection of airway. The second step is directed at localizing the site and cause of bleeding and final step is the application of definitive and specific treatments to prevent recurrent bleeding.

Table 3: Presenting clinical manifestations.

Category	Feature	Disorder
History	Smoking, asbestos exposure	Bronchogenic carcinoma
	Risk factors for aspiration (alcohol, swallowing disorder, level of consciousness)	Lung abscess, pneumonia, foreign body (FB) aspiration
	Recent chest trauma or procedure	Traumatic or iatrogenic lung injury
	Previously diagnosed pulmonary cardiac, or systemic disease	Important clue
Symptoms	Hoarseness of voice	Bronchogenic carcinoma
	Purulent sputum	Pneumonia, lung abscess, bronchiectasis, bronchitis
	Paroxysmal nocturnal dyspnea (PND)/Orthopnea	Mitral stenosis (MS)/left ventricular failure (LVF)
	Dyspnea and pleuritic chest pain	Pneumonia Pulmonary embolism
	Weight loss, night sweats, cough, fever	Tuberculosis Bronchogenic carcinoma
Signs	Localized decreased breath sounds, Localized wheeze, stridor	Bronchogenic carcinoma FB aspiration Tracheal tumor
	Bronchial breath sounds	Pneumonia
	Pleural rub	Pneumonia, pulmonary embolism
	Diastolic murmur	Mitral stenosis
	Clubbing	Suppurative lung disease, bronchiectasis, bronchogenic carcinoma
	S3 gallop	Left ventricular failure
	Oral aphthous ulcers, genital ulcers, and uveitis Saddle nose, rhinitis, and septal perforation	Behçet's disease in which arteriovenous malformations (AVMs) are present Wegener's granulomatosis

First Step

A quick history and physical examination followed by chest radiograph. Airway, breathing, and circulation (ABC) approach should be started. All patients with massive hemoptysis must be monitored in ICU.

Airway Protection

Patency of the airway should be the first priority to prevent exsanguination. To achieve immediate control of the airway, patient should be intubated with large single-lumen endotracheal tube (ETT) for proper suctioning, it will also help in initial diagnostic and therapeutic bronchoscopy. Double-lumen ETT can be placed to isolate and ventilate the lung if bleeding from one side. If the bleeding can be localized from one side then with the help of bronchoscope, ETT tube can be placed in normal lung side to protect it from aspiration. Double-lumen ETT tube should be placed by experienced person with the help of pediatric bronchoscope to confirm the tube position.

Breathing

The patient must lie in lateral decubitus position toward the bleeding side to prevent the normal lung from exsanguination, and supplement the oxygen to maintain saturation of peripheral oxygen (SpO_2) greater than 95%.

Circulation

A large bore intravenous (IV) cannula or central venous line should be inserted and IV fluid started. Intra-arterial catheter is necessary for more accurate monitoring of blood pressure. If the general condition of the patient is rapidly deteriorating, O-positive (in childbearing women O-negative) should be transfused while waiting for blood grouping and crossmatching. Arterial blood gas (ABG) should be sent immediately.

Laboratory Investigations

The following investigations are essential in all patients:

Complete hemogram, coagulation profile, renal function test, liver function test, ABG, D-dimer, urine analysis, and any other specialized tests needed according to the suspected underlying disease.

Chest X-ray: It helps in localizing the bleeding in 33–82% of cases and underlying cause in 35% like tuberculosis or tumors; however, found inconclusive in about 20–60% cases but rarely normal in massive hemoptysis.

Sputum and bronchoalveolar lavage should be sent for examination of Gram stain, aerobic culture, acid-fast bacilli (AFB), fungus culture, and *contrast-enhanced computed tomography (CECT) chest* can be ordered before bronchoscopy. It gives clue for type and site of lesion and can also detect bronchial and nonbronchial arterial vascular lesions like arteriovenous malformations (AVMs).

Multidetector computed tomography (MDCT): MDCT angiography is more useful in localizing the site, source of bleeding, and underlying lung pathology. With the help of MDCT, mapping of thoracic vasculature can be done and a detailed study of bronchial and nonbronchial circulation can be seen. Contrast CT was found accurate in 84% of patients to find feeding vessels in massive hemoptysis. However, it is not wise to shift an unstable patient from ICU to CT unit, unless some therapeutic intervention is planned. In such patients, bedside bronchoscopy should be performed initially.

Bronchoscopy

The ideal time for bronchoscopy is controversial; however, general consensus is to perform it early in rapidly deteriorating patients, delayed bronchoscopy, that is within 24–48 hours of admission can be done in stable patients. Rigid bronchoscopy is ideally recommended in massive hemoptysis for better suctioning and maintenance of airway. Flexible bronchoscopy [fiberoptic bronchoscopy (FOB)] is a very friendly tool for pulmonologist that can be done bedside without the use of general anesthesia. Overall accuracy in localizing the site of bleeding is 10–50%. FOB can reach up to the upper lobe and lesions located distal up to the sixth bronchial generation. The disadvantage of FOB is nonvisualization and clogging of channel by blood clots. Due to limitations with both flexible and rigid bronchoscopy, they can be combined to achieve maximum bleeding control and evaluation.

In case of blood clot seen in a segment, it is advisable not to remove it as it may restart massive hemoptysis.

Various therapeutic measures can be done with FOB to control bleeding:
- Lavage with 4°C cold saline in the involved lung.
- Lavage with cold saline up to 1,000 mL in 50 mL aliquots at the bleeding site.
- Administration of topical hemostatic agents like diluted epinephrine (1:20,000) or thrombin fibrinogen. Topical epinephrine should be used with caution as it can precipitate tachyarrhythmias and accelerate hypertension. Newer agents like antidiuretic hormone (ADH) derivatives like ornipressin have been successfully used.

Bronchoscopy-guided topical hemostatic tamponade (THT): Oxidized regenerated cellulose mesh, a sterile knitted fabric is used. It saturates in contact with blood and swells up to form a brownish gelatinous mass clot and can immediately stop bleeding with success rate of up to 98%.

In life-threatening hemoptysis, endobronchial tamponade using balloon catheter (4 Fr 100 cm Fogarty balloon catheter) has a good success rate to prevent aspiration to the contralateral normal lung and preserve gas exchange, they can be inserted through working channel of FOB. A double-lumen balloon catheter with detachable valve at proximal end can be passed through working channel of bronchoscope and can leave the catheter in bronchus by removing detachable valve. They can be used as bridge therapy before embolization and surgery. Disadvantages are that they can cause ischemic mucosal injury and postobstructive pneumonia.

Endobronchial airway blockade (silicone spigot) can be placed with the help of flexible bronchoscope to control bleeding and stabilize the patient before embolization or surgery.

Endobronchial biocompatible glue N-butyl cyanoacrylate which has prothrombin activity is commonly used in mild hemoptysis. It is injected into the bleeding airway through a catheter via flexible bronchoscope. It solidifies on contact with humidity.

Neodymium-doped yttrium aluminum garnet (Nd:YAG) or argon plasma coagulation (APC) is also used in tumors in which chemotherapy and radiotherapy have been exhausted with success rate up to 60%. APC is a noncontact electrocoagulation tool.

SPECIFIC MEDICAL THERAPY

On the basis of history, physical and laboratory examination, specific therapy should be started to correct the cause because invasive therapeutic interventions do not help to control bleeding secondary to coagulopathies, immunologically mediated disorder like Goodpasture's syndrome. Specific therapies like antibiotics, correction of coagulopathies with platelet, fresh frozen plasma (FFP), cryoprecipitates, blood transfusion, steroids, immunosuppressive therapies or plasmapheresis are mandatory to control the precipitating factor. Vitamin K supplements and tranexamic acid are also used to control bleeding. IV vasopressin has also been used but caution is advised in patients with coexistent coronary artery disease or hypertension. Vasoconstriction of the bronchial artery may also hamper effective bronchial artery embolization (BAE) by obscuring the site of bleeding, leading to difficulties in cannulation of the artery. Recombinant activated factor VII (rFVIIa) has been used in hemoptysis with community-acquired pneumonia. Danazol or gonadotropin-releasing hormone (GnRH) has been used in catamenial hemoptysis. Systemic antifungal agents have been tried in the management of hemoptysis related to mycetoma, but results are not satisfactory. However, percutaneous or bronchoscopic direct instillation of these drugs in cavity are having promising results. This technique is useful in cases bleeding after failed BAE and in those who are not fit for surgery. Radiation therapy has been used in vascular tumor or mycetoma-related massive hemoptysis by necrosis of feeding vessel and vascular thrombosis due to perivascular edema.

BRONCHIAL ARTERY EMBOLIZATION

This procedure was first reported by Remy and colleagues in 1973 and has been found very useful in massive hemoptysis. Once the bleeding bronchial artery is identified and cannulated, particles of polyvinyl alcohol foam, isobutyl-2-cyanoacrylate, Gianturco steel coils or absorbable gelatin pledgets are infused into the artery. The immediate success rate is 64–100%, although the recurrent nonmassive bleeding has been reported in 16–46% of patients. 13% technical failure are reported and caused by nonbronchial artery collaterals from systemic arteries like internal mammary, subclavian, intercostal, and phrenic arteries. Complications of BAE include vessel perforation, intimal tears, chest pain, pyrexia, hemoptysis, systemic embolization, and neurological complication. When anterior spinal artery is identified as originating from bronchial artery, embolization should be avoided to prevent infarction and paraparesis. With newer coaxial microcatheter, selective catheterization and embolization of bronchial artery can be achieved and occlusion of anterior spinal artery can be avoided.

Bronchial artery embolization is time-buying procedure so definitive diagnosis and definitive treatment should be given. In AVM, BAE is the definitive treatment. In case of normal bronchial artery angiography, pulmonary angiogram should be obtained to investigate pulmonary circulation.

SURGICAL MANAGEMENT

With the development of different endobronchial tamponade and BAE techniques and higher success rates, practice of thoracic surgery has decreased. Recently however surgical resection is indicated when BAE is unavailable or the bleeding is unlikely to be controlled by embolization. It remains the treatment of choice for the management of life-threatening hemoptysis due to a leaking aortic aneurysm, hydatid cyst, iatrogenic pulmonary rupture, chest injuries, bronchial adenoma, selected case of AVMs, or hemoptysis related to mycetoma-resistant to other treatments. Surgery is considered the treatment of choice for the localized lesions. Surgical

Flowchart 1: Algorithm for management of massive hemoptysis.

mortality ranges from 1% to 50% in different series depending upon surgical criteria. Surgery is contraindicated in patients with inadequate respiratory reserve or those with inoperable lung cancer due to direct thoracic spread, inability to lateralize the bleeding site, diffuse disease like vasculitis, multiple AVMs, cystic fibrosis. In patients with poor respiratory reserve or extensive pleural adhesions, physiological lung exclusion strategy has been used. Here the bronchus and pulmonary artery to the involved lobe or segment are surgically ligated and the pulmonary veins left intact and without lung resection.

RADIATION THERAPY

It has been used in hemoptysis due to vascular tumor or mycetoma. It acts by inducing vascular necrosis of feeding vessel or vascular thrombosis due to perivascular edema.

SUMMARY

Due to unpredictable course of massive hemoptysis, quick resuscitation, airway protection and correction of coagulopathy are required. Timely confirmation of diagnosis by history, physical examination and investigations and interventions and appropriate management can save the patient. Early bronchoscopy is recommended. BAE is now treatment of choice in massive hemoptysis where conservative treatment fails. Surgical resection is for selective conditions where bleeding site is localized and patient is fit for surgery.

Algorithm for management of massive hemoptysis has been shown in **Flowchart 1**.

Hemorrhoids

Ashok Puranik

INTRODUCTION

Hemorrhoidal disease is one of the most chronic diseases in the history of mankind. Ancient texts dates back to Babylonian, Egyptian, Greek, and Hebrew cultures. Although very few people have died after hemorrhoids, many people wish they had. It is hoped this chapter will guide the practitioners in more humane approach to treat hemorrhoidal disease patients.

ETIOLOGY AND RELATED ANATOMY

Hemorrhoids are submucosal cushions containing venules, arterioles, and smooth muscle fibers in the anal canal. These cushions are primarily located at right anterolateral (11 o'clock), right posterolateral (7 o'clock), and left lateral (3 o'clock) positions. Hemorrhoids are thought to have a role in anal continence and they aid in complete closure of anal canal at rest.

Hemorrhoidal disease occurs as a result of abnormality in the constituents of these cushions leading to bleeding which may or may not be associated with the prolapse of the hemorrhoidal tissue. This can occur as a result of excessive strain, chronic constipation due to low-fiber diet and increased internal anal sphincter tone.

CLASSIFICATION OF HEMORRHOIDS

External Hemorrhoids

External hemorrhoids are located distal to dentate line and are covered by anoderm and because anoderm is highly innervated, the thrombosis of external hemorrhoids can be extremely painful. So, external hemorrhoids should not be ligated or excised without adequate anesthesia. Skin tag at anal verge often represents the thrombosed, fibrotic external hemorrhoids. Skin tag can cause itching and difficulty in maintaining hygiene. Treatment of external hemorrhoids and skin tag is only indicated for symptomatic relief.

Internal Hemorrhoids

Internal hemorrhoids are located proximal to the dentate line and are covered by insensate anorectal mucosa. Internal hemorrhoids can bleed and prolapse but are rarely painful. They can become painful if severe thrombosis and necrosis occurs which is usually related to severe prolapse, incarceration, and strangulation.

The standard classification of internal hemorrhoids is as follows:
Grade 1: Bleeding only
Grade 2: Prolapse with spontaneous reduction
Grade 3: Prolapse requiring manual reduction
Grade 4: Prolapsed and cannot be reduced (are at high risk for strangulation).

Combined Internal and External Hemorrhoids

They are located at the dentate line and have features of both external and internal hemorrhoids. Hemorrhoidectomy is often needed for this type of hemorrhoids.

CLINICAL FEATURES

Bleeding and protrusion are the most important symptoms of hemorrhoids. Bleeding from hemorrhoids is typically bright red either on toilet paper or actually into the commode after bowel moments, this is usually painless. If it is painful then most of the time it is associated with fissure-in-ano. Although bleeding is the most common symptom, anemia is rare in these patients.

EXAMINATION

The preferred position for examination is left lateral position with knees drawn up toward the chest as high as possible. This approach allows patient relative comfort and the ability to clearly inspect the perineal skin, perform digital rectal examination (DRE) unless they are thrombosed. On proctoscopy, hemorrhoids are seen as masses prolapsing into the scope.

Treatment

Medical Management/Conservative Management

Bleeding from Grades 1 and 2 often improve by giving bulk laxatives like isabgol (Psyllium), stool softeners, and avoidance of straining. It is very important to increase the daily water intake along with fibers. Failure of conservative management is an indication for some surgical intervention.

Sclerotherapy

It was first advocated by Mitchell in 1871. The principal of sclerotherapy is scaring of submucosa which results in atrophy and fixation of the hemorrhoidal complex to the wall of the anal canal. Variety of solutions are available like 5% phenol, sodium morrhuate, sodium tetradecyl sulphate (STD). The procedure is performed in patient with left lateral decubitus position. An anoscope is inserted to identify symptomatic hemorrhoids then 1-2 mL of sclerosant is injected into the submucosal plane using 25 gauge spinal needle. Before injection, syringe should be aspirated to avoid intravascular injection. Accidental injection into prostate in male is very painful as it causes chemical prostatitis. Not more than two hemorrhoids should be injected in one sitting to avoid anal stenosis.

Rubber Band Ligation

Barron was the first to describe hemorrhoidal banding using rubber band in 1963. It is often applied in patients with Grade 2 and 3 hemorrhoids. Mucosa over the hemorrhoids 1-2 cm above the dentate line is grasped and pulled into the rubber band applicator. The procedure is usually well tolerated if the band is applied above dentate line. It is important to ask the patient if they experience any pain during placement of the bander before deployment of the band. If they have pain before deployment of band, it will worsen after banding. Other complications of banding include urinary retention, infection, and bleeding. Urinary retention occurs in nearly 1% of patients. Necrotising infection is an uncommon but life-threatening complication. Severe pain, fever, and urinary retention are early signs of infection and should prompt immediate evaluation of the anal canal under anesthesia. Treatment includes debridement of necrotic tissue, drainage of associated abscess, and broad spectrum antibiotics. Bleeding may occur 7-10 days after banding when ligated pedicle necrosis and sloughs. Bleeding is usually self-limiting but persisted bleeding may require examination under anesthesia and outer ligation of pedicle.

Infrared Coagulation and Ultroid (Direct Current) Therapy

Infrared coagulation technique uses tungsten halogen lamp that generates heat for 1.5 seconds leading to destruction of mucosa and submucosal hemorrhoids. Ultroid uses direct current and is applied for 10 minutes over hemorrhoidal complex.

Excisional Hemorrhoidectomy

The decision for excisional hemorrhoidectomy requires mutual decision by the physician and patient. Physician must explain that medical and nonexcisional options are either not appropriate or law failed. The usual clinical symptoms that require surgical excision are frequent prolapse and anal seepage or hemorrhoids making anal hygiene difficult to maintain.

Milligan and Morgan Hemorrhoidectomy (Open Hemorrhoidectomy)

It was originally described in 1973 and is widely practiced in Europe. In this procedure, the entire enlarged hemorrhoidal complex is excised with ligation of the vascular pedicle and preservation of the intervening anoderm. While dissecting, internal anal sphincter should be brushed away to preserve them. Wound is left open and allowed to heal by secondary intention.

Ferguson Hemorrhoidectomy (Closed Hemorrhoidectomy)

This technique was proposed as an alternative to open hemorrhoidectomy as open hemorrhoidectomy has prolonged discomfort and morbidity. In this technique, an hour glass-shaped excision of internal and external hemorrhoids is done with ligation of the vascular pedicle. The center of the hour glass is anoderm. After excision, wound is closed by absorbable suture. It is crucial to identify the internal and external anal sphincter and preserve them. In this technique, all the primary hemorrhoids can be removed in single sitting by this technique, although care should be taken to avoid resecting a large area of perianal skin to avoid postop anal stenosis.

Whitehead Hemorrhoidectomy

This technique was devised in 1982 to excise internal hemorrhoids circumferentially and relocate the prolapsed dentate line which is often a component of prolapsed hemorrhoids. In this technique, the enlarged internal hemorrhoids are excised circumferentially just proximal to the dentate line and after excision the rectal mucosa is advanced and sutured to dentate line. But this technique has been abandoned by most surgeons because of its complications like anal stenosis and mucosal ectropion (Whitehead's deformity).

Procedure for Prolapsed Anal Hemorrhoids or Stapled Hemorrhoidectomy

The term PPH has largely replaced the term SH because in this procedure, hemorrhoid tissue is not excised instead the redundant mucosa is fixed above the dentate line. In this procedure, a short segment of rectal mucosa proximal to dentate line is removed circumferentially using circular stapler. This causes the ligation of feeding venules of hemorrhoid plexus along with fixation of redundant mucosa higher in anal canal. But this technique is only appropriate for internal hemorrhoids and cannot be used for external or combined hemorrhoids.

Complications of Hemorrhoidectomy

Postoperative pain is the most common complication following hemorrhoidectomy. It is usually managed by oral/IV narcotics, nonsteroidal anti-inflammatory drugs (NSAIDs), muscle relaxants, topical analgesics, and comfort measures like sitz bath.

Urinary retention is another common complication after hemorrhoidectomy and occurs in 10–50% of patients. The incidence can be reduced by minimizing the intraoperative and perioperative IV fluids and providing adequate analgesics.

Fecal impaction is also a complication of postoperative pain which can be minimized by adequate analgesia and liberal use of laxatives.

Bleeding is also a common complication after hemorrhoidectomy. Small amount of blood with stool is suspected but massive bleed requires urgent examination and pedicle ligation under anesthesia in operation theater (OT). Bleeding can occur after 7–10 days when necrotic mucosa overlying the vascular pedicle sloughs, although some of the patients can be safely observed but if the bleeding is massive may require examination and suture ligation of vessel on OT.

Infection is a rare complication after hemorrhoidectomy but necrotizing soft tissue infection mostly in immunocompromised individuals can be devastating. Severe pain, fever, and urinary retention are the early signs of such infection. In this condition, emergency examination and debridement should be done under anesthesia. Long-term complications include anal stenosis and ectropion (after Whitehead's hemorrhoidectomy).

CHAPTER 52

Headache

Alireza Baratloo

INTRODUCTION

Headache is one of the most prevalent patients' complaints, whether as chief or ancillary, in emergency departments (ED), consist of millions of ED yearly visits. Despite of uncertainty and major knowledge gaps, it was estimated that percentage of the adult population with an active headache disorder is almost 50% in general, with minor difference in various societies. It is a functionally disabling disorder leading to considerable years living with disability (YLDS), and has been experienced at least once by almost everyone. Therefore, it has taken into consideration by World Health Organization (WHO) as a public-health priority, in 2000. Although most of the cases are benign in nature, but needs some special attention regarding various aspects including primary pain management, diagnostic approach, disposition, and outpatient follow-up.

ETIOLOGY/CAUSES

When it comes to etiology, most acceptable categorization for headache is primary versus secondary causes, based on presence or absence of a pathologic structure justifying the symptoms. The first recorded classification system was published by "Aretaeus," the ancient Greek physician, active during 1st century CE. Today, the third edition of the international classification of headache disorders is available that has been released by Classification Committee of International Headache Society (HIS) in 2018 (was published in 2013 in a beta version ahead of the final version) showed in **Table 1**. More than 200 types of headaches have been defined till now, so for better understanding, WHO ICD-10NA and IHS ICHD-II codes have been defined in this regard which is available via the link: http://www.ihs-klassifikation.de/en/02_klassifikation/00.00.00_icd10table.html.

PATHOPHYSIOLOGY OF THE CONDITION

The brain parenchyma has no pain receptors, so is not sensitive to pain itself. But some other components, adjunct to it such as meninges, blood vessels, skin, etc. has nociceptors that could be stimulated from traction to or irritation by. It usually defines the pathophysiology of secondary type headache. But, unlike secondary causes, the pathophysiology of primary headache disorders is not well understood and proposed theories were changed during the

Table 1: The international classification of headache disorders, 3rd edition.

Part 1: The primary headaches
Migraine
Tension-type headache (TTH)
Trigeminal autonomic cephalalgias (TACs)
Other primary headache disorders
Part 2: The secondary headaches
Headache attributed to trauma or injury to the head and/or neck
Headache attributed to cranial or cervical vascular disorder
Headache attributed to nonvascular intracranial disorder
Headache attributed to a substance or its withdrawal
Headache attributed to infection
Headache attributed to disorder of homoeostasis
Headache or facial pain attributed to disorder of the cranium, neck, eyes, ears, nose, sinuses, teeth, mouth or other facial or cervical structure
Headache attributed to psychiatric disorder
Part 3: Painful cranial neuropathies, other facial pains, and other headaches
Painful lesions of the cranial nerves and other facial pain
Other headache disorders

time. For example, it was long assumed that some vascular involvement is explaining the migraine pathophysiology. This vascular theory, which was settled and progressed in the 20th century, is no longer accepted. It seems that the literatures are yet nonconclusive in this era and more studies are still required to understanding the pathophysiology of primary headache disorders.

CLINICAL PRESENTATION

Headache is the sensation of pain anywhere in the region of the head or neck. Depending on the type, it could present with various manifestations. The presentation process is so important for the in-charge physicians. Some may present with new onset rapid progressive headache raise the attention to critically important underlying cause; on the other hand, some present with chronic pain not responded to their regular treatment. The details were discussed in the following sections.

RED FLAGS

Although most of headaches are benign, but there are still some life-threatening causes. Red flags are highly important points that careful attention to them by rapid reviewing in dealing with each patient, help the physician to differentiate the serious cause require further emergent investigations. Overall, complaining of first or worst headache, progressively worsening headache, headache triggered by exertion or started while engaged in sexual intercourse or after a recent traumatic event, presence of focal neurological findings or papilledema on physical examination, and any alteration in mental status warrant further work up in ED. To remember of the red flags for recognizing a secondary type headache, the American Headache Society recommends using of "*SSNOOP*" mnemonic abbreviated for the items below:

- *S*ystemic symptoms (fever or weight loss)
- *S*ystemic disease [human immunodeficiency viruses (HIV) infection, malignancy]
- *N*eurologic symptoms or signs
- *O*nset sudden (thunderclap headache)
- *O*nset after age 40 years
- *P*revious headache history (first, worst or different headache).

EVALUATION (A: HISTORY; B: PHYSICAL EXAMINATION)

As obviate from the mentioned points in previous section, all the red flags were assessed through a detailed history taking and focused physical examination.

For a confident history taking, patient should ask for 10 important points about the pain including location, pattern and onset, activity at the onset (during marked exertion or coitus), characteristics (throbbing, steady, or tension), exacerbating or alleviating factors, history of trauma, risk factors (HIV or another immunocompromised state), prior history of headache, intensity, and associated symptoms (blurred vision, fever, nausea, vomiting, or syncope).

Physical examination also including of general appearance assessment, checking the vital signs, head and neck evaluation (acute red eye, poorly reactive, or nonreactive pupils, or third nerve palsy), and precise neurological examination (even the least change in mental status, any focal neurologic deficit or alteration in cerebellar tests). Ophthalmoscopy is also necessary for demonstrating or ruling out the possible loss of venous spontaneous pulsation or presence of papilledema. Evaluation of patient with Headache is summarized in **Flowchart 1.**

INTERPRETATION OF FINDING

It is expected that the primary evaluations reveal some findings that their interpretation leads to suggesting appropriate differential diagnosis which will be the basis for the next steps of patient evaluation process and proper decision-making in fact. Those life-threating diagnoses which need treatment interactions right after confirming the diagnosis or even before are called as critical diagnosis. Subarachnoid hemorrhage, carbon monoxide (CO) poisoning, temporal arthritis, meningitis or encephalitis are among the most important critical diagnosis of a patient presenting with headache. Space occupying lesions including brain abscess and hemorrhagic events, cerebral vein thrombosis (CVT), glaucoma, hypertensive crisis, and mountain sickness are also considered as emergent diagnosis.

INVESTIGATIONS

Considering the suggested differential diagnosis, the patient may undergo some para-clinical procedures including laboratory and/or imaging. Complete blood count (CBC), and

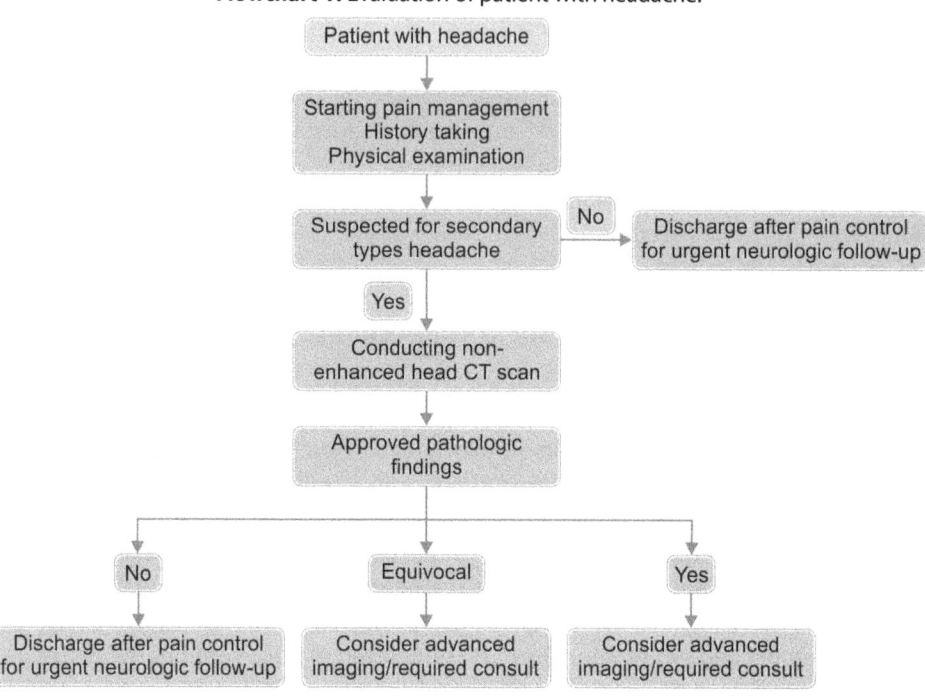

Flowchart 1: Evaluation of patient with headache.

a coagulation profile by all required laboratory tests. Cerebrospinal fluid (CSF) analysis in those with impression of meningitis/encephalitis following lumbar puncture (LP) and erythrocyte sedimentation rate (ESR) in those suspected as giant cell arteritis are also required. Requesting for common biochemical profile is usually unnecessary.

Major parts of the patients, suspected for secondary causes almost always need to perform a nonenhanced head computed tomography (CT) scan as soon as possible. Almost all the hemorrhagic causes are diagnosed by this imaging. It also revealed some findings pointing to other intracranial lesions such as brain abscess or tumors, that may require contrast enhanced magnetic resonance imaging (MRI) in next step.

Advanced imaging techniques including magnetic resonance angiography (MRA) and magnetic resonance venography (MRV) also may necessitate in suspicion of vascular disorders including intracranial aneurysm and CVT, respectively.

TREATMENT

Along with diagnostic approach, pain management is always necessary in all patients. Since benign primary disorders are the most frequent diagnosis, that is the only intervention in most cases as well. There are frequent guidelines for management of acute headaches that generally recommended several different agents. Intravenous (IV) acetaminophen, nonsteroidal anti-inflammatory drugs (NSAIDs), and opioids are common first choice. Corticosteroids,

Table 2: Common pain killer agents used for parenteral administration in emergency department (data were extracted from Medscape).

Agent	Dosage
Acetaminophen	• <50 kg: 12.5 mg/kg IV q4hr or 15 mg/kg IV q6hr; not to exceed 750 mg/dose or 3.75 g/day infuse IV over at least 15 minutes • ≥50 kg: 650 mg IV q4hr or 1,000 mg IV q6hr; not to exceed 4 g/day infuse IV over at least 15 minutes
Ketorolac	• IV: 30 mg as single dose or 30 mg q6hr; not to exceed 120 mg/day • IM: 60 mg as single dose or 30 mg q6hr; not to exceed 120 mg/day
Ibuprofen	• 400–800 mg IV infused over 30 minutes q6hr PRN; not to exceed 4,200 mg/day
Morphine	• SC/IM (opioid-naïve patients): 5–10 mg q4hr PRN; dose range, 5–20 mg • IV (opioid-naïve patients): 2.5–5 mg q3–4hr PRN, infused over 4–5 minutes; dose range, 4–10 mg

(IM: intramuscular; IV: intravenous; SC: subcutaneous)

magnesium sulfate, caffeine, ergotamine, and sumatriptan may also be required. Serotonin antagonist (granisetron), intranasal lidocaine, and high-flow oxygen were also studied in this regard but have reported conflicting results. There is an interest about using IV ketamine as a treatment option for acute pain but does not provide significant relief. Despite huge number of randomized clinical trials (RCTs), there is not an agreement on a single approved guideline. Overall, it is likely that investigators have tried to reduce using opioids and replace them by nonopioid agents that assumed have less side effects, but opioids administration remains still prevalent in the ED. **Table 2** shows the dosage of some more frequent agents used as parenteral pain killer in ED. More detailed information is available at https://reference.medscape.com/drugs/pain-management.

All secondary type headaches require specific intervention depending on the exact diagnosis, whether surgical or nonsurgical. Surgical interventions are usually conducted in cases of intracranial hemorrhagic insults, brain mass, and abscess. Nonsurgical treatments are also include antibiotic therapy in meningitis, antiviral therapy in encephalitis, corticosteroid in temporal arteritis, oxygen therapy in CO poisoning, topical treatment to lower intraocular pressure (IOP) in glaucoma, and anticoagulation in CVT (even hemorrhagic ones).

SUMMARY

In dealing with a patient complaining of headache, ruling out the critical and emergent diagnosis in ED is far more important than ruling in an exact benign diagnosis. Therefore, the physician should make his/her effort in this regard. Pain management should be considered for all types of headaches whether primary or secondary. Further investigation in ED should also be considered for those suspected for secondary types based on history and physical examination findings.

CHAPTER 53

Hiccups

Hatinderjeet Singh Sethi, Nimarpreet Kaur

INTRODUCTION

Hiccups as a symptom is very commonly seen in clinical practice and is usually a transient condition affecting almost all people in their lifetime. Intractable hiccups and complications from hiccups are rarely seen.

What are Hiccups?

Hiccups are sudden inspiratory activities generated due to contraction of intercostal muscles and diaphragm; contractions are intermittent, involuntary, and spasmodic in nature with the frequency of 5–50/minutes.

On the basis of duration, hiccups can be divided into three groups:
1. A "hiccup bout" is an episode of hiccups lasting up to 48 hours
2. "Persistent hiccups" are hiccups that continue longer than 48 hours and up to 1 month
3. "Intractable hiccups" are hiccups that continue longer than 1 month.

EPIDEMIOLOGY

The precise epidemiology of hiccups, including severe intractable hiccups, is uncertain in the general population as well as the palliative care population.

Most people have experienced hiccups at some point in their life, and these hiccups are generally self-limited. Hiccups can, however, become chronic and persistent in rare cases.

Hiccups may be associated with comorbid conditions:
- Vascular
- Chronic kidney disease (CKD)
- Postoperative
- Central nervous system (CNS) disease
- Duodenal ulcer
- Reflux esophagitis
- Advanced cancer

Hiccups can cause significant adverse effects which include:
- Dehydration
- Malnutrition
- Fatigue

- Weight loss
- Insomnia
- Nervous stress
- Poor quality of life.

PATHOPHYSIOLOGY

The exact mechanism which provokes the hiccups including severe intractable hiccups, remain unclear. In majority of the patients, hiccups involve unilateral contraction of the left hemidiaphragm.

Several neural pathways make up the hiccup reflex:
- Gamma-aminobutyric acid (GABA) appears to be the most important mediator for neural connections in the hiccup reflex arc.
- Other mediators may include dopaminergic, muscarinic, and serotonergic pathways (i.e. 5-HT1A receptors).

ETIOLOGY

Common and benign causes of hiccups are overeating, carbonated drinks, stress emotional changes, spicy, and alcohol ingestion. Intractable hiccups may reflect serious underlying disease, such as an infection (e.g. meningitis, encephalitis) or a structural lesion (e.g. intracranial neoplasm, hydrocephalus). Potential causes of persistent and intractable hiccups are given in **Box 1**.

Box 1: Causes of persistent and intractable hiccups.

Vascular:
Ischemic/hemorrhagic stroke, arteriovenous (AV) malformations, temporal arteritis
Infections:
Encephalitis, meningitis, brain abscess, neurosyphilis, subphrenic abscess
Structural:
Head trauma, intracranial neoplasms, brainstem neoplasms, multiple sclerosis, syringomyelia, hydrocephalus
Vagus and phrenic nerve irritation:
Goiter, pharyngitis, laryngitis, hair or foreign body irritation of tympanic membrane, neck cyst or other tumor
Gastrointestinal disorders:
Gastric distention, gastritis, peptic ulcer disease, pancreatitis, pancreatic cancer, gastric carcinoma, abdominal abscesses, gallbladder disease, inflammatory bowel disease, hepatitis, aerophagia, esophageal distention, esophagitis, bowel obstruction
Cardiovascular disorders:
Myocardial infarction, pericarditis
Thoracic disorders:
Enlarged lymph nodes secondary to infection or neoplasm, pneumonia, empyema, bronchitis, asthma, pleuritis, aortic aneurysm, mediastinitis, mediastinal tumors, chest trauma, pulmonary embolism
Toxic and metabolic:
DM, alcohol, hypocalcemia, hyponatremia, herpes zoster, hypocapnia, tuberculosis, malaria, uremia
Postoperative drugs:
Alpha-methyldopa, short-acting barbiturates, diazepam, dexamethasone
Psychogenic:
Anorexia nervosa, schizophrenia, stress, malingering, conversion reaction

EVALUATION

Hiccup bouts are common and most of the individuals do not need thorough evaluation or medical attention. While intractable hiccups required thorough evaluation to ascertain the underlying causes.

The history should include:
- Severity and duration of hiccups
- Any associated medical conditions and previous surgery
- Drug abuse or alcohol intake
- A complete list of medications
- The persistence of hiccups during sleep suggests an organic rather than psychogenic etiology.

In the physical examination:
- Examination of external auditory canals to rule out infection or foreign body which may be a potential irritant of tympanic membranes
- A detailed head and neck examination is important to exclude an enlarged thyroid and lymphadenopathy
- Neurological examination (including cranial nerve assessment)
- Auscultation of the chest
- Per abdominal examination to palpate for any mass lesions.

LABORATORY TESTS

To obtain in patients with persistent or intractable hiccups include:
- Complete blood count
- Renal function test (RFT)
- Liver function test (LFT)
- Serum electrolytes
- Serum calcium
- Serum amylase/lipase
- Electrocardiography (ECG)
- Radiological investigations
- X-ray chest
- Contrast-enhanced computed tomography (CECT).

A chest radiograph or computed tomography (CT) scan is helpful to detect pulmonary and mediastinal abnormalities irritating the vagal or phrenic nerves or the diaphragm in patients presenting with dyspnea. Patient with esophageal symptoms, dysphagia should undergo upper gastrointestinal (GI) endoscopy for evaluation to find out esophagitis stricture or malignancy.

In patients with advanced malignancy, the cause of intractable hiccups is often multifactorial, and an exhaustive evaluation is required.

TREATMENT

Most of the patients' hiccups are self-limiting and not required any treatment. Treatment of underlying illness is required if it is due to any medical illness.

Treatment of intractable hiccups requires pharmacological or nonpharmacological management for persistent or intractable hiccups.

1. If a specific pathology is found to be potentially causing the hiccups, the choice of treatment should be directed toward treating the illness. As an example, treatment with a proton-pump inhibitor or an H_2 blocker should be given if gastroesophageal reflux disease (GERD) is a likely cause.
2. If the cause is idiopathic, empiric therapy with physical maneuvers is first-line treatment. These maneuvers are easy to perform and have a low risk of complications.
3. Physical maneuvers: Common maneuvers are suggested—breath holding, Valsalva maneuver sipping cold water, gargling with water, swallowing a teaspoon of dry sugar, compression over the eyeballs, pulling knees to chest, leaning forward to compress the chest.

Pharmacologic Therapy

Drug therapy should be reserved for treatment of hiccups when physical maneuvers have failed.

If hiccups subside following treatment, drug treatment can usually be stopped the day after cessation of hiccups. Most drug treatments can be used for 7–10 days. If hiccups persist, it is reasonable to consider another pharmacologic or nonpharmacologic treatment option.

Chlorpromazine

Chlorpromazine is centrally acting dopamine, acts by antagonism in the hypothalamus, remained the drug of choice for many years, and is the only medication approved for hiccups by the US Food and Drug Administration. Intravenous administration may be more effective, although the drug must be infused in 500–1,000 mL saline with the patient in the supine position to avoid hypotension, the lower dosing for hiccups is generally well-tolerated. Generally, it is not recommended as first drug of choice due to serious side effects, also contraindicated in older people.

Metoclopramide

Metoclopramide also has central dopamine antagonism but slightly weaker than chlorpromazine. The usual oral dose is 10 mg three or four times daily for up to 7–10 days. Metoclopramide is also associated with tardive dyskinesia, especially at high doses and with chronic use.

Other Drugs

Other drugs effective in hiccups are:
- Baclofen
- Haloperidol

- Anticonvulsants
- Nifedipine
- Methylphenidate
- Midazolam
- Lidocaine
- Antidepressants (e.g. amitriptyline)
- Antiarrhythmic drugs (e.g. quinidine)
- Olanzapine
- Amantadine
- Oral viscous lidocaine (2%) solution.

Surgery

Surgical approach, including phrenic nerve crushing or blocking with a local anesthetic, may be successful in refractory cases.

CHAPTER 54

Hyperventilation

Bhawana Sharma

INTRODUCTION

Hyperventilation is one of the common presentations in clinical medicine which always troubles family physician, emergency physician, respiratory physician, cardiologist, psychiatrist, neurologist, and intensivist. Main complaint of patient is shortness of breath. Dizziness, weakness, chest pain, tingling numbness are other associated features of hyperventilation. Patient breathing is more quickly but shallow. High index of suspicion is required for diagnosis along with reassurance and management of anxiety is the key for management.

DEFINITION

Ventilation in excess of metabolic requirements (CO_2 production) leading to a reduction in PCO_2. There is increased alveolar ventilation and a drop in PCO_2 to approximately 20 mm Hg.

In some patients, hyperventilation occurs frequently and they seek medical advice regularly, frequent occurrence of this condition termed as hyperventilation syndrome.

Anxiety and panic are associated with hyperventilation but these are not synonymous with hyperventilation.

CAUSE AND PHYSIOLOGICAL EFFECTS OF HYPERVENTILATION

Anxiety, fear, anger, and stress are the triggering factors in most of the patients, though the reason behind this is unclear, but possible theory of adrenergic drive in response to flight of fight reaction works behind the rapid respiration.

Hypocapnia and respiratory alkalosis are the important physiological changes during hyperventilation and produce variety of signs and symptoms. Patient may present with wheezing, bronchoconstriction. Pre-existing asthma can be worse during this period.

Careful history should be obtained to rule out other causes of hyperventilation like fever, left ventricular failure, and pulmonary emboli. In this chapter, discussion is limited to hyperventilation due to anxiety and stress.

SYMPTOMS OF HYPERVENTILATION

Symptoms can be so diverse that patients usually present to a variety of health care provider including emergency physicians, neurologist, respiratory physicians, cardiologists,

Table 1: Symptoms of hyperventilation.

Respiratory	Cardiac	Neurological	Gastrointestinal	General
Shortness of breath	Palpitation	Dizziness	Nausea	Spasm, cold hand and feet, tremors in hand, tingling in fingers
Chest tightness	Tachycardia	Faintness	Abdominal pain	
Rapid and shallow breathing	Chest pain (atypical)	Headache		
		Blurred vision		Anxiety, stress
				Fatigue, lethargy, insomnia

psychiatrists or psychologists. Onset of chest pain, dyspnea, paresthesia or altered sensorium can be alarming signs. Various symptoms are described in **Table 1**.

DIAGNOSIS

- High index of suspicion is required because increased minute ventilation can be difficult to detect on physical examination.
- Arterial blood gas (ABG)—compensated respiratory alkalosis with a near normal pH, low $PaCO_2$, and low calculated bicarbonates are necessary to confirm the diagnosis of chronic hyperventilation.

Other causes of respiratory alkalosis—mild asthma and systemic illnesses such as diabetic ketoacidosis can present with respiratory symptoms associated with acute hyperventilation.

At first, evaluate the serious causes for acute hyperventilation like acute myocardial infarction, pneumothorax, and pulmonary embolism. Diagnosis of hyperventilation syndrome must be ascertain by excluding above causes, otherwise adverse event may occur.

Once hyperventilation syndrome is established a sustained 10% increase in alveolar ventilation and is enough to perpetuate hypocapnia. This increase can be accomplished with subtle changes in the respiratory patterns, such as occasional sigh breaths or yawning two to three times per minute.

TREATMENT

- Reassurance and frank discussion
- Identify and eliminate habits that perpetuate hypocapnia (such as frequent yawning or sigh breathing can be helpful)
- Breathing exercises and diaphragmatic retraining may be beneficial in some patients
- In cases with palpitations or tremors—beta-blockers may be helpful
- Pharmacological approach for underlying anxiety by benzodiazepines, antidepressant, and cognitive behavioral therapy
- There are very less well-controlled treatment studies on hyperventilation and hyperventilation syndrome due to its diverse features and lack of a universally accepted diagnostic process

- Considerable time is spent in identifying initiating factors, excluding alternative diagnosis, and discussing the patient's concern and fears.

SUMMARY

Hyperventilation is rapid and shallow breathing episode usually triggered by anxiety, stress anger, leading to reduction in pCO_2. Patient presents with variety of symptoms. Frequent occurrence of hyperventilation is known as hyperventilation syndrome. Diagnosis is by exclusion. Management includes reassurance, breathing exercise, pharmacological therapy for anxiety.

CHAPTER 55
Inflight Medical Problems

Rajeev Kapur

INTRODUCTION

Air travel has made it possible to travel longer distances in shorter times. Economic development has enabled people from different socioeconomic strata to travel by air. Some of them have pre-existing diseases and conditions that may get aggravated while flying.

Human beings were designed by nature to live on ground and not fly in the air. Air travel has challenges in the form of *a drop in atmospheric pressure, low oxygen, low temperature, vibration, and unusual motion environment* due to atmospheric turbulence and the movements of aircraft at high speeds. Pressurization and the design of the aircraft reduce these challenges considerably, but not completely. Most civil airliners restrict the cabin altitude to 5,000–7,000 feet above earth even when the aircraft is flying at 33,000 feet atmospheric altitude. However, the medical problems that exist in general population are often exacerbated during air travel due to being confined to a small space with restricted mobility, dry cabin air, and travel across the time zones.

Though precise data on incidence of inflight medical emergencies is not available or limited, the common medical symptoms encountered are chest pain, breathlessness, dizziness, giddiness, fainting, loss of consciousness, fits (seizures), vomiting, loose motions and minor cuts/wounds, high blood pressure, acute pain abdomen, high blood pressure, low or high blood sugar, urinary retention due to prostate enlargement, bleeding per vaginal (PV) due to menorrhagia or abortion. Rarely, childbirth may occur on board. The range is from trivial to serious events like cerebral stroke, myocardial infarction, cardiac arrhythmias, cardiac arrest, and death. Fortunately, most of the symptoms are due to trivial reasons and can be managed on board with the available first aid and medical kits.

OTITIC BAROTRAUMA

Earache

It is common to hear infants cry as the aircraft descends before touchdown. All air passengers experience a popping sensation in the air when the aircraft takes off and some experience pressure or pain in the ears during descent. Change in the cabin altitude is responsible for these. During ascent air in the middle ear cavity comes out of the eustachian tube, through its opening in the throat, as cabin pressure decreases with increasing altitude. This causes the popping sensation. During descent the cabin pressure increases while that inside the middle ear cavity is low so air tries to get back into the middle ear through the same eustachian tube, but is restricted by the valve like action of eustachian tube that tends to prevent entry of anything into the middle ear. This is exaggerated if there is an infection in the nose and throat region. Even a common cold can block the eustachian tube opening and cause severe pain in the ear during descent. In a few cases the *eardrum may be perforated*.

Feeding an infant or giving a soother to suckle, movements of jaw, swallowing of saliva or taking small sips of water, and gently breathing out against a close nostril can help open the valve of the eustachian tube that equalizes the pressure between middle ear and the cabin. The practice of giving sweets to all passengers during ascent and descent was meant to deal with anxiety and to prevent pain in the ears. Unfortunately this has been stopped as a cost-saving measure. Also, the experienced pilots use a slow, gradual descent that allows easier equalization of pressure in the middle ear.

In a few cases the pain in ear may persist after landing, which may require being examined and treated by a doctor.

DECOMPRESSION SICKNESS

Aircraft systems are designed to be very safe with each component designed to have very low risk. However, failure of cabin pressurization can occur due to various external factors. Cracking of a window or small hole in cabin structure can result in decompression of cabin exposing the passengers to low atmospheric pressure. Pilots descend down rapidly if such a rare event happens on their flight. That would prevent most of the effects of decompression sickness. In case of prolonged exposure to low atmospheric pressure while flying in an unpressurised aircraft or that with a failure of cabin pressure to altitude above 25,000 feet, the following symptoms may occur. Flying soon after deep sea diving or working in a mine can increase the chances of decompression sickness. If caused by altitude, pain can occur immediately or up to many hours later after landing.

Bends

Severe pain in knee and hip joints or other large joints of the body due to bubbling of nitrogen may occur. These symptoms are similar to those reported by mine workers, deep sea divers, and caisson workers as they come out of high-pressure environment to low-pressure environment.
- Localized deep pain, ranging from mild to excruciating. Sometimes a dull ache, but rarely a sharp pain
- Active and passive motion of the joint aggravates the pain
- The pain may be reduced by bending the joint to find a more comfortable position.

Chokes

Irritation in throat, dry cough, and retrosternal chest pain/burning sensation may occur on sudden or prolonged exposure to low atmospheric pressure. Air embolism may occur with sudden onset of breathlessness.

Creeps

Tingling, insect crawling sensation, irritation, itching, and redness may occur on the skin in any part of the body. Itching may occur on arms, around ears, face, and neck. There may be mottling of skin on arms and upper torso. Pitting edema may be noted on the skin of the affected parts.

Staggers

If central nervous system (CNS) is affected dizziness, giddiness, vomiting, disorientation, altered sensorium (paresthesia or hyperesthesia) may occur. Confusion, loss of memory, changes in mood or behavior, visual disturbances, convulsions, and loss of consciousness may occur. Deafness and loss of balance may also occur. Fecal and urinary incontinence and ascending paralysis may occur in a few cases. A general sense of malaise or not feeling well, fatigue, and headache may be the only symptom in some.

Treatment for decompression sickness is rest, oxygen and descent, and symptomatic treatment. On landing back the mainstay of treatment for decompression sickness is hyperbaric chamber along with appropriate supportive therapy.

HYPOXIA

The relative lack of oxygen may aggravate the existing respiratory and cardiovascular diseases like chronic bronchitis, asthma, and coronary artery disease. Those with anemia are more affected by prolonged exposure to the dry cabin air with lower partial pressure of oxygen at cabin altitude of 5,000–7,000 feet whereas healthy passengers do not get affected at all. In case of pressurization failure, supplemental oxygen is supplied to each passenger through automatic drop down masks. The elaborate oxygen mask drill that is demonstrated by cabin crew before each takeoff can be a lifesaver though most passengers tend to ignore it as a routine "nuisance." Dry cabin air can aggravate eye irritation; nose and throat dryness; and those wearing contact lenses may have discomfort and redness of eyes.

TEMPERATURE

Most airliners fly at an altitude of 33,000–35,000 feet above sea level and are exposed to temperatures around minus 51°C. Crew and the passengers are well protected by the pressurization and air conditioning systems that maintain a comfortable cabin temperature. Elderly and others not in peak health may feel cold even at 22–24°C cabin temperature and may need blankets or hot fluids. Overheating of cabin may lead to thirst, dryness of mouth, and muscle cramps especially in hot weather. This is frequently experienced if the aircraft is held up on ground for any reason after the passengers have boarded the aircraft. Inflight such an event rarely occurs, but may happen due to technical fault or inadvertent higher setting by the pilot.

VIBRATION AND UNUSUAL MOTIONS

Those susceptible to motion sickness and vertigo may get nausea, vomiting, and giddiness during takeoff and turning of aircraft in air. Air turbulence can adversely affect anyone with these symptoms. Severe, sudden turbulence may lead to lacerations, cuts and contusions if the passenger is not wearing seat belt properly or is hit by any loose object or luggage that may act as a missile in the air. People with low backache, intervertebral disk prolapse, and other joint conditions may experience pain on being confined to seat for a long time. This is more likely to happen in a crowded economy class seat with narrow leg space and elbowroom. Patients on intravenous (IV) drip may get their IV lines dislodged—if not properly secured preflight—due to vibration and buffeting caused by air turbulence.

PSYCHOLOGICAL

Anxiety, fear of accident, and fear of being confined in a crowded space may be encountered in first time flyers and in also in some experienced flyers. Excessive consumption of alcohol and slight hypoxia with anxiety may lead to air rage wherein the flyer may behave in an inappropriate and aggressive manner. Cabin crew has to manage such passengers tactfully. Restricting the supply of alcohol, identifying nervous passengers, and reassuring them helps. The captain of the aircraft has the authority to order restraint and confine any person on board to the seat if he/she is considered a threat to safety. Informed consent is not required in such a case.

DEEP VEIN THROMBOSIS AND PULMONARY THROMBOEMBOLISM

Deep vein thrombosis (DVT) is a potentially life-threatening condition that may occur in susceptible persons after prolonged immobilization due to travel (by air, sea, and train) and sickness leading to enforced bed rest. It may be asymptomatic till thromboembolism occurs in a few cases. In most cases the symptoms could be any of the following: swelling of foot, ankle or leg usually on one side, cramping pain, which typically begins in the calf, severe, unexplained pain in the foot or ankle, a patch of skin that feels warmer to the touch than skin surrounding it, a patch of skin that turns pale, or turns a reddish or bluish color.

Signs of a pulmonary thromboembolism (PE) may include dizziness, sweating, chest pain that becomes worse after coughing or deep inhales, rapid breathing, coughing up blood, and rapid heart rate.

Symptoms of DVT and PE, collectively referred to as venous thromboembolism (VTE) may not occur for several weeks after a flight.

Connection between Deep Vein Thrombosis

Sitting for extended periods of time in cramped airplane may slow blood circulation and increase your risk for DVT. Prolonged inactivity and dry cabin air seem to contribute to the risk. While there is some debate as to the connection, some studies have found evidence that the prevalence of DVT within 48 hours of flying on a plane is 2–10%. That is the same rate that people in hospitals develop DVT. Staying in a hospital is another risk factor for DVT. The risk, however, varies greatly among passengers. In general, the longer the flight, the higher is the risk. Flights lasting for more than 8 hours are thought to pose the most risk.

CHAPTER 56

Immunization for Adults and Travelers

Sara Nooruddin Kazim, Nisreen Hamza Maghraby, Azza Omar Yousif

■ INTRODUCTION

Immunization is the process of stimulating the bodies' own immune system to produce specific proteins called antibodies against specifically selected bacteria or viruses in order to prevent illness. To achieve this process, substances called vaccines are used; hence, the process is either referred to as immunization or vaccination.

Where the patient lives, what vaccines where received during childhood, where he/she is planning to travel, how long the trip will last, and the activities planned to be carried out, are all factors that will determine which vaccines are recommended. Usually vaccines prevent the disease lifelong, in some situations specially if given during childhood, some vaccines need a second dose, which is referred to as a booster dose.

There are different types of vaccines, active, passive, and toxoids. Regardless of the type, the process is similar. Unlike immunity gained naturally by getting the disease and becoming ill, this process is based on weakening the substances used, to a point where they are sufficient to stimulate the immune system to create antibodies against the bacteria or virus without yet actually causing the disease. Active vaccination refers to using the specific bacteria or virus that causes the disease in order to stimulate the immune system to generate its own antibodies. Another form of active immunization are toxoids, which are used for diseases where the bacterium itself does not cause the disease but a specific toxin that it releases does, e.g. diphtheria and tetanus. Similarly, a weakened form of this toxin is used to stimulate the immune system to generate its own antibodies. On the other hand, passive vaccination or immunization refers to giving the patient preformed antibodies from donors that have generated these antibodies against specific organisms. Unlike active immunization, passive immunization is a weaker process, which is not recommended for healthy adults but may be required in certain situation such as immunocompromised individuals.

As a general rule, vaccines are mostly considered safe. They have a long history of preventing death and saving lives all over the world, with a good safety profile. In very rare instances like with any other medical substance, they can cause an allergic reaction or some form of encephalopathy or encephalitis leading to seizures. The more common effects are mild and include local redness, soreness, or a low-grade fever.

In the next section, we will summarize the most common vaccines recommended. For each vaccine, we will review the etiology/causes, clinical presentation, investigations, vaccine/

treatment, and we will end with special considerations (immunocompromised, pregnancy/breastfeeding, healthcare professionals, travelers).

■ INFLUENZA

Etiology/Causes
Viral infection highly contagious commonly referred to as the flu.

Clinical Presentation
Fever lasting 2-5 days, headache, myalgia, runny nose, and sore throat.

Investigations
Clinical diagnosis, testing is sometimes done for documentation in a new outbreak or in patients at risk of complications.

Vaccine/Treatment

Vaccine

The vaccine is available in three different forms: (1) intramuscular (IM), (2) intradermal (ID), or (3) nasal spray. The ID vaccine and nasal spray use a smaller dose. For elderly or patients with risk of severe infection, the IM higher dose is recommended or the vaccine with an adjuvant, which increases the effectiveness of the vaccine.

Treatment

Mostly symptomatic, antiviral medications are used either for treatment or prevention of illness. For treatment, they decrease the duration of illness by approximately 1 day. They are not recommended, if symptoms more than 48 hours. Usually used for elderly patients or patients with chronic medical illnesses who are at risk of developing severe complications. For prevention, they are used for the same group of patients mentioned above after exposure who did not take the vaccine.

Special Considerations
- Immunocompromised—recommended
- Pregnancy/breastfeeding—inactive form recommended (preferably before if possible)
- Healthcare professionals—recommended
- Travelers—depending on the session of travel (spreads in the winter).

■ HAEMOPHILUS INFLUENZAE TYPE B

Etiology/Causes
Haemophilus influenzae serotype b (Hib) bacteria.

Clinical Presentation (History and Physical Examination)

Prior to vaccination *H. influenzae* has the leading cause of bacterial meningitis. Due to its vascular invasion tendency, it has the ability to cause other disease such as epiglottitis, pneumonia, empyema, pericarditis, bacteremia, and septic arthritis.

Clinical presentation will depend on the area involved.

Investigations

Mainly a clinical diagnosis and treatment are started empirically. For invasive disease, microbiological testing with cultures is required from sterile sites for confirmation.

Vaccine/Treatment

Vaccine

Active vaccination with 2-3 primary doses and a booster dose as part of childhood vaccination has a protection efficacy against ~95% of the disease.

Treatment

Beta-lactam agents (e.g. amoxicillin or a second- or third-generation cephalosporin) are the preferred antimicrobial agents. Alternative agents include fluoroquinolones, macrolides, tetracyclines, and aminoglycosides.

Special Considerations

- Immunocompromised—recommended (specifically postsplenectomy)
- Pregnancy/breastfeeding—no specific recommendation as long as it was taken as part of childhood vaccine, no specific contraindications if needed, preferably during third trimester.
- Healthcare professionals—no specific recommendation as long as it was taken as part of childhood vaccine.
- Travelers—no specific recommendation as long as it was taken as part of childhood vaccine.

PERTUSSIS

Etiology/Causes

Bordetella pertussis bacteria.

Clinical Presentation (History and Physical Examination)

Results in a protracted illness, presenting with paroxysmal coughing, affecting daily function. Serious complications, including failure to thrive, apnea, pneumonia, respiratory failure, seizures, and death threat younger patients.

Investigation (Suspected Laboratory Abnormalities)

Clinical diagnosis, although cultures or molecular testing can be used for suspicious cases. Due to the duration, treatment is started on clinical suspicion to prevent spread of the disease.

Vaccine/Treatment

Vaccine

Pregnant women who have been previously immunized with a full three-dose series of tetanus/diphtheria (Td) vaccine should receive a single dose of tetanus, diphtheria, and pertussis (Tdap), ideally during the early part of the 27–36-week gestational age range.

Treatment

For suspected cases of pertussis and cough less than or equal to 3 weeks, antibiotics are recommended. Macrolides are the antibiotics of choice. Azithromycin or clarithromycin have a better compliance profile and are better tolerated than erythromycin. For who macrolide intolerance, trimethoprim-sulfamethoxazole is an acceptable alternative. Cough persistent for 3-6 weeks, antibiotic may not affect the cough duration or severity but are used to reduce the likelihood of transmission to others. Therefore, for pregnant women, healthcare workers, and individuals working with infants, antibiotic are recommended for persistent cough up to 6 weeks.

Special Considerations

- Immunocompromised—no specific recommendations
- Pregnancy/breastfeeding—recommended booster for 27–36 weeks, if previously immunized. If not full 3 dose series.
- Healthcare professionals—no specific recommendations
- Travelers—no specific recommendations.

DIPHTHERIA

Etiology/Causes

Gram-positive bacillus *Corynebacterium diphtheriae*.

Clinical Presentation (History and Physical Examination)

Infection may lead to respiratory disease, cutaneous disease, or an asymptomatic carrier state. Classical throat examination demonstrates adherent gray pseudomembrane that bleeds with scraping.

Investigations (Suspected Laboratory Abnormalities)

Definitive diagnosis requires culture of *C. diphtheriae* with specimens collected from respiratory tract secretions or cutaneous lesions and a positive toxin assay. Routine laboratory results are usually nonspecific and may include a moderately elevated white blood cell count and proteinuria.

Vaccine/Treatment

Depending on the location and severity of infection, a combination of antitoxin and antibiotics is required. In general, erythromycin or procaine penicillin G is the antibiotic used. Antibiotics are used to decrease the growth preventing further toxin production, slows local spread, and reducing transmission.

Special Considerations

- Immunocompromised—no recommendations
- Pregnancy/breastfeeding—recommended
- Healthcare professionals—no recommendations
- Travelers—no recommendations.

TETANUS

Etiology/Causes

Toxin-producing anaerobe *Clostridium tetani*.

Clinical Presentation (History and Physical Examination)

Tetanus can present in one of four clinical patterns: (1) generalized, (2) local, (3) cephalic, and (4) neonatal. The most common and severe clinical form of tetanus is generalized tetanus. Generalized tetanus characteristically has tonic contraction of their skeletal muscles and intermittent intense muscular spasms. Since patients with tetanus have no impairment of consciousness or awareness, both the tonic contractions and spasms are intensely painful.

Investigations (Suspected Laboratory Abnormalities)

Clinical diagnosis based on typical presentation.

Vaccine/Treatment

Vaccine

Since tetanus is one of the few bacterial diseases that does not confer immunity following recovery from acute illness, all patients with tetanus should receive active immunization with a total of three doses of tetanus and diphtheria toxoid spaced at least 2 weeks apart, commencing immediately upon diagnosis. Tetanus toxoid should be administered at a different site than tetanus immune globulin.

Treatment

Treatment is usually in the intensive care unit, symptomatic management with airway observation and management as needed.

Special Considerations

- Immunocompromised—no specific recommendations
- Pregnancy/breastfeeding—recommended
- Healthcare professionals—no specific recommendations
- Travelers—no specific recommendations.

PNEUMOCOCCUS

Etiology/Causes

- Bacterial infection caused by gram-positive diplococci: *Streptococcus pneumoniae*
- *Pneumococcal disease*:
  - *Noninvasive*: Ear and sinus infections and pneumonia
  - *Invasive*: Bacteremia and meningitis.

Investigations (Suspected Laboratory Abnormalities)

- *Invasive*: Isolation of the organism from blood or other normally sterile body sites like cerebrospinal fluid (CSF)
- *Noninvasive*: More than 25 white blood cells and fewer than 10 epithelial cells per high-power field, and a predominance of gram-positive diplococci on gram stain. There is also the urinary antigen test based on an immunochromatographic membrane technique to detect the C-polysaccharide antigen of *Streptococcus pneumoniae*.

Vaccine/Treatment

- Vaccination is recommended for:
  - Infants and children below 2 years and adults 65 years and older and special groups:
    - *Special groups*: People 2–64 years with chronic illness, with cochlear implants or CSF leaks, or smoke cigarettes.
- *Treatment*:
  - *Noninvasive*: Antibiotics in penicillin and erythromycin groups
  - *Invasive*: Wide-spectrum antibiotic. Once the sensitivity of the bacteria is known, a more targeted antibiotic may be selected.
  - *S. pneumoniae* has developed resistance to drugs. Drug-resistant *S. pneumoniae* (DRSP) depends in the country of residence and introduction of vaccine. Two types of vaccine

are available: *(1) pneumococcal conjugate vaccine (PCV13) and (2) pneumococcal polysaccharide vaccine (PPSV23).*

Special Considerations
- Immunocompromised—recommended
- Pregnancy/breastfeeding—not recommended
- Healthcare professionals—no specific recommendation
- Travelers—no specific recommendation.

MENINGOCOCCUS

Etiology/Causes
Neisseria meningitidis bacteria

Clinical Presentation (History and Physical Examination)
- *Meningococcal meningitis*: Fever, headache, and stiff neck (nausea, vomiting, photophobia), altered mental status (confusion), lethargy poor feeding and irritability in newborn
- *Meningococcemia*: Sepsis and rash, fever, fatigue, vomiting, cold hands and feet, cold chills, severe aches or pain in the muscles, joints, chest or abdomen, rapid breathing, diarrhea.

Investigations (Suspected Laboratory Abnormalities)
Isolation and identification of *Neisseria meningitidis* with a Gram stain of the CSF sediment or by detection of specific antigens in the CSF by a latex agglutination test or using rapid diagnostic test (RDTs). Positive results for any of these tests can rapidly provide evidence of infection, even if cultures fail to grow.

Vaccine/Treatment

Vaccines
Meningococcal conjugate vaccines and serogroup B meningococcal vaccines.

Treatment
- Prompt treatment with antibiotic upon clinical suspicion, cardiopulmonary support, and wound care as needed.
- *11-12-year-old*: Should be vaccinated
- *16 years*: May give a booster dose
- *16-23 years*: To be vaccinated with a serogroup B meningococcal vaccine, if they have complemented component deficiency, functional or anatomic asplenia, they are living with HIV, they are a 1st-year college student living in a residence hall or they are a military recruit.

Special Considerations

- Immunocompromised—recommended
- Pregnancy/breastfeeding—if high risk, no contraindication to administration
- Healthcare professionals—they are a microbiologist who is routinely exposed to *Neisseria meningitidis*
- Travelers—recommended for those traveling or residing in countries in which the disease is common.

■ HERPES ZOSTER (VARICELLA)

Etiology/Causes

Varicella zoster virus (VZV).

Clinical Presentation (History and Physical Examination)

Fever malaise, painful rash with dermatomal distribution.

Investigations (Suspected Laboratory Abnormalities)

Polymerase chain reaction (PCR).

Vaccine/Treatment

Vaccine

Live vaccine recombinant zoster vaccine recommended for people aged 50 years and older.

Treatment

Antiviral medication acyclovir, valacyclovir, and famciclovir to shorten duration, analgesia.

Special Considerations

- Immunocompromised—no specific recommendation
- Pregnancy/breastfeeding—not recommended, postexposure for nonimmune pregnant ladies varicella-zoster immune globulin
- Healthcare professionals—no specific recommendations
- Travelers—no specific recommendations.

■ HUMAN PAPILLOMAVIRUS

Etiology/Causes

Human papillomavirus (HPV), sexually transmitted disease.

Clinical Presentation (History and Physical Examination)

Causes common warts, persistent infection can lead to—cervical, vaginal, and vulvar cancers in women; penile cancers in men; and oropharyngeal and anal cancers in both men and women.

Investigations (Suspected Laboratory Abnormalities)
- *Pap test*: Looks for precancer changes
- *HPV DNA test*: Looks of HPV.

Vaccine/Treatment
- *Vaccine*: 9-valent HPV given to all adolescent at 11-12 years up to 15 years of age in two doses regimen, second 6-12 month from first dose.
- Inactivated HPV.

Special Considerations
- Immunocompromised—three dose regimens is recommended (0, 1-2, and 6 months)
- Pregnancy/breastfeeding—not recommended, limited safety profile
- Healthcare professionals—no specific recommendations
- Travelers—no specific recommendations.

TUBERCULOSIS (BACILLUS CALMETTE-GUÉRIN)

Etiology/Causes
Bacterium called *Mycobacterium tuberculosis*.

Clinical Presentation (History and Physical Examination)
Fever, chills, night sweats, weight loss, cough, gastrointestinal (GI) symptoms, bone pain depending of affected area.

Investigations (Suspected Laboratory Abnormalities)
Tuberculosis (TB) skin test (Mantoux) tells if person is infected, TB blood test (interferon-gamma release assays or IGRAs or T spot) tells if person has latent TB infection (LTBI), acid-fast bacilli (AFB) on sputum smear along with chest X-ray diagnosis TB disease.

Vaccine/Treatment
- *Vaccine*: Bacillus Calmette-Guérin (BCG) vaccine given to infants' countries where TB is common.
- *Treatment*:
  - For TB latent infection: Four treatment regimens for latent TB infection (LTBI) use isoniazid (INH), rifapentine (RPT), or rifampin (RIF). Modified if drug resistant.
  - For TB disease: Isoniazid (INH), rifampin (RIF), ethambutol (EMB), pyrazinamide (PZA).

Special Considerations
- Immunocompromised—contraindicated
- Pregnancy/breastfeeding—not recommended
- Healthcare professionals—recommended for high percentage or continuous transmission or exposure with isoniazid and rifampin resistant TB
- Travelers—no specific recommendations.

MEASLES/MUMPS/RUBELLA

Etiology/Causes
- *Measles*: Ribonucleic acid (RNA) virus from genus *Morbillivirus*
- *Mumps*: RNA mumps virus
- *Rubella*: RNA virus classified as a *Rubivirus*.

Clinical Presentation (History and Physical Examination)
- *Measles*: Fever, cough, maculopapular skin rash, conjunctivitis with serious illnesses like pneumonia and encephalitis
- *Mumps*: Fever, headache, muscle aches, tiredness, loss of appetite, tender swollen salivary glands, deafness, and in severe cases encephalitis
- *Rubella*: Fever, sore throat, conjunctivitis, arthritis in women, miscarriages, and birth defects in pregnant women.

Investigations (Suspected Laboratory Abnormalities)
Measles: Detection of measles-specific IgM antibody and measles RNA by real-time polymerase chain reaction (RT-PCR) in nasopharyngeal swaps.

Vaccine/Treatment
- *Vaccine*: Live-attenuated vaccine recommended for:
  - *Two doses*: First at 12–15 months of age and second at 4 to 6 years of age
  - Two doses, 28 days apart for teenagers without evidence of immunity
  - One dose at least for adults without evidence of immunity.
- *Treatment*: Supportive and wound care.

Special Considerations
- Immunocompromised—not recommended
- Pregnancy/breastfeeding—not recommended, IV immunoglobulin for postexposure within 6 days (measles)
- Healthcare professionals—if no evidence of immunity
- Travelers—unvaccinated adults and infants 6 to 11 months.

CHICKENPOX

Etiology/Causes
Varicella zoster virus.

Clinical Presentation (History and Physical Examination)
Varicella zoster infection manifest early as a nonspecific viral illness followed by a vesicular rash. Patient's condition can progress to more serious pneumonia and encephalitis.

Investigations (Suspected Laboratory Abnormalities)
Direct virology or PCR detection from body fluids and vesicles scraping.

Vaccine/Treatment
- *Vaccine*: Live attenuated virus vaccine. Routine vaccination is recommended for all patients:
  - Age above 60 years of age
  - Previous history of chickenpox
  - Chronic medical condition.
- *Treatment*: Antiviral reduces the duration and severity of illness, if the patient received it within 24-48 hours after new vesicle formation. Supportive treatment and management of complications.

Special Considerations
- Immunocompromised—varicella vaccine is recommended for patients with mild-to-moderate immune suppression. Varicella vaccine is recommended for patients at least 14 days before receiving immunosuppressive therapy.
- Pregnancy/breastfeeding—varicella vaccine is not recommended to be administered during pregnancy. Pregnant women suspected to be at risk of varicella zoster infection are given two vaccines postpartum. One immediately in the postpartum period and the second vaccine at 4-8 weeks postpartum.
- *Healthcare professionals*—no specific recommendations
- *Travelers*—no specific recommendations.

HEPATITIS A

Etiology/Causes
Hepatitis A virus (HAV)

Clinical Presentation (History and Physical Examination)
Fever abdominal pain, loss of appetite, vomiting, and jaundice.

Investigations (Suspected Laboratory Abnormalities)
Detection of anti-hepatitis A virus (HAV), IgM antibodies, and the determination of total anti-HAV by enzyme immunoassay.

Vaccine/Treatment
- *Vaccine*: Inactivated (killed) vaccine, routinely given to children 12 to 23 months of age.
- *Treatment*: Supportive care.

Special Considerations
- Immunocompromised—no specific recommendation
- Pregnancy/breastfeeding—no specific recommendation
- Healthcare professionals—no specific recommendation
- Travelers—recommended for high-risk areas.

HEPATITIS B

Etiology/Causes
Hepatitis B virus (HBV).

Clinical Presentation (History and Physical Examination)
Fever, hepatitis, liver cirrhosis, liver cancer, liver failure, and death.

Investigations
Check anti HBs status

Vaccine/Treatment
Children and adults: Three-dose vaccine series administered intramuscularly, the second and third administered 1 and 6 months after the 1st month.

Special Considerations
- Immunocompromised—recommended, if not vaccinated
- Pregnancy/breastfeeding—no contraindication, if high risk of exposure and no travelers—no specific recommendation.
- Previous vaccination schedule is given in **Table 1**.
- A seroprotective (adequate) level of anti-HBs after completion of a vaccination series is defined as anti-HBs more than or equal to 10 mLU/mL; a response less than 10 mLU/mL is inadequate and is not a reliable indicator of protection.

Table 1: Vaccination schedule of hepatitis B vaccines

Vaccination and antibody response status of exposed person	Treatment		
	Source HBsAg-positive	Source HBsAg-negative	Source not tested or status unknown
Unvaccinated	HBIG × 1; initiate HB vaccine series	Initiate HB vaccine series	Initiate HB vaccine series
Previously vaccinated			
Known responder	No treatment	No treatment	No treatment
Known nonresponder			
After three doses	HBIG × 1 and initiate revaccination	No treatment	If known high-risk source, treat as if source were HBsAg-positive
After six doses	HBIG × 2 (separated by 1 month)	No treatment	If known high-risk source, treat as if source were HBsAg-positive
Antibody response unknown	Test exposed person for anti-HBs. If adequate, no treatment. If inadequate, HBIG × 1 and vaccine booster	No treatment	Test exposed person for anti-HBs. If adequate, no treatment. If inadequate, initiate revaccination

(HBIG: hepatitis B immune globulin; HBsAg: surface antigen of the hepatitis B)

YELLOW FEVER

Etiology/Causes

Single-stranded RNA virus and a member of *Flavivirus* family.

Clinical Presentation (History and Physical Examination)

- Mosquito-borne viral hemorrhagic fever
- Signs and symptoms vary from mild nonspecific febrile illness to severe life-threatening hemorrhage with multiorgan failure.

Investigations (Suspected Laboratory Abnormalities)

- Nucleic acid amplification test (NAAT) to detect yellow fever virus (YFV) in various body fluids (urine, serum, cerebrospinal fluid—CSF).
- Yellow fever virus-specific IgM or fourfold raise in IgG levels.

Vaccine/Treatment

- *Vaccine*: Single live attenuated virus vaccine is recommended for:
  – Person more than 9 months of age traveling to or living in areas with high risk of virus transmission.

- *Treatment*: Mainly supportive treatment and management of complications. Antivirals and steroids are of no proven benefit in treating yellow fever.

Special Considerations
- *Immunocompromised*: Patients require revaccination every 10 years before traveling to endemic areas with YFV.
- *Pregnancy—Breastfeeding*—Patients require revaccination regardless of the trimester before traveling to endemic areas with YFV.
- *Healthcare professionals*: Workers dealing with live YFV require revaccination every 10 years.
- *Travelers*: Travelers who have their vaccination more than 10 years and are traveling to high-risk areas and intend to stay for prolonged periods require revaccination.

POLIO

Etiology/Causes
- Poliovirus is a member of Enterovirus family that colonizes the gastrointestinal tract.
- Transmission is mainly through the fecal-oral rout.

Clinical Presentation (History and Physical Examination)
- *Mucocutaneous and respiratory manifestations*: Nonspecific febrile illness followed by maculopapular rash on palms and soles and upper and lower respiratory tract infection.
- *Neurologic and systemic manifestations*: Present as aseptic meningitis, acute flaccid paralysis, and encephalitis.

Investigations (Suspected Laboratory Abnormalities)
Nucleic acid amplification test to detect poliovirus in various body fluids (urine, serum, cerebrospinal fluid—CSF). Poliovirus-specific IgM antibodies in the CSF or serum.

Vaccine/Treatment
- *Vaccine*:
    - Inactivated polio vaccine (IPV): Incorporated into routine vaccination schedule given at age of:
        - 2 months
        - 4 months
        - 6-8 months
        - 4-6 years
    - Oral polio vaccine (OPV): Life attenuated, oral drops. Given during polio eradication campaigns.
- *Treatment*: Mainly supportive treatment and management of complications. Antivirals and immunoglobulins are of no proven benefit in treating poliovirus infection.

Special Considerations
- *Immunocompromised*: IPV is recommended for patients traveling to high-risk areas.
- *Pregnancy and breastfeeding*: IPV is not contraindicated in breastfeeding mothers. IPV is recommended for patients traveling to high-risk areas.
- *Healthcare professionals*: IPV is indicated in personnel in close contact with patients who traveled to area with high risk of polio.
- *Travelers*: IPV is indicated for travelers to high-risk areas.

■ TYPHOID

Etiology/Causes
- *Salmonella enterica* Typhi and Paratyphi A, Paratyphi B, and Paratyphi C
- Transmission is through the fecal–oral rout.

Clinical Presentation (History and Physical Examination)
Typhoid and paratyphoid fever have an incubation period from 6 days to 30 days. Symptoms onset is insidious with gradually increasing fever, fatigue, and abdominal pain. Complications causing death include gastrointestinal hemorrhage and perforation.

Investigations (Suspected Laboratory Abnormalities)
Bone marrow can blood culture for detecting *Salmonella* species.

Vaccine/Treatment
- *Indications*:
    - Travelers to areas endemic with *Salmonella typhi*.
    - Person with close contact with a documented *Salmonella typhi* carrier.
    - Microbiologists and laboratory working with cultures of *Salmonella typhi*.
- *Treatment*: Mainly supportive treatment and management of complications in addition to early antibiotic treatment. Chloramphenicol or amoxicillin is currently associated with significant resistance rate. Quinolones and third-generation cephalosporins are associated with higher cure rates.

Special Considerations
- *Immunocompromised*: Life-attenuated vaccine is contraindicated and the oral vaccine is of limited efficacy.
- *Pregnancy and breastfeeding*: Oral live attenuated virus is contraindicated while there is no evidence that parenteral form is contraindicated.
- *Healthcare professionals*: No specific recommendations
- *Travelers*: Travelers to endemic areas require immunization to be completed at least 2 weeks prior to exposure.

JAPANESE ENCEPHALITIS

Etiology/Causes
Japanese encephalitis virus (JEV) is a mosquito-borne *Flavivirus*. This virus occurs in Asia and parts of the western Pacific at agricultural areas with Rice farming.

Clinical Presentation (History and Physical Examination)
Japanese encephalitis' (JE) incubation period ranges from 5 days to 15 days. JE prodromal phase starts as a nonspecific febrile illness (fever, nausea, vomiting, headache, and malaise). This phase is followed by the encephalitis phase. Encephalitis present with altered mental status, focal neurological deficit, and abnormal movements. Status epilepticus and motor neuron weakness are poor prognostic signs.

Investigations (Suspected Laboratory Abnormalities)
- JEV-specific IgM antibodies in the cerebrospinal fluid (CSF) or serum.
- Nucleic acid amplification test (NAAT) to detect viremia is insensitive to diagnose JE.
- Detection of virus-specific IgM antibodies CSF or serum.

Vaccine/Treatment
- *Vaccine*: Preventive measure to prevent JE include mosquito control, animal immunization, and human immunization.
  - *Recommended for*:
    - Residents of endemic areas
    - Laboratory workers exposed to live infectious JEV
    - Travelers who plan to stay more than 1 month in endemic areas during JE outbreaks.
  - *To consider for*:
    - Travelers who plan to stay less than 1 month in endemic areas during JE outbreaks.
    - Travelers to areas with ongoing JE outbreaks.
  - *Not recommended for*:
    - Short-term travelers whose visits are restricted to urban areas or areas outside a JE outbreak areas.
- *Treatment*: Mainly supportive treatment and management of complications. Antivirals and steroids are of no proven benefit in treating JE.

Special Considerations
- *Immunocompromised*: No specific recommendations for vaccination in immunocompromised patients.
- *Pregnancy and breastfeeding*: JE vaccine is recommended for pregnant women traveling to endemic areas and planning to stay for long period. JE vaccine is not contraindicated in breastfeeding women.

- *Healthcare professionals*: JE is recommended for laboratory workers dealing with live infectious JEV.
- *Travelers*: JE is recommended for travelers intending to stay for more than 1 month in an endemic area with JE.

RABIES

Etiology/Causes

An RNA in the Rhabdoviridae family. Transmission occurs via saliva of an infected host to an uninfected victim through bites.

Clinical Presentation (History and Physical Examination)

Rabies infection in human present in five phases:
1. *Incubation period:* The incubation period ranges between 1 month and 2 months but can be as early as 7 days postexposure and up to more than 6 years postexposure.
2. *Prodromal phase*: Nonspecific symptoms including nausea, vomiting, fever, and paresthesia at the bite site.
3. *Acute neurological phase:*
   - *Encephalitic (furious) rabies:* Hyperactive symptoms aggravated by thirst, fear, light, or noise. During this phase, characteristic phobic spasms occur, mainly aerophobia and hydrophobia.
   - *Paralytic (dumb) rabies*: Ascending paralysis that is difficult to diagnose since it resembles other neurological diagnosis that present with progressive paralysis.
4. *Coma*: Common precipitants include respiratory muscles spasm, nodal dysrhythmia, and cardiogenic shock.
5. *Recovery*: It is noted mainly in patients who received immediate postexposure prophylaxis (PEP).

Investigations (Suspected Laboratory Abnormalities)

- *Animal*: Direct fluorescent antibody (DFA) on two samples from brain tissue.
- *Human*: Anti-rabies virus antibody detection in serum, CSF, and saliva. Reverse transcriptase followed by polymerase chain reaction (RT-PCR) in saliva or nuchal biopsy, for detecting rabies virus RNA. Direct fluorescent antibody testing (DFA), for detecting rabies virus.

Vaccine/Treatment

- *Vaccine*: Inactive vaccine can be given as pre-exposure prophylaxis or as PEP **(Table 2)**. Rabies immunoglobulin is administered postexposure in high-risk groups.
  - *Pre-exposure prophylaxis is indicated for*:
    - Personnel at risk of exposure to live rabies virus (laboratory staff, veterinarians, animal handlers, and wildlife officers).

Table 2: Post exposure prophylaxis in dog bite

Category of exposure	Description	Postexposure prophylaxis
Category I	Touching or feeding a potentially rabid animal Licks on intact skin	Not clinically relevant exposures No PEP indicated
Category II	Licking uncovered skin Minor scratches or abrasions without bleeding	Wound disinfection Antirabies vaccine only
Category III	Single or multiple transdermal bites Contamination of exposed skin or mucus membranes with saliva	Wound disinfection Antirabies vaccine Rabies immunoglobulin

(PEP: postexposure prophylaxis)

- Children living or visiting rabies endemic areas.
- Travelers to rabid endemic areas.
- *Dose regimen*:
  - Rabies vaccine is administered intramuscularly on days 0, 7, and 21 or 28.
- *Postexposure prophylaxis steps*:
  - *Wound treatment*: Immediate wound washing and flushing in addition to disinfection with detergent.
  - *Avoid suturing the sound*: Rabies vaccine and immunoglobulins (RIG) are administrated according to the category of exposure.
- *Dose regimen*:
  - Rabies vaccine is administered intramuscularly on days 0, 3, 7, and 14.
  - Rabies immunoglobulin, 20 IU/kg body weight is infiltrated around and into the wound. Remaining volume is administered intramuscularly at anatomically distant site from the vaccination area.
- *Treatment*: Wound cleansing and supportive care. Antirabies vaccine and immunoglobulins for bites from infected animals.

Special Considerations

- *Immunocompromised*:
  - *Pre-exposure prophylaxis*: Rabies vaccination is deferred until immunosuppression status resolves. If not possible, then pre-exposure regimen is administered and antibody response if checked in 2–4 weeks.
  - *Postexposure prophylaxis*: Wound cleansing. RIG administration for category II and III exposures. Rabies vaccine regimen is changed from the four-dose regimen to the five-dose regimen (0, 3, 7, 14, and 28). If possible, withhold other immunosuppressant agents during PEP.
- *Pregnancy and breastfeeding*: Pregnancy and breastfeeding are not contraindications for PEP.

- *Healthcare professionals*: Pre-exposure prophylaxis is indicated for personnel at risk of exposure to live rabies virus (laboratory staff, veterinarians, animal handlers, and wildlife officers).
- *Travelers*: Pre-exposure prophylaxis is indicated for travelers to rabid endemic areas.

SMALLPOX

Etiology/Causes
Variola virus, a member of the Orthopox family. Transmission occurs through person-to-person contract and saliva droplets.

Clinical Presentation (History and Physical Examination)
Signs and symptoms occur after an incubation period. This is followed by a prodromal phase (2–3 days), which is characterized by high-grade fever (40°C). This is followed by the most contagious stage, which starts with red spots in the mouth and tongue followed by vesicular or pustular rash spreading down from face to limbs and trunk that finally scabs off 3 weeks after the appearance of rash.

Investigations (Suspected Laboratory Abnormalities)
- *Electron microscopy*: Done at WHO smallpox biological safety level 4 laboratory.
- *Polymerase chain reaction*: Detects variola virus DNA.

Vaccine/Treatment
- *Vaccine: Vaccinia virus vaccine*: Live attenuated virus against viruses within the *Orthopoxvirus* genus including the smallpox virus and other viruses causing infection in humans. Vaccinia vaccine is not recommended for the general population, its use is indicated for laboratory personnel in direct contact with cultures or animals contaminated with Orthopox viruses causing infection in humans (variola, monkeypox, and cowpox).
- *Treatment*: The mainstay of treatment is supportive in addition of antivirals (Tecovirimat, Brincidofovir, or Cidofovir) in outbreak cases.

Special Considerations
- *Immunocompromised*: Vaccinia vaccine is an absolute contraindication unless there is a smallpox outbreak.
- *Pregnancy and breastfeeding*: Vaccinia vaccine is an absolute contraindication unless there is a smallpox outbreak.
- *Healthcare professionals*: Vaccination is contraindicated unless, the patient is in close contact with Orthopox virus infected humans, tissue, or animals.
- *Travelers*: Vaccination is usually not indicated unless patient will be at close contact with poxvirus family.

ANTHRAX

Etiology/Causes
- A zoonotic disease caused by gram-positive, spore-forming bacteria *Bacillus anthracis*. Although *B. anthracis* spores are used as a biological weapon, outbreaks of the infection are not uncommon.
- Humans exposed to *B. anthracis* spores by direct contact or inhalation develop anthrax.

Clinical Presentation (History and Physical Examination)
Symptoms related to anthrax exposure are nonspecific and resemble other viral infections. Patients can exhibit itchy blisters that progress to painless ulcers with black center (ESCHAR). Other nonspecific features include dyspnea, chest tightness, nausea, vomiting, fever, and abdominal pain.

Investigations (Suspected Laboratory Abnormalities)
Diagnosis of *B. anthracis* depends on history of exposure to an infected animal, the presence of prodromal symptoms in addition of demonstrating gram-positive bacilli in tissue cultures or bloodstream. Tissue cultures might be negative in patients who receive antibiotics prior to sample retrieval.

Vaccine/Treatment
- *Vaccine*: Vaccination against *B. anthracis* is not routinely recommended for the general population. *B. anthracis* vaccines are given as pre-event or postevent vaccination.
  - *Pre-event vaccination*: *B. anthracis* vaccination is only recommended for high-risk population at increased risk of occupational exposure. Recommended dose is 5 IM doses administered at days 0, week 4, and months 6, 12, and 18. The population at high risk of exposure includes:
    - Laboratory workers who are at high risk of repeated exposure to virulent *B. anthracis*.
    - Military personnel at risk of exposure to aerosolized *B. anthracis*.
    - Environmental investigators who repeatedly enter contaminated areas with *B. anthracis* spores.
    - Emergency response personnel who are at risk of encountering aerosolized *B. anthracis*.
- *Postexposure prophylaxis*: The Center for Disease Control and Prevention (CDC) recommends PEP with 60 days of appropriate antibiotics in addition to three subcutaneous doses of *B. anthracis* vaccine.
  - The PEP is recommended for unvaccinated personnel after exposure to *B. anthracis*.
- *Treatment*: The main stay of treatment is supportive care in addition to early antibiotic initiation. Ciprofloxacin and doxycycline are preferred antibiotic choices for anthrax PEP.

Special Considerations

- *Immunocompromised*: Not recommended
- *Pregnancy and breastfeeding*: Pre-event vaccination is not recommended in low-risk exposures. PEP is recommended following exposure to *B. anthracis* and breastfeeding is not a contraindication for vaccine administration.
- *Children*: Pre-event vaccination is generally not recommended. PEP is recommended following exposure to *B. anthracis*.
- *Healthcare professionals*: Pre-event vaccination is generally not recommended. PEP is recommended following exposure to *B. anthracis*.
- *Travelers*: Pre-event vaccination is generally not recommended. PEP is recommended following exposure to *B. anthracis*.

CHAPTER 57

Immunization in Pregnancy and Children

Ashok Mishra

INTRODUCTION AND BACKGROUND

Immunization is one of the most cost-effective public health interventions. Various foreign particles, e.g. proteins, virus, pathogens, parasitic worms, chemicals, toxins are trying to gain access into the body. Our immune system readily separates them from natural healthy tissues, its cells, and proteins. When this immune system is sensitized with the milder infective form of disease, this same immune system helps protect the body from subsequent attack of disease causing agent. Immunization is the process whereby a person is made immune or resistant to an infectious disease, typically by the administration of a vaccine. Vaccines stimulate the body's own immune system to protect the person against subsequent infection or disease [World Health Organization (WHO)].

The most important elements of immune system are T-cells, B-cells and the antibodies B-cells, while memory T-cells and memory B-cells are responsible for swift action at the time of second encounter with the disease causing agents. This whole process is known as active immunization. When readymade antibodies are inoculated into the body of a person without its being produced by body itself it is known as passive immunization.

World Health Organization estimates that vaccination averts 2–3 million deaths per year (in all age groups), and up to 1.5 million children die each year due to diseases which could have been prevented by vaccination.

During 2016, 116.5 million infants worldwide received three doses of diphtheria–tetanus–pertussis (DTP3) vaccine, protecting them against infectious diseases that can cause serious illness and disability. There was 84% drop in measles deaths between 2000 and 2016 worldwide, due to measles vaccination. Polio cases have decreased by over 99% since 1988. Today, only three countries (Afghanistan, Nigeria, and Pakistan) remain polio-endemic, down from more than 125 in 1988.

In 2016, an estimated 19.5 million infants worldwide were not reached with routine immunization services such as DTP3 vaccine. Around 60% of these children live in 10 countries: Angola, Brazil, the Democratic Republic of the Congo, Ethiopia, India, Indonesia, Iraq, Nigeria, Pakistan, and South Africa.

The Global Vaccine Action Plan (GVAP) was launched with a roadmap to prevent millions of deaths through more equitable access to vaccines by 2020. To date, progress toward the GVAP targets is off track. In May 2017, Ministers of Health from 194 countries endorsed a new resolution on strengthening immunization to achieve the goals of the GVAP.

Vaccination is a miracle of modern medicine. In the past 50 years, it saved more lives worldwide than any other medical product or procedure. Modern medicine knows Edward Jenner as the father of immunology/vaccination, an English physician and scientist who was the pioneer of smallpox vaccine, the world's first vaccine and also coined the term vaccine and vaccination. But the story of vaccine does not begin here; rather Chinese were pioneer in variolation for smallpox as early as 1000 AD.

HISTORICAL ASPECT OF VACCINATION

Buddhist monks drank snake venom to confer immunity to snake bite and variolation (smearing of a skin tear with cowpox to confer immunity to smallpox) was practiced in 17th century China. The earliest documented examples of vaccination are from India and China in the 17th century, where vaccination with powdered scabs from people infected with smallpox was used to protect against the disease. The mention of inoculation in the *Sact'eya Grantham*, an *Ayurvedic text*, was noted by the French scholar Henri Marie Husson in the journal Dictionaire des Sciences Médicales. However, the fascinating story of vaccination goes back all the way to Ancient Greece.

BRIEF HISTORY OF VACCINATION

429 BC	The Greek historian Thucydides observed that those who survived the smallpox plague in Athens did not become reinfected with the disease.
1554 AD	Some 8,000 children died in Goa, India, from a smallpox epidemic most likely introduced by the Portuguese.
1718	Variolation in Turkey, Lady Mary Wortley Montagu (1689-1762) had her son variolated in Constantinople by Dr Charles Maitland (April 1718)
1721	Lady Mary Montagu brought the practice of variolation to England, where she had Dr Charles Maitland variolate her two-year-old daughter.
1796	On May 14, 1796, Edward Jenner inoculated eight-year-old James Phipps with matter from a cowpox sore on the hand of milkmaid Sarah Nelmes and from the basis of vaccination.
1813	US Vaccine Agency established signed by James Madison.
1853	The United Kingdom Vaccination Act of 1853 made smallpox vaccination mandatory in the first three months of an infant's life.
1881–85	Louis Pasteur presented the success of rabies vaccine and successfully used them on 350 people later, only one died as vaccination was started late. Anthrax vaccine was developed by Louis Pasteur in 1881.
1923	Diphtheria toxoid vaccine developed
1926–27	Pertussis, BCG vaccination
1963	Oral Polio Vaccine

Chapter 57: Immunization in Pregnancy and Children

Prior to 1974 and expanded program on immunization, child vaccination coverage for tuberculosis, diphtheria, pertussis, tetanus, polio, and measles was estimated to be fewer than 5%.

The WHO initiated the Expanded Programme on Immunization (EPI) in May 1974 with the objective to vaccinate children throughout the world. But the vaccination schedule for EPI was formulated by WHO in 1984 and included bacillus Calmette-Guérin (BCG), DPT, oral poliovirus vaccine (OPV), and measles. With the advent of newer vaccines, EPI was expanded and included hepatitis B (HepB), *Haemophilus influenzae* type B (Hib), and yellow fever vaccine in endemic areas. Subsequently in 1999 Global Alliance for Vaccines and Immunization (GAVI) was created to increase the access of EPI in the farthest and poorest countries. Inspired from WHO, India launched the EPI in 1978 which was expanded in 1985 as Universal Immunization Programme (UIP) which became part of Child Survival and Safe Motherhood in 1992. UIP then became important component of National Reproductive and Child Health Programme in 1997, currently UIP is part of NHM since 2005. At present, 12 vaccine preventable diseases are covered under UIP, i.e. TB, diphtheria, pertussis, tetanus, polio, measles, hepatitis B, diarrhea, Japanese encephalitis (JE), rubella, pneumonia (*H. influenzae* type B), and pneumococcal diseases (pneumococcal pneumonia and meningitis). Hepatitis B and pneumococcal diseases were added to the UIP in 2007 and 2017, respectively. Inactivated poliovirus vaccine (IPV), rotavirus vaccine (RVV), MR, and JE were the addition in the UIP recently.

To strengthen routine immunization planning and delivery mechanism, the Ministry of Health and Family Welfare, Government of India, launched its flagship program "Mission Indradhanush" in December 2014 to achieve more than 90% full immunization coverage in the country.

VACCINATION IN PREGNANCY

Fetal development and its fate depend on mother's health and wellbeing. Her contracting the disease affects the fetus in womb. Hence proper immunization of "to be mother" plays a significant role in preventing untoward incidences during pregnancy and at term. Vaccinated mother passes disease protecting antibodies to fetus having immature adaptive immune system, which then protects both mother and fetus from vaccine preventable diseases during pregnancy and later life as "to be born baby" is highly susceptible for various disease causing agents.

Live virus poses a threat to developing fetus in womb hence it is generally contraindicated for giving live vaccines to women planning conception within 4 weeks (in preconception phase) and already pregnant women. Toxoids, killed/inactivated bacteria or virus vaccines have not shown any untoward incidences to both mother and fetus hence it is very important to vaccinate a mother if she is at high risk of being exposed to vaccine preventable disease or if infection poses a great threat to the lives of fetus or mother or both.

It is very imperative to assess the risk versus the protective benefits provided by the vaccination in each situations, regardless of its being live or inactivated vaccine. UIP by Government of India recommends two doses of tetanus toxoid to all pregnant women at an interval of 4 weeks as soon as pregnancy is detected.

All live attenuated vaccines are not routinely recommended for immunization schedule. Vaccines which are contraindicated in pregnant women are human papilloma virus, measles, mumps, rubella, varicella, oral typhoid vaccine, live attenuated Japanese encephalitis vaccine, zoster vaccine. Others not recommended in routine immunization schedule can be given in exceptional circumstances where benefits of vaccination surpass the associated risk.

VACCINATION FOR PREGNANT WOMEN AS PER NATIONAL IMMUNIZATION SCHEDULE

Tetanus Toxoid Vaccine

Exotoxin produced by *Clostridium tetani* causes tetanus which is an acute, often fatal disease. This is due to low levels of antitetanus antibody in neonates transferred passively from mother.

TT vaccine was first produced in 1924 and used extensively for the first time among soldiers during World War II. Since then, immunization program using TTs have been highly successful in preventing maternal and neonatal tetanus (MNT) as well as injury-associated tetanus.

World Health Organization estimates that there were 59,000 neonatal tetanus deaths in 2008, a 92% reduction from the late 1980s and an indicator of how widely maternal TT immunization is being used. It is estimated that at least 100 million doses of TT vaccine were given to pregnant women in 2011 (compared with 64 million women between 1995 and 2004).

A WHO position paper on tetanus, published in 2006, suggested that three doses of DTP vaccine should be given in infancy, with boosters in childhood and adolescence and a sixth dose at first pregnancy as TdaP (tetanus diphtheria and acellular pertussis). If a good immunization history is not available pregnant women should receive two doses of vaccine 4 weeks apart and at least 2 weeks (preferably 4 weeks) before delivery.

Optimal timing for TdaP/TT administration is between 27 and 36 weeks of gestation although Tda/TTP may be given at any time during pregnancy.

A search of the vaccine adverse events reporting system (VAERS) database for 2005–2010 did not identify any concerns about maternal, infant, and fetal outcomes following vaccination with a reduced amount of diphtheria toxoid, tetanus toxoid, and acellular pertussis vaccine.

Recently, vaccination with TdaP combined with IPV has been recommended for pregnant women in the United Kingdom.

The American Congress of Obstetricians and Gynecologists also recommends giving diphtheria toxoid, tetanus toxoid, and acellular pertussis vaccine to pregnant women.

VACCINATION FOR PREGNANT WOMEN UNDER SPECIAL CIRCUMSTANCES

Influenza Vaccine

Pregnant women are at increased risk of influenza disease. Its severe complications included small for gestational age and preterm birth for fetus, both are at increased risk of mortality. Pregnant women with underlying medical conditions develop increased incidence of seasonal influenza disease with severity. Benefits associated with influenza vaccination particularly in second and third trimester with transplacental transfer of protective antibodies providing indirect protection against illness in mothers and their infants have outnumbered the risk factors. These benefits have made many countries all over the world to incorporate influenza vaccines in their national immunization schedule and policies. A single dose of 0.5 mL I/M is to be given.

Though live attenuated influenza vaccine (LAIV) is not recommended for use during pregnancy.

Japanese Encephalitis Vaccine

JE vaccine should not be routinely administered during pregnancy. Pregnant women who must travel to an endemic area during the transmission season where risk of JE is high and if staying for more than 30 days should be vaccinated. Vaccination should be considered if she is visiting a rural area with extensive outdoor activities and even if staying for less than 30 days, as the theoretical risks of immunization are outweighed by the risk of infection to the mother and developing fetus. Dose is 1 mL SC on 0, 7, and 30 days. Booster doses of 1.0 mL may be administered after 2 years.

Hepatitis A Vaccine

Not routinely recommended for immunization in pregnant lady. Hepatitis A vaccine (HAV) is produced from inactivated HAV; the theoretical risk to the developing fetus is expected to be low. The risk associated with vaccination should be weighed against the risk for hepatitis A in pregnant women who might be at high risk for exposure to HAV. Live vaccine is contraindicated in pregnancy.

Hepatitis B Vaccine

Pregnant women who are identified as being at risk for hepatitis B vaccine (HBV) infection during pregnancy (e.g. having more than one sex partner during the previous 6 months, been evaluated or treated for a sexually transmitted disease (STD), recent or current injection drug use, or having had a HBsAg-positive sex partner) should be vaccinated. Dose of vaccination is 1 mL I/M at 0, 1, and 6 months interval.

Meningococcal Vaccines

Meningococcal conjugate vaccines may be given to pregnant women who are at increased risk, e.g. complement component deficiency, e.g. C5–C9, properdin, factor H, factor D, etc. or functional or anatomic asplenia (including sickle cell anemia), human immunodeficiency viruses (HIV), etc. Two primary doses of meningococcal conjugate vaccines are required with booster doses every 5 years.

Serogroup B meningococcal vaccines should only be given to pregnant or breastfeeding women who are at increased risk for Serogroup B meningococcal disease if the benefits of receiving the vaccine outweigh the risk. Dose is 0.5 mL I/M.

Haemophilus influenzae Type B

Pregnant women with certain high-risk conditions, e.g. lack of a functioning spleen, need vaccination with Hib. It is safe to receive it at any time during pregnancy though not routinely recommended in immunization schedule.

Pneumococcal Polysaccharide Vaccine (PPSV23)

PPSV can be given in pregnant women if she is having high risk of getting pneumococcal infection/disease, i.e. DM, chronic lung disease, chronic cardiovascular diseases, cochlear implants, immunocompromising conditions, and functional or anatomic asplenia (e.g. sickle cell disease and other hemoglobinopathies, congenital or acquired asplenia, splenic dysfunction, or splenectomy).

Rabies Vaccine

If a pregnant lady gets exposed to category 2 or 3 bites by a wild animal/rabid dog or untraceable dog/cat she should get five doses of ARV I/M on 0, 3, 7, 14, 28 days with or without rabies immunoglobulin as per schedule without delay. If the risk of exposure to rabies is substantial, preexposure prophylaxis also might be indicated during pregnancy on 0, 3, 21 days or 0, 7, 21 days.

As an alternative to IM regimen, ID route can be used. Dose is 0.1 mL ID on both shoulders on 0, 3, 7, 28 days.

Yellow Fever Vaccine

Vaccines are live attenuated viral vaccines from the 17D lineage. As far as possible it should be avoided in pregnant women. Pregnant women should be advised against going to the rural areas of yellow fever endemic areas (and to urban areas of West African countries as well). However, where travel to an at-risk country is unavoidable, such women should be vaccinated. YF vaccines are given as a single dose (0.5 mL) injected either subcutaneously or intramuscularly.

■ VACCINATION IN CHILDREN

Every year vaccination prevents 2.5 million deaths globally. All the children immunized against vaccine preventable diseases can thrive and have better chances of survival with full potential. Hence immunization is, and should be recognized as, a core component of the human right to health. As part of a comprehensive package of interventions for disease prevention and control, vaccines and immunization is an essential investment in a country's—indeed, in the world's—future.

Now is the time for showing commitment to achieving the full potential of immunization. The vision for the Decade of Vaccines (2011–2020) is of a world in which all individuals and communities enjoy lives free from vaccine-preventable diseases. The mission of the Decade of Vaccines is to extend, by 2020 and beyond, the full benefit of immunization to all people, regardless of where they are born, who they are or where they live.

VACCINATION FOR CHILDREN AS PER NATIONAL IMMUNIZATION SCHEDULE

Vaccines routinely recommended for children as per National Immunization Schedule from birth onward are given here.

Bacillus Calmette-Guérin Vaccine

Bacillus Calmette-Guérin vaccine is a suspension of a live attenuated strain of mycobacterium. Reconstituted vaccine contains $8-32 \times 10^6$ colony forming units per mL and monosodium glutamate 1.5% w/v. BCG vaccination probably has little effect on preventing infection per se, or reactivation among those already infected with TB. However, there is strong evidence that BCG vaccination in infancy provides greater than 70% protection against severe disseminated forms of TB disease in young children, including miliary TB and tubercular meningitis. BCG vaccine should be stored at 2–8°C, not to be frozen and should be protected from light. Reconstituted vaccine is very unstable and must be stored at 2–8°C and used within one working session preferably of 4 h. Diluent of BCG vaccine is normal saline. Dose is 0.05 mL for infants less than 1 month, 0.1 mL for more than 1 month till 1 year by intradermal route, using 26–27 gauge needle as a single dose on left deltoid region only. Generally within 2–3 weeks of vaccination a small red papule forms and eventually ulcerates, it heals subsequently. Moderate-to-late preterm infants (gestational age > 31 weeks) and low-birth weight infants (<2,500 g) who are healthy and clinically stable can receive BCG vaccination at birth, or at the latest, upon discharge. Infants born to mothers treated with disease modifying anti-rheumatic drugs (DMARDS) (e.g. TNF-alpha blocking monoclonal antibodies) in the third trimester of pregnancy frequently have detectable antibodies for several months and they should not be vaccinated. Infants exposed to immunosuppressive treatment in utero or via breastfeeding should not receive BCG.

Precaution can be taken for neonates who are medically unstable or born of mothers who are HIV positive and HIV status of infant is not ascertained yet, till then it should be avoided.

Hepatitis B Vaccine

Monodose vial (0.5 mL) or prefilled syringe of hepatitis B vaccine contains 10 µg HBsAg protein, adsorbed onto 0.25 mg aluminum as aluminum hydroxide and it may contain yeast proteins also. Hepatitis B is given at birth along with OPV and BCG, as birth dose of hepatitis B, followed by three doses of a hepatitis B containing combination vaccine (e.g. pentavalent) at 6, 10, 14th week of life. As per UIP, birth dose is to be given within 24 h of birth only, if missed need not be given later, only three doses at 6, 10, 14th week can be given. For older children less than 20 years, if hepatitis B is missed earlier, a three dose schedule of pediatric formulation can be given at 0, 1, 6th month interval. For those more than 20 years, 1 mL I/M dose can be given at 0, 1, and 6th month.

Oral Poliovirus Vaccine

Two drops of Zero dose bivalent OPV is to be given to infant at birth or as soon as possible within 15 days followed by bOPV at 6, 10, and 14th week along with other vaccines. To ensure early protection a schedule of two fractional intradermal doses of inactivated polio vaccine administered at 6 and 14 weeks is added in the National Immunization Schedule. Site is right upper arm. There was a planned global switch from tOPV to bOPV in April 2016. A booster dose is given at 16–24 months of age.

GOI launched the Pulse Polio Abhiyan in 1995 as an immunization campaign by vaccinating all children under 5 years of age till poliomyelitis is eliminated from India. Since almost all the cases of polio come under 5 years, the upper age limit for vaccination in the campaign is 5 years for bOPV. The age range of polio might go up in well-immunized communities, due to the retardation of circulation of the causative wild polioviruses. The World Health Organization recommends to monitor all cases of acute flaccid paralysis in children up to 15 years and to investigate them for poliovirus etiology.

Pneumococcal Vaccine

The vaccine contains 0.02% polysorbate 80 (P80), 0.125 mg of aluminum as aluminum phosphate (AlPO4) adjuvant, 5 mL of succinate buffer, and no thiomersal preservative. Except for the addition of six serotypes, P80, and succinate buffer, the formulation of PCV13 is the same as that of PCV7. Dose is 0.5 mL I/M on anterolateral aspect of mid-thigh at 6 and 14th week followed by booster dose at 9 months of age or alternately as three primary doses 4/8 weeks apart.

Pentavalent Vaccine

Contains combination of five vaccines, i.e. diphtheria toxoid, pertussis, tetanus toxoid, Hib, and HepB vaccine. In 2000, before widespread introduction of Hib vaccine in resource-poor countries, Hib caused 8.13 million cases of serious disease in children aged 1–59 months with 371,000 deaths.

When Hib is given to a child greater than 12 months of age for the first time (who has not received pentavalent vaccine), only one dose is recommended. Hib vaccine is not required for healthy children after 5 years of age.

Pentavalent vaccine is given in a dose of 0.5 mL I/M on anterolateral aspect of mid-thigh at 6, 10, and 14th week of age. The need for early infant vaccination with DTP-containing vaccine, i.e. pentavalent vaccine is principally to ensure rapid protection against pertussis, because severe disease and death from pertussis is almost entirely limited to the first weeks and months of life. Despite high vaccination coverage (in 2014, 86% coverage with three doses of a pertussis containing vaccine) pertussis remains endemic in all countries and continues to be a public health concern. Pertussis containing vaccine (DPT, pentavalent vaccine, etc.) should be started as soon as 6 weeks of age and WHO recommends that primary series of immunization should ideally be completed by 6 months. It provides protection for at least 6 years. Only aP (acellular pertussis) containing vaccines should be used for vaccination of persons aged greater than or equal to 7 years.

Pentavalent vaccine is a freeze sensitive vaccine, and should be stored and transported at 2–8°C in ice lined refrigerators and vaccine carriers with conditioned ice packs.

From 2011-2015, India had the largest number of reported cases of diphtheria (18,350 cases) followed by Indonesia and Madagascar (3,203 and 1,633 cases, respectively). The first dose of vaccine should be given as early as 6 weeks of age, and the third dose completed by 6 months of age, i.e. 4-week interval between doses. DPT is given at 16-24 months of age as 1st booster and at 5-7 years as second booster dose.

Tetanus can be protected for life if at least six doses (three primary plus three booster doses) are provided to all people through routine childhood immunization schedules. WHO recommends three TT booster doses, ideally with at least 4 years between booster doses. These should be given at: 12-23 months of age; 4-7 years of age; 9-15 years of age.

In National Immunization Schedule, TT is given as pentavalent vaccine at 6, 10, 14 weeks, then as DPT vaccine at 16-24 months and at 5-7 years of age. Then, TT is given at 10 and 16 years of age. Pentavalent vaccine is not given beyond 1 year of age.

Rotavirus Vaccine

Rotaviruses (RVs) are globally the leading cause of severe, dehydrating diarrhea in young children. Two rotavirus vaccines are available. RV1 originates from a human strain, whereas RV5 contains five reassortants developed from rotaviruses of human and bovine origin. It is a live, oral, attenuated rotavirus vaccine. National Immunization Programme recommends three doses at 6, 10, and 14th week. Five drops are given orally along with pentavalent vaccine and OPV. Healthy children aged over 2 years are not considered necessary. Precautions for use of rotavirus vaccination include a history of intussusceptions or intestinal malformations, chronic gastrointestinal disease, and severe acute illness. Vaccination should be postponed when the child has ongoing acute gastroenteritis or fever with moderate to severe illness.

Measles Vaccine

Measles is one of the most contagious disease of humans, and in the absence of vaccination, about 95% of individuals would be infected with measles virus by 15 years of age. In 2000, measles was the fifth leading cause of childhood morbidity and mortality worldwide. There were an estimated 770,000 deaths, with more than half of these occurring in Africa. In 2015, there were an estimated 134,200 measles deaths globally, representing a 79% decline since 2000. All six WHO regions have measles elimination goals before or by 2020, and the GVAP, endorsed by the WHO, has a goal to eliminate measles in five of the six WHO regions by 2020.

Measles vaccination is a cost-effective measure in preventing morbidity and mortality with measles. Dose recommended is 0.5 mL S/C at 9-12 months of age and booster to be given at 16-24 months of age. Vaccinating infants before or at the age of 6 months often fails to induce seroconversion due to the immaturity of the immune system as well as the presence of neutralizing maternal antibodies. WHO recommends vaccination of infants from 6 months during a measles outbreak/epidemic, here the risk of measles among infants lesser than 9 m is high; infants travelling to countries experiencing measles outbreaks; infants known to be HIV infected or exposed. Measles administered before 9 months of age should be considered a supplementary dose and recorded as "Measles 0 (Zero)" dose, these infants should be immunized at recommended age as per schedule. Diluent for measles vaccine is double distilled water and reconstituted vaccine should be used within 2 h to prevent toxic shock syndrome due to contamination with *Staphylococcus aureus*.

VACCINATION FOR CHILDREN UNDER SPECIAL CIRCUMSTANCES (TABLES 1 AND 2)

Mumps Vaccine

The initial dose is recommended between the age of 12 and 18 months of age. The second dose is then typically given between 2 and 6 years of age. Usage after exposure in those not already immune may be useful. Combined vaccine in the form of MR, MMR, and MMRV can be given with minimum 4 weeks interval between two doses.

Rubella Vaccine

Usually a mild self-limited illness, rubella during early pregnancy may result in miscarriage, fetal death, or congenital defects known as Congenital Rubella Syndrome (CRS). Before introduction of rubella vaccine, the incidence of CRS varied from 0.1 to 0.2 per 1,000 live births during endemic periods and from 0.8 to 4 per 1,000 live births during rubella epidemics.

Most rubella vaccines are based on the live, attenuated RA 27/3 strain. Ninety-five to hundred percent of susceptible persons aged greater than or equal to 12 months develop rubella antibodies after a single dose of the vaccine. Dose schedule is 0.5 mL, S/C or I/M at 12–15 months of age.

Japanese Encephalitis Vaccine

JE virus is the leading cause of viral encephalitis in Asia, currently and estimated 3 billion people live in the 24 countries mainly in the WHO South East Asia and Western Pacific Regions, considered at risk of JE. It is estimated that 67,900 severe clinical cases of JE occur annually despite widespread availability of vaccine with approximately 13,600–20,400 deaths.

JE vaccines fall into four classes: inactivated mouse brain-derived vaccines, inactivated vero cell-derived alum-adjuvanted vaccine (SA14-14-2 strain) requires two intramuscular doses at 4-week intervals, starting at greater than or equal to 6 months of age in endemic settings. The dose is 0.5 m, IM.

Live attenuated vaccines with single dose of 0.5 mL SC at greater than or equal to 8 months of age.

Live recombinant (Chimeric) vaccines single dose at greater than or equal to 9 months of age. A single booster dose can be given 12–24 months later for those less than 18 years of age as booster for adults are not recommended as of now.

In our national immunization schedule 2 doses of live attenuated JE vaccine (SA-14-14-2) are given at 9–12 months and at 16–24 months of age in high endemic areas, e.g. in selected endemic districts of UP, Bihar, Assam, Karnataka, West Bengal. Diluent used for JE vaccine is phosphate buffer.

Chapter 57: Immunization in Pregnancy and Children

Table 1: National Immunization Schedule for children and pregnant women endorsed by IAPSM.

Vaccine	Dose and site	Schedule for children	Schedule for pregnant women
Tetanus toxoid (TT)	0.5 mL, IM	At 10 years and 16 years as boosters.	First dose as soon as pregnancy is diagnosed. Second dose, 4 weeks later. Only one booster if present pregnancy is within 3 years of the previous pregnancy with full immunization.
Bacillus Calmette-Guerin (BCG)	0.05 mL or 0.1 mL, ID	As soon as possible after birth till 1 month of age. If missed can be given till 1 year of age.	
Hepatitis B	0.5 mL, IM	Birth dose within 24 hr. Then as pentavalent vaccine at 6, 10, 14 weeks.	
bOPV	Two drops orally	At birth as zero dose, then 6, 10, 14 weeks. 16–24 months as booster. Also as a part of Pulse Polio Campaign.	
Pentavalent vaccine*	0.5 mL, IM	At 6, 10, 14 weeks.	
Fractional inactivated poliovirus vaccine (IPV)	0.1 mL, ID	At 6, 14 weeks.	
Rotavirus	5 drops orally	At 6, 10, 14 weeks.	
Measles	0.5 mL, SC	First dose at 9–12 months and second dose at 16–24 months.	
Vitamin A	1 lakh IU (1 mL) 2 lakh IU (2 mL)	At 9–12 months. Second dose at 16–24 months then repeated every 6 months till 5 years of age.	
Diphtheria, pertussis, tetanus (DPT)	0.5 mL, IM	At 16–24 months, and at 5 years of age, can be given upto 7 years.	
Pneumococcal conjugate vaccine	0.5 mL, IM	6, 14 weeks then booster at 9 months.	
Japanese encephalitis: Live attenuated vaccine	0.5 mL, SC	Two doses at 9–12 months then 16–24 months of age (in selected endemic states).	

*Contains diphtheria toxoid, pertussis, tetanus toxoid, hepatitis B, and *H. influenzae* type B.

Table 2: Other vaccines recommended under special circumstances.

Vaccine	Dose	Recommended in children under special circumstances*	Recommended in pregnant women under special circumstances*
TdaP	0.5 mL IM		Ideally at 27 and 36 weeks of pregnancy. But can be given at any time in pregnancy.
Hepatitis B	0.5 mL IM	0, 1, 6 months if not received earlier.	Pregnant women with increased risk can get 1 mL IM at 0, 1, 6 months.
Mumps	0.5 mL IM	12–18 months then second at 2–6 years of age.	
Rubella	0.5 mL IM, SC	12–15 months as single dose.	
Pneumococcal polysaccharide vaccine	0.5 mL IM, SC		Can be given as single dose.
Japanese encephalitis (JE) (inactivated vero cell)	0.5 mL SC	Two doses 4 weeks apart.	All should be vaccinated if travelling to high risk areas. 1.0 mL SC, on 0, 7, 30 days.
Inactivated influenza vaccine	0.5 mL IM		Single dose in pregnant women. 0.5 mL, IM.
Hepatitis A: inactivated	0.5 mL IM	Greater than 1 year age children then second at an interval of 6–12 months.	Single dose 0.5 mL, IM.
Hepatitis A: live	0.5 mL SC	Single dose.	
Meningococcal conjugate vaccine (quadrivalent)	0.5 mL IM	High risk children. Greater than 2 years as 0.5 mL single IM dose. 9–23 months should get two doses 3 months apart.	High risk pregnant women should get two primary doses with booster every 5 years depending on the conditions.
Meningococcal polysaccharide	0.5 mL IM Not recommended in less than 2 years children	High risk greater than 2 years old, booster 3–5 years later.	High risk pregnant women should get a dose with booster every 5 years.
Hib (*Haemophilus influenzae* type b)	0.5 mL IM	Greater than 1 year of age, only single dose.	High risk pregnant women should get single dose.

Contd...

Contd...

Vaccine	Dose	Recommended in children under special circumstances*	Recommended in pregnant women under special circumstances*
Typhoid vaccine (live attenuated Ty21a) Ty21a also as an oral capsule	0.5 mL IM Enteric-coated capsule	Greater than 6 months as a single dose. Three doses on alternate days (oral capsule).	
Typhoid vaccine unconjugated Vi polysaccharide (ViPS)	0.5 mL IM, SC	Greater than 2 years as a single dose.	
Cholera vaccine	Oral vaccine	2–5 years, three doses, 1–6 weeks apart. Greater than 5 years, two doses, 1–6 weeks apart recommended.	High risk pregnant women. Two doses, 1–6 weeks apart to help prevent spread.
Varicella vaccine	0.5 mL SC	Preferably starting at 12–18 months of age. Two doses, 4–12 weeks apart.	
Rabies vaccine	0.5/1 mL IM 0.1 mL ID	Depending on exposure/risk 0, 3, 7, 14, 28 days of schedule. 0, 3, 7, 28 days on both shoulders.	Depending on exposure/risk 0, 3, 7, 14, 28 days of schedule. 0, 3, 7, 28 days on both shoulders.
Human papilloma virus vaccine	0.5 mL IM	9–14 years age 0, 6 months or 0, 1–2, 6 months. 15–26 years age should get 0, 2, 6 months.	
Yellow fever vaccine	0.5 mL IM, SC	9–12 months of age.	

*All vaccines which are recommended in special circumstances must be given after consultation with qualified doctor.

Yellow Fever Vaccine

Vaccines are live attenuated viral vaccines from the 17D lineage. YF vaccines are given as a single dose (0.5 mL) injected either subcutaneously or intramuscularly at age 9–12 months at the same time as the measles vaccine. All unvaccinated travelers aged greater than 9 months and asymptomatic HIV-infected persons with CD4 T-cell counts greater than or equal to 200 cells/mm should get yellow fever vaccine. YF vaccine is contraindicated in children aged less than 6 months. It is not recommended for those aged 6–8 months, except during epidemics.

Typhoid Vaccine

Typhoid fever is an acute generalized infection, caused by a highly virulent and invasive enteric bacterium, *Salmonella typhi*. Global estimates of typhoid fever burden range between 11 and 21 million cases and approximately 128,000–161,000 deaths annually. The majority of cases occur in South/South-East Asia, and sub-Saharan Africa.

Currently three types of typhoid vaccines are licensed for use: (i) typhoid conjugate vaccine (TCV); (ii) unconjugated Vi polysaccharide (ViPS); and (iii) live attenuated Ty21a vaccines. The second and third types have been recommended by WHO since 2008 for the control of typhoid in endemic and epidemic settings. Typbar-TCV was first licensed in India in 2013 for intramuscular administration of a single dose (0.5 mL) in children aged 6 months and older. Each vaccine dose comprises 25 µg of purified Vi-capsular polysaccharide conjugated to tetanus toxoid. ViPS is licensed for use in individuals aged 2 years and older, to be administered subcutaneously or intramuscularly as a single dose of 0.5 mL. But booster dose may be given after 3 years.

The Ty21a vaccine is currently only available as enteric-coated capsules for oral administration on alternate days in a three-dose regimen (or a four-dose regimen in Canada and the USA).

Cholera Vaccine

Cholera is a rapidly dehydrating diarrheal disease caused by ingestion of toxin producing strains of serogroup O1, or less commonly, serogroup O139, of the bacterium *Vibrio cholerae*. Approximately 1.3 billion people are at risk of cholera in endemic countries. An estimated 2.86 million cholera cases (uncertainty range 1.3–4.0 m) occur annually in endemic countries. Among these cases, there are an estimated 95,000 deaths. About half of the cholera cases and deaths are estimated to occur in children less than or equal to 5 years of age. WC vaccines (Shanchol, Euvchol, and mORCVAX) (killed modified whole cell bivalent (O1 and O139) vaccine without the B subunit), two doses should be given 14 days apart to individuals greater than or equal to 1 year of age.

For WC-rBS vaccine (Dukoral) (killed whole cell monovalent (O1) vaccines), three doses should be given to children 2–5 years of age, and two doses to children aged greater than or equal to 6 years and adults, with an interval of 1–6 weeks between doses in both groups.

Rabies Vaccine

If a child gets exposed to category 2 or 3 bites by a wild animal/rabid dog or untraceable dog/cat he/she should get five doses of ARV IM on 0, 3, 7, 14, 28 days with or without rabies immunoglobulin as per schedule without delay. If the risk of exposure to rabies is substantial, pre-exposure prophylaxis also might be indicated on 0, 3, 21 days or 0, 7, 21 days.

As an alternative to IM regimen, ID route can be used. Dose is 0.1 mL ID on both shoulders on 0, 3, 7, 28 days.

Human Papilloma Virus Vaccine

Persistent infection by oncogenic HPV types is a prerequisite for the development of cervical cancer, which each year hits about 528,000 women and causes 266,000 deaths worldwide. The viral types 16 and 18 HPV are the most common types in invasive cervical cancer, accounting for about 70% of all cervical cancers. In total, 85% of cervical cancer cases occur in the less developed regions and mortality rates vary as much as 18-fold between industrialized and developing countries. Other manifestations of HPV infection include vaginal, vulvar, penile, oropharyngeal, and anal cancers. In addition, HPV types 6 and 11 cause anogenital warts and recurrent respiratory papillomatosis. HPV is mainly transmitted sexually.

Recommended target population for the prevention of cervical cancer is females aged 9-14 years, prior to becoming sexually active.

Three prophylactic HPV vaccines are in use directed against high-risk HPV types. The quadrivalent vaccine (e.g. Gardasil) was first licensed in 2006. It contains noninfectious protein antigens for HPV 6, 11, 16, and 18. The bivalent vaccine was licensed in 2007 and contains noninfectious protein antigens for HPV 16 and 18. The nonavalent vaccine (e.g. Gardasil 9) licensed in 2014 contains noninfectious protein antigens for HPV 6, 11, 16, 18, 31, 33, 45, 52, and 58.

Dose is 0.5 mL, I/M. Two dose schedule for 9-14 years old children are 0, 6-12 months. Three dose schedules for 9-14 years are 0, 2, 6 months. For more than 15 years old, three dose schedule is recommended at 0, 2, 6 months interval.

Varicella Vaccine

Varicella (chickenpox) is an acute, highly contagious disease with worldwide distribution caused by the varicella zoster virus (VZV). In temperate climates, most cases occur before the age of 10 years. Based on conservative estimates, the global annual varicella disease burden would include 4.2 million severe complications leading to hospitalization and 4,200 deaths. In the prevaccine era in high-income developed countries, case fatality rates for varicella were approximately 3 per 100,000 cases.

Two doses of varicella vaccine are recommended and should be administered at 12-18 months of age as 0.5 mL S/C dose 3 months apart till 12 years of age. For more than 12 years, two doses of 0.5 mL each can be given as S/C injection 4 weeks apart.

COLD CHAIN

Vaccines are sensitive biological products. Some vaccines are sensitive to freezing, some to heat and others to light. Vaccine potency, meaning its ability to adequately protect the vaccinated patient, can diminish when the vaccine is exposed to inappropriate temperatures. Once lost, vaccine potency cannot be regained if it is lost anytime between manufacturing site to administration site.

The storage and transportation of vaccine from the site of manufacturing to the site of utilization under optimum temperature (2–8°C) in known as cold chain.

Freeze sensitive vaccines are: cholera DTP, hepatitis B, Hib, IPV (hexavalent), pentavalent, human papillomavirus (HPV), inactivated poliovirus, influenza, pneumococcal, rotavirus (liquid and freeze-dried), tetanus, DT, Td.

Vaccines that are as sensitive to light as they are to heat include BCG, measles, measles–rubella, measles–mumps–rubella, and rubella. These vaccines are often supplied in dark glass vials.

A vaccine vial monitor (VVM) is a label containing a heat sensitive material which is placed on a vaccine vial to register cumulative heat exposure over time.

ADVERSE EVENTS FOLLOWING IMMUNIZATION

Immunization is among the most cost-effective public health interventions. It has led to the global eradication of smallpox as well as the elimination of poliomyelitis in regions of the world. Immunization currently averts an estimated 2–3 million deaths from diphtheria, tetanus, pertussis (whooping cough), and measles every year in all age groups. Unlike drugs, the expectations from vaccinations are much higher and problems arising from the vaccine or vaccination are less acceptable to the general public. Allegations that vaccines/vaccination cause adverse events must be dealt with rapidly and effectively as it can undermine confidence in a vaccine and ultimately have dramatic consequences for immunization coverage and disease incidence long after proof is generated that the adverse event was not caused by vaccine (e.g. autism and MMR, encephalopathy and pertussis). Adverse event following immunization (AEFI): This is defined as any untoward medical occurrence which follows immunization and which does not necessarily have a causal relationship with the use of the vaccine. The adverse event may be any unfavorable or unintended sign, an abnormal laboratory finding, a symptom or a disease.

All vaccines should be given under medical supervision after consultation with a qualified medical practitioner. Before starting any immunization session, kindly ensure the availability of emergency tray with all necessary drugs and equipment.

CHAPTER 58

Insect Bite (Arthropods: Bites, Stings, and Other Contacts)

Au Kin Heng Constantine

INTRODUCTION

An arthropod is an invertebrate animal with a segmented body and paired, jointed appendages, and an exoskeleton. The name *arthropod* is based on the Greek *arthr-*, meaning joint, and *pod*, meaning foot. Arthropods comprise 84% of all animal species on Earth (**Fig. 1**). Entomologists classify arthropods into classes, orders, families, genera, and species. Common orders include Blattaria (cockroaches), Coleoptera (beetles), Diptera (flies and mosquitos), Ephemeroptera (mayflies), Hemiptera (wasps, ants, and bees), Isoptera (termites), Lepidoptera (butterflies and moths), Odonata (dragonflies and damselflies), Orthoptera (grasshoppers and crickets), Phthiraptera (lice), and Siphonaptera (fleas). As health care professionals, it is often not necessary to be aware of this detailed classification. A description of the morphology of arthropods may be good enough for clinical practice. The following are some arthropods

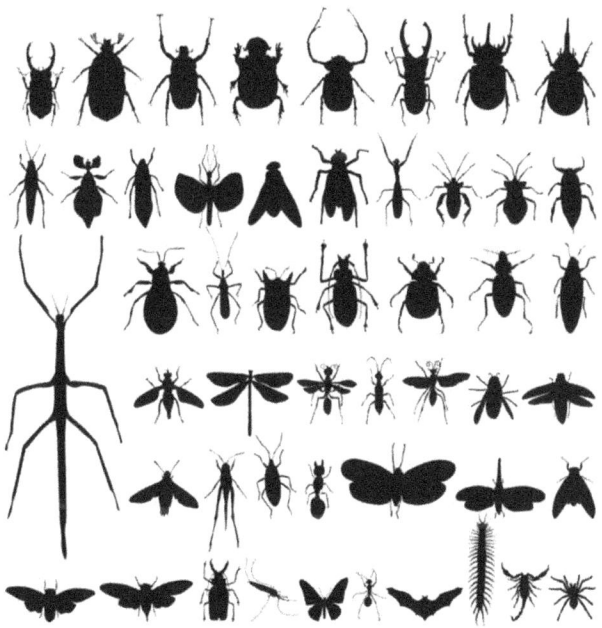

Fig. 1: Different types of arthropods.

that have medical significance. Adult insects consist of six legs and three body regions (head, thorax, and abdomen), and some insects have wings. Adult spiders have eight legs and two body regions (cephalothorax and abdomen). Adult mites and adult ticks have eight legs and one body region but no true mouth (with mouthparts only). Adult scorpions have eight legs with a broad flat body region and a tail with a stinger. Adult centipedes have a pair of legs in each body segment. The number of body segments is numerous and the shape is usually flat. Adult millipedes have two pairs of legs in each body segment and the number of body segments is numerous and the shape is usually cylindrical. Because millions of arthropod species exist on Earth, this chapter can only include common ones that have medical significance. Stress is put on the general principles. Travel has become very popular and many exotic regions have become accessible. In managing a patient who has a recent travel history, clinicians should think about the possibility of arthropod-related diseases of the destinations. Delusion of parasitosis and other psychiatric diagnoses like amphetamine bugs must be excluded.

ETIOLOGY

Commonly Encountered Arthropods

Because millions if not billions of different arthropod species exist on Earth, the following discussion only includes those ones that people commonly encounter. Adult arthropods may look very different from larval/developmental stages. Please consult a biologist, entomologist, veterinary surgeon, or poison center if needed.

PATHOPHYSIOLOGY

Exposure to arthropods can be experienced via bites, stings, local irritation causing local infection, systemic hypersensitivity, anemia, ingestion, and arthropod-borne diseases. Venom and irritating chemicals complicate the condition. The proceeding section is a brief summary of the common contacts (**Table 1**).

Locally

Blockages of Orifices and Skin Attachment

Small arthropods may enter and block any orifices of our body. Sometimes arthropod body parts remain lodged. A tick may stick strongly on the skin.

Local Wounds

Bites, stings, and even scratching by arthropod feet might result in local wounds. The wounds are usually small. Some wounds may carry foreign bodies. Bees leave their stings behind. Mouthparts may be broken. Soil or other dirt may be present. Local inflammation with increased blood flow, increased capillary permeability, and increased white cell count are common. The severity of a rash can range from local pain, itchiness, and swelling that lasts for a few hours to extensive swelling that lasts for days. As with every wound, local infection by superimposed bacteria can happen. Cellulitis, necrosis, and sepsis may follow.

Table 1: Common arthropods that have contact with humans.

Arthropod	Nature of contact/wounds and harm	Transmission of diseases	Remark
Ants			
Ants (worldwide)	Bite and sting. Skin lesion is erythematous with a central wheal. Later, pustules may develop.	Not known	
Fire ants (worldwide), harvester ants (USA), and velvet ants (USA)	Painful sting. Skin lesion is erythematous with a central wheal. Later, pustules may develop. Re-exposure can lead to serious systemic reactions.	Not known	
Bees			
Bees (worldwide)	Sting. The wound shows local swelling with a central white spot with erythematous halos. Re-exposure can lead to serious systemic reactions.	Not known	
Honey bees (worldwide), bumble bees (worldwide), and Africanized honey bees (in Central and South America, Mexico, and USA)	Painful stings. The wound shows local swelling with a central white spot with erythematous halos. Re-exposure can lead to serious systemic reactions.	Not known	
Beetles			
Beetles (worldwide)	Most are benign (except blister beetles).	Not known	
Blister beetles (worldwide)	Secrete irritating chemicals causing kidney failure, cardiovascular collapse, coma, and even death.	Not known	Cantharidin penetrates the skin and pederin causes blisters
Bugs			
Bed bugs (worldwide)	Bite and suck blood from humans. Red blotches grouped in linear pattern with urticarial wheals and sometimes bullous.	Suspected	

Contd...

Contd...

Arthropod	Nature of contact/wounds and harm	Transmission of diseases	Remark
Conenose bugs (in the Americas)	Bite at night. Feed on human blood. Variable lesions.	Vectors for *Trypanosoma cruzi* that causes Chagas disease via fecal contamination of the bite.	
Wheel bugs (USA)	Painful bite. Lesion shows swelling, inflammation, and induration.	Not known	
Caterpillars			
Urticating caterpillars (worldwide)	Venomous hairs or spines that can sting or irritate the skin with immediate burning sensation. Variable lesions. Burning sensation.	Not known	The venom of *Lonomia* in South America contains anticoagulants
Centipedes			
Centipedes (worldwide)	Painful bite. Typical lesions show two hemorrhagic punctures.	Not known	Cytolysin-based venom
Cockroaches			
Cockroaches (worldwide)	Food contamination and possibly allergy. Bite occasionally. Blocking orifices.	Many bacteria, fungi, or viruses mechanically	
Earwigs			
Earwigs (worldwide)	Relatively harmless. Abdominal cerci of larger ones may pinch human skin. Trivial lesion.	Not known	Some live in water wells
Fleas			
Adult fleas (worldwide)	Bite and feed on blood. The lesions varies from one species to another.	Plague (*Yersinia pestis*), rickettsial diseases (murine typhus, *Rickettsia typhi*). An intermediate host of dog tapeworm (*Dipylidium caninum*).	

Contd...

Contd...

Arthropod	Nature of contact/wounds and harm	Transmission of diseases	Remark
Flies			
Flies (biting)			
Black flies (worldwide)	The lesion has variable patterns with systemic reactions.	Onchocerciasis	
Congo floor maggot (sub-Sahara Africa and Cape Verde Islands)	Myiasis. Nocturnal bite blood-feeding larvae. The lesion is usually a pinprick.	Not known	
Deer flies (worldwide)	Painful bites. The lesion is deep and singular; cellulitis.	Tularemia (deer fly fever/rabbit fever) and loiasis (Loa loa)	
Horse flies (worldwide)	Painful bites. The lesion is deep and singular; cellulitis.	Not known	
Biting midges (worldwide)	Bite. The lesion is minute papular in pattern with erythematous halo. Wheals may occur.	Oropouche fever (a virus in the Simbu group of *Bunyaviridae*)	
Sand flies (worldwide)	Bite and suck blood. Lesions may be red papules or wheals.	Leishmaniasis (*Leishmania donovani*), bartonellosis (*Bartonella bacilliformis*), and sand fly fever	
Stable flies (worldwide)	Bites. The lesions are small evanescent vesicles.	Not known	
Tsetse flies (tropical Africa)	Bites. The lesions are small punctures with hemorrhaging.	African trypanosomiasis (*Trypanosoma brucei*)	
Flies (nonbiting)			
House flies/filth flies (worldwide)	Do not bite. They may contaminate food and water and may cause myiasis.	Transmission of disease is mainly carried out mechanically. More serious examples include typhoid, cholera, and dysentery.	

Contd...

Contd...

Arthropod	Nature of contact/wounds and harm	Transmission of diseases	Remark
Eye gnats (almost worldwide)	Do not bite but may scratch the eyes.	Yaws (*Treponema pertenue*) and pinkeye are transmitted by eye gnats.	
Nonbiting midges (worldwide)	Hypersensitivity reactions in the eyes or respiratory tract.	Not known	Mass emergence of nonbiting midges may cause traffic accident and other nuisances.
Flies (nonbiting) and myiasis			
Human bot flies (Central and South America and Mexico)	Do not bite but may cause myiasis. Superficial, painful, swollen with a central opening.	Not known	
The larvae of screwworm flies (Central and South America, South Pacific region, and tropical Africa)	Extensive damage to human tissues and cause pocket-like sinuses. Fatal myiasis.	Not known	
Tumbu flies (tropical Africa)	Red or shiny nodules and furuncular myiasis.	Not known	
Wohlfahrtia flies consist of *W. magnifica* (Arabian Peninsula, Asia, North Africa, and southern Europe)	Myiasis. Causes deep lesions.	Not known	
W. vigil (Canada and Northern USA).	Myiasis. Causes papules or pustules.	Not known	
Lice			
Body lice (worldwide)	Bites and feeds on human blood. The lesion are red papules, 3–4 mm in diameter, with purpuric halo.	Epidemic typhus (*Rickettsia prowazeki*), trench fever (*Bartonella quintana*), and louse-born relapsing fever (*Borrelia recurrentis*)	Not the bite but crushing the lice and their feces into skin transmits these diseases.

Contd...

Contd...

Arthropod	Nature of contact/wounds and harm	Transmission of diseases	Remark
Head lice (worldwide)	Irritate the skin and may cause secondary infection. Itchy scalp is the common presentation.	Not known	
Pubic lice (worldwide)	Irritates the skin and may cause secondary infection. The lesion is variable and may present as blue spots.	Not known	
Millipedes (worldwide)	May burn the skin. The lesions range from yellow to brown. Blisters may be present.	Not known	
Mites			
Chigger mite (worldwide)	Irritation and itchiness on the skin. The lesion is variable and may present as a red, dome-shaped papule.	Scrub typhus in Asia	
House dust mites (worldwide)	Do not bite but cause allergies, especially in the respiratory tract.	Not known	
Biting mites (worldwide)	Painful bites. The lesions vary.	May possibly transmit rickettsial pox.	
Scabies mites (worldwide)	Intense itchiness and secondary infection. Burrows and papules are formed on the skin.	Not known	
Follicle mites (worldwide)	Live on human skin and are usually harmless.	Not known	
Mosquitos (worldwide)	Bite and cause puncture, hemorrhages, popular lesions or wheals with edema.	Malaria (*Plasmodium vivax, Plasmodium ovale, Plasmodium malariae,* and *Plasmodium falciparum*), yellow fever (*flavivirus*), dengue fever (DEN-1, DEN-2, DEN-3, and DEN-4), Rift Valley fever, Ross River virus disease, and chikungunya fever. Mosquitos transmit	

Contd...

Contd...

Arthropod	Nature of contact/wounds and harm	Transmission of diseases	Remark
		lymphatic filariasis (*Brugia malayi*), and many other filarial worms. Encephalitides transmitted by mosquitos include Eastern equine encephalomyelitis, Western equine encephalitis, Venezuelan equine encephalitis, Japanese encephalitis, St. Louis encephalitis, West Nile encephalitis (West Nile virus), and La Crosse encephalitis.	
Moths			
Moths (worldwide)	Stinging hairs or spines cause skin irritation. Some body parts may detach and cause irritation in the respiratory system. Skin lesions vary.	Not known	
Pentastomes/tongue worms			
Pentastomes/tongue worms (worldwide)	Reside in human liver, spleen, lungs, throat, and eustachian tubes. They are benign and may cause irritation in the throat.	Not known	
Scorpions			
Scorpions (worldwide)	Sting painfully and some species give fatal venomous sting to humans. Lesions vary.	Not known	
Spiders			
Violin spider (Africa, Australia, South America, and USA)	Bites cause variable lesions plus necrotic wounds and possible hemolytic anemia.	Not known	

Contd...

Contd...

Arthropod	Nature of contact/wounds and harm	Transmission of diseases	Remark
Widow spiders (worldwide)	Bite causes two small puncture wounds, and neurotoxic venom may be fatal. Myocarditis and dyspnea can occur as well.	Not known	
Hobo spiders (Europe and USA)	Bite is usually painless at first. Induration followed by expanding erythema and blister. Necrosis may develop with eschar formation.	Not known	
Sydney funnel web spiders (Australia)	Bite site may be extremely painful. Death within 1 hour.	Not known	The venom acts on the somatic and autonomic nerves, quickly causing hypotension and apnea.
Tarantula spiders (USA)	Painful bites. The urticating hair may cause much irritation on the skin and mucosal surfaces.	Not known	
Ticks			
Ticks (worldwide)	Bite and feed on human blood. The lesion is a red papule with erythema. Hypersensitivity to tick saliva causes erythematous ring. Tick-paralysis is caused by the neurotoxin in tick saliva.	Babesiosis (protozoan; Europe and USA), Colorado tick fever (virus; Canada and USA), Crimean-Congo hemorrhagic fever (virus; Africa, Asia, and Europe), Kyasanur Forest disease (virus; India), Lyme disease (spirochetes; Australia, China, Europe, Japan, and USA), relapsing fever (spirochetes worldwide), *Rickettsiae* (many diseases, e.g. African tick bite fever in sub-Saharan Africa;	

Contd...

Contd...

Arthropod	Nature of contact/wounds and harm	Transmission of diseases	Remark
		American boutonneuse fever/maculatum fever in the Americas; boutonneuse fever/Mediterranean fever in Africa; ehrlichiosis and anaplasmosis in the USA; Japanese spotted fever in East Asia, Japan, Mediterranean, and the Middle East; North Asian tick typhus/Siberian tick typhus in Central Asia, Mongolia, and Siberia; Queensland tick typhus in Australia; Rocky Mountain spotted fever in the western hemisphere; tick-borne lymphadenopathy in Europe), tick-borne encephalitis (virus in Europe), and tularemia (bacterium in Canada, Europe, Japan, Mexico, Russia, USA)	
Wasps			
Yellow jackets (worldwide), hornets (worldwide), and paper wasps (worldwide)	Give painful stings and may cause allergic reactions. The lesion is central white spot with erythematous halo. The degree of local swelling varies. Re-exposure can lead to serious systemic reactions.	Not known	

Invasion of Human Tissues: Myiasis

Myiasis means infestation of larvae of flies in the organs or tissues of humans or other animals. Myiasis can be classified into intentional therapeutic myiasis, accidental myiasis, facultative myiasis, and obligate myiasis. Therapeutic myiasis is to use larvae for wound debridement. The use was very common before the antibiotics era. Accidental myiasis occurs when eggs are ingested accidentally. The larvae may survive for a short while, which is considered a relatively benign condition. The patient may complain of stomach pain, nausea, and vomiting, which is also known as pseudomyiasis because of the lack of full development of a fly. In facultative myiasis, a larva leaves the necrotic tissue and invades the healthy tissue, causing pain and damage. Screwworm flies and human bot flies may develop in human tissue. Tissue damage and occasional death may occur.

Systemic
Allergic Reaction or Hypersensitivity

Allergic reaction or hypersensitivity is usually classified into Type I (IgE-mediated), Type II (cytotoxic reaction), Type III (antibody–antigen complex), and Type IV (T-lymphocytes and macrophages). Type I, II, and III are usually immediate in onset, whereas Type IV usually has a delayed onset of a few hours to days. The venom, protein substances, and foreign bodies infiltrated by stings and bites can certainly cause allergic reaction. Beware that a simple contact by an arthropod on the skin or mucous area can cause allergy.

Local allergic reaction is usually irritating and may subside in a few hours. However, if the site involved is the throat or head and neck region, a severe local reaction can compromise the airway. Severe systemic allergic reaction can occur if the allergens reach the blood or lymphatic circulation and different organs are involved. Anaphylaxis is one of the worst forms of systemic presentation of hypersensitivity. It is usually quick in onset, with obstruction in the upper airway and the lower airway. Swelling in the lips and tongue, dyspnea, and wheezing may be found. Pruritus, urticaria, erythema, and angioedema are found on the skin. Cardiovascular collapse may occur due to peripheral vasodilation, increased vascular permeability, and possibly arrhythmia.

Anemia

Anemia, ranging from mild to severe, may occur depending on the number of bites and duration of bites.

Ingestion and Food Contamination

For some readers, eating arthropods may be an alien idea. However, people do eat arthropods. For example, scorpions are roasted or cooked in other ways in China. It is believed that the venom of scorpions is heat liable. Some may consume scorpions raw with the tail and stinger removed. If the preparation is not perfect, the venom may enter the body via the gastrointestinal tract. Gastric acid and other enzymes may denature the venom though. Some players of survival games eat scorpions and black widow spiders. Ingestion of the arthropods, their body parts, or chemicals may be accidental as well. Cockroaches, flies, and other arthropods may contaminate food by their body parts, fluids, feces, etc.

Venom and other Irritating Chemicals

Arthropods have many venoms and irritating chemicals. Here are some common examples.

Necrotic Venom

The venom in bees and wasps has phospholipase A. The venom in violin spiders has lipase and hyaluronidase. Possibly, the lipase induces neutrophil chemotaxis, causing tissue necrosis.

Neurotoxic Venom

Tick paralysis is caused by a neurotoxin and the presentation resembles Guillain–Barré syndrome. The venom in widow spiders is a kind of neuromuscular-damaging protein. It affects ion transport, leading to sweating, muscular spasm, weakness, paralysis, and convulsions. Scorpion venom contains multiple low-molecular weight proteins, salts, mucus, and some other organic compounds. The low-molecular weight proteins increase the permeability of the sodium channel in the neuromuscular junction and the autonomic nervous system. Presentation includes blurred vision, paralysis, abnormal eye movement, excessive salivation, convulsion, respiratory paralysis, myocarditis, and death.

Other Venoms

In the bites of blister beetles, cantharidin penetrates the skin and pederin causes the blisters. *Lonomia* (a caterpillar in South America) venom contains anticoagulants and may cause severe bleeding. Centipedes bite with a cytolysin-based venom.

Respiratory Tract Reaction

House dust mites cause allergic reaction presented as asthma-like attacks. Other arthropods can cause allergic reaction in the respiratory tract as well.

CLINICAL PRESENTATION

Local

In terms of skin or scalp presentation, arthropod contact ranges from no obvious sign to mild rash, papules, nodules, and necrotic tissue. The patient may have minimal complaints like light itchiness, light pain to severe itchiness, and pain.

Systemic

Anaphylaxis, fever, sepsis, anemia, weight loss, and other signs may be present. Alternation in consciousness, coma, and even death. They may be caused by the contact alone or by the diseases transmitted.

RED FLAGS

More signs and more diseases may be present on top of the wound or rash after arthropod contact.

Patients may not recall any bites, stings, or contact with an arthropod. Skin signs or wounds may not be obvious even for a poisonous widow spider. Clinicians are encouraged to seek more information about the arthropods that resided in their regions of practice.

A patient may correctly recall an overseas trip, but details of a local trip may not be recalled as vividly. Offer hints like any contacts with wild or domestic animals, any local parks, woods, etc.

For any patients with fever of unknown origin, unaccounted symptoms or signs, exposure to arthropods must be excluded.

Warn a patient about delayed hypersensitivity, which may have an onset in terms of days.

A skin rash, wound, nodule, ulcer, etc. with a history of arthropod contact can be caused by other diseases. Exclude allergic reaction against an antigen other than an arthropod. Exclude melanoma, basal cell cancer, and squamous cell cancer. Think of other causes of anemia. Sometimes tests for allergens and biopsy may be needed. Psychiatric illness, substance abuse, and withdrawal should be excluded.

EVALUATION

History

Bites are common in many regions, especially in tropical and subtropical areas, but a patient may not be aware. Ask for any possibility of arthropod contact. If there was an arthropod contact, ask what, where, when, and how the contact was made. Check the arthropod identity—the body shape, wings, number of legs, mouth parts, stingers, etc. Adult arthropods may look very different from larval/developmental stages. **Figure 1** may help in identification. Characteristics of the place like plants may help. Travel history must be checked. In addition to overseas travel, a hiking trip in the neighborhood may result in arthropod contacts. Ask for details of the trip like the location, water source, plants, etc. Check the photos taken during the trip, they may give some hints. Change in occupation, residence, hobbies, or recent cleaning of lodgings may give rise to arthropod contact. Ask for similar presentation in family members and friends because they may share the same exposure.

Physical Examination

Do not take arthropod bites or contact lightly. More signs and more diseases may be present on top of the wound or rash.
- Beware of life-threatening signs, either present or in progression. Look for signs of severe allergic reaction like difficulty in breathing and hypotension.
- Do not focus only on the wound. Do a general examination. In the general examination, look for pallor, jaundice, edema, lymph nodes, and splenomegaly. Look for signs of possible diseases transmitted. Check for fever. A simple contact does not usually cause fever.

- Check the wounds. Note the severity of swelling and the location. A swelling in the head, neck, and throat regions demand special care.
- The pattern and distribution of the rash, if any, may give a hint of the culprit.

INTERPRETATION OF FINDING

It is important to grade the result of the contact. Do not miss any life-threatening conditions. Think about the possibility of transmitted diseases. Think of the differential diagnosis. A skin rash, wound, nodule, ulcer, etc. with a history of arthropod contact can be caused by other diseases, even malignant ones. Psychiatric illness, substance abuse, and withdrawal should be excluded.

INVESTIGATIONS

Most arthropod-related cases do not need any investigation. For those severe cases, use the white blood cells (WBCs), blood film (e.g. malaria and other parasites), and viral titer, e.g. dengue virus (usually two titers are needed to see the trend). For patients with possible organ failure, check the renal function and liver function. For suspected myocarditis, arrange cardiac enzymes and echocardiogram.

A skin rash, wound, nodule, ulcer, etc. with a history of arthropod contact can be caused by other diseases. Exclude melanoma, basal cell cancer, and squamous cell cancer. Think of other causes of anemia. Sometimes tests for allergens and biopsy may be needed.

TREATMENT

Treatment includes prevention of bites, prevention of arthropod-borne infection, local wound care, supportive care, allergy (mild-to-severe), and antivenom.

Prevention

As in every aspect of medicine, prevention plays an important role. Avoid contact with arthropods.

Personal Protection

Avoid using perfume in the wild because perfume may attract arthropods. Similarly, sweat may attract arthropods.

Avoid contact with ants because they may be fire ants. Do not go near bee hives.

Avoid contact with wild animals. For domestic animals like pet dogs, use tick and flea collars or other products to repel ticks and fleas. Regular washing with antiarthropod shampoo helps to remove fleas and ticks. For other domestic animals like horses, seek advice from veterinary surgeons for prevention of arthropods. Do not handle any sick or dead animals, even pets, unprotected. Always wear gloves, etc. For bedbugs, professional pest control may be needed.

Wear long sleeves, long pants, etc. to protect the skin. Proper use of repellents like DEET or the use of insecticides in the garden may help. Beware of allergies caused by repellents and insecticides. Beware that many commercial insect repellents or folk remedies may not work.

Arthropods may hide in shoes, socks, pockets of shirts, blankets, bed linens, etc. Flip and check before use.

The Environment

General hygiene and proper handling of food and wastage can reduce the chance of survival of cockroaches, flies, and other arthropods. The mosquito *Aedes aegypti* can spread dengue fever, yellow fever, Zika virus, and chikungunya. Avoid stagnant water so that its eggs cannot develop properly. *Aedes aegypti* are most active just after sunrise and just before sunset but can bite at night. Anopheles mosquitoes, the vector for malaria, are active at dusk or dawn and active at night. Plan the activities accordingly. Mosquito nets, window screens, and bed nets can reduce the chance of mosquito contact. Dust mites can be prevented by regular and proper mattress cleaning. Furniture can be treated with both heat and steam. Isolation, either of a patient or others, is needed for scabies and hair lice until treated.

Vaccines and Prophylaxis

A vaccine is available for yellow fever. Prophylaxis against malaria is also available. Advice from a travel clinic will be useful. Make sure to receive a consultation as early as possible. Some vaccines or prophylaxes need repeated doses. For yellow fever, usually only government agencies have the drugs and appointments may be tight.

Food Storage and Preparation

Food, raw or cooked, should be stored properly to prevent contamination by arthropods. Food must be properly cooked before consumption.

After Exposure

Do not Crush the Arthropod

Crushing a mosquito while it is biting on the skin may be a second reflex for many people. Crushing a mosquito is relatively safe. For some arthropods, it may not be that safe. Epidemic typhus (*Rickettsia prowazeki*), trench fever (*Bartonella quintana*), and louse-born relapsing fever (*Borrelia recurrentis*) are transmitted by crushing the lice and their feces on the skin. Crushing also destroys the identity of the arthropod. Take a photo of the culprit, if safe. Take note of the number of legs, color, shape, etc. of the arthropod.

Local Wound

The usual wound care must be conducted. Check for foreign bodies. Look for unusual swelling, necrosis, or sign of infection. In terms of treatment of local wounds, think of AI's: antihistamine, analgesics, antibiotics, antitetanus, (adrenaline/epinephrine (for anaphylaxis)), ice, and steroid. The possible route of administration can be topical, oral, intramuscular, subcutaneous, and intravenous. Local antihistamine cream may work for simple itchiness. Oral analgesics are usually good enough. Consider local antibiotics cream. Oral or even intravenous (IV) antibiotics may be needed for infected wounds. Because bites or stings may carry soil, the antitetanus status of the patients should be checked. Adrenaline is included here so as to stress the importance to exclude anaphylaxis. Steroid cream may be needed for severe itchiness. Beware of the adverse effects of treatment especially for ice and steroid.

Blockage of Orifice

If an arthropod blocks an orifice, removal must be done carefully. Light may sometimes guide an arthropod to exit an orifice. Olive oil may float an arthropod out of the orifice. Removal of embedded arthropods like maggots must be planned carefully. Breakage of the maggots may lead to hypersensitivity. Consult a clinical microbiologist, entomologist, a poison center, or a veterinary surgeon for the necessary precaution and prophylaxis before removal.

Remaining Stings and Ticks

Removal of a remaining sting must be done carefully so as not to squeeze remaining toxin and chemicals into the skin. Consider using a card to scrub the sting out. Ticks can be removed with a forceps or a tweezers with gentle traction. Consult experts if in doubt.

Systemic

Look for signs and symptoms of allergic reaction. Antihistamine local or oral is usually enough for mild reaction. Add steroid, if needed, but with caution. IV antihistamine (e.g. diphenhydramine 1 mg/kg) and IV steroid are necessary for moderate reaction. Adrenaline, subcutaneous (SC), IM, or IV is needed for severe life-threatening reaction. Some patients carry an Epi-pen with them. In the prehospital setting, these patients may need help in the administration of Epi-pens. Ventolin puff can relieve bronchospasm. Support the airway, breathing, and circulation with oxygen supply, intubation, IV fluid, and inotropes as the conditions require. Anaphylaxis means intensive care unit (ICU) care.

Always think of delayed hypersensitivity. If in doubt or because of a relatively high number of bites or stings, admit the patient for observation.

Specific Treatment

Permethrin can kill *Sarcoptes scabiei* (scabies) and lice. Other treatments are also available. Isolation, conduct contact tracing and treat all the contacts. Careful surgical exploration and removal may be needed in some types of myiasis. Bursting of the maggots must be avoided. Infested tissues may be cleansed with nitrofurazone. Antivenoms exist for certain bites and stings (e.g. for certain species in scorpions and black widow spiders). Please contact a local poison center for advice. Professional pest control may be needed for certain arthropods. Please refer to the relevant chapters of this book for the treatment of the diseases transmitted. Please consult a microbiologist, entomologist, veterinary surgeon, or poison center if needed.

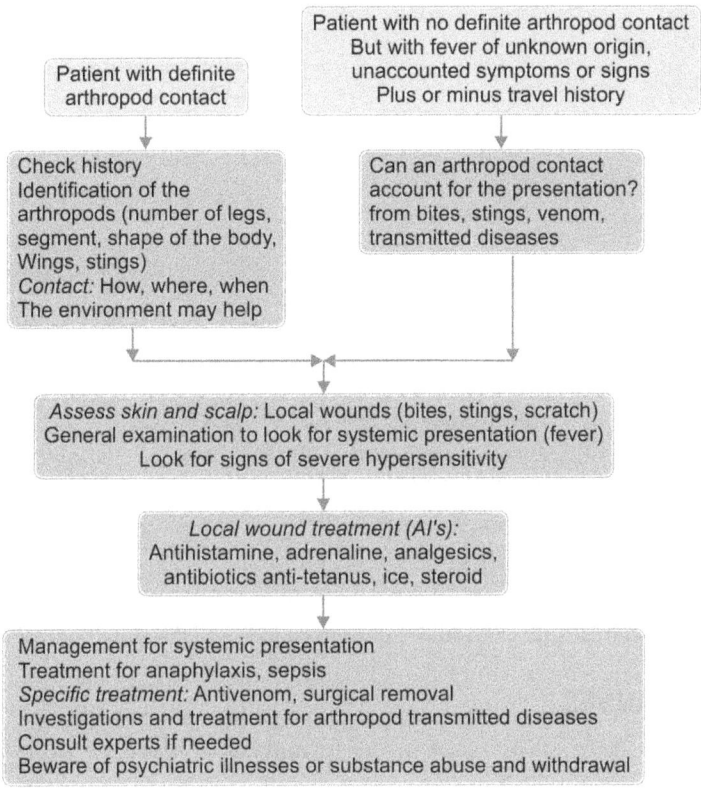

Flowchart 1: Summary of approach to patient with insect bite.

Follow-up

For most bites, follow-up is not necessary. Arrange follow-up if there is any worry about wound infection. Check for similar contacts with family members or colleagues. Arrange treatment if needed.

SUMMARY

Arthropod contact is common. Contact may cause local wound, systemic presentation, and infection (local and systemic). Chapter is summarized in **Flowchart 1**.

ACKNOWLEDGMENT

Thanks to Dr Quintin Kwok of the Accident and Emergency Department of Queen Elizabeth Hospital, Hong Kong for his comments on the draft of this chapter.

CHAPTER 59

Jaundice in Adult

Anukalp Prakash, Amit Mittal

INTRODUCTION

Jaundice (icterus) is a clinical condition characterized by yellow discoloration of the skin, conjunctivae and mucous membranes as a result of widespread tissue deposition of the pigmented metabolite bilirubin. Involvement of the sclera helps distinguish jaundice from other causes of cutaneous pigmentation such as melanin, hypercarotenemia, and mepacrine therapy. Jaundice is not a disease, but rather a sign that occurs in different diseases. The implications of jaundice in certain conditions can be life threatening (e.g. cholangitis) and thus a timely diagnosis is important. After immediate life-threatening causes of jaundice have been excluded, a systemic approach to the patient helps to make the diagnosis.

ETIOLOGY/CAUSES

Jaundice can result from an increase in the formation of bilirubin or a decrease in the hepatobiliary clearance of bilirubin. Jaundice is classified in three categories as described in **Figure 1**. Causes of different categories are given in **Table 1**.

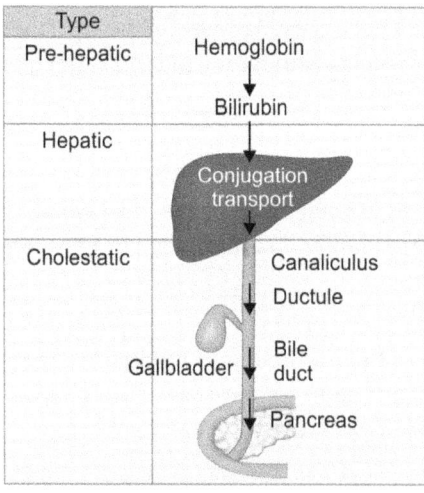

Fig. 1: Types of jaundice.

Table 1: Causes of prehepatic, hepatic, and posthepatic jaundice.

Prehepatic	
Unconjugated hyperbilirubinemia	Hemolysis, ineffective erythropoiesis, drugs, e.g. rifampicin, Gilbert's syndrome Crigler–Najjar syndrome
Conjugated hyperbilirubinemia	Dubin–Johnson syndrome, Rotor's syndrome
Hepatic	
Hepatocellular dysfunction	*Acute*, e.g. Toxins (Ethanol, Amanita), drugs (isoniazid, phenytoin, paracetamol), ischemia (hypotension, Budd–Chiari syndrome), viral
	Chronic, e.g. autoimmune hepatitis, ethanol, viral, Wilson's disease, hereditary hemochromatosis
Liver disorders with prominent cholestasis	Granuloma (tuberculosis, lymphoma, sarcoidosis, malignancy), primary biliary cirrhosis, total parenteral nutrition, benign recurrent intrahepatic cholestasis (BRIC), cholestasis of pregnancy
Posthepatic (common bile duct/hepatic duct)	
Luminal	Worm, e.g. ascariasis, stone, hydatid cyst
Wall involvement	Stricture/stenosis, choledochal cyst, infection of bile duct (e.g. HIV), cholangiocarcinoma
Extrinsic compression	Lymph node at porta hepatis, vascular enlargement (aneurysm, portal cavernoma), chronic pancreatitis, carcinoma head of pancreas, ampullary adenoma

PATHOPHYSIOLOGY

Bilirubin is an end product of heme catabolism, the majority (80–85%) of which is derived from hemoglobin and only a small fraction from other heme containing proteins such as cytochrome P450, myoglobin, and immature bone marrow cells **(Fig. 2)**. Approximately, 300 mg bilirubin is formed daily. The enzyme that converts heme to biliverdin is microsomal heme oxygenase. Biliverdin is converted to bilirubin by biliverdin reductase in the reticuloendothelial system. Bilirubin binds to albumin and taken up at the sinusoidal membrane of hepatocytes via organic anion transport protein (OATP). Bilirubin is conjugated via microsomal bilirubin uridine-diphosphate glucuronosyltransferase (UGT) to form bilirubin mono- and diglucuronides. Biliary excretion of the glucuronide is mediated by the adenosine triphosphate (ATP)-dependent multidrug-resistance protein-2 (MRP-2) at the canalicular membrane and is the rate-limiting factor in the transport of bilirubin from plasma to bile. Bilirubin diglucuronide is not reabsorbed from the small intestine but in the colon may be hydrolyzed by bacterial β-glucuronidases, producing urobilinogens and urobilin, which are excreted in the stool or urine. In cholangitis, bacterial hydrolysis of bilirubin glucuronide in the biliary tree produces unconjugated bilirubin, which may result in production of pigment gallstones.

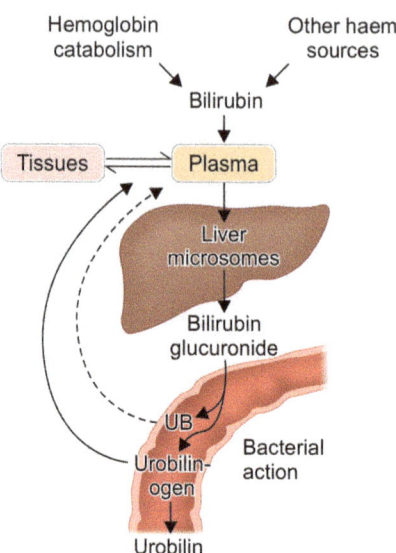

Fig. 2: The metabolism of bilirubin. (UB: unbound bilirubin).

CLINICAL PRESENTATION

A patient can be totally unaware of jaundice at the onset especially if it is mild. Friends or relatives often notice jaundice and inform the patient. Initially yellowish discoloration of the eyes and discoloration of urine is noted by the patient and in some time the jaundice can involve the whole body in progressive disease. Hemolytic jaundice presents with recurrent episodes of anemia, cola-colored urine, and mild jaundice (bilirubin less than 5). Hepatic jaundice can present with prodromal symptoms in case of viral hepatitis. Cholestatic jaundice can manifest in form of itching (severe itching can limit activity, cause anxiety, disturb sleep), clay-colored stools, skin pigmentation, and cholangitis in some cases.

RED FLAGS

- Look for the key indicators of life-threatening causes of jaundice: acetaminophen overdose, massive hemolysis (e.g. falciparum malaria, clostridium perfringens sepsis), ascending cholangitis, fulminant hepatic failure, pancreatic mass.
- No role of myths (e.g. sugarcane juice is the best treatment of jaundice, avoidance of yellow-colored food, black magic).
- In cholestasis, patients have been treated for a decade or more on the basis of a mistaken diagnosis of skin disease when itching is not accompanied by jaundice.
- Differential diagnosis includes acute pancreatitis, amyloidosis, biliary obstruction, cholangitis, cholecystitis, hemorrhagic shock, miliary tuberculosis, sarcoidosis, and tricuspid regurgitation.

EVALUATION

History

- *Onset* (rapid in hemolysis, cholangitis, renal failure), *precipitants* (dehydration, fasting in Gilbert's syndrome)
- *Duration* of jaundice
- *Awareness* (who noticed? relative/patient), *depth* (maximum recorded level of bilirubin)
- *Progression* (advanced end-stage liver disease, malignant obstruction), *fluctuation* [hemolysis, common bile duct (CBD) stone, worm, periampullary carcinoma], *intermittent* [hemolysis, Gilbert's syndrome, benign recurrent intrahepatic cholestasis (BRIC)]
- *Prehepatic jaundice*: Normal-colored (acholuric) or cola-colored urine in hemolysis, recurrent episodes, recurrent anemia, no prodromal symptoms, no cholestasis, normal stools, history of gallstones/stunted growth/leg ulcers
- *Hepatic jaundice*: History of prodromal symptoms (nausea, vomiting, anorexia, myalgia, skin rash, fever in viral infections), drugs (antibiotics/azathioprine/antitubercular/herbal), toxins, injections, blood transfusion, alcohol, contact with other jaundiced patients, ascites (decompensation of chronic liver disease)
- *Cholestasis*: Accumulation of biliary constituents, e.g. itching (site, severity, nocturnal symptoms, and progression), mustard oil like urine, clay-colored stools, skin darkening, xanthomas; deficiency of bile acids in intestine presenting as fat-soluble vitamin deficiency (night blindness, dry skin, leg cramps, bleeding), steatorrhea; cholangitis (pain abdomen, fever with rigors, and jaundice); pain abdomen (biliary colic is steady and increases in 15 minutes to 1 hour; pancreatic pain is dull, continuous and radiates to back); awareness of lump in abdomen, weight loss
- *Past history*: Recurrent jaundice (relapsing viral hepatitis A), right upper quadrant surgery (postcholecystectomy biliary stricture), cholestasis during pregnancy, and recurrent biliary colic (cholelithiasis)
- *Occupation, place of origin, family history* (hemolysis, congenital hyperbilirubinemia)
- *How are the symptoms now*? Progression or improvement.

Physical Examination

Look for nutrition, anemia, depth of jaundice, lymphadenopathy, spider angioma, purpura, scratch marks, body hair, liver and spleen size, ascites, flapping tremors, pigmentation and ulcers in legs, pedal edema, Bitot spots in eyes.

INTERPRETATION OF FINDING

- *Age and sex* (type A viral hepatitis in young patients, drugs and alcohol in adults, gallstone in obese female, and malignant biliary obstruction in old age)
- *General examination*: Anemia, weight loss (malabsorption, cancer), skin signs of cirrhosis in alcoholics, palmar creases, bruising, purpura, loss of secondary sexual hair, lymphadenopathy, clubbing, xanthoma, mental state (fetor hepaticus, flapping tremors,

Table 2: Differences between benign [common bile duct (CBD) stones] and malignant causes (cancer periampullary/head of pancreas) of biliary obstruction in clinical practice.

		CBD stones	Cancer periampullary/head of pancreas
Age		30–50 years approximately	50–70 years approximately
Sex		Females > Males	Females < Males
Duration		Long	Short
Symptoms			
	Jaundice	Intermittent	Progressive
	Fever	Present	+In sever obstruction
	Pain	Intermittent	Progressive, not colicky
	Pruritis	Mild	Severe
	Loss of appetite	Not significant	Significant
	Loss of weight	No	Significant
	Clay-colored stools	No	Yes
Signs			
	Pallor	No	Yes
	Icterus	Deep yellow	Green yellow
	Abdomen	Liver—smooth, firm	Liver—sharp, hard
		Gallbladder not palpable	Gallbladder palpable
Secondaries		No	Yes

intellectual deterioration in hepatocellular jaundice, and hepatic coma), multiple venous thrombosis (cancer of pancreas)
- *Abdominal examination*: Small liver (hepatitis, cirrhosis), large nodular liver (cancer), tender liver (congestive heart failure, alcoholism), palpable enlarged gallbladder (pancreatic cancer), splenomegaly (hemolysis, portal hypertension), ascites (cirrhosis, malignancy).

Differentiating features of benign and malignant causes of biliary obstruction are described in **Table 2**.

INVESTIGATIONS

- Complete blood count provides complimentary information concerning the cause of jaundice. The presence of anemia leaves opens the possibility that a hemolytic disorder is responsible for bilirubin overload. Leukocytosis may be clue to biliary tract obstruction or inflammation (cholangitis, alcoholic hepatitis, underlying malignant disease). Thrombocytopenia is a characteristic finding in cirrhosis because of reduced platelet production from decreased hepatocyte synthesis of thrombopoietin or from

increased platelet consumption from splenic sequestration associated with portal hypertension. Look for peripheral smear and reticulocyte count, if hemolysis is suspected [Wilson's disease, G6PD (glucose-6-phosphate dehydrogenase) deficiency, and parvovirus infection].
- *Serum biochemical tests*: Bilirubin to confirm jaundice and know its depth, transaminases (much raised in hepatitis and low in cholestasis, ALT > AST in hepatitis but AST > ALT in alcoholism), alkaline phosphatase (elevated in cholestasis and biliary obstruction). Prothrombin time is elevated in obstructed biliary tree (10 mg vitamin K corrects prothrombin time within a few hours in cholestasis).
- *Serological testing*: Viral serologies for hepatitis B and C, iron, transferrin (for hemochromatosis), ceruloplasmin (for Wilson disease), antinuclear antibodies of antimitochondrial antibodies (for primary biliary cirrhosis).
- *Radiology*:
    - Chest film to look for tumor and elevation of diaphragm due to enlarged liver.
    - To visualize bile ducts the first procedure should be ultrasound (inexpensive, noninvasive, and portable), which allows distinction between intrahepatic and extrahepatic biliary obstruction, identifies cholelithiasis, intrahepatic space occupying lesion (SOL), and ascites. The disadvantage is that it is operator dependent and difficult to interpret in obesity and gaseous distension of abdomen.
    - Abdominal computed tomography (CT) scan can detect small SOL, which is expensive and needs intravenous contrast (needs normal renal function).
    - Magnetic resonance cholangiopancreatography (MRCP) is the procedure of choice, if ultrasound shows dilated ducts. It provides the road map before going for endoscopic retrograde cholangiopancreatography (ERCP), which is reserved for additional diagnostic modalities, e.g. biliary cytology or therapy to relieve obstruction caused by stones or strictures.
    - If access to duodenal papilla is impossible (duodenal stenosis, previous hepaticojejunostomy or failed ERCP), percutaneous cholangiography (PTC) should be undertaken to drain an obstructed and potentially infected biliary system.
- *Liver biopsy*: In suspicion of drug or infiltrative liver disease (after correction of prothrombin time with vitamin K).

TREATMENT

The optimal treatment of jaundice is directed toward the underlying etiology (cessation of ethanol, antiviral, stoppage of drugs, etc.). For cholestasis, medical options include ursodiol, cholestyramine (time difference in ingestion among ursodiol and cholestyramine to be kept is 2 hours), rifampicin, naloxone, antihistamine. Biliary decompression (papillotomy, balloon dilatation of biliary strictures, and placements of drains or stents) is aimed at relieving the biliary obstruction. If malignant obstruction is inoperable or unresectable, stent can be inserted through percutaneous route. A laparotomy for bypass with hepaticojejunostomy and Roux-en-Y is the alternative.

Flowchart 1: Differential diagnosis of the jaundiced patient.

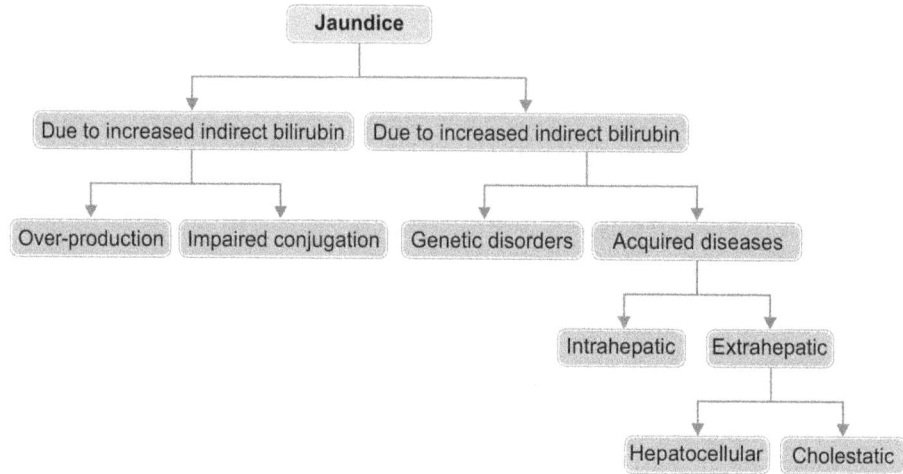

Flowchart 2: Evaluation and management of jaundice.

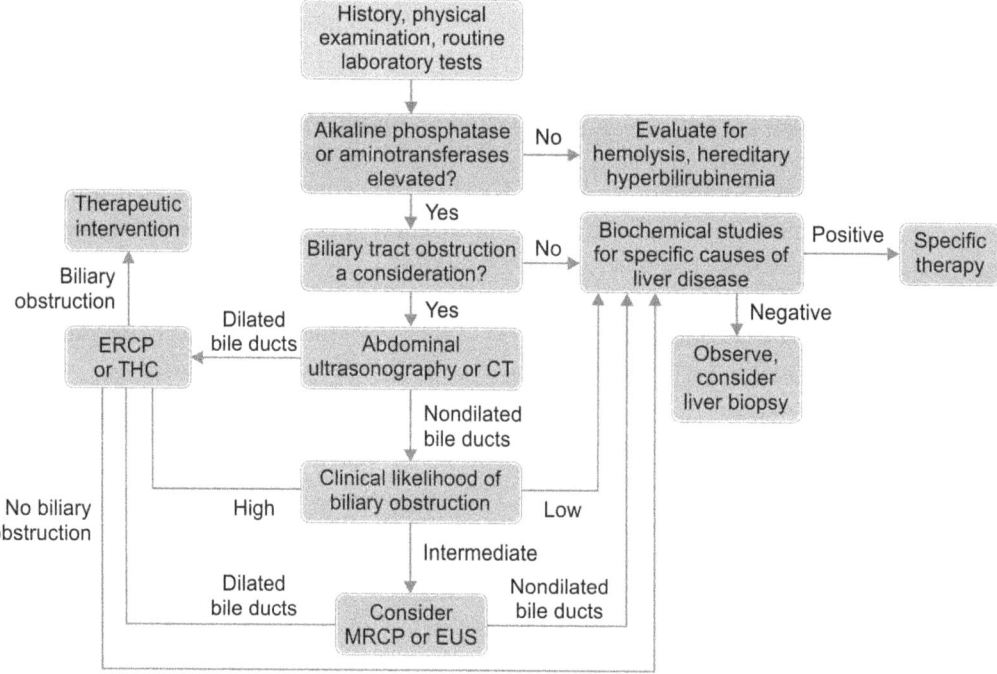

(CT: computed tomography; ERCP: endoscopic retrograde cholangiopancreatography; EUS: endoscopic ultrasound; MRCP: magnetic resonance cholangiopancreatography)

SUMMARY

Chapter can be summarized by identifying the type of jaundice (**Flowchart 1**) and evaluation and management of jaundice (**Flowchart 2**).

- Bilirubin is an end product of heme catabolism, the majority (80–85%) of which is derived from hemoglobin.
- For clinical purposes, serum bilirubin is fractionated to classify hyperbilirubinemia into different categories—increased production, impaired uptake, impaired conjugation, obstruction, hepatocellular injury, or cholangitis.
- Multiple clues to the etiology of jaundice can be obtained from the history and examination.
- Jaundice is not a constant finding in cholestasis. Prominent features of cholestasis, both acute and chronic, are itching and malabsorption of fat and fat-soluble nutrients.
- Involvement of the sclera helps to distinguish jaundice from other causes of cutaneous pigmentation.
- Identify life-threatening causes of jaundice.
- Higher values of transaminases may be found in acute bile duct obstruction due to a stone.
- Which imaging study should be ordered first? Differentiate extrahepatic (dilated CBD and intrahepatic biliary radicals) from intrahepatic biliary obstruction.
- Treat the cause of jaundice.
- Prolonged cholestasis may cause deficiency of vitamin A, D, E, or K and require parenteral replacement therapy for prevention and treatment of complications.
- Exogenous administration of vitamin K normalizes prolonged prothrombin time in extrahepatic biliary obstruction, but not in liver disease caused by hepatocellular injury.
- The treatment approach depends upon the patient, the facilities and the expertise available.

CHAPTER 60

Jaw Dislocation

Harshil Mehta

INTRODUCTION

Jaw (mandible) dislocation results due to the displacement of mandibular condyles from articular groove in temporal bone. Most of the dislocations can be managed and reduced in emergency department.

ANATOMY

The temporomandibular joint (TMJ) is formed by articular surface between the mandibular condyles and the temporal bone. It is lined by synovial membrane and acts by hinge as well as sliding mechanism. It is supported by various ligaments.

PATHOPHYSIOLOGY

Dislocation of mandible can happen in four positions: (1) anterior, (2) posterior, (3) superior, and (4) lateral.

Anterior Dislocation

This is the most common type of position amongst all and results in displacement of the condyle anterior to the articular eminence of the temporal bone. This condition is classified as acute, chronic recurrent, and chronic.

Anterior dislocations happen due to dissociation between muscular actions of jaw muscles (masseter, temporalis, lateral pterygoid).

Etiologies of anterior dislocation are most often the result of low energy trauma (e.g. tooth extraction) or secondary to a medical condition that affects the stability of the joint (seizures, ligamentous laxity, degeneration of joint capsule, dystonia, general anesthesia). Even after endoscopic procedure, anterior dislocation has been reported.

Posterior Dislocation

It usually occurs due to a blow directly to chin. Due to blow to mandible, its condyles are pushed backward to toward mastoid.

Lateral Dislocation

The most common reason of such dislocation is mandibular fracture. The condylar head can be palpated in temporal space as it migrates laterally away from skull.

Superior Dislocation

It occurs due to direct blow to a half open mouth. It is also known as central dislocation. With such kind of injury, fracture of glenoid fossa can occur with mandibular condyle displacement into middle skull base.

Risk factors for mandibular dislocations are as following:
- Shallow mandibular fossa
- Dystonia
- Convulsions
- Hypermotility syndrome
- Previous history of TMJ dislocation.

CLINICAL PRESENTATION

Jaw pain or trismus after extreme mouth opening or direct blow to the jaw are the most common presenting features of jaw dislocation. Immediately after dislocation, a loud crunch noise can be heard against the eardrum. Apart from these, other symptoms are not able to close mouth completely, drooling from mouth, difficulty with speaking, swallowing, and malocclusion.

Previous history of similar kind of dislocation or hypermotility syndrome or any injury to TMJ should be elicited.

Physical examination is needed to rule out other pathologies apart from jaw dislocation as pain and jaw movement difficulty is present in all patients with mandibular pathologies.

Anterior dislocation will have a palpable and/or visible periauricular depression from displacement of condyle. Deviation of jaw to any one side is evident in unilateral jaw dislocation of the opposite side. In bilateral anterior dislocations, patients generally show an underbite or prognathism with pain over both TMJ.

Oral cavity examination is necessary to rule out any laceration that may suggest open injury.

Examination of external auditory canal is also necessary to assess any injury.

Thorough examination of V and VI cranial nerves are mandatory to rule damage to them while dislocation.

DIFFERENTIAL DIAGNOSIS

- Condylar fracture
- Trismus
- Mandible fracture
- Dystonic reaction
- TMJ dysfunction
- Traumatic hemarthrosis.

DIAGNOSIS

Before relocation of any joint, a plain X-ray must be done to rule out any fracture. Likewise, X-ray of mandible also must be done to rule out anterior mandible fracture especially in traumatic dislocation.

Orthopantomogram is the view of choice in case of jaw dislocation. It is a panoramic view that is acquired with camera planning around the patient.

Computed tomography (CT) scan is more sensitive in diagnosing mandibular dislocations and other abnormality hence its use is increasing in traumatic dislocations. It is acceptable now-a-days to do CT scan as initial imaging modality in traumatic mandibular pathologies.

Primarily, magnetic resonance imaging (MRI) is not ordered for acute management. However, it is a useful tool to detect soft tissue injury along with complications of mandibular injuries. It is informative for planning of long-term management in chronic recurrent dislocations.

Laboratory tests are not required in healthy patients with isolated jaw injury.

MANAGEMENT

In emergency department, initially assessment of airway, breathing, and circulation (ABC) is to be done primarily. If every sign and investigation is suggestive of isolated acute mandibular dislocation, then it is to be decided whether close reduction in emergency is appropriate or not.

Maxillofacial surgeon opinion is required in complicated as well as chronic mandibular dislocations.

Close reduction can be done in emergency under proper analgesia and muscle relaxants. Local anesthesia can be five in TMJ as well as masseter and deep temporal nerve block. By reducing spasm and pain, it aids to successful reduction. Systemic benzodiazepine, i.e. intravenous midazolam also helps in reduction by pain relief and reducing muscle spasms.

Various methods are used routinely to reduce anterior jaw dislocation. Eliciting gag reflex may be useful in reducing jaw dislocation according to some case reports.

Classical Technique (Fig. 1)

This is the most commonly used technique. While doing this maneuver physician stands in front of sitting patient and places gloved thumbs on inferior molars a deep as possible and fingers are curved beneath the body and angle of mandible. Backward and downward pressure is to be given through thumb and fingers with slight mouth opening. This help to reposition the condyles back into fossa by disengaging them from anterior eminences. Sometimes it is difficult as the strength of masseter contractions has to be overcome. A risk of fingers bitten or disease transmission is involved in such procedures.

Recumbent Approach (Fig. 2)

Standing behind the recumbent patient, physician places both thumb on inferior molars and gives downward and backward pressure until condyles reaches back to normal position.

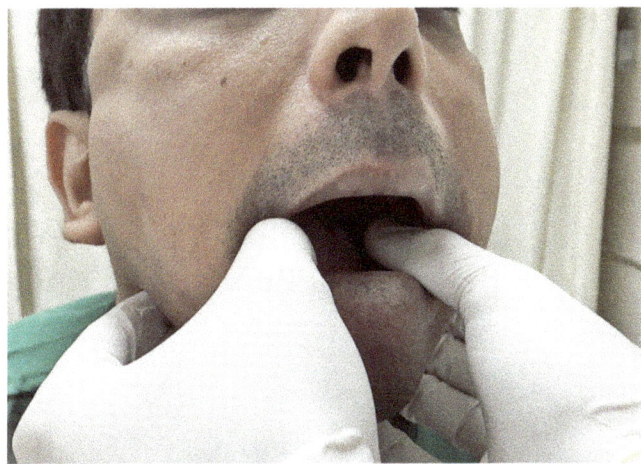

Fig. 1: Classical technique.

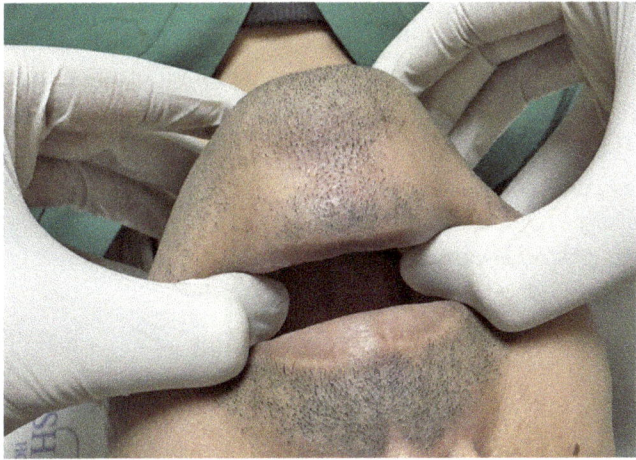

Fig. 2: Recumbent approach.

Wrist Pivot Method

With same position as classical method, cephalad pressure on tip of mentum by thumb and caudal pressure on inferior molars by fingers as shown in **Figure 3** is to be given to reduce displaced mandible.

After successful relocation, no specific medicines are required. Sometimes soft collar may be prescribed to support TMJ.

Patients must be advised not to open mouth very wide or yawn forcefully. Patients with history of recurrent dislocation or with other complications are requested to follow-up with specialists.

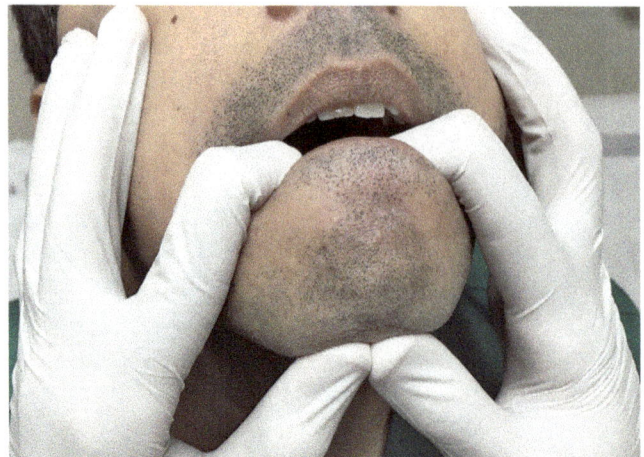

Fig. 3: Wrist pivot method.

Those patients who are suffering from chronic dislocations may get help initially from Barton bandage (elastic fabricated bandage that wraps around the top of the head and mandible). Further surgical management is required for permanent solution of chronic dislocation.

■ COMPLICATIONS

Complications due to dislocation are as follows:
- Degenerative disease of joint structures
- Injury to facial and external carotid nerve
- Injury to external auditory canal
- Deafness.

Complications of reduction are as given here:
- Fracture of mandible
- Physician thumb may get injured.

■ CONCLUSION

Jaw dislocation is not uncommon to treat for emergency physician. Prompt action and accurate maneuver can relocate mandible without much efforts to its normal location. Patients can be discharged after correction with follow-up with specialist, oral analgesics, and safety instructions.

CHAPTER 61

Joint Pain

Sourabh Malviya

INTRODUCTION

Joint pain is one of the most common presentations in emergency ward. Thorough initial assessment always helps to differentiate and characterize joint pain. All emergency practitioners should be well versed in the evaluation of the "red, hot joint." Rarely it can be life-threatening and may be sole manifestation of serious systemic diseases and infections. So "red flags" of joints should be in the mind of every emergency department (ED) clinician if he/she encounters any patient of acute joint pain. These "red flags" are septic arthritis, acute gout, and fracture. On the other hand, inflammatory arthritis can present with acute joint pain and swelling and if not diagnosed and treated on time can lead to long-term deformity and disability. So through clinical examination and then evaluation should be done for any joint pain. Below are the history, symptoms of red flags (**Table 1**) and examination (**Table 2**) to suggest differential diagnosis.

CLINICAL HISTORY

Detail clinical history may help in evaluation whether patient has articular or periarticular disease.

Table 1: Red flag history.

History	*Probable diagnosis*
Fever, history of infection recently	Septic arthritis
History of immunosuppression	Septic arthritis
Elderly, diabetic	Septic arthritis
IV drug abuser	Septic arthritis
History of hyperuricemia	Gout
History of trauma	Fracture
Cancer	Pathologic fracture
History of inflammatory back pain	Spondyloarthritis
History of uveitis/psoriasis/inflammatory bowel disease (IBD)	Spondyloarthritis

Table 2: Examination.

Examination clues	Probable diagnosis
Sick look or toxic	Septic arthritis
Limited range of motion	Fracture or septic arthritis
Single red hot swollen joint	Septic arthritis
Pustular skin lesion	Gonococcal arthritis
Heart murmur	Endocarditis
Urethritis/cervicitis/conjunctivitis	Reiter's syndrome
Firm hepatosplenomegaly	Malignancy
Multiple joints involved	Inflammatory arthritis
Malar rash, Raynaud's phenomenon	Systemic lupus erythematosus (SLE)
Psoriasiform rash	Psoriatic arthritis
Tophi	Gouty arthritis

Table 3: Differential diagnosis as per number of joint involved.

Monoarticular	Oligoarticular	Polyarticular	Periarticular
Septic arthritis	Reiter's syndrome	Acute rheumatic fever	Bursitis
Hemarthrosis	Sarcoidosis	Drug-induced arthritis	Cellulitis
Osteoarthritis	Juvenile idiopathic arthritis	Gonococcal arthritis	Tendonitis
Gout/Pseudogout	Lymphoreticular malignancy	Systemic lupus erythematosus (SLE)	
Trauma	Oligoarticular-onset polyarthritis	Rheumatoid arthritis	
Monoarticular-onset polyarthritis	Seronegative spondyloarthropathies	Seronegative spondyloarthropathies	
	Reiter's syndrome	Viral arthritis	

If articular, then type, number and areas of joints involved can give information of probable disease (**Table 3**).

Location of Pain

Articular pain may be described as generalized sensation of joint pain. On the other hand, periarticular pain is localized to a specific site of inflammation.

Acute or Chronic

Injury, infection or inflammatory process, or acute exacerbation of a chronic arthritis can give rise to acute joint pain. History of recurrent acute pain could be due to chronic arthritis.

Worsening Factor

Joint pain is often exacerbated by both active and passive motion of the joint, can also occur at rest, as seen in acute inflamed joint (inflammatory or infective arthritis). If muscles or tendons are actively or passively moved then periarticular pain can be exacerbated, commonly seen with overuse conditions.

Involvement of Number of Joints

Bursitis/tendinitis or any periarticular problem usually involves single joint. Arthritis should be differentiated into monoarticular (septic and gouty arthritis), oligoarticular [juvenile idiopathic arthritis (JIA), sarcoidosis, seronegative spondyloarthritis (SpA)] or polyarticular [acute: viral arthritis, or gonococcemia; chronic: rheumatoid arthritis (RA), systemic lupus erythematosus (SLE), psoriatic arthritis, or dermatomyositis].

Symmetric or Asymmetric

If it is polyarthritis then it should be looked whether it is symmetric (e.g. drug-induced arthritis, RA, SLE) or asymmetric (e.g. psoriatic arthritis, gonococcal arthritis, acute rheumatic fever).

Distribution of Joints

Location of joint pain may be characteristic of some forms of arthritis. Proximal interphalangeal (PIP) is commonly involved in RA, SLE, osteoarthritis (OA) and distal interphalangeal (DIP) joints of the hand in psoriatic arthritis, OA or sarcoidosis. Metacarpophalangeal (MCP) is commonly affected in RA. Gout commonly affects the great toe metatarsophalangeal (MTP) joint (known as podagra). Ankle and knee are commonly affected in OA or seronegative SpA. Hip joint is usually involved in JIA, OA, or SpA.

Associated Clinical Findings

Extra-articular signs and symptoms should be elicited in a patient of joint pain to reach proper diagnosis. High-grade fever can be a symptom of septic arthritis whilst low-grade of inflammatory arthritis or connective tissue diseases (CTDs). Other constitutional features like Raynaud's phenomenon, malar rash, erythematous skin rash, recurrent hair fall, and recurrent oral ulcer may suggest SLE while dryness of mouth or eyes more likely of Sjögren's syndrome. Track marks in skin may be of injection drug users in endocarditis. Ocular findings can also give some clues like episcleritis may points toward RA or anterior uveitis for ankylosing spondylitis. Tophi in the skin or uric acid stones in kidneys may be associated with gouty arthritis. Purulent urethritis suggests infective etiology like gonococcal disease. The combination of palmoplantar skin lesions, conjunctivitis and urethritis suggests Reiter's syndrome.

Past Medical History

One should always inquire about past history of chronic inflammatory arthritis—other autoimmune disease, gout, hemophilia, and malignancy. Drug history should be taken as few drugs do have joint or skin manifestations. Thiazide diuretics increase uric acid levels and may precipitate gout. Isoniazid, procainamide, and hydralazine therapy may lead to a lupus-like syndrome. Family history is important in diagnosing few arthritis especially seronegative SpA. Inquiries about overuse activities, sports, injection drug use and sexual history should also be made. History of infections like tuberculosis or leprosy should be elicited to look for infective arthritis related to said diseases.

■ PHYSICAL EXAMINATION

To reach into differential diagnosis of joint pain in ED after history and thorough physical examination should be conducted.

General Examination

With mere general appearance, sometimes clinician can make out what patient could be having, like if infective or septic arthritis patient will have sick look. Abrasions or contusions may be there in case of traumatic joint.

Infective or traumatic conditions may give rise to tachycardia or hypotension. Inflammatory arthritis or CTD typically presents with a normal temperature or low-grade fever, and possibly mild tachycardia or tachypnea due to pain.

Examination of Joints

Joint swelling may be secondary to hemorrhagic fluid from an injury, infection (purulent fluid), or due to synovitis, excessive amounts of synovial fluid. Initial look to be given to number of joints involved. If monoarticular, predominantly large joints lower of lower limb then it could be crystal arthritis. If nearby skin is indurated and some signs of cellulitis are there along with red swollen joint then infection will be more likely. In case of knee pain if both joints are involved, looks swollen, may be one more than other then one should think of OA. OA of hands commonly involves first carpometacarpal (CMC) and DIP joints. While inflammatory arthritis like RA mainly small joints of hands (PIP/MCP) are affected. Joints will be swollen in RA are mostly symmetrical. In RA, there can be deformities of hands involved but in CTD like lupus there may not be the same. Tophi anywhere in the skin or joint line can suggest gouty arthritis.

Typical signs of inflammation would be there in case of inflammatory arthritis or infective arthritis or crystal arthritis like redness, warmth, tenderness, and range of motion will be reduced. These findings should always be compared to opposite joint. These palpatory examination findings can also take examiner toward diagnosis, can delineate if it is a particular joint structure (ligament or tendon) or whole joint. Swelling, particularly due to a joint effusion, may be palpable if not easily visualized on inspection.

Range of motion may be decreased secondary to pain from degenerative joint disease, inflammation, infection, or injury or with increasing age. Hypermobile joints may occur with joints that are unstable from ligamentous injury, or in association with joint hypermobility syndrome like benign hypermobile joint syndrome, Ehlers-Danlos syndrome, etc.

Few tests can help examiner to look for subtle effusion in joint like patellar tap test or wave test in the knee joint.

Patellar Tap Test

The patient is lying in supine with the leg extended. Examiner puts pressure on the proximal side of the knee in an effort to squeeze the fluid out of the suprapatellar pouch. The fluid can be moved under the patella while maintaining the pressure on the suprapatellar pouch; the examiner uses his/her other hand to press up on the medial and lateral recesses forcing the fluid under the patella. Tapping down the patella with the index to create an upward and downward movement and a palpable "click" as the patella hits the underlying femur. If the test is negative, the femur and the patella are already in contact. A positive test is when the patella can be felt to move down through the fluid and rebounds on the patella. The test can be false positive; therefore, we must always test both sides to compare.

Fluid Wave Test

It is used when the effusion is less than 30–50 cc. The patient lies supine and examiner presses his/her fingers in both parapatellar gutters. Because there is a pressure from below upward, the gutters are emptied. The patient is asked to stand while the examiner keeps his/her fingers in the parapatellar gutters. If examiner releases his/her fingers and the fluid comes back in the parapatellar gutters, it is a positive sign.

Also weight-bearing cases of more pain suggest arthritis. Periarticular structural problem commonly results in pain during active range of motion.

Detail General and Systemic Examination

Detail general and systemic examination should be done in presence of other patient complaints, signs or symptoms (**Table 4**). A detailed examination will help identifying an underlying systemic like skin tightening in scleroderma, heart murmur of endocarditis, pharyngitis or eye findings of associated arthritides, or skin rashes of SLE or of dermatomyositis. Reduced salivary pool in oral cavity or reduced tear secretion points toward Sjögren's syndrome. Hypoesthetic patch with dactylitis may suggest leprosy. Chronic cough with chest findings like localized crepitations with history of tuberculosis can guide to us diagnosing Poncet's arthritis.

■ EVALUATION OF JOINT PAIN

Laboratory Tests

Evaluation through blood tests is not of very much significance in reaching diagnosis, but clinical examination. Leukocytosis may suggest infective etiology of joint pain, while anemia may point toward chronic arthritis like RA. Inflammatory markers [erythrocyte sedimentation rate (ESR) or C-reactive protein (CRP)] may be elevated in infection or inflammatory arthritis but may be nonspecific sometimes. Hyperuricemia can be there in up to 5% patient in normal individual but in case of acute gout, serum uric acid levels are often normal. Any

Table 4: Differential diagnosis describes causes of joint pain.

Diagnosis	Symptoms	Signs	Evaluation
Osteoarthritis	Monoarticular acute flares within chronic arthritis without any systemic findings. First CMC, DIP, PIP joint and knees and first MTP joints are most commonly affected	Generally elderly age groups are affected. Joint examinations have crepitus and swelling in the affected joints. Bouchard's nodes (PIP) and Heberden's nodes (DIP) often present in the hands	CBC and biochemistry is often normal; inflammatory markers (ESR/CRP) typically normal. Plain radiographs demonstrate formation of osteophytes and joint space narrowing
Gout	Monoarticular symptoms, with MTP joint of the great toe. At onset pain may be severe. Systemic symptoms are uncommon. Tophi can be there on examination in few cases, mostly in polyarticular involvement	Patients are generally afebrile. Affected joints are erythematous, warm, and painful on movement	Serum uric acid may be normal in acute attacks. Synovial fluid analysis demonstrates negatively birefringent, needle-shaped crystals and high WBC counts in the fluid If turbid or purulent fluid then associated septic arthritis must be ruled out by joint fluid Gram stain and culture
Pseudogout	Can be seen in osteoarthritic joint. Monarticular arthritis usually occurring in the knee, wrist, ankle, and elbow. More than one joint may be involved. Typically less acute and less severe than gout	Affected joints are erythematous, warm and painful to touch or movement. Systemic systems typically absent	CBC and biochemistry is often normal; inflammatory markers (ESR/CRP) typically normal. Radiographs sometimes show calcifications (chondrocalcinosis) in joints, tendon insertions, ligaments, and bursae. Synovial fluid examination under polarized microscopy will reveal rhomboidal, weakly positive birefringent crystals of calcium pyrophosphate dihydrate
Septic arthritis	Mostly monoarthritis, erythema, warmth, and swelling. More than 70% of cases involve large joints. Associated symptoms may be fever with chills, loss of appetite, malaise	Affected joints are erythematous, warm, and exquisitely sensitive to touch or movement. Fever may be present	Leukocytosis may be there. ESR is commonly elevated. CRP may be disproportionately higher than ESR. Blood cultures may grow etiologic agents (about half). Synovial fluid analysis shows marked polymorphonuclear leukocytosis. Gram stain may demonstrate organisms (50–70%), although synovial culture is the gold standard. Plain radiographs could suggest soft tissue swelling only
Rheumatoid arthritis	Polyarticular, usually symmetric, arthritis with acute flare-ups occurring in the context of chronic disease. The hands (MCP and PIP joints), wrists, elbows and feet (MTP joints) are most often affected. Constitutional/extra-articular symptoms may be there with joint pain lasting months	Joints are warm, tender, and swollen. Deformities such as *swan neck* and *boutonniere* deformities in the hand, and muscle atrophy and subcutaneous nodules may be present	Synovial fluid is typically inflammatory. ESR/CRP is often elevated Hemoglobin may be low due to anemia of chronic disease. Rheumatoid factor, an antibody against IgG, is positive in 70–80% of patients but is nonspecific. Radiographs demonstrate soft tissue swelling, periarticular osteopenia, erosions in joints or joint space narrowing

Contd...

Contd...

Diagnosis	Symptoms	Signs	Evaluation
Seronegative spondyloarthropathies	Polyarticular, symmetric arthritis, often associated with other symptoms such as psoriatic rash, low back pain from sacroiliitis, urethritis, or uveitis. Family history of similar illnesses (ankylosing spondylitis, psoriatic arthritis, arthropathy of IBD, Reiter's syndrome and other reactive arthritides) often presents. Onset is subacute (may occur over several months). Morning stiffness may be a component of all of these	In addition to polyarticular, symmetric arthritis, a variety of clinical signs related to the underlying condition (psoriatic rash or uveitis) may be present	Laboratory analysis shows a negative rheumatoid factor, although CBC may show mild anemia with elevated WBC. ESR is often elevated. 80% of patients have HLA-B27 marker. Radiographs may demonstrate sacroiliitis and "bamboo spine" in ankylosing spondylitis. Synovial fluid is typically inflammatory
Trauma/hemarthrosis	Monoarticular joint pain and swelling, with history of known trauma. In the case of coagulopathy, a history of trauma may be absent, although a personal or family history of bleeding diatheses may be present in patients with coagulopathy	Pain and swelling in the affected joint. Signs of inflammation are minimal acutely. Systemic signs such as fever are typically absent	Laboratory testing (PT, PTT, bleeding time, platelet count) may demonstrate evidence of coagulopathy if the hemarthrosis is atraumatic. Radiographs may demonstrate fracture if there is traumatic etiology. The synovial fluid is bloody, with fewer than 10,000 WBC mm^3; presence of marrow elements possible in trauma
Viral arthritis (immune complex disease)	Polyarticular (symmetric or asymmetric) concomitantly or following viral syndrome, typically rubella, hepatitis B, parvovirus, mumps, or adenovirus. Typically, the PIP, knee, ankle, and MCP joints are most commonly affected. Other symptoms dependent on the temporal relationship of the arthritis to the primary viral infection; fever with swollen lymph nodes may be the only other symptoms	Fever may be present, and signs of hepatitis or other specific viral illness may be noted. The arthritis is typically severe	Elevated WBC count may be noted. Liver function tests may be abnormal in hepatitis, and should be followed with serologies for specific viral etiologies. The synovial fluid is typically noninflammatory, with cell counts—2,000 cells/mm^3. May develop inflammatory characteristics as the disease progresses

patient presented to ED if has polyarthritis, few tests to be done, routine tests like complete blood count (CBC), liver function tests (LFTs), kidney function tests and also subjected to rheumatoid factor (RF) if symptoms are more than 6 weeks duration. In RA, RF has sensitivity of around 80–95% but specificity 55–60%. Anti-cyclic citrullinated peptide (CCP) antibody can also be done if RF is negative or for prognostication and in some cases of diagnostic dilemma if clinical profile suggests RA. Anti-CCP has 50–60% sensitivity and 95–98% specificity in RA. If some other features are there apart from joint pain which are mentioned for CTD then antinuclear antibody (ANA) can be ordered. Gold standard method of ANA is by indirect immunofluorescence rather than enzyme-linked immunosorbent assay (ELISA). For further characterization of CTD, extractable nuclear antigen (ENA) profile may help in further delineating diagnosis. In case of acute onset polyarthritis associated with fever, then viral etiology like chikungunya fever should be suspected especially if it is short duration of less than 6 weeks. Routine blood tests should be done like CBC, LFT, parvovirus, etc. and so few viral markers like human immunodeficiency virus (HIV), hepatitis B surface antigen (HBsAg), and anti-hepatitis C virus (HCV). If clinical possibility of infection is there than blood culture do guide us if there is hematogenous spread. In case of trauma hemarthrosis can be suspected but if not, then coagulation disorders should be ruled out with routine coagulation profile like prothrombin time (PT), partial thromboplastin time (PTT), bleeding time, and platelet count.

Synovial Fluid Analysis (Table 5)

Synovial fluid analysis is a very useful tests to march toward diagnosis especially in case of septic arthritis, crystal arthritis or to differentiate between inflammatory versus infective arthritis and also in a case of joint effusion if diagnostic dilemma. These can be done through arthrocentesis. Synovial fluid analysis includes routine like cell count and differential, sugars or glucose and microscopy like Gram stain and culture. Also crystal analysis should be done. Gram stain and cultures should be sent to microbiology laboratory once aspirated. Crystal analysis is performed using polarizing microscopy, with monosodium urate crystals in gout appearing as, needle-shaped crystals that are negatively birefringent. In contrast, calcium pyrophosphate crystals in pseudogout appear as polymorphic (often rhomboid) positively birefringent crystals.

IMAGINGS

In ED setting, X-rays are indicated for patients with a history of significant trauma looking for fractures, deformities, neoplasm, osteomyelitis, avascular necrosis, or other bone disease or foreign bodies. Radiographs may show loss of joint space, periarticular osteopenia, or erosions. In infective or septic arthritis, one may find subchondral bone destruction, erosions or periosteal new bone formation. Ultrasonography may be useful in confirming a joint effusion, tendinitis or tenosynovitis and can also be used to guide joint aspiration. For further confirmation of findings, computed tomography can be done for better bony anatomy, whereas magnetic resonance imaging (MRI) is extremely useful for defining soft tissue pathology.

Table 5: Synovial fluid analysis.

Characteristics	Normal	Noninflammatory	Inflammatory	Septic	Traumatic
Color	Colorless	Yellow	Yellow	Yellow	Red
Appearance	Clear	Clear	Cloudy	Cloudy	Cloudy
WBC/mL	<200	<2,000	2,000–100,000	>100,000	
Percentage of polymorphonuclear neutrophils (PMNs)	<25	<25	>50	>95	
Crystals	None	None	May be present	None	None
Cultures	Negative	Negative	Negative	Positive	Negative
Conditions		Trauma, osteoarthritis, viral infections	Inflammatory arthritis like RA, spondyloarthritis, SLE, acute rheumatic fever, reactive arthritis, crystal-induced arthritis	Bacterial arthritis, tubercular arthritis	Fractures, coagulopathies

TREATMENT

Treatment should be based on differential diagnosis of any patient presenting with joint pain. But few general principles should be followed immediate immobilization of joint, adequate analgesia, joint aspiration in case of septic arthritis, appropriate antibiotics as per suspected antibiotics, and proper referral to concerned specialty as per differential diagnosis.

When to Give Analgesia?

Step ladder approach should be followed for analgesia like if suspected of degenerative arthritis then begin with paracetamol first, maximum 1 g 6 hourly can be given. If no response, then opioid analgesia might help like codeine, tramadol or morphine in severe cases if no contraindication.

In cases of inflammatory arthritis, paracetamol or opioids may give mild relief. Nonsteroidal anti-inflammatory drugs (NSAIDs) are often helpful in relieving pain in inflamed joint. Steroids can be added judiciously if pain does not get relieved with NSAIDs as former can reduce synovitis and thereby pain.

In cases of crystal arthropathies like gouty arthritis, first line of treatment is NSAIDs in adequate dosages. Secondly colchicine (a microtubule inhibitor to reduce inflammation) may be added to reduce synovitis. In resistant cases or in patients where NSAIDs are contraindicated, steroids can be given in tapering schedule. Sometimes intra-articular steroids can also be given if there is large synovitis which reduces joint inflammation significantly. There is no role of urate-lowering therapy (ULT) (uric acid lowering agent) in acute setting. If patient is already on ULT then it should be continued.

Is There Any Role of Immobilization?

Immobilization of affected joint might help in reducing pain by not stimulating stretch receptors in synovium. Measures like rest, ice fomentation, compression, and elevation of affected joint can reduce pain. Patients should be encouraged to begin range-of-motion exercises to avoid the loss of function, stiffness, and muscle atrophy once pain relief with all measures (both pharmacologic and nonpharmacologic).

Arthrocentesis: Is It Important?

In case of acute onset arthritis, especially monoarthritis, joint aspiration, and drainage with lavage help for diagnostic and therapeutic purposes. In cases of septic or infective arthritis, this is most important if large joint like knee or hip is involved. If large joint even has moderate effusion, then aspiration and drainage is always better than medical management.

Do Antibiotics have Any Role?

In case of septic arthritis, antibiotic should be started as soon as diagnosis is being made. It could be life threatening if not treated on time and patient improves with administration of appropriate intravenous antibiotics and should be broad-spectrum covering major organism like *Staphylococcus aureus*, *Streptococcus*, *Escherichia coli*, etc. If organism is methicillin-resistant *S. aureus* (MRSA), then intravenous vancomycin is the drug of choice. In case of gonococcal infection intravenous ceftriaxone could be ideal. Acute rheumatic fever is best treated with injectable benzathine penicillin G, or oral penicillin V for 10 days.

In case if suspicion is of tuberculosis, then joint fluid should be sent for demonstration of acid-fast bacilli (AFB) and culture, appropriate drugs should be started as soon as diagnosis is made.

Steroids: Where Does It Stand in ED for a Patient with Joint Pain?

It is very tricky situation regarding usage of corticosteroids in ED. On one hand, it can worsen septic arthritis but on the other hand, it helps in improving patients of inflammatory or crystal arthritis. It should be used if one has ruled out infective cause. Because of its beautiful anti-inflammatory action, steroids do improve synovitis although temporarily. It can be given either intramuscular, intravenous or even high-dose pulse therapy in very severe cases. In cases of diabetes mellitus, it should be used with caution or with strict glucose monitoring or control.

When to Start Disease-Modifying Anti-Rheumatic Drugs?

Disease-modifying anti-rheumatic drugs (DMARDs) are the main stay and anchor-sheet drugs in case of inflammatory arthritis like RA. But it may take few weeks to show its action so sometimes steroids can be used as a bridging therapy. Different DMARDs are methotrexate, sulfasalazine, leflunomide, hydroxychloroquine, azathioprine, cyclosporine, etc. These drugs should be used for long term but need frequent monitoring of laboratory tests like CBC, LFTs, and renal function tests for its side effects. If a patient of inflammatory arthritis is already on this drug then it should be continued in ED. DMARDs are true disease modifiers, control long-term disease activity and complications of primary disease.

What is the Role of Surgery?

In cases of traumatic or fracture in the joint or joint line or septic arthritis then urgent orthopedic consultation should be sought. Septic arthritis may need lavage of joint or debridement and fracture may need corrective surgery.

CHAPTER 62

Knee Problems

Attique Vasdev, Govind Sharma

INTRODUCTION

Knee is complex joint consists of synovial capsule, bony articular surfaces, menisci, ligaments tendons, and muscles. Knee joint has important role in weight bearing, ambulation, and every day activities. Knee is susceptible for various injuries like ligament tear, meniscus injury, patella dislocation and patella fracture, and knee dislocation. Knee pain is common presentation after trauma. Physician should be aware of these knee injuries due to various forces and their evaluation and management.

ANATOMY OF KNEE JOINT

Knee is a hinge joint. In the sagittal plane, knee has the movement from 3 degrees of hyperextension to 155° of flexion. Thigh-calf contact limits flexion. Normal gait requires a range of 0–70° of flexion in the knee. Unlike the elbow, due to the shape of femoral and tibial condyles, flexion, and extension of the knee is not a simple hinge movement.

KNEE STABILITY

Four ligaments are responsible for knee joint stability. They are anterior and posterior cruciate ligaments and medial and lateral collateral ligaments.

The lateral collateral ligament (LCL) is the stabilizer of the knee during varus stress. Superficial portion of the medial collateral ligament (MCL) stabilizes the knee during valgus stress whereas the tibial spines provide mediolateral stability to an extended knee.

Anterior cruciate ligament (ACL) is a primary stabilizer for anterior translation. ACL is attached to the posteromedial aspect of lateral femoral condyle and anteriorly between the intercondylar eminences of the tibia. ACL has an anteromedial bundle which is tight in flexion and a posterolateral bundle which is tight in extension. ACL also has a role in axial rotation.

Posterior cruciate ligament (PCL) is a primary stabilizer for posterior translation. PCL is attached to anterolateral aspect of medial femoral condyle and distally to the tibial sulcus about 14 mm below the articular surface. PCL has an anterolateral bundle which tight in flexion and a posteromedial bundle which is tight in extension.

CLINICAL EXAMINATION OF KNEE JOINT

History

Patient with knee problem due to trauma can present with various sign and symptoms like joint pain, restricted motion effusion, and inability to walk. A detailed clinical examination is mandatory. The opposite knee should also be examined as it serves as a comparative standard. History from the patient and symptoms described are a must to ascertain the mechanism of injury. Previous history of knee injury or surgery should be obtained.

Physical Examination

Soon after the injury, detailed physical examination of knee should be done, before starting the assessment patient should be pain free. Any deformity, effusion, erythema, ecchymosis, abrasion, and laceration over the knee should be noted. Effusion appears in intra-articular injuries and ACL tear. All major joint structure should be palpated like quadriceps, ligaments, and tendons. Patellar motion should be assessed.

Lachman test, anterior drawer test, and pivot shift test are performed to demonstrate ACL injury.

The posterior cruciate ligament, collateral ligaments, and the posterolateral corner (PLC) structures provides restraint to the posterior translation of the tibia on the femur. Injuries of the PCL may occur in sports and dashboard injuries. Hyperextension injuries to the PCL may be associated with damage to the other structures and or dislocation of the knee joint. Patients usually complaining of pain, stiffness, and knee swelling. Posterior drawer, Lachman, posterior sag, and quadriceps active tests are tests to determine PCL deficiency.

KNEE DISLOCATION

Dislocation of the knee is defined as complete disruption of the tibiofemoral joint. Mechanism of injury is usually severe high-energy trauma to the knee (vehicular accidents) and account for the majority of knee dislocations. These are more destructive to the soft tissue envelope of the knee and have a higher incidence (32%) of associated vascular injury. Sports related and lower energy trauma like soccer and wrestling also lead to knee dislocations but the incidence of vascular complications here is low (4.6%). Knee dislocation not only damages the intra-articular and stabilizing structures of the knee but may also damage the neurovascular bundle resulting in a limb-threatening situation. The various structures can be damaged when a knee dislocates: like cruciate ligaments, collateral ligaments, menisci, articular cartilage, medial and lateral capsular structures, popliteal artery, tibial, and peroneal nerves.

These injuries require a timely and accurate diagnosis, stabilization, and treatment to minimize disability. Treatment of a vascular injury takes precedence over the dislocation and a vascular surgeon along with an orthopedic surgeon should be involved at the outset. Delay in vascularization of more than 8 hours from the time of injury increases the amputation rates from 13% to 86%.

The surgeon in the emergency focuses on the inspection of the limb, skin integrity, color, vascular assessment, and visual and tactile joint examination. A neurovascular examination must be done and documented prior to and after reducing a dislocated knee. Vascular surgery consultation must be sought immediately if the pulses are absent or decreased and/or the post-reduction ankle brachial index (ABI) is more than 0.9. Sensation in the distribution of both superficial and deep peroneal nerves should be assessed and peroneal nerve motor function documented. Radiographs are obtained to determine the direction of dislocation and assess the presence of any fractures. After the reduction radiographs are obtained again to verify the reduction and if the joint is grossly unstable some form of splint or external fixation may be deemed essential. Once the patients are medically stabilized a magnetic resonance imaging (MRI) scan of the knee is done to evaluate the integrity of the ligaments, menisci, and cartilage in the knee joint.

Urgent surgical intervention is required in case of a vascular injury, open dislocations, or irreducible dislocations (most commonly a posterolateral dislocation with button holing of the medial femoral condyle through the medial joint capsule with subsequent invagination of the capsule into the joint). Fractures associated with knee dislocations ought to be fixed urgently.

THE LOCKED KNEE

The locked knee may be divided into:
- True-locked knee
- Pseudo-locked knee.

Causes of true-locked knee include: Meniscal tears especially bucket handle tears which may be caused by a force causing twisting or rotating of the knee while full weight bearing. The patient may give history of swelling, stiffness, a popping sound or sensation followed by inability to extend the knee after that. Loose bodies, osteochondral fragments following an injury may also lead to locking of the knee.

Causes of pseudo-locking include: Knee injuries due to fractures, subluxations, tendinitis, tendon ruptures, bursitis, and inflammation due to degenerative joint disease, synovitis, and plica syndrome. Here, the knee is not physically locked but the patient is unable to move the knee because of pain. There is nothing in the knee preventing the knee from moving.

PATELLAR DISLOCATION

Patellar dislocation is a common injury in athletes especially in basketball players and when external force on medial or anterior patella leads to patella dislocation. Patient complains of pain and unable to bear weight with inability to flex or extend the knee. In patient with history of patellar dislocation, spontaneous reduction is common. Radiography usually not required to establish the diagnosis. Treatment includes analgesics, closed reduction by gently extending the knee and guiding patella medially.

PATELLAR FRACTURE

Patellar fracture typically occurs due to trauma or if direct blow to patella by bat or by fall. Pain and swelling are the presenting features in patellar fracture. Extension of knee may be possible. Radiology confirmation by anterior posterior lateral and sunrise view is required. If fracture is minor and extensor mechanism is preserved, a long leg cast is applied for 4-6 weeks. Open reduction and internal fixation is performed if fracture is displaced by more than 2-3 mm.

SUMMARY

Knee injuries are common either sport related or due to trauma. Relevant history, physical examination along with neurovascular examination should be performed. Appropriate radiology and RICE (rest, ice, compression, and elevation) therapy initially in acute injuries is usually helpful. Each injury being unique, requires different treatment options and decisions depend on function expectations like a torn ACL in a young patient usually requires surgery but may be treated nonoperatively in an older patient and each patient needs to be assessed individually.

CHAPTER 63

Lower Extremity Pain, Edema, and Ulcers

Ayşegül Bayır

INTRODUCTION

Acute leg pain, edema, and ulcers are common complaints at emergency clinics. The underlying cause may be induced by a life-threatening problem or it may prevent the lower limb from continuing its vitality. Lower extremities include muscles, bones, joints, tendons, nerves, vascular structures, skin, and subcutaneous tissue. Pain, ulcers, and edema may occur due to traumatic or nontraumatic damage of these structures, infection or inflammation, and obstruction of vascular structures.

Differential diagnosis of the causes that can threaten the life of the patient or cause permanent organ dysfunction in patients with lower extremity pain, edema, and/or ulcer admitted to emergency services should be done first and should be treated rapidly.

LOWER EXTREMITY PAIN AND EDEMA

Causes

- *Traumatic causes*:
  - Fractures in bone structures forming lower limb
  - Joint dislocation or subluxation
  - Tendon rupture
  - Sprains
  - Muscle ruptures or injuries
  - Joint or intramuscular hematomas
  - Compartment syndrome
  - Rupture Baker's cyst.
- *Nontraumatic causes*:
  - Deep vein thrombosis
  - Peripheral artery embolism
  - Peripheral artery disease
  - Varicose veins
  - Tendinitis—bursitis
  - Arthritis (bacterial or reactive)
  - Osteoarthritis

- Disc hernia
- Osteomyelitis
- Malignant or benign tumors related to bone or cartilage
- Rheumatoid arthritis
- sacroiliitis
- Sciatica
- Spinal stenosis
- Perthes disease
- Osgood-Schlatter disease
- Psoriatic arthritis
- Pseudogout
- Cellulitis
- Thrombophlebitis
- Lymphangitis
- Post herpetic neuralgia.

Edema in the lower extremity can be unilateral or bilateral. Edema is not sometimes accompanied by the pain. In such cases, different etiologic reasons should be considered. Congestive heart failure, chronic liver disease, renal failure, vena cava inferior obstruction, myxedema, drugs, malnutrition (hypoproteinemia), pregnancy, and hormonal changes should also be investigated mainly if painless and bilateral edema is present. In such cases edema is not usually accompanied by the pain. Unilateral lower extremity edema usually suggests causes such as deep and superficial venous thrombosis, ruptured Baker's cyst, cellulitis, and lymphangitis.

The main drugs leading to edema in the lower extremities can be counted as; oral contraceptives, steroids, calcium channel blockers, gabapentin, pregabalin, nonsteroidal anti-inflammatory agents, and thiazolidinediones (pioglitazone and rosiglitazone).

Pathophysiology

Pain in the lower extremity may occur due to the stimulation of nerves as a result of press. Some mediators such as infections, inflammation, and trauma released from the damaged tissue in this area also cause pain. The pain can be sharp, blunt, stabbing, or burning depending on the underlying condition. The pain can be continuous or intermittent. Depending on the underlying pathology, the site may be in a specific area or may spread. The patient may also mention complaints such as numbness, tingling, increased local temperature, and loss of power. Pain may vary according to the reason; it may be new and sudden onset (e.g. trauma) or long-lasting (e.g. peripheral artery disease).

The main pathophysiological mechanisms for the formation of edema in the lower extremity include increased capillary permeability, high capillary hydrostatistical pressure, low plasma oncotic pressure due to hypoalbuminemia, ingestion of water and sodium taken intravenously or dietary by the kidneys, disturbance of the lower extremity lymphatic drainage, regional infection or local dropsy secondary to inflammation.

Clinical Presentation

The complaints of pain in the patient may also be accompanied by localized temperature increase or systemic fever (infection, septic arthritis, cellulitis, osteomyelitis, and thrombophlebitis), coldness in the extremity (peripheral arterial embolism), edema (deep vein thrombosis, trauma, infection, and compartment syndrome) paleness (peripheral arterial embolism), motor loss (peripheral arterial embolism), empurpling (deep vein thrombosis and venous insufficiency), ecchymosis (trauma), deformity-crepitation (bone fracture), numbness-tingling (peripheral arterial disease, peripheral arterial emboly, and disk hernia), and motor loss (peripheral arterial emboly and disk hernia).

Systemic diseases can be accompanied by complaints of underlying disease in case of secondary edema. For example, dyspnea, orthopnea, and decrease in effort capacity in cardiac insufficiency may be secondary symptoms to acute pulmonary edema.

In cirrhotic patients, lower extremity edema may be accompanied by acid, consciousness blur, and coagulopathy.

Red Flags

- The age of the patient is less than 20 years and greater than 55 years
- History of trauma
- Loss of motor with pain in lower extremity, not feeling the pulse
- History of malignancy
- Immobilization
- High fever or localized fever
- Sudden onset and severe pain
- Exacerbation of pain by passive movements
- Rectal or urinary incontinence
- Pregnancy
- The extremity is cold and pale or purple
- Prolonged capillary filling time.

Evaluation

History

First, a detailed story should be obtained from the patient. The patient is questioned about when the pain starts, the characteristic of the pain, whether the pain increase or not with movement, the trauma story, whether the pain is continuous or intermittent, and other accompanying symptoms (fever, edema, numbness, motor loss, and urinary-stool incontinence). Information about the medical resume of the patient should be obtained. Cancer, diabetes, atherosclerosis, heart disease, past pulmonary embolism, and medications that they are using should be questioned and noted.

Physical Examination

Physical examination begins with obtaining vital parameters. Arterial blood pressure, pulse, fever, and respiration rate are measured. The patient's cardiovascular system, respiratory system, and gastrointestinal system are examined. Musculoskeletal examination and neurological examination should be done in detail.

The lower extremity is inspected first. It is examined whether there is color change (pale or bruise), deformity-malformation, edema, and ecchymosis. By palpating the limb with pain; crepitation, local temperature increase or coldness, whether pain increases or not with passive movements and whether movement is restricted are determined. Lower extremity pulses (femoral, popliteal, dorsalis pedis, and tibialis posterior) are palpated. The diameters of both lower extremities are measured at the same level. Homan's test should be done in all cases. Straight leg lift test is performed and nerve root pressure is assessed.

Deep tendon reflexes are evaluated and whether pathological reflexes exist or not are examined. A sensory examination of the extremity is performed.

Interpretation of Findings

In patients with history of trauma crepitation, ecchymosis, hematomas, limitation of movement, and bone fracture are suggested together with pain and local edema. Peripheral artery embolism or peripheral artery disease is considered in patients with cold, pale, no distal pulse, sensation disorder or paresthesia. Deep venous thrombosis usually occurs with findings such as unilateral leg pain, swelling of the legs, temperature increase, and redness.

Joint pain, edema, joint effusion, joint pain aggravated by movement, redness, temperature increase, and accompanying systemic symptoms (lassitude and exhaustion) support septic arthritis. In addition to clinical findings, some risk factors for septic arthritis are also present in patients. These factors include advanced age (>80 years), diabetes mellitus, immunosuppression [chemotherapy and human immunodeficiency virus (HIV) infection], osteoarthritis, rheumatoid arthritis, history of previous bone or joint prostheses, intravenous drug dependence, and current skin infection. Systemic fever is an important finding in infections such as cellulitis, osteomyelitis, and septic arthritis, which cause swelling and pain in legs. Positive Homan's test can also be detected in ruptured Baker's cyst except deep vein thrombosis.

Cellulitis is usually characterized by local edema, redness, tenderness, and increased temperature that rapidly develop within 24 hours, secondary to a skin lesion such as eczema, usually present in people with one or more risk factors such as diabetes mellitus. Usually local findings are accompanied by fatigue, exhaustion, widespread muscle soreness, and sweating. Especially in patients in risk group (HIV, diabetes mellitus, oncologic patients receiving chemotherapy, and immunosuppressed patients), cellulitis may mutate to necrotizing fasciitis progressing in deep facial layers. In this case, blisters filled with hemorrhagic fluid in the skin, cyanotic lesions pointing to necrosis in some places, ulcer, systemic infection (sepsis) findings, rapid deterioration in general condition, and anaerobic infection findings (edematous infected skin and crepitation in subcutaneous tissue in palpation, malodorous dark-colored flow) may be present. Necrotizing fasciitis may lead to death progressing rapidly.

Blunt or crush trauma or severe physical exercise history in compartment syndrome are referred to diagnosis. The extremities are cold and pale together with complaints of increased pain with severe, continuous, and passive movements in patients. Paresthesia or sensory abnormality is detected as in peripheral artery embolism. In the last phase of compartment syndrome, circulation in the extremity stops completely and peripheral pulses cannot be palpated.

Lymphangitis is a bacterial infection of the lymphatic drainage pathways. Generally, patients have a small, if any, trauma, abrasion or cutoff story to the skin. Pain, tenderness, and swelling in the nearby lymph nodes, fatigue, systemic fever, tachycardia, abscess in the infected area or infected wound together with tenderness, redness, and edema along the path of the lymph may be seen.

Diagnostic Studies

Laboratory Tests

Laboratory tests may support prediagnosis when evaluated with clinical findings. The high white blood cell and platelet levels in the whole blood count support acute infection, inflammation or sometimes malign diseases. Apart from malign diseases, acute phase reactance, erythrocyte sedimentation rate, antistreptolysin O (ASO), and C-reactive protein (CRP) levels are measured high in infections such as cellulitis, osteomyelitis, septic arthritis, and problems secondary to inflammation.

Procalcitonin levels are high in patients suspected of necrotizing fasciitis and sepsis. In these patients, blood culture and culture, if available, from material obtained from wound or abscess formation should be sent. For the diagnosis of septic arthritis, joint puncture must be performed absolutely and cell counting, gram staining, culture, and biochemical examination should be performed on the obtained material. The fluid obtained by arthrocentesis in septic arthritis is blurred. The cell count has a leukocyte count of between 50,000 and 100,000 and more than 75% of the polymorphonuclear leukocyte (PNL) weight. In patients with neonatal synovitis, the synovial fluid is straw—colored and clear. The cell count has a leukocyte count between 5,000 and 15,000 and a PNL ratio is below 25%.

In patients suspected of deep venous thrombosis, the risk score for deep vein thrombosis and pulmonary embolism is found using clinical probability tests (modified Geneva or Wells scoring systems) in evidence-based medical practice. D-dimer testing is required for patients with moderate risk scores. The D-dimer test is also important for the decision to start anticoagulant treatment. The high sensitivity D-dimer test is significant above 500 ng/mL in individuals up to 50 years of age. If the patient is over 50 years of age, the age-related normal limit should be determined by calculating the D-dimer added with age (age × 10 ng/mL) as the D-dimer value will also increase with age.

Radiological Diagnostic Methods

Direct X-rays: In patients with trauma history, anterior-posterior and lateral direct X-rays should definitely be taken of the area with clinical findings. Fractures and dislocations can be seen on direct radiographs. In trauma patients, direct radiographs are diagnostic at high rates. In addition, if there is a penetrating trauma story on the lower extremity with edema, painful and open wound, contrasting foreign bodies or objects can be detected on the direct graph. Oblique radiographs may also be necessary for some patients.

Malignant bone lesions, osteoporotic changes, degenerative bone and joint changes, and pathological fractures are also lesions that may be seen on direct graph.

Ultrasonography: It is the most commonly used radiological diagnostic method at emergency. Fractures and dislocations in lower extremity traumas can usually be diagnosed by direct radiography. However, ultrasonography (USG) is a radiological diagnostic method that may be preferred to detect fractures in patients with lower extremity trauma as the patient is not exposed to radiation and its bedside application. The USG examination, however, largely depends on clinical experience. In USG, the presence of steps in cortex is diagnostic.

Foreign bodies, necrotizing fasciitis, abscess formation, inflamed or infected tendons that cannot be seen on direct graph can also be detect with USG. A linear probe with 7.7 MHz and higher frequency should be used to detect these lesions. A curvilinear probe with lower frequency is suitable to examine deeper structures. Intra-articular effusions can also be seen with USG.

Ultrasonography is not only used for diagnostic purposes, but also for joint puncturing, drainage of abscess and foreign body removal.

Compression USG has a high sensitivity and specificity for the diagnosis of lower extremity deep vein thrombosis. With the help of the portable USG, the whole leg should be examined at 5–7 MHz frequency with a linear transducer at the bedside. All veins are scanned downward starting from the femoral vein in the examination. If there is normal venous flow, the lumen is easily compressed. There is no venous compression in the vein with thrombus in the lumen and the thrombus inside can be seen easily. Venous Doppler USG is required to see the blood flow pattern and obstruction site.

The arterial Doppler USG is an important method for the diagnosis of lower extremity arterial embolisms and peripheral arterial diseases. Convex probe is used at 9–15 MHz. From the region where the embolus is located, the flow at the distal side is slowed down or absent.

Ultrasonography is also a diagnostic technique for patients suspected of lower extremity vascular injuries.

Lower extremity computed tomography angiography: It can be used in vascular injuries secondary to trauma and diagnosis of peripheral arterial diseases.

Magnetic resonance imaging: It can be used for diagnosis of muscle, cartilage, and joint pathologies, especially for differential diagnosis of benign or malign tumors, cysts and abscess, and medulla spinalis lesions.

Treatment

Treatment is cause oriented. If pathology leading to edema and pain in the lower extremity is a pathology that should be initiated under emergency conditions and treatment can be performed in an emergency clinic, immediate treatment should be started. Consultation from the relevant clinic is requested if the treatment cannot be performed under emergency conditions. For the treatment of benign or malignant lesions involving the lower extremity muscle, cartilage and bone tissues, the patient should be firstly consulted with an orthopedic clinic and, if necessary, the patient should undergo analgesic treatment.

Treatment of Problems related to Traumatic Causes

First, fracture or dislocation reduction is performed in patients with fracture or joint dislocation. Sedoanalgesia should be performed before reduction. Verification should be done by taking a direct X-ray after reduction, the circulation of the extremity should be controlled, and peripheral nerve examination should be performed. Immobilization is achieved by applying a splint after reduction. If reduction is not available, if the fracture is related to the joint, if vascular or nerve injury is present, the patient is consulted with orthopedic clinic for operative treatment.

Extremities are relaxed in soft tissue traumas and in tendinitis. If necessary, splint is applied, extremity elevation is provided, cold application is made on the edema area, and nonsteroidal anti-inflammatory agent is given.

Septic Arthritis

Parenteral antibiotic treatment should be given for at least 2 weeks. Initially, antibiotic therapy is applied empirically and replaced with specific antibiotic according to culture results. Antibiotic treatment can be extended to 4 weeks according to the effect (*Staphylococcus aureus*). Initially, joint immobilization and analgesic treatment may be required for pain control. The fever of the patients with systemic fever should absolutely be reduced by peripheral cooling and antipyretics. Physical therapy is necessary to maintain the postinfectious function of the joint. Septic arthritis treatment requires joint drainage and washing. Patients with septic arthritis are treated by hospitalizing at the orthopedic clinic. The needle drainage is performed 2–3 times a day. Surgical drainage is performed in patients who require more frequent drainage.

Lower Extremity Peripheral Arterial Embolism

The main treatment is the restoration of circulation by noninvasive or invasive embolectomy. Antithrombotic agents (anticoagulant and thrombolytic therapy) may be administered. Antiplatelet agents (aspirin, clopidogrel, and ticlopidine) and anticoagulants (heparin and warfarin) prevent the formation of new clots. Thrombolytics dissolve the clot. Thrombolytics are administered intra-arterially via a flexible catheter directly over the clot. Vasodilators and analgesics may also be given.

Deep Vein Thrombosis

The main goal in the treatment of deep vein thrombosis is to prevent pulmonary embolism to prevent or minimize the risk of post-thrombotic syndrome development. Anticoagulants [low molecular weight heparin (LMWH) and warfarin], mechanical thrombolysis or endovascular treatments may be used for treatment. Catheter thrombolytic therapy is preferred to systemic thrombolytic therapy because of the risk of bleeding. Low-risk patients for pulmonary emboly can be monitored as ambulant patients by prescribing LMWH. After reaching effective international normalized ratio (INR) levels with oral anticoagulants to be started during LMWH treatment, LMWH is discontinued and oral anticoagulant therapy is continued for 3-12 months. Endovascular intervention is recommended for patients with anticoagulation and thrombolysis contraindications. For this, it is necessary to consulate the patient to interventional radiology. Surgical thrombectomy may be required for patients with massive deep vein thrombosis. These patients must be evaluated with a cardiovascular surgeon. If the treatment is inadequate despite adequate anticoagulation, if the systemic venous circulation thrombus fragments are involved, a vena cava filter may be considered for these patients. A prosthetic valve may be required to prevent the development of post-thrombotic syndrome.

Elastic compression stockings are recommended to reduce edema in the leg, restore microcirculation, and prevent venous ischemia and post-thrombotic syndrome. Anticoagulation therapy is recommended along with early ambulation and effective compression on day 2 after the initiation of therapy. Without elastic compression stock, ambulation can cause movement of thrombus components and fatal pulmonary embolism.

Cellulitis

Generally, *S. aureus* or streptococcus group are the bacterial agents and antibiotics to which these agents are sensitive (tetracycline, trimethoprim-sulfamethoxazole, methicillin, vancomycin, linezolid, penicillins, ampicillin, amoxicillin, ampicillin-sulbactam combination, amoxicillin-clavulanate combination or cephalosporins) are used. Depending on the severity of the infection of the patient, the treatment can be done either orally at home or intravenously by hospitalizing. Patients with risk factors (diabetes mellitus and immunosuppressive diseases) should be hospitalized and intravenous antibiotic therapy should be started. The antibiotic regimen can be administered with a combination of different groups. Patients in this group may require gram staining and culture from the swab taken from the infected area. Antibiotic treatment is changed according to the culture result.

Edema can also be reduced by elevation of the leg and cold application. If purulent flow on the infected area is present, it must be cleaned with saline in sterile conditions. In the first day after the treatment started, erythema may temporarily increase a little due to antibiotic-induced lysis. If symptoms persist despite antibiotic treatment and systemic infection findings such as tachycardia and hypotension occur, they should be followed in the hospital and treatment should be reconsidered.

Necrotizing Fasciitis

It is one of the surgical emergencies. It is necessary to take the patient to the surgical intensive care unit as soon as the diagnosis is made and to apply widespread debridement to the infected necrotic tissue urgently. Hemodynamic support should be provided to the patient in a toxic condition. Amputation of the lower extremity may be required if the profound tissues are severely affected. Antibiotic therapy should be started concurrently. When choosing antibiotics, gram (-), gram (+) and antibiotics effective on anaerobes (penicillin G and aminoglycoside combination) should be preferred. Vancomycin can be used in patients suspected of methicillin-resistant *Staphylococcus aureus* (MRSA). Hyperbaric oxygen therapy can be applied after emergency surgical debridement.

Lymphedema and Lymphangitis

Some drugs for lymphedema treatment can contain benzopyrene that include coumarin and some flavonoids. Drug therapy should be accompanied by complex physical therapy. Diuretics are ineffective in treatment. Lymph drainage is relieved by treating the underlying cause in the secondary lymphedema (caused by neoplasia or infection). During the day, compressive socks which will not disturb the circulation should be worn. Intermittent pneumatic pump compression therapy may be applied to the patients without congestive heart failure, active infection, and deep vein thrombosis. Manual lymphatic drainage (Leduc technique and Vodder technique) is a treatment method that can be applied. Palliative surgical treatments can be applied to relieve lymph drainage.

Intravenous administration of analgesics and anti-inflammatory agents to patients with lymphedema decreases edema, pain, and inflammation in the legs. Since group A beta-hemolytic streptococci and *S. aureus* are the most common agents, antibiotics against these agents (dicloxacillin, cephalexin, cefazolin, cefuroxime, trimethoprim/sulfamethoxazole, clindamycin, and nafcillin) are administrated. Elevation of the leg reduces the spread of the infection, pain, and edema. If abscess formation occurs, surgical drainage should be performed.

■ LOWER EXTREMITY ULCERS

Lower extremity ulcers are not a disease, but symptoms of an underlying disease. These ulcers can be acute or chronic. Despite not being seen frequently (0.18–2%), they are major health problems because of the money and time spent on treatment, serious complications that could lead to death resulting from inadequate treatment. The incidence also increases with increased age. The incidence of over 65 years old is around 5%.

Causes

- Ulcers arising from inadequate arterial circulation
- Venous insufficiency ulcers
- Infectious ulcers (necrotizing fasciitis, pyoderma gangrenosum, and erysipelas)
- Neurotrophic ulcers (diabetic foot ulcers)
- Lymphatic insufficiency ulcers
- Malignant ulcers
- Inflammatory ulcers
- Ulcers caused by drugs (steroid ulcers, granulocyte stimulating factor, methotrexate, hydroxyurea, halogens, and vaccines)
- Acute or chronic trauma-related ulcers (pressure ulcers).

Pathophysiology

Chronic venous pump or valve failure results in abnormal retrograde flow or pooling of venous blood. Venous hypertension leads to the increase of capillary pressures and accumulation of macromolecular deposits such as fibrin in the pericapillary region. As a result, oxygen and nutrients cannot be diffused into the tissue and ulcers develop.

Diabetic foot ulcers are caused by nephropathy and peripheral arterial disease secondary to diabetic. Peripheral neuropathy is a major risk factor for the development of diabetic foot ulcers. Sensory neuropathy reduces perception of pressure, pain, and heat sensation of foot. An ulcer develops after an insidious trauma. Ulcers may develop in the bony prominences exposed to high pressures. Autonomic neuropathy leads to the skin dehydration. This problem triggers drying, crack growth, and infection in the skin.

Long-term pressure, especially at the point where the bone protrudes, disturbs the perfusion of this region and leads to local tissue damage. Ulcers develop easily even with minor traumas, especially in elderly skin with impaired perfusion which is suffering from loss of elastin. Frictional forces lead to superficial erosion and blister development. The most important causes of the development of arterial ulcers are the peripheral arterial diseases and occlusions in peripheral arteries. Tissue perfusion deteriorates and ulcer develops.

Evaluation

History

The risk factors that will lead up to the development of the ulcer should be questioned in the story. These risk factors [advanced age (over 55 years), male sex, history of venous insufficiency, deep vein thrombosis and pulmonary embolism, history of previous ulcers, history of venous insufficiency-ulcer or edema in lower extremities in the family, number of pregnancies in women and whether still pregnant or not, the history of skeletal-muscle-joint disease in the lower extremity, physical inactivity, diabetes mellitus, heart failure, current medicine used, hypertension, hyperlipidemia, other systemic diseases, diagnosed vasculitis and anemia, cigarette and other drug addictions] are questioned. Recently trauma or travel stories should be taken.

In addition, a history of ulcers should be taken in order to help differential diagnosis. How long the ulcer is present is questioned. Concomitant systemic symptoms such as fever, fatigue, weight loss, and altered consciousness are questioned. Ulcer related discharge, local fever, edema, coldness and loss of power in the extremity, tingling, loss of sensation, and color change around the ulcer are questioned. The patient is asked whether he has diseases such as Factor V Leiden gene mutation, protein S or C deficiency, and antithrombin III deficiency.

Physical Examination

First of all, vital parameters (fever, pulse, arterial blood pressure, and respiratory rate) are obtained and noted. All systems are thoroughly examined in order to obtain findings related to a systemic disease that may cause ulcer. Then the extremity where the wound is located and the wound area are examined.

The color of ulcer and skin, the depth and size of ulcer, whether there is discharge, the color and smell if there is discharge, local temperature increase or coldness on extremity, and circulation status of extremity are evaluated. Sensory and motor examinations are performed. The shape and the color of the extremity are examined, the duration of capillary recycling is evaluated, and whether edema or diameter increases or not is assessed. Muscle atrophy and local infection findings are evaluated. A joint examination is performed.

Clinical Presentation

Along with the complaints of ulcer in the lower extremity, complaints about underlying systemic disease symptoms (diabetes mellitus, heart failure, and peripheral artery disease) may be present. The ulcer is usually seen in the distal part of the lower extremity, especially on the bony protrusions, in the toes and in the pressure-affected areas. The ulcer may be deep or superficial, sometimes with a stitched margin to give a stapled image, and in some cases its border may be irregular. Necrotic tissue or granulation tissue may be present on the ulcer. Infected ulcers may contain purulent material. Yellowish serous discharge is detected on some ulcers.

Especially in ulcers due to arterial occlusion, the extremity is cold and pale. Peripheral pulses cannot be felt or weak. The patient may complain of motor loss, sensory loss, and paresthesia on the limb. Skin and hair atrophy is visible, capillary retraction time is prolonged. Dry, increased callus texture, and insensitive skin are seen especially in diabetic foot ulcers.

Interpretation of Findings

Venous ulcers are the ulcers on the medial malleol, flat-superficial, mild-to-moderate exudate, and crusted granular tissue on the base. The patient's thick, fibrotic, eczematous, hemosiderin-containing itchy leg skin, and the normal period of capillary retraction support the venous ulcer.

Arterial ulcers are deep ulcers that look like punctured by staples in areas of compression, on toes, feet, lateral malleolus, and tibia. The fact that the wound floor is covered with dark necrotic tissue and irregularly margin appearance suggest arterial ulcer. If these ulcers are not infected, they contain minimal exudate. Thin and pale skin and weak hair growth are yet again findings supporting arterial ulcers.

Diabetic neuropathic ulcers are usually seen on the soles of the feet, on the plantar side of the foot, and laterally in the fifth metatarsal. Weak or nonpalpable pulse, prolonged capillary retraction, and gangrene accompany arterial ulcer.

The pressure ulcers are seen in the lateral and medial malleolus and the heel of foot, which are more exposed to press. Sometimes it is deep, necrosis ulcer that reaches to the bone tissue. Atrophic muscle mass and skin suggest pressure ulcer.

Diagnostic Studies

Laboratory tests directive for diagnosis and treatment (full blood count, ASO, CRP, procalcitonin, sedimentation rate, biochemical parameters, gram staining, and culture from the exudate or discharge from the wound) should be sent.

Duplex USG is a cheap, simple, and fast method to detect vascular causes. Venous insufficiency may indicate venous thrombosis, arterial embolism, and aneurysmatic problems. Plethysmography is a technique that can be used for the qualitative diagnosis of arterial and venous vascular problems. CT angiography (CTA) can quickly scan the whole arterial tree of the lower extremity. CTA diagnoses peripheral artery disease and arterial embolism. CT venography (CTV) is also an important diagnostic tool for proximal venous thrombosis. CT is also the most important diagnostic tool for the diagnosis of aneurysms. Magnetic resonance arteriography (MRA) is a noninvasive method for the diagnosis of vascular problems. It is an important diagnostic method in distinguish local arterial obstruction from long-segment arterial obstruction. In addition, proximal venous thrombosis can be diagnosed with magnetic resonance venography (MRV), and acute thrombosis and chronic thrombosis can be distinguished. If invasive imaging methods cannot be helpful in diagnosis, invasive radiological methods such as plethysmography, contrast arteriography, and intravascular USG can be used. Contrast arteriography is the gold standard in the differential diagnosis of arterial diseases. However, it is expensive and may cause complications such as embolization, pseudoaneurysm, arteriovenous fistula, hematoma, dissection, and renal failure.

Treatment

Treatment of Venous Ulcers

The goal is to remove venous hypertension, to heal the wound, to reduce edema, and pain. The leg is elevated above the heart level several times a day for 30 minutes to reduce the edema. Patients with severe illness symptoms need venous compression treatment. With this treatment, venous flow and lymphatic drainage are improved, leakage in the superficial veins and venous pressure are reduced. The volumetric load in the venous system decreases. The optimal pressure of the compression bandage should be 35-40 mm Hg. Arterial embolism, deep vein thrombosis, and congestive heart failure are contraindications for bandage. In the meantime, wound care should be done regularly, topical and/or systemic antibiotics should be started if infected.

Treatment of Arterial Ulcers

First of all, circulation should be re-established. Analgesics are given to the patient and the extremity is prevented from going to amputation. If the patient is not a candidate for revascularization, if ulcer does not lead to ischemic pain or gangrene, the patient is followed by medical treatment. In these patients, anticoagulant therapy is started and complications are prevented by modifying cardiovascular risk factors.

Treatment of Diabetic Foot Ulcers

Pressure is reduced as much as possible. Necrotic tissues are debrided and topical and/or systemic antibiotic therapy is initiated for cultured infected ulcers. Daily wound dressing should be done. Blood sugar regulation is vital.

Treatment of pressure ulcers: The patient's position needs to be frequently changed and turned in order to distribute and reduce the pressure. Nutritional status and anemia which are effective on wound healing should be improved. Necrotic tissues are cleared from the wound surface. Cultures should be taken from infected injuries, topical and/or systemic antibiotics should be initiated. The ulcer area should be followed by daily dressing.

CONCLUSION

The rapid and accurate diagnosis of the lower extremity pain, edema, and ulceration leads to the application of the required treatment for the patient without delay, both reduces the cost of diagnosis and treatment and prevents the complications that can threaten the patient's life or cause permanent organ damage and limb loss.

CHAPTER 64

Low Back Pain

Devendra Richhariya

INTRODUCTION

About 80–90% of individuals experience low back pain at some point in their lifetime. Back pain is common usually self-limiting within 4–6 weeks in most of the cases, and few patients require diagnostic interventions like X-ray, computed tomography (CT), or magnetic resonance imaging (MRI). Most of the causes of low back ache are benign and self-limiting so that this is very important to follow systematic approach toward each and every patient to identify red flags of the serious causes that can have significant morbidity and mortality.

CAUSES

Nonserious and serious causes of low back pain are listed in **Table 1**.

EVALUATION OF LOW BACK PAIN

History

Low back pain can be divided into three categories: (1) acute pain (resolve within 6 weeks), (2) chronic pain (persists > 12 weeks), and (3) subacute pain (persists for 6–12 weeks). History

Table 1: Nonserious and serious causes of low back pain.

Nonserious causes	Serious causes	Nonspinal causes	Trauma
Muscular strain	Malignancy	Aortic dissection	Minor trauma
Ligamentous strain	Epidural and intradural metastatic diseases	Aortic aneurysm	Major trauma
Sprains	Intramedullary tumors	Ureteric colic	
Uncomplicated sciatica	Infections	Renal infarction	
Spinal stenosis	Spinal abscess	Prostatitis	
	Osteomyelitis	Renal tumors	
		Pancreatitis	
	Central disk herniation causing cauda equina syndrome	Pancreatic malignancy	
		Cholecystitis, cholangitis	
		Retroperitoneal hemorrhage	

of duration of pain is important because pain longer than 6 weeks is red flag and needs close attention and further evaluation.

Benign low back pain is usually dull, worsens with movement and relieves with rest. If pain increases at night not rending to analgesia and rest, rule out infections and tumors. Pain due to herniated disk is aggravated by coughing, sitting and relieved by lying supine. Spinal stenosis is sciatic pain of bilateral limbs increased by standing and backward extension and relieved by rest and forward flexion.

Back pain in patient of less than 18 years of age group has congenital and bony abnormalities, while spinal stenosis, ruptured abdominal aortic aneurysm are causes of low back pain in older patient.

Localized pain in back is generally due to muscular or ligamentous strain or from degenerative disk disease. If pain radiates into the legs (below knee) is a red flag for a herniated disk and nerve root compression below L3 nerve root. At this point of time, important to differentiate between low back pain and sciatica. Sciatica is a radicular pain with primarily leg symptoms in lumbar and sacral nerve root area and associated with sensory and motor deficit. Sciatica may be associated with low back pain but only in 1–2% of cases.

Most of the patients with the low back pain do not have any neurological deficit. If any rapidly progressive neurological deficit with bowel and bladder incontinence is present, serious etiologies like spinal cord compression, cauda equina syndrome, and conus medullaris syndrome should be ruled out.

History of any trauma even minor in elderly is a red flag and needs evaluation for fracture. History of cancer is important in low back pain evaluation. Malignancies of breast, lung, thyroid, kidney, and prostate are frequently metastasized to spine.

History of fever, chills, night sweats, and weight loss should raise the suspicion of infections of malignancy, especially important in immunocompromised patient and diabetics.

History of referred pain to back is important for serious illnesses like ruptured abdominal aortic aneurysm, pancreatitis, posterior lower lobe pneumonia, renal infarcts, and nephrolithiasis.

Physical Examination

Physical examination for low back pain should be simple and completed in a short duration of time with the main objective to rule out any red flags and identifying neurological deficit. Important points for examination are listed in **Table 2**.

LABORATORY TESTS

Complete hemogram, erythrocyte sedimentation rate (ESR), C-reactive protein, and blood cultures should be ordered when suspecting infection malignancy and rheumatological disease. Urine analysis is required to rule out urinary tract infections.

DIAGNOSTIC IMAGING

For most patients with low back pain, MRI is preferred modality. Best resolution and excellent visualization are obtained for vertebral bodies, soft tissues, spinal canal, spinal

Table 2: Important point to be examined in low back pain patient.

Vitals signs	Fever strongly suggestive of infection
General appearance	Patients comfortable in supine position with nonserious cause of back pain
Abdomen	Abdomen examination essential for any mass tumor
Back	Examine back for any tenderness, discharge, in case of infections and contusions, swelling in cases of trauma
Straight leg raising test	Positive test suggestive of L4-L5 and L5-S1 herniated disk
Neurological examination	Most important part of physical examination
	Light touch pinprick temperature should be tested. Muscle strength reflexes and specific nerve root examination should be performed

Table 3: Treatment for low back pain with serious causes.

Condition	Steps	Definitive treatment
Metastatic epidural tumor	Early referral to oncologist, radiation oncology, dexamethasone (empirical)	Steroid, chemotherapy, radiotherapy, and surgery
Spinal epidural abscess	Blood culture before antibiotics	Antibiotics and surgery
Central disk herniation		Surgery

cord and disk disease. MRI can be used as routine or urgent basis when low back pain is more than 8-week duration. Plain radiograph of spine in anterolateral and lateral position is required if fracture is suspected. CT scan is also useful in evaluating the fracture and when MRI is not available.

MANAGEMENT OF SIMPLE BACK PAIN

Nonpharmacological Modalities

Heat or ice may provide symptomatic relief. Better outcome if early resumption of normal activities in comparison to bed rest. Very short duration of bed rest (2 days) is recommended if required. Spinal manipulative therapy has no beneficial effects on low back pain treatment.

Pharmacological Therapy

Nonsteroidal anti-inflammatory drugs (NSAIDs) are efficacious and first-line therapy for acute low back pain. Acetaminophen, opiate analgesics, and muscle relaxants are as effective as NSAIDs.

Management of Low Back Pain due to Serious Causes

Treatment for low back pain with serious causes is listed in **Table 3**.

SUMMARY

Low back pain is common symptom. Most of the patients recover within 4–6 weeks. Simple musculoskeletal pain required short course of NSAIDs with or without opioids and muscle relaxants. Encourage the patient to resume normal activities earliest. Imaging is required if serious etiology is suspected and back pain persists more than 6- to 8-week duration. MRI is gold standard diagnostic imaging.

CHAPTER 65

Lymphadenopathy

Ritin Mohindra, Praveen Aggarwal

INTRODUCTION

Lymph nodes are a group of specialized cells that represent a division of the defense system in the human body. The body has approximately 600 lymph nodes, and their locations are scattered around portals of entry as well as major blood vessels. Lymph nodes in children are being constantly exposed to newer antigens inciting immune responses, and are thereby larger than those found in adults. Lymph passes through at least one lymph node in the body before getting back into the bloodstream. **Figure 1** shows the different lymph node regions in the body.

DEFINITIONS

Lymphadenopathy is defined as lymph nodes that are abnormal in size, consistency or number. It is said to be localized if only one group of lymph nodes is involved, limited if two to three

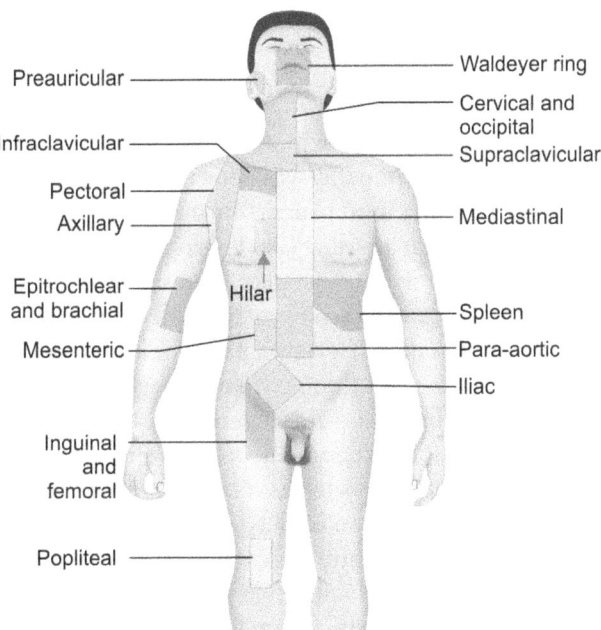

Fig. 1: Lymph node regions.

contiguous groups are involved and generalized if more than three contiguous or more than one noncontiguous groups are involved. In localized or limited lymphadenopathy, the clinician should assess the lymphatic drainage areas, whereas in generalized lymphadenopathy, evaluation should focus on systemic signs and symptoms.

The enlarged lymph nodes may show the following patterns on microscopy:
- *Follicular hyperplasia*: Due to increase in size and number of B-cells
- *Paracortical hyperplasia*: Due to extension of T-cells in the paracortical region
- *Sinus hyperplasia*: Due to expansion of the histiocytes in the medullary and cortical sinuses
- *Granulomatous inflammation*: Due to formation of histiocytic granuloma in the lymph nodes
- *Acute lymphadenitis*: Due to follicular hyperplasia, infiltration by polymorphonuclear cells and necrosis
- *Metastatic infiltration*: Due to infiltration of lymph nodes by malignant cells.

ETIOLOGY

The causes of generalized and localized lymphadenopathy are given in **Tables 1 and 2**.

CLINICAL EVALUATION

A detailed history and meticulous physical examination will identify a readily diagnosable cause of lymphadenopathy such as upper respiratory tract infection, pharyngitis, conjunctivitis, periodontal disease, recent vaccination, cat-scratch disease or dermatitis. Detailed evaluation is needed where the cause and course of lymphadenopathy is not obvious.

History

The history in a patient with lymphadenopathy should focus on the age of the patient, duration of the lymphadenopathy and associated symptoms, underlying comorbidities and the circumstances in which the lymphadenopathy was detected. The precise time of the onset of lymphadenopathy is however elusive as most patients are unable to tell with certainty as to when the enlargement started. Lymphadenopathy that lasts less than 2 weeks or more than 1 year with no progressive size increase is less likely to be neoplastic. Presence of painful lymphadenopathy is commonly reassuring; as it is usually indicative of an underlying benign pathology such as an inflammatory process or suppuration. However, pain does not always necessarily suggest a benign cause and can sometimes occur due to hemorrhage into the necrotic center of a neoplastic node, or immunologic stimulation of pain receptors, or rapid tumor expansion.

Family history may raise suspicion for certain neoplasias such as carcinomas of the breast and melanoma. Environmental exposures such as tobacco, alcohol, and ultraviolet radiation as well as occupational exposures to silicon or beryllium may raise suspicion for metastatic carcinoma of the internal organs, the head and neck, and skin. Furthermore, a history of animal exposure, ingestion of certain drugs and foods, high-risk behaviors, and history of recurrent infection and immunodeficiency can help the diagnosis.

Table 1: Causes of generalized lymphadenopathy.

Infections	• *Bacterial*: Mycobacterial infections, miliary tuberculosis, typhoid fever, syphilis, tularemia, brucellosis, plague, leptospirosis • *Fungal*: Disseminated histoplasmosis • *Protozoal*: Toxoplasmosis, leishmaniasis • *Viral*: Infectious mononucleosis, cytomegalovirus infections, measles, rubella, hepatitis B, dengue fever, HIV
Connective tissue disorders	• Churg-Strauss syndrome • Dermatomyositis • Rheumatoid arthritis • Sjögren's syndrome • Still's disease • Systemic lupus erythematosus
Drugs/Medications	• Allopurinol • Atenolol • Captopril • Carbamazepine • Cephalosporins • Gold • Hydralazine • Penicillin • Phenytoin • Primidone • Pyrimethamine • Quinidine • Sulfonamides • Sulindac
Malignancy	• Lymphomas • Leukemias • Metastaic
Lymphoproliferative disorders	• Angioimmunoblastic T-cell lymphoma • Castleman's disease • Progressive transformation of germinal centers
Metabolic storage diseases	• Gaucher's disease • Niemann-Pick disease
Miscellaneous causes	• Amyloidosis • Chronic granulomatous disease • Langerhans cell histiocytosis • *Penicillium marneffei* infection • Reticuloendotheliosis • Sinus histiocytosis • Sarcoidosis

- A triad of moderate to high fever, pharyngitis, and moderately tender lymph node with or without splenomegaly characterizes classic infectious mononucleosis. Cytomegalovirus, toxoplasmosis, human immunodeficiency virus (HIV), and human herpes virus type 1 can cause mononucleosis-like syndrome.

Table 2: Causes of localized lymphadenopathy.

Head and neck	Oropharyngeal infections (e.g. staphylococcal infection, group A streptococcal infections viral infections), upper respiratory tract infections, viral infections (e.g. infectious mononucleosis, herpes virus, Coxsackievirus infection, cytomegalovirus infection, HIV), mycobacterial lymphadenitis (tuberculous and atypical mycobacteria), dental abscess, conjunctivitis, otitis media, facial cellulitis, cat scratch disease, Hodgkin's lymphoma, non-Hodgkin's lymphoma, thyroid cancer, squamous cell carcinoma of the head and neck, Kawasaki disease, Kikuchi disease, Kimura disease, sinus histiocytosis, autoimmune lymphoproliferative disorders
Supraclavicular	Abdominal/thoracic neoplasm, thyroid cancer, Hodgkin's lymphoma, non-Hodgkin's lymphoma, breast carcinoma, bronchogenic carcinoma, mycobacterial infections, fungal infections
Axillary	Arm/chest wall infection (staphylococcal and streptococcal), cat-scratch disease, tularemia, brucellosis, sarcoidosis, breast cancer, lymphomas, metastatic melanomas, leukemias
Inguinal	Benign reactive lymphadenopathy, urinary tract infections, sexually transmitted diseases (e.g. syphilis, chancroid, genital herpes, lymphogranuloma venereum), perineal infections, lower limb cellulitis, plague squamous cell carcinoma of the penis and vulva, lymphomas, metastatic melanomas
Epitrochlear	Local infections in upper extremity, sarcoidosis, lymphoma, infectious mononucleosis, sporotrichosis, cat-scratch disease, secondary syphilis, HIV
Hilar/Mediastinal	Tuberculosis, histoplasmosis, sarcoidosis, blastomycosis, coccidioidomycosis, silicosis, leukemias, lymphomas, metastasis, Castleman's disease
Abdominal	Mesenteric adenitis (e.g. tuberculosis, measles, yersiniosis, Group A streptococci), lymphomas, gastrointestinal malignancies

- Significant fever, night sweats, and unexplained weight loss (>10% in <6 months) are the "B symptoms" of lymphoproliferative disorders, but they may also be seen in tuberculosis or collagen vascular diseases. Petechiae and purpura associated with lymphadenopathy and splenomegaly may be detected in myeloproliferative disorders.
- Presence of oral ulcers, photosensitivity, joint pains, early morning stiffness, muscle weakness, or butterfly rash indicates the possibility of an autoimmune pathology.
- A recent travel to an endemic area or exposure to an infected patient with active tuberculosis along with painless, gradually progressive, single or matted lymph nodes can suggest mycobacterial infection.
- A history of animal contact or raw milk ingestion may suggest brucellosis.

Clinical Examination

The peripheral groups are the ones which are readily palpable by clinical examination and routinely looked for. The search for enlarged lymph nodes must be carried out in a systematic manner; otherwise, lymph nodes that are only minimally enlarged or embedded in tissue may be missed. The examination should begin with visual inspection of the area, looking for asymmetry or erythema which is followed by systematic palpation of all accessible lymph nodes.

The lymph nodes of the head and neck are always palpated from behind with the patient sitting or standing with the head bending forward to relax the anterior neck muscles. If one side of the neck is palpated at a time, the neck should be flexed to that side. Starting from the top of the neck and going down, all of the various cervical lymph node chains, i.e. preauricular, posterior auricular, occipital, superior cervical, posterior cervical, submandibular, submental, inferior deep cervical, and supraclavicular should be examined.

- The preauricular lymph nodes lie in front of the tragus and may become enlarged in localized infections of the face.
- The postauricular or the retroauricular lymph nodes are located just beneath the ear on the mastoid insertion of the sternocleidomastoid muscle and may become enlarged in mastoiditis.
- The occipital lymph nodes can be palpated at the back of the head close to the insertion of the trapezius muscle in infections of the head and scalp.
- Supraclavicular lymphadenopathy is almost always abnormal and carries the highest risk of malignancy. The patient should be asked to perform a Valsalva's maneuver during palpation of the supraclavicular fossa. Right-sided supraclavicular nodes drain parts of the lung and mediastinum and are signals of intrathoracic lesions, particularly in the lung and esophagus. Left-sided supraclavicular nodes (Virchow's nodes) may indicate pathology in the testes, ovaries, kidneys, pancreas, prostate, stomach or gallbladder. Patients with supraclavicular lymphadenopathy should be examined for dullness over the manubrium sterni indicating concomitant hilar or mediastinal lymphadenopathy.
- Scalene nodes present above and behind the head of clavicles, deep to the sternocleidomastoid on either side of the neck may become enlarged in bronchogenic carcinoma.

The patient should then be examined for axillary lymphadenopathy in the sitting or supine position. The patient's arm, supported by one of the examiner's hands, should be held in a slightly flexed position and adducted. The examiner's right hand is used to examine the patient's left axilla, and the left hand for the right axilla. All the five groups, i.e. (1) central group, (2) apical group, (3) lateral group, (4) anterior group, and (5) the posterior group of axillary nodes should be examined sequentially. The posterior (subscapular) group is better assessed from behind. Axillary lymphadenopathy may be part of a generalized process or may be localized and secondary to infection in the limb. Concomitant epitrochlear, axillary, and supraclavicular lymphadenopathy should raise the question of cat-scratch fever. In patients with underlying breast carcinoma, sometimes axillary lymphadenopathy (sentinel node) may be the only presenting symptom before a breast lump becomes clinically apparent.

Epitrochlear nodes are best palpated with the patient's elbow slightly flexed and forearm supinated. The right epitrochlear area is approached by inserting the examiner's left hand from behind the patient's elbow while the examiner's right hand grasps the right wrist of the patient, supporting the forearm. Epitrochlear node enlargement is usually secondary to infections of the hand and forearm especially in manual laborers. Occasionally, neoplastic processes may present with isolated epitrochlear lymphadenopathy. Enlarged epitrochlear nodes occur frequently in infectious mononucleosis.

Presence of a paraumbilical (Sister Mary Joseph's) node although rare indicates significant intra-abdominal lymphadenopathy and may be a sign of an abdominal or pelvic neoplasm.

The presence of significant inguinal lymphadenopathy may be seen in conditions like syphilis, chancroid, and lymphogranuloma venereum. Unilateral inguinal lymphadenopathy is usually a response to ipsilateral lower extremity infection. Sometimes, inguinal lymphadenopathy can be a part of systemic processes such as lymphoma or leukemia. Femoral lymph nodes can be palpated in the femoral triangle. Their enlargement is also secondary to chronic infection and trauma, but carries much more pathologic significance than inguinal lymphadenopathy. Occasionally lymphadenopathy can be found in the popliteal fossa as part of a generalized process or can be localized secondary to infection or trauma of the lower extremity.

The following additional points may be noted in the assessment of lymphadenopathy:

- *Size*: Lymph nodes in the axillary and cervical region up to 1 cm in diameter, and those in the inguinal region up to 1.5 cm in diameter are considered normal. Palpable supraclavicular, iliac, popliteal nodes and epitrochlear nodes greater than 0.5 cm, and inguinal nodes greater than 1.5 cm are abnormal. The nodes in other areas are considered as abnormal if their diameter is greater than 1 cm. The term "shotty" is sometimes used for multiple small nodes that do not carry any diagnostic significance.
- *Consistency*: Acute inflammation by infiltrating the node may make it firm in consistency with concomitant tenderness, due to the tension on the capsule. Chronic inflammation also leads to fibrotic changes, making the node hard on palpation. Painless stony-hard nodes are usually signs of metastatic cancer. Firm irregularly shaped rubbery nodes can imply lymphoma. "Matted" lymph nodes are described in benign (mycobacterial infection and sarcoidosis) or malignant (lymphoma and metastatic carcinoma) disorders when a group of nodes are conglomerated.
- *Mobility*: Lymphadenopathy resulting from infections and collagen vascular diseases are usually freely mobile in the subcutaneous tissue. Rubbery mobile nodes are associated with lymphoma. Nodes that are associated with malignancy are often fixed to the skin or surrounding tissues.
- *Tenderness*: Tenderness in a node suggests recent rapid enlargement that has caused capsular stretching. It is normally associated with an inflammatory process but can also result from hemorrhage into a node, immunological stimulation and malignancy.

Many important lymph node groups cannot be evaluated by the physical examination. Whenever there is evidence of generalized lymphadenopathy, these groups should be evaluated carefully. Hilar and mediastinal lymphadenopathy can compromise regional structures such as the superior vena cava or trachea and potentially cause a life-threatening complication. There are multiple lymph node groupings in the abdomen, including mesenteric, para-aortic, celiac, and retrogastric. Bulky abdominal lymphadenopathy can also compromise structures, including the ureters and inferior vena cava, and can cause complications such as renal failure.

Organomegaly (especially splenomegaly) is sometimes associated with lymphadenopathy, as in infectious mononucleosis, acute leukemia, Hodgkin's disease, non-Hodgkin's lymphoma, and sarcoidosis. Skin involvement can be in the form of unusual lesions suggesting malignancy such as melanoma, and for traumatic lesions that potentially can be an inoculation site for microbial germs. Therefore, it is pertinent for all patients with lymphadenopathy to undergo a complete and systematic physical examination.

Investigations

If history and physical examination findings suggest a benign or self-limited process, the patient can be reassured and asked to follow-up if lymphadenopathy persists. Findings suggestive of infectious or autoimmune etiologies may require specific testing and treatment as indicated. If there is low suspicion of malignancy on clinical evaluation, localized lymphadenopathy can be observed for 4 weeks. Generalized lymphadenopathy should prompt laboratory testing to look for systemic causes.

Laboratory Diagnostic Methods

The workup in patients with lymphadenopathy should start with complete and differential blood counts, erythrocyte sedimentation rate (ESR), C-reactive protein (CRP), and a peripheral blood smear. Anemia and other cytopenias may indicate a serious underlying cause like leukemias, systemic lupus erythematosus (SLE), and HIV. Increased neutrophil count can be seen in acute bacterial infections whereas an extreme increase ($\geq 50,000/mm^3$) is a leukemoid reaction in response to infections or inflammation and is rare in myeloproliferative disorders. Lymphocytosis can be seen in leukemias, infectious mononucleosis, chronic granulomatous diseases, and autoimmune diseases. Raised lactate dehydrogenase (LDH) and serum uric acid levels indicate a rapid cell turnover as seen in malignancies. Bone marrow examination may be warranted in the presence of atypical lymphocytosis on peripheral smear. HIV serology should be done in patients presenting with generalized lymphadenopathy. If autoimmune diseases are suspected, antinuclear antibody, double-stranded DNA (dsDNA) antibody, and complement level should be checked.

Imaging

Imaging is superior to physical examination when it comes to assessment of lymph node characteristics. The imaging assessment is done in terms of the number, size, site, shape, margins, and the internal structure of the lymph nodes. Ultrasonography (USG) can readily assess these nodal characteristics in case of peripheral lymphadenopathy whereas computed tomography (CT) scan and magnetic resonance imaging (MRI) are more useful in assessment of lymphadenopathy in the thorax and the abdominopelvic cavity. Color Doppler US can further evaluate the vascular pattern, displacement of vascularity, vascular resistance, and pulsatility index (PI) which can be used to differentiate an old lymphadenopathy from a recent lymphadenopathy which is still active. A normal or reactive node is usually oval and is isoechoic with the adjacent structures with a long axis to short axis ratio (Solbiati index) more than 2 and has prominent hilar vascularity whereas metastatic nodes may be round with sharp borders and a long axis to short axis ratio (Solbiati index) of less than 2, hypoechoic in comparison to the adjacent structures and often have a peripheral perfusion pattern and a poorly preserved hilum. The vascular resistance indices, i.e. resistive index (RI) and the PI measured by spectral Doppler US can sometimes differentiate between benign and malignant nodes. Benign nodes have a low RI (<0.8) and a low PI (<1.5) whereas in case of malignancies in nodes, there is high RI (>0.8) and a high PI (>1.5).

Newer techniques like endoscopic ultrasound (EUS) and endobronchial ultrasound (EBUS) are minimally invasive but highly effective procedures in differentiating between various diseases causing enlarged lymph nodes in the abdomen and chest. Additionally, EBUS also allows the physician to obtain tissue or fluid samples from the enlarged lymph nodes using a technique known as transbronchial needle aspiration (TBNA). Positron emission tomography (PET) scanning is not helpful as a screening tool to distinguish between benign and malignant conditions as both may cause intense uptake. It is however helpful in staging of some malignancies, once the diagnosis is confirmed.

Tissue Diagnosis

Tissue diagnosis is the gold standard in the evaluation of lymphadenopathy. Fine-needle aspiration cytology (FNAC) is a safe, simple, and cost-effective technique which provides rapid results directing further approach to a patient presenting with lymphadenopathy. It is most useful when looking for the recurrence of a previously diagnosed cancer. The cytomorphological features collaborate with histopathology and have qualities of a microbiopsy. The diagnostic yield of FNAC of deep-seated lymph nodes can be improved by radiological guidance like USG and CT scan. The limitations of FNAC remain in the lack of proper tissue sample to run special studies including cytogenetics, flow cytometry, electron microscopy, and special stains. There is also a potential risk of seeding a tract with malignancy during this procedure.

Core needle biopsy provides more specimen from the tissue than FNAC for special studies in addition to providing information on nodal architecture and is extremely useful in the diagnosis and classification of lymphomas. Open biopsy allows histological examination of intact tissue and provides information about the presence of abnormal cells and abnormal node architecture.

If multiple node groups are involved, one of the larger, firmer, and most recently enlarging nodes should be biopsied. If no single node predominates, the supraclavicular node is selected followed by nodes of the neck, groin, and axilla in that order. The chance of infection and damage to neurovascular structures is greatest in the groin and axilla as is the possibility of a nonspecific result. The high tissue yield in cases of open biopsy allows the pathologist to do smears, strains, cultures, immunohistochemical, cytogenetic, and molecular genetic techniques. The development of newer minimally invasive endoscopic and percutaneous techniques and the widespread application of molecular genetic techniques may limit the need for open biopsy in the evaluation of lymphadenopathy in the near future.

A common dilemma that the clinician faces is to differentiate between a benign and a malignant lymph node enlargement. Certain features that can aid the clinician in differentiating between a benign and malignant lymph node enlargement are given in **Table 3**.

Table 3: Differences between benign and malignant lymph nodes.

	Benign	*Malignant*
History: • Age • Duration • Rate of growth • Pain • Type	<40 years <4–6 weeks Slow Painful Localized	>40 years >4–6 weeks Rapid Painless Generalized
Examination: • Size • Location • Tenderness • Consistency • Mobility • Surroundings	<2 cm Inguinal/Submandibular Tender Soft Mobile Not attached	>2 cm Supraclavicular/Epitrochlear Nontender Firm/Hard/Rubbery Fixed Attached
Biomarkers: • Serum soluble IL-2 receptor • Serum LDH	Normal Normal	Raised Raised
Imaging: • Shape • Border • Hilum • Internal echogenicity • Blood flow distribution • Solbiati index • Resistive index • Pulsatility index	Ovoid Regular Hyperechoic Isoechoic Hilar High (>2) Low (<0.8) Low (<1.5)	Round Variable Loss of echogenic hilum Hypoechoic Peripheral Low (<2) High (>0.8) High (>1.5)
Histopathology: • Cells with neoplastic appearance • Nuclear atypia • Mitosis • Necrosis • Ulceration • Capsular invasion • Structural differentiation • Functional differentiation • Retention of specialization • Molecular aberrations • Immunohistochemistry markers for malignancy	Absent Absent Normal Absent Absent Absent Present Present Present Absent Negative	Present Present Abnormal Present Present Present Absent Absent Absent Present Positive

COMPLICATIONS

Complications can result from the lymphadenopathy itself or the underlying etiology. Management of local compressive symptoms due to the enlarged lymph nodes like airway or bronchial obstruction requires emergency airway management. Erosion of a node into a bronchus or trachea can result in hemoptysis which may require angiographic embolization. Mediastinal lymphadenopathy can cause superior vena cava syndrome with obstruction of the blood flow which is treated with chemotherapy and possibly radiation therapy. Abdominal lymphadenopathy leading to intestinal obstruction caused by intussusceptions requires emergency surgery. Serious metabolic complications like uric acid nephropathy, hyperkalemia, hypercalcemia or hypocalcemia, hyperphosphatemia, and acute renal failure due to underlying malignant etiology should be searched for and managed promptly.

TREATMENT

The treatment of lymphadenopathy depends on the underlying etiology. A short course of oral antibiotics may be warranted before aspiration or biopsy is performed especially in patients with a high suspicion of an underlying infection. Therapy with glucocorticoids should be avoided until a definitive diagnosis is made as they may mask and delay the diagnosis of certain malignancies. Patients may also become ineligible for certain treatment protocols if they have received glucocorticoids. Antitubercular treatment is recommended for documented diagnosis of lymph node tuberculosis. With the availability of newer molecular techniques for the diagnosis of lymph node tuberculosis, empiric antitubercular therapy is no longer recommended. The diagnosis of HIV requires prompt initiation of antiretroviral therapy. Autoimmune conditions like SLE or sarcoidosis may require corticosteroids and other immunosuppressants while the diagnosis of a malignancy may require surgery, chemotherapy, and radiotherapy.

CHAPTER 66

Melena

Shashank Karale, Uday Sanglodkar

INTRODUCTION

Melena is the term used for black stool. Melena indicates about the bleeding from the upper gastrointestinal (GI) tract. As the blood passes through the ileum and the colon, iron in the hemoglobin oxidizes and stool become black. Immediate resuscitation and hemodynamic stability are the important measures in the patient with melena followed by diagnostic studies and treatment of specific disorder.

CAUSES

- Peptic ulcer disease
- Erosive gastritis
- Esophageal and gastric varices
- Mallory-Weiss tear
- Dieulafoy lesion
- Upper GI malignancy.

CLINICAL FEATURES

- Peptic ulcer-epigastric and right upper quadrant pain
- Erosive gastritis—dysphagia, reflux
- Mallory-Weiss tear—retching emesis
- Variceal bleeding, jaundice, weakness, fatigue, anorexia
- Gastrointestinal malignancy, dysphagia, cachexia.

RED FLAGS

- Symptoms that suggest severe bleeding
- Orthostatic hypotension
- Dizziness
- Confusion
- Palpitation
- Cold clammy extremities.

INITIAL EVALUATION

History

Every patient with history of black stool should be evaluated as soon as possible to assess the severity of bleeding, to ascertain source of the bleeding. Information collected from the initial evaluation helpful in resuscitation, diagnostic, and treatment. Mostly melena occurs if GI bleeding proximal to ligament of Treitz.

Past medical history about hematemesis, abdominal pain, dyspepsia, and dysphagia should be obtained. History of smoking, alcohol, and liver disease should be documented. History of use of nonsteroidal anti-inflammatory drug (NSAID), antiplatelets and anticoagulants or iron tablets are important.

Physical Examination

In cases of upper GI bleed (hematemesis, melena), physical examination is the key to check hemodynamic status. Signs of hypovolemia like low pulse pressure, tachycardia, cold clammy extremities, postural hypotension should be addressed on priority basis. Palmar erythema, jaundice, spider angioma, and gynecomastia give clue for existing liver disease. Abdominal examination is performed for any tenderness organomegaly mass and ascites. Rectal examination may also give some clue for diagnosis.

INVESTIGATIONS

Initial laboratory workup starts with complete hemogram, knowing the status of baseline hemoglobin and obtaining the blood grouping and typing, other tests helpful are lactate level, coagulation profile, liver function test, kidney function test. Patient with upper GI bleed usually has raised blood urea nitrogen (BUN):creatinine or urea:creatinine ratio. Electrocardiograph, cardiac enzyme should be obtained in the high-risk group patient like elderly.

MANAGEMENT

Triage

Hemodynamic stabilization is the key for initial management. Aggressive resuscitation in patient with hemorrhagic shock. Two large bore cannulas should be inserted immediately, typed and cross-matched blood transfusion as soon as possible. Airway management should be considered in patient with respiratory difficulties and altered mental status. Elective intubation further decreases the risk of aspiration.

Fluid Resuscitation and Blood Transfusion

Patient with active bleeding and/or with the unstable hemodynamic parameters should receive intravenous fluid (normal saline or Ringer's lactate 500 mL in 30 minutes) till the blood is arranged. Initially baseline hemoglobin level should be obtained later hemoglobin level is diluted by movement of extravascular fluid to vascular space and also by intravenous fluid during resuscitation. Most of the guidelines suggested to keep the hemoglobin level greater than 7 g in active bleeding patient and greater than 9 g in patient with unstable coronary artery disease. Avoid transfusing the blood in variceal bleed patient as it can worsen the bleeding from the varices. Platelet and fresh frozen plasma transfusion should be considered in patient with low platelet count and deranged coagulation profile [international normalized ratio (INR) >1.5]. Platelet transfusion should also be considered in patient on antiplatelet therapy.

Nasogastric Lavage

Nasogastric lavage is not beneficial in all patient of upper GI bleed. Nasogastric lavage is helpful in removing the particulate matter, blood clot, fresh blood from the stomach which facilitates the endoscopy.

Endoscopy

For upper GI bleed, endoscopy is diagnostic modality of choice. Endoscopy is helpful in identifying in bleeding lesion and after that hemostasis can also be achieved in bleeding lesion by therapeutic endoscopy. Early endoscopy is recommended in patient with upper GI bleed.

Medications

Medications used in upper GI bleed have been shown in **Table 1**.

Table 1: Medications used in upper gastrointestinal bleed.

Acid suppression	Proton pump inhibitors (PPIs) Pantoprazole, Omeprazole, Esomeprazole	Intravenous PPIs are started and decision for further continuation is taken after endoscopy. Benefits of PPIs are decrease risk of rebleeding incidence, shorter length of hospital stay.
		Bolus dose 80 mg followed by infusion 8 mg/h continued for 72 hours then patient can be switched to oral dose if no further bleeding
Somatostatin and its analog	Octreotide	Used in variceal bleeding also lowers the risk of bleeding in nonvariceal bleeding. It should not be used as routine in nonvariceal bleeding. Intravenous bolus dose 50 µg followed by 50 µg/h
Prokinetics	Erythromycin Metoclopramide	Prokinetic agents helpful in gastric clearance (of blood, clot, food residue) and provide better visualization during endoscopy
		Erythromycin 3 mg/kg intravenous over 30 minutes (60–90 minutes prior to endoscopy)
		Metoclopramide single dose intravenous 60–90 minutes prior to endoscopy

Consultation

Consultation by gastroenterologist should be obtained for all patients with upper GI bleed (hematemesis and melena).

Other Diagnostic Tests

- Angiography
- Tagged red blood cell scan
- Capsule endoscopy.

SUMMARY

Careful history taking and physical examination is important to assess the severity, identify the possible source of bleeding. Resuscitation with intravenous fluid and blood product in hemodynamic unstable patient should be started as soon as possible. Further information may be obtained by blood tests and endoscopy. Therapeutic endoscopy can be used to achieve the hemostasis. Medications like proton pump inhibitors, somatostatin and its analog, prokinetics are also helpful. Gastroenterologist opinion should be taken as early as possible.

CHAPTER 67

Muscle Cramps

Sayuri Enriquez Saenz

INTRODUCTION

Contraction and relaxation are the important function of muscles, and any disruption in this mechanism causes muscle cramps. Common causes of muscle cramp are dehydration due to hot weather, exercise or standing for prolonged period. Calf muscles of leg is the most commonly involved muscles. Muscle cramp is a temporarily troublesome but harmless situation where it is very difficult to use the affected muscle.

ETIOLOGY

Underlying causes are inadequate blood supply, nerve compression, and mineral depletion.
- *Dehydration*: Diarrhea, alcohol
- *Electrolyte*: Hypocalcemia, hypokalemia, hypomagnesemia
- *Endocrine*: Hypothyroidism, hyperthyroidism
- Respiratory alkalosis
- *Peripheral arterial disease*: Arterial occlusive disease
- *Trauma*: Muscle, spinal injuries, fractures.

RISK FACTORS
- Elderly population
- Athletes/sports participation in hot weather
- Comorbidities like diabetes, chronic kidney disease, chronic liver disease, and thyroid disorder.

CLINICAL PRESENTATION

Muscle cramps are usually infrequent but in elderly and some individual are frequent. Duration of cramps lasts between few seconds to minutes. Night cramps usually occur in Legs while resting at night times. History about timing, severity and location of the spasm should be obtained from the patient. Intermittent claudication, aching and cramping mostly in calf muscle during walking or exercise but symptoms relieved by rest are the main symptoms of the peripheral arterial disease. In this case, a specific history should be taken about how far they

can walk without symptoms. Pain swelling and involvement of soft tissue and decreased range of motion are the common symptoms for cramps, sprain, and strain.
- *Spasm*: It is sudden involuntary contraction of muscle which further progresses to chronic spasm and shortening of the muscle and finally decreased range of motion.
- *Sprain*: It is overstretching of ligaments which cause weakening and tearing of ligaments. Any joint can be affected but ankle joint most commonly affected.
- *Strain*: It is overstretching of muscle or tendon also known as pulled muscle.

INVESTIGATIONS

- Complete blood count, serum sodium, potassium, magnesium, calcium, thyroid function tests, electrocardiography, arterial blood gases, carbon dioxide level, and arteriography.

MANAGEMENT

First aid: Avoid heat, apply ice packs for 20–30 minutes, every hour this will relax the muscles, reduce the pain and inflammation. Stretching and massaging the muscle also helpful in relieving the muscle pain.

Emergency interventions: Start the treatment measures to reduce the inflammation so the range of motion can be increased. If symptoms persist, check signs of hypocalcemia, evaluate for respiratory functions, if these signs are present suspect hypocalcemia, obtain blood for investigations, and prepare for intravenous administration of calcium.

Heat cramps occur due to taking water without adequate salts which causes hypernatremia and muscle cramps. Treatment started with fluid (normal saline) and electrolytes.

Oral potassium supplementation is recommended in the mild to moderate deficiency of hypokalemia muscle cramps.

Hypomagnesemic muscle cramps have similar symptoms like hypokalemia, muscle weakness and cramps. Hypomagnesemia and hypokalemia share common etiologies like diuretics, diarrhea, alcoholism, and aminoglycosides. Many conditions refractory to potassium replacement until magnesium is replaced.

TREATMENT

Symptomatic relief—by narcotics, benzodiazepines muscle relaxant. Suggested drugs for treatment of cramps are magnesium, calcium, vitamin B complex, vitamin E, quinine. Intravenous fluid and diazepam can be used for very severe cramp. Magnesium sulfate (intravenous) can also be used for severe cramp.

SUMMARY

Muscle spasms are common in population mostly are self-limiting or relieved by simple stretching. Few needs intravenous fluid and electrolyte replacement (potassium, calcium and magnesium).

CHAPTER 68

Muscle Wasting

Praveen Aggarwal, Ritin Mohindra

INTRODUCTION

Muscle wasting is a clinical syndrome characterized by a progressive loss of skeletal muscle mass with/without loss of function. The term "muscle wasting" is a broad term which does not take into account the onset, i.e. whether the muscle wasting is acute or chronic, or the underlying pathophysiology of the muscle wasting. Of late, a new term "myopenia" has been suggested when there is a clinically relevant degree of muscle wasting that is associated either with impaired functional capacity and/or with increased risk of morbidity and mortality.

Muscle wasting is said to be "localized" if it occurs in specific muscles as a result of denervation or inactivity, or "generalized" if there is global muscle wasting secondary to diseases like sepsis, cancer, renal, and cardiac failure. The etiology of muscle wasting is multifactorial and involves an imbalance between the anabolic and catabolic pathways that determine muscle mass. These factors include genetic influences, disuse atrophy or immobility, nutritional deficiencies and hormonal imbalances.

PATHOPHYSIOLOGY

Muscle wasting occurs when the rate of muscle protein breakdown exceeds the rate of protein synthesis. The major anabolic pathway that leads to increased muscle protein synthesis is the Akt-mammalian target of rapamycin (mTOR) pathway. Insulin-like growth factor 1 (IGF-1), branched chain amino acids, testosterone, aerobic activity, and β2-adrenergic agents promote muscle growth by upregulating this pathway. The major catabolic pathway involved in muscle wasting acts by activating the ubiquitin-proteasome system (UPS) pathway and calpain and caspases which are under the control of transcription factors Forkhead box O and nuclear factor (NF)-κB. The myostatin pathway has also been implicated in muscle wasting as it downregulates the Akt-mTOR pathway. Most muscle proteins, especially the myofibrillar components, are degraded by the UPS, and the reduction in muscle strength is attributed to this loss of contractile machinery. The cell organelles like mitochondria are also degraded by autophagy, and their loss accounts for decreased endurance of the wasted muscles. Certain proinflammatory cytokines like tumor necrosis factor-α (TNF-α), interferon-γ (IFN-γ), and interleukin (IL)-6 which are elevated in catabolic conditions like sepsis, burns, and cancers may also trigger muscle wasting by increasing the expression of other cytokines and NF-κB.

CLINICAL EVALUATION

History

At the outset, it is important to distinguish true muscle wasting/weakness from lassitude as patients with a variety of systemic disorders may have a perception of weakness due to functional limitation, but may have normal muscle power and muscle bulk on testing. The weakness associated with muscle wasting disorders is usually persistent and may be generalized, as in myasthenia gravis, long-standing periodic paralysis, advanced disuse atrophy from prolonged bed rest or long-standing motor neuron disease. If not generalized, the patient may present with muscle wasting which is symmetric or asymmetric.

Symmetric patterns of wasting can have proximal, distal or specific distributions.

- Proximal muscle wasting involves the axial muscle groups, deltoids, and hip flexors. The patient usually complains of difficulty rising from a chair (hip muscles) or combing his/her hair (shoulder girdle). In majority of the myopathies including polymyositis and dermatomyositis, and myasthenia gravis, the proximal muscles are weaker than the distal muscles and the involvement is usually symmetric. The facial muscles are usually spared in most of myopathies (limb-girdle involvement). This pattern of involvement is also seen in muscular dystrophies except myotonic dystrophy type 1 (facial and distal limb weakness).
- Distal muscle wasting is characterized by reduced grip strength and difficulty doing fine work with the hands (intrinsic hand muscles). The patient may also complain of difficulty in standing on his/her toes (gastrocnemius/soleus). It is found in early motor neuron diseases and peripheral neuropathies.
- Specific distributions of muscle wasting involving specific muscle groups usually suggest a dystrophy. Facial involvement and winging of scapula are characteristic of facioscapulohumeral dystrophy. Presence of ptosis or extraocular muscle weakness (cranial nerve involvement) is seen in neuromuscular junction disorders (e.g. myasthenia gravis), oculopharyngeal muscular dystrophy and mitochondrial myopathy.

Asymmetric muscle wasting most likely reflects diseases of the central or peripheral nervous system. Asymmetric involvement of flexor forearm muscles and quadriceps muscles is virtually diagnostic of inclusion body myositis. Selective neck extensor muscle involvement (dropped head syndrome) can be seen in myasthenia gravis, hyperparathyroidism, focal myositis, etc.

Muscle pain is usually not associated with muscle wasting disorders. Localized muscle pain is often secondary to trauma or infection or neoplastic infiltration of the muscle. Myopathies are usually painless. Generalized myalgias are seen in fibromyalgia syndrome and polymyalgia rheumatica. Infectious myopathies such as trichinellosis and viral myositis and certain drugs like cimetidine, cocaine, cyclosporine, labetalol, and statins are also implicated in myalgias. The long-term use of these drugs, if continued, can lead to muscle wasting.

Muscle cramps or spasms are painful, involuntary, localized muscle contractions with visible and palpable muscle hardening and occur during pregnancy, neurogenic disorders, and polyneuropathies. It is rarely seen in primary muscle disorders. Myotonia is a condition of prolonged muscle contraction followed by slow muscle relaxation and is seen in muscular dystrophies and some channelopathies. Muscle stiffness different from the one caused due to inflammation of joints and periarticular surfaces is seen in stiff person syndrome and neuromyotonia.

In muscle wasting disorders due to myopathies, muscle tissue is often replaced by fat and connective tissue, but the apparent size of muscle is unaffected. However, some patients with limb-girdle myopathies may have enlarged calf muscles.

Age at onset and sex of the patient may point to some muscle dystrophies. A history of recurrent episodes of exertion-related pigmenturia and weakness suggests a metabolic myopathy. Endocrinopathies such as thyroid dysfunction or Cushing's syndrome may be the cause of true muscle weakness and wasting.

Clinical Examination

The first step in the clinical examination of muscle wasting is to carefully search for disorders that can cause the perception of weakness. This helps to distinguish true muscle weakness and wasting from lassitude or motor impairment not due to loss of muscle power. The examiner should then try to localize the site of the lesion in the neuromuscular system which is producing the wasting. The sites include motor cortex, corticospinal tracts, anterior horn cells, spinal nerve roots, peripheral nerves, neuromuscular junction, and finally the muscle. The distribution of weakness, presence or absence of deep tendon reflexes, associated sensory defects, presence of clonus and fasciculations, and the Babinski sign all help to localize the lesion in the neuromuscular system. Once the neuromuscular site has been identified, the cause of the lesion (genetic/inflammatory/immunological/infectious/neoplastic/toxic/metabolic) should be determined.

A preliminary general inspection should be done to compare the shape and size of the limbs and to detect deformities. The patient should be examined in the lying, sitting, and later in the standing position, placing the limbs in symmetrical positions. Any apparent differences in size must be checked by careful measurement which can be due to congenital maldevelopment, long-standing neurological lesions or due to acquired lesions of local structures. This should be followed by examination of the shoulder girdles, upper arms, forearms, hands, hip girdles, thighs, and calf muscles to detect wasting. If wasting is observed, inspect the each group of muscle carefully. Sometimes, the wasted limb muscles may be superficially obscured by subcutaneous fat and felt on palpation only. Conversely, loss of subcutaneous tissue can be mistaken for muscle wasting. Different disease processes presenting with different patterns of muscle wasting are shown in **Table 1**.

Muscle tone, defined as the degree of tension present in a muscle at rest should be assessed after asking the patient to relax. The muscles should always be compared with their counterparts on the other side and tone should be evaluated in both the upper limbs and the lower limbs. The strength of each muscle can be assessed by determining how much force is required by the examiner to overcome maximal contraction by the patient and can be graded from 0 to 5 as per the Medical Research Council grading system.

Table 1: Types of muscle wasting.

Generalized wasting	• Human immunodeficiency virus (HIV) • Malignancies • Thyrotoxicosis • Motor neuron diseases • Myopathies • Chronic obstructive pulmonary disease (COPD)
Individual muscle group wasting	• Compressive/Traumatic nerve root lesion • Vascular/Traumatic lesion of peripheral nerve • Peripheral nerve lesions in metabolic or toxic neuropathy • Local trauma to muscle

Proximal muscle wasting	• Muscular dystrophies
	  – Facioscapulohumeral dystrophy
	  – Limb-girdle syndromes
	  – X-linked muscular dystrophies
	• Motor neuron disease
	• Syringomyelia
	• Inflammatory lesions
	  – Neuralgic amyotrophy
	  – Old poliomyelitis
	  – Inflammatory myopathies
	• Compressive lesions
	  – Cervical spondylosis
	  – Cervical cord tumors
	  – Cauda equina lesions
	  – Massive disk prolapse

Distal muscle wasting	• Muscular dystrophies
	  – Myotonic dystrophy
	  – Muscular dystrophy of Welander
	• Motor neuron disease
	• Inclusion body myositis
	• Syringomyelia
	• Old poliomyelitis
	• Traumatic lesions of nerves/brachial plexus
	• Compressive lesions
	  – Cervical rib
	  – Cervical spondylosis
	  – Cervical cord tumors
	  – Cervical glandular enlargement
	  – Superior pulmonary sulcus tumors

Peripheral wasting in both proximal and distal muscles	• Inclusion body myositis • Peroneal muscle atrophy (Charcot-Marie-Tooth disease) • Chronic polyneuropathies

Facial, ocular, and neck muscles are affected early in certain muscle wasting diseases, and must be examined in all patients with muscle wasting. Additionally, changes in the tongue and bulbar region must be looked for as their involvement can also serve to distinguish between myopathies, motor neuron diseases, and other forms of progressive muscle diseases. At the end

Table 2: Localization of muscle weakness.

Functional impairment	Muscle weakness
• Impaired eye closure	Upper facial muscles
• Impaired pucker	Lower facial muscles
• Inability to raise head from prone position	Neck extensor muscles
• Inability to raise head from prone position	Neck flexor muscles
• Inability to raise hands above head	Shoulder muscles
• Inability to get up from a chair	Hip muscles
• Inability to get up from the floor without climbing up the extremities	Hip/thigh/trunk muscles
• Back-kneeing	Knee extensor muscles
• Steppage gait	Leg muscles (anterior compartment)
• Waddling gait	Hip muscles
• Toe walking	Achilles muscle (tendon)

of the clinical examination, if the patient is well enough, he should be made to walk in a straight line, then turn and walk back to the starting point. This may reveal a lordotic posture caused by combined trunk and hip weakness, frequently exaggerated by toe walking. A waddling gait is caused due to weakness of the hip muscles; hyperextension of the knee (back-kneeing) is characteristic of quadriceps muscle weakness. Distal muscle wasting in the lower limbs is accompanied by a steppage gait due to a foot drop. The functional impairment caused by the different muscle groups is represented in **Table 2**.

Investigations

Laboratory studies: Plasma enzymes (creatine kinase, aldolase, lactate dehydrogenase, and the aminotransferases) can be elevated in muscle diseases. Amongst these, creatine kinase is the preferred muscle enzyme to measure in myopathies. Damage to muscles causes it to leak into serum. The MM isoenzyme predominates in the skeletal muscle while the MB isoenzyme is a marker for cardiac muscle. Raised levels of aldolase, lactate dehydrogenase, and aminotransferases may be erroneously attributed to liver disease, when in fact muscle may be the cause. If the level of γ-glutamyl transferase level is also raised, it helps to establish a hepatic origin of the other enzymes as γ-glutamyl transferase is not found in muscles. Absence of red blood cells (RBCs) in the urinary sediment with a positive test for urine blood suggests myoglobinuria.

Serological tests like antinuclear antibody (ANA), antineutrophil cytoplasmic antibody (ANCA), anti-Ro/SSA, anti-La/SSB, anti-Sm, hepatitis B and C serologies, and cryoglobulins should be obtained in patients with suspected inflammatory myopathy, connective tissue disorders, and vasculitis. Specific tests for drugs, toxins, metabolic or endocrine disorders can be ordered if these are suspected on the basis of clinical evaluation.

Electrodiagnostic studies: Electrodiagnostic tests can help to differentiate whether the site of lesion is in the peripheral nervous system, the neuromuscular junction or the muscle itself. These include electromyography (EMG), sensory and motor nerve conduction, F response, and

H reflex. The EMG of a patient who has muscle wasting due to a myopathy shows a decreased amplitude and duration of response as compared to a patient who has muscle wasting due to a neuropathic cause. Increased spontaneous activity and fibrillations may also be seen in the former on EMG. The nerve conduction studies help in determining the extent of sensory motor deficits and categorizing demyelinating (prolonged terminal latency, slowing of nerve conduction velocity, dispersion, and conduction block) and axonal (marginal slowing of nerve conduction) neuropathies. EMG may also be useful in directing the site of muscle biopsy.

Imaging: In routine practice, very few tools are available to detect muscle loss or even muscle wasting in affected patients. Magnetic resonance imaging (MRI) can reveal underlying muscle edema, muscle atrophy or a mass in the muscle and can also give a clue to whether biopsy is required in muscle wasting diseases. It may even be better than EMG in choosing the site of muscle biopsy. X-ray absorptiometry is the standard method of assessing lean mass including the muscle. However, bioelectrical impedance analysis when available is a better alternative because of its mobility and rapid technical application, without use of radiation. New isotope-based invasive method using deuterium oxide (D_2O) has been recently validated in quantifying muscle anabolism before any changes in muscle mass become detectable. Another method allows measurement of a stable (nonradioactive) isotope of creatine (D_3-creatine) that reflects total muscle mass in a single urine sample. These methods seem to be suitable for the assessment and monitoring of muscle mass in patients with muscle wasting diseases.

Muscle biopsy: Muscle biopsy helps to determine the precise cause of muscle wasting. The biopsy is usually obtained from quadriceps or biceps brachii muscle and less commonly from the deltoid muscle. Evaluation includes a combination of techniques—light microscopy, histochemistry, immunochemistry, and electron microscopy. Western blot analysis and antibody testing against abnormal muscle proteins like dystrophin and merosin are also available, which can help to diagnose certain dystrophies.

Genetic testing: Genetic testing serves as an important tool for the definitive diagnosis of many muscle disorders and in the categorization of certain heritable myopathies.

■ TREATMENT

Despite extensive research efforts in the field of muscle wasting in the last few decades, no effective treatment of muscle wasting exists. Despite differences in their pathophysiology, it is widely believed that these diseases may respond to interventions and/or drugs that increase muscle mass and strength. Till date, exercise training is the only validated treatment for muscle wasting. Endurance training has been shown to decrease systemic inflammatory markers and improve endothelial function which helps to overcome anabolic resistance. On the other hand, light-load resistance training is known to cause muscle hypertrophy. Together, both promote skeletal muscle angiogenesis and increase muscle growth and mass by downregulating the myostatin pathway. However, exercise is not a practical option for bed-ridden, frail, older patients or those with acute illnesses. Disuse atrophy can often be treated with restoration of appropriate exercise. Depending on severity, physical rehabilitation may be advised.

In addition, patients' nutrition should be optimized to prevent nutritional lack of proteins and micronutrients. The provision of nutritional supplements incorporating essential amino acids combined with exercise training has been suggested to be the best method of attenuating muscle wasting. Muscle wasting caused by nerve damage may require musculoskeletal manipulations, anti-inflammatory medications such as corticosteroids, and even surgery to reduce pressure on injured nerves. Low-voltage electric stimulation has also been used to stimulate denervated muscles in individuals with peripheral nerve damage. Pulsed focused ultrasound, by stimulating the activation and propagation of neural signals in the targeted neurons, may also have a beneficial role in muscle atrophy.

The use of most of the drugs for muscle wasting has not progressed beyond the development phase. This is because, for the use of these agents as therapies for muscle wasting, it requires much more than simply the demonstration of increased muscle mass by them. It is difficult to demonstrate the efficacy of these drugs in vivo, while ensuring safety. Also, the improvements in quality of life are difficult to quantify. Also, such therapies that build muscle are liable to be misused to enhance athletic performance. All these are major roadblocks in the development and licensing of these newer agents.

Despite all these limitations, a number of candidate drugs have shown promise in treating muscle wasting diseases. Ghrelin agonists like anamorelin which are growth hormone secretagogues have been shown to stimulate appetite and food intake, improve body composition and muscle wasting in malnourished patients. Selective androgen receptor molecules (SARMs) are in late stage clinical development for muscle wasting and cancer cachexia. SARMs modulate the same anabolic pathways targeted with classical steroid androgens but are devoid of the side effects commonly seen with the latter. These have been shown to increase muscle mass and improve physical function in patients with muscle wasting and cancer cachexia. Tirasemtiv, a fast skeletal muscle troponin activator has also been shown to increase muscle function and performance in animal models, by sensitizing the sarcomere to calcium even when nerve input is reduced. Myostatin inhibition in the form of myostatin antibodies, anti-myostatin peptibodies, anti-myostatin adnectin, etc. is also being attempted, since myostatin has now been recognized as the endogenous inhibitor of muscle growth. The myostatin inhibitor stamulumab has shown marked therapeutic benefit in patients with muscle wasting, but the results need to be validated in large clinical trials.

Although considerable challenges still remain in our understanding and development of these new agents for treatment of muscle wasting, the potential medical benefits of such therapies are likely to be substantial.

CHAPTER 69

Multiple Trauma

Behcet Al, Mustafa Sabak

INTRODUCTION

Emergency physicians play a crucial role in the management of multiple trauma patients and a systemic approach is required to reduce morbidity and mortality. Trauma care providers should be in a team work with surgical branches as well as leadership and clinical skills in the stabilization of multiple trauma patients.

According to 2016 statistics from the National Center for Health Statistics, 231,991 injury-related deaths occurred. Unintentional injuries (69.6%) ranked as the first most common cause of death. The leading causes of death by mechanism of injury and their percentages in 2016 were shown in **Figure 1**.

In 2016, the American College of Surgeons (ACS), National Trauma Data Bank, reported that the motor vehicle related events are peaking at the age of 14–29, reaching the second peak in the 40–50 age range (**Fig. 2**). If we look at age and gender distribution; 70% of the cases up to the age of 70 were males, and after the age of 71 were largely females.

Injury mortality was defined as a trimodal distribution which is categorized immediately, early and late by Trunkey in 1983. The timing distribution of trauma deaths is shown in **Figure 3**.

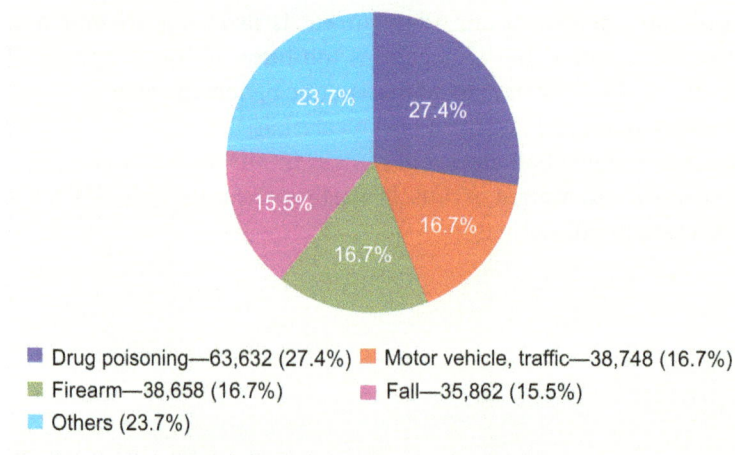

Fig. 1: Injury-related causes of death.

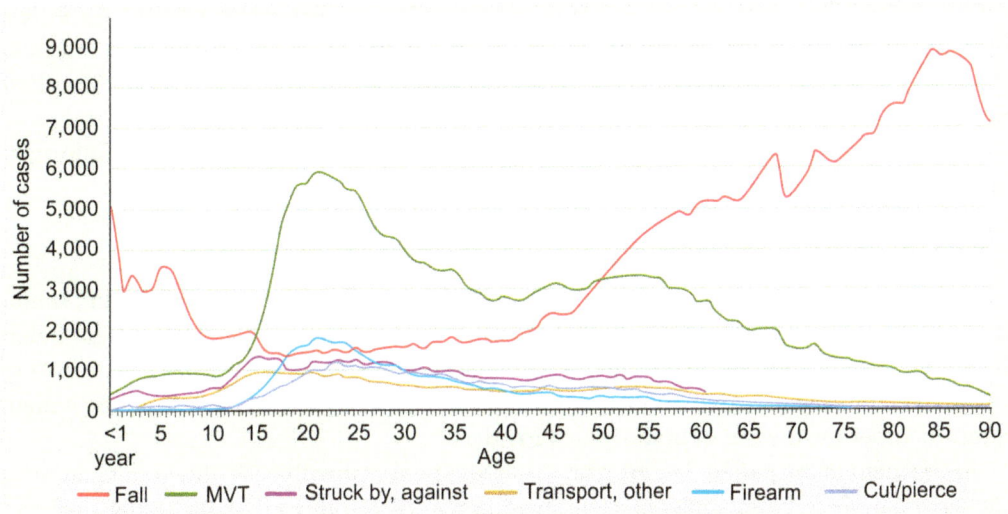

Fig. 2: Events by mechanism of injury and age.

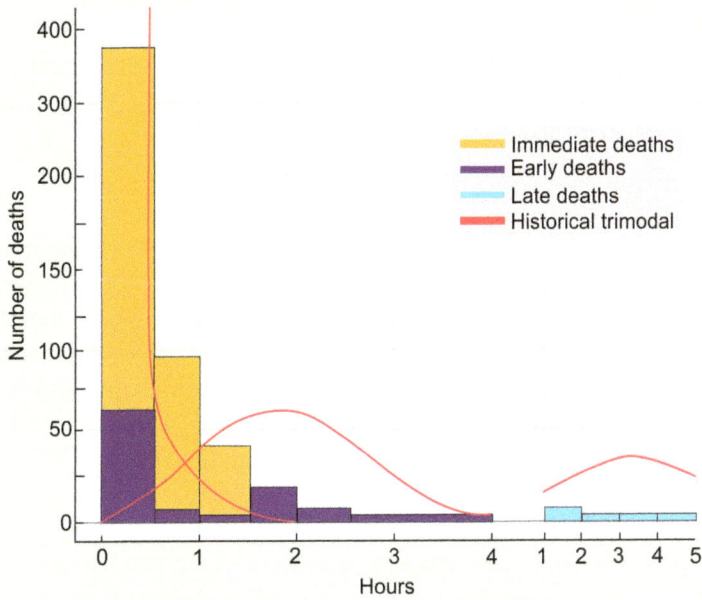

Fig. 3: Timing distribution of trauma deaths.

In the immediate period time, causes of death are usually caused by severe brain or high brain cord damage, cardiac, and major vascular injuries. In this period, the most effective way of reducing the death rate is to improve the protection methods.

The causes of death in the second peak period are generally caused by severe intracranial bleeding, hemopneumothorax, exsanguination (i.e. spleen and liver injuries). Rapid assessment and resuscitation are needed at this time, which is defined as the golden hour.

Late deaths occur days to weeks after trauma and usually cause deaths from multiple organ failure and sepsis.

INITIAL RESUSCITATION IN THE EMERGENCY DEPARTMENT

Information about the patient, vital signs, clinical findings, and the mechanism of injury should be provided by the Emergency Medical Services (EMS) providers to the trauma team before the trauma patient admitted to the emergency department. The physician must obtain history, ingestion of intoxicants, pre-existing medical condition, and medication use from the patient, family members, witnesses or prehospital providers.

Assessment of the patient begins with the assessment of possible life-threatening injuries. Management of the trauma patient as outlined in the ATLS 10th edition, including a primary survey, a secondary survey and definitive care.

PRIMARY SURVEY

The purpose of the primary survey is to ensure rapid diagnosis and treatment of life-threatening injuries. The physicians have to comply with the **A**irway (cervical spine protection is crucial while maintaining patent airway), **B**reathing, **C**irculation, **D**isability, **E**xposure/Environmental control (**ABCDE**) sequence to achieve a saving the life (**Box 1**).

Airway

Traumatic causes such as such as maxillofacial and neck injuries; accumulated blood and secretions can compromise the airway (**Fig. 4**). The priority must be maintained patency of the airway. If possible, the airway should be managed by two trauma team members. One of them provides cervical stabilization while the other one provides airway management. If the patient's consciousness alters or the Glasgow Coma Scale (GCS) is equal or less than 8, the patient is considered to be in coma or has a severe brain damage. This kind of patients' needs definitive airway intervention.

Box 1: Primary survey.

- Airway—assess and secure the airway. While assessing the airway, protect the cervical spine with cervical collar
- Breathing—listen to the lungs bilaterally and treat if there are tension/open pneumothorax, hemothorax
- Circulation—assess and control the bleeding, check the pulse of upper and lower extremities bilaterally, hemodynamic status, obtain intravascular and intraosseous access
- Disability—assess patient's neurologic status (i.e. GCS score, pupillary size and reaction, level of spinal cord injury)
- Exposure/environmental control—the patient must be completely understand ensure a warm environment because hypothermia is one of the death triad

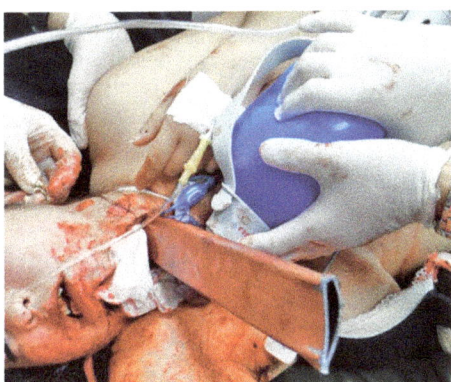

Fig. 4: Neck injury after a traffic accident.
Source: Adapted with permission from Gaziantep University Faculty of Medicine Emergency Department archive.

Breathing

In some studies, it has been showed that 20–25% of deaths due to chest trauma are by reason of inadequate oxygenation and ventilation. Injuries that may cause early mortality such as tracheobronchial injury, tension pneumothorax, massive hemothorax, open pneumothorax, fail chest should be detected and treated as earlier as possible to obtained adequate breathing and ventilation.

Life-threatening thoracic injuries are shown in **Table 1**.

Circulation

Assessment of the patient's hemodynamic status is crucial during managing the multiple trauma patients. The recognition of post-traumatic bleeding and rapid control and initiation of resuscitation constitute the most important steps in preventing hemorrhagic deaths. States of consciousness, skin perfusion, and pulse features are the element of clinical observation. When circulating blood volume is reduced, changing of these elements helps the clinician to making decision on the patient's hemodynamic status.

Clinician must identify the source of bleeding as external or internal. Five important locations of blood loss resulting in hemorrhagic shock are shown in **Box 2**.

External bleeding can be controlled by direct manual pressure on the wound or tourniquet during primary survey. According to ACS, blind clamping is not recommended due to damaging to neurovascular structures.

The cause of internal hemorrhage is generally identified by physical examination or imaging. Diagnostic tests are essential such as chest X-ray (CXR), pelvic X-ray, focused assessment with sonography for trauma (FAST) or diagnostic peritoneal lavage (DPL) for detecting the bleeding sources. During primer survey, immediate interventions can be done

Table 1: Life-threatening thoracic injuries.

Conditions	Diagnosis and treatment
Tracheobronchial tree injury *Introduction*: Most tracheobronchial injuries are within 2 cm of carina, rare, high mortality rate, hard diagnosis. Pain, soft tissue crepitus, ecchymosis on the injured side of the neck or chest by penetrating or blunt injuries *Clinic presentations*: Dyspnea or respiratory distress and hoarseness or dysphonia *Signs*: Pneumothorax, subcutaneous emphysema, hemoptysis	*Diagnosis*: CT, bronchoscopy (*gold standard*) *Treatment*: Surgical repair, removable stent
Tension pneumothorax *Introduction*: "One-way valve" leak occurs from the lung or through the chest wall. As a result, collapsing the affected lung. It may cause a shock due to decreased venous return to the heart *Clinic presentations*: Chest pain, shortness of breath *Signs*: Tachycardia, hypoxia, hypotension, tracheal deviation, unilateral absence of breath sounds, neck vein distention, cyanosis	*Diagnosis*: Physical examination, focused assessment with sonography for trauma (FAST) *Treatment*: Requires immediate decompression. A large, over the needle catheter (≥14 gauge) at the 5th interspace, finger thoracostomy, tube thoracostomy (at least 32 French in diameter)
Open pneumothorax *Introduction*: Large injuries to the chest wall (sucking chest wound). Rib fractures and penetrating trauma are the most common causes *Clinic presentation and signs*: Respiratory distress and other manifestations of pneumothorax (pain, difficulty breathing, tachypnea, decreased breath sounds on the affected side)	*Diagnosis*: Clinically and requires inspecting the entire chest wall surface *Treatment*: Cover the wound with three-sided occlusive dressing, chest tube placement (36–40F)
Massive hemothorax *Introduction*: Chest cavity can hold 40% of circulating blood volume. The accumulation of ≥1/3 of the patient's blood circulation to the chest cavity *Clinic presentation and signs*: Decreased/absent breath sounds on the affected side, no chest movement, dullness with percussion on the affected side	*Diagnosis*: Chest X-ray (CXR), USG, CT (gold standard) *Treatment*: Simultaneously restoring blood volume and decompressing the chest cavity by chest tube (28–32F) at the 5th intercostal space, evacuation of >1,500 mL of blood immediately or 200 mL/hr4hr: require thoracotomy
Flail chest *Introduction*: Trauma associated with multiple rib fractures (in ≥2 locations on same ribs) of ≥3 adjacent ribs, can cause respiratory failure *Clinic presentation and signs*: Decrease respiratory effort, paradoxical chest movement, hypoxia, palpation of crepitus from rib/cartilage fractures	*Diagnosis*: Physical examination (paradoxical movement of affected side), CXR *Treatment*: Adequate ventilation and oxygenation, analgesia, consider intubation

Box 2: Locations of possible life-threatening bleeding.

- Thoracic cavity
- Retroperitoneum
- Femur fracture
- Peritoneal cavity
- External hemorrhage

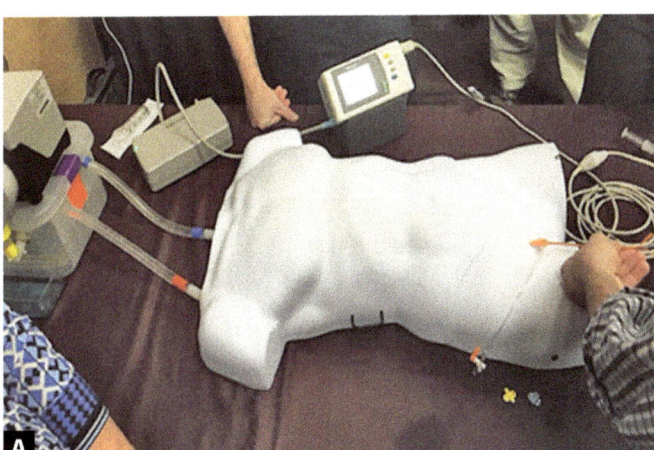 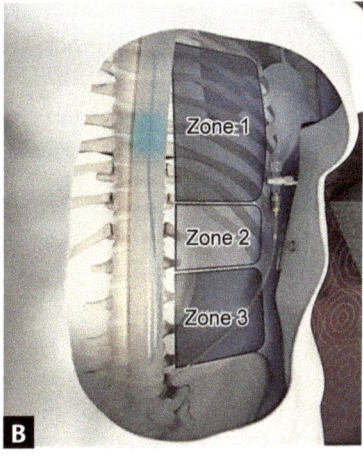

Figs. 5A and B: Placement of REBOA catheter and its appearance within the aorta.
Note: Figures 5A and B show that the inserting REBOA catheter and the position of the balloon (blue color) at the end of the catheter in zone 1 on simulator. The balloon should not be used in zone 2.
Source: Adapted with permission from Gaziantep University Faculty of Medicine Emergency Department archive.

such as chest decompression, pelvic stabilization device or bed sheet, extremity splints, resuscitative endovascular balloon occlusion of the aorta (REBOA) (**Figs. 5A and B**) which is used temporarily to stop intra-abdominal and retroperitoneal bleeding via catheter placed in the aorta along with replacement of intravascular volume.

Vascular access can be obtained via two large-bore peripheral venous catheters or intraosseous (IO) catheter (**Fig. 6**)—an alternative route that is commonly used to provide rapid fluid and blood products replacement in trauma resuscitation (maximal infusion rate of the common cannulas is showed in **Table 2**). Blood samples must have obtained for baseline hematologic studies, blood type, cross matching, blood gases (for learning the presence or degree of shock), lactate, and pregnancy test (if there is an indication).

Aggressive fluid resuscitation is not recommended by ACS because of increased mortality and morbidity. At the beginning of the fluid resuscitation of adult trauma patients can begin with warm (37–40°C) 1 L normal saline. If the patient is unresponsive, despite the initial fluid bolus, should receive a blood transfusion and definitive control of bleeding sources. If transfusion is required, give the patient *1:1:1 (plasma, platelets, and red blood cells)* ratio of

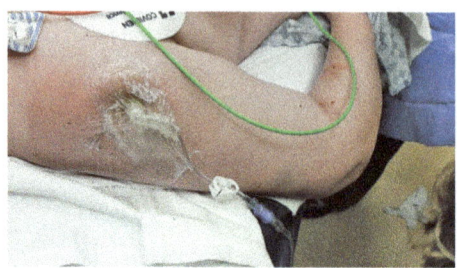

Fig. 6: Humoral intraosseous access.
Source: Adapted with permission from Dr Wael Hakmeh archive.

Table 2: Maximal infusion rate of the common cannulas.

Cannulas	mL/min
Humeral intraosseous (IO)	80
Tibial IO	15
14G IV	325
16G IV	215
18G IV	110
20G IV	63

blood products. In the CRASH 2 trial found that trauma patients requiring transfusion can benefit from tranexamic acid within 3 hours after trauma. It is recommended that 1 g of tranexamic acid is given within 10 minutes and the other 1 g is given within 8 hours.

Disability

The neurological examination of the trauma patient should include GCS which is used to determine the level of consciousness, pupil reactivity and size, motor and sensory function. All pathologic findings of detected on physical examination should be noted. Immobilization of the spine should be maintained in case of possible spinal cord injury. If there is a depressed level of consciousness in the trauma, patient should be considered of low blood sugar, alcohol intake, and possible poisoning as well.

Exposure and Environmental Control

The trauma patient's clothes should be removed and examined all his/her entire body so that the possible injury is avoided during the primary survey. Cover the patient's body with warm blanket to avoiding hypothermia. Hypothermia has been considered as the significant contributors to coagulation manifestations following trauma, known as the lethal triad. Additionally, the fluids that we used them during resuscitation and the heat of the resuscitation room are also important for protecting the trauma patient from hypothermia.

Additional parameters (**Box 3**) can be used before proceeding to the secondary survey. Vital signs (body temperature, pulse rate, respiration rate, and blood pressure), urinary output and arterial blood gas levels reflect the adequacy of resuscitation.

Box 3: Adjuncts to the primary survey with resuscitation.

• Electrocardiography	• Urinary and gastric catheter
• Pulse oximetry	• Blood lactate
• CO_2 monitoring	• X-ray (chest, pelvic, etc.)
• Ventilatory rate	• Focused assessment with sonography for trauma
• Arterial blood gas	• Extended focused assessment with sonography for trauma (eFAST)
	• Diagnostic peritoneal lavage (DPL)

SECONDARY SURVEY

All trauma patients are thoroughly examined from head-to-toe to avoid missed injuries and a complete history is obtained after the primary survey is completed.

Tertiary survey is also very important for detecting missed injuries such as diaphragmatic rupture, ureteral injury, esophageal perforation, compartment syndrome, so it should be completed in all trauma patients admitted to an intensive care unit. According to Chen et al.'s study, the most frequently missed injuries of the body region are *head/neck*, thorax and extremities, respectively.

The physicians should obtain a complete history of the patient from the prehospital personnel or family members. The AMPLE (**A**llergies, **M**edications, **P**ast illnesses/**P**regnancy, **L**ast meal, **E**vents/**E**nvironment-related injury) history is very useful mnemonic for it. The physician can obtain mechanism of injuries such as blunt and penetrating trauma from the prehospital staff.

The use of anticoagulants and antiplatelet agents especially in the elderly is increasing day by day and increased mortality and mobility in trauma the patients. Whether or not patients are using it should be questioned and possible situations should be taken into consideration. Rapid reversal can potentially decrease mortality.

Nonaccidental trauma such as child abuse, neglect and intimate partner violence should be considered when evaluating the trauma patients.

The goal of physical examination is to identify the injuries during secondary survey.

Physical examination of each part of system has been shown in **Table 3**.

Diagnostic Tests and Additional Imaging

Adjunct specialized diagnostic test during the secondary survey shows in **Box 4**.

All significantly injured patients underwent portable, plain radiographic imaging of their cervical spine, chest, and pelvis.

Plain Radiographs are used for detecting spine, pelvis and extremities fractures, foreign bodies, dislocations during the secondary survey. It is insufficient to demonstrate the occult hemothorax and pneumothorax; therefore, plain CXR should be used as an initial screening tool more carefully.

Focused assessment with sonography for trauma is noninvasive, cost-effective, easy and a crucial tool for detecting the intraperitoneal, pericardial and pleural-free fluid while evaluating the trauma patient.

Table 3: Complete physical examination on completion of secondary survey.

Head and face	<ul><li>Tenderness, deformity, bleeding</li><li>Scalp laceration</li><li>Foreign bodies</li><li>Sign of basilar skull fractures (hemotympanum, Battle's sign, and raccoon's eyes)</li><li>Nasal septum hematoma</li><li>Sign of eye globe rupture, intraocular bleeding, pupillary size, shape, reactivity, and extraocular movement</li></ul>
Neck	<ul><li>Check the cervical spine (can ruled out the fractures by using NEXUS rules or X-ray/CT)</li><li>Inspect and palpate the whole of the neck</li></ul>
Chest	<ul><li>Sternum and clavicles fractures (suggest the presence of further injury, if present)</li><li>Small hemothorax, pneumothorax, pericardial effusion can missed</li></ul>
Abdomen	<ul><li>Inspect laceration, contusions, ecchymosis</li><li>Palpate for tenderness and rigidity</li><li>Pay attention specifically to the elderly, patient with altered mental status and pregnant</li></ul>
Rectum and genitourinary	<ul><li>Inspect the perineum</li><li>Digital rectal and vaginal examination</li></ul>
Musculoskeletal	<ul><li>Inspect and palpate the whole of the extremities and pelvis for deformity, tenderness, penetrating injuries</li><li>Check neurovascular status of each extremity</li></ul>
Skin	<ul><li>Sign of lacerations, abrasions, ecchymosis, hematoma</li><li>Pay special attention to back, gluteal region, posterior scale</li></ul>
Neurological examination	<ul><li>Assess the patient's GCS score</li><li>Evaluation of the extremities' sensory and motor functions</li><li>Status of consciousness</li><li>Pupillary size, shape and reactivity and eye movements</li><li>Protect the spinal cord</li></ul>

Box 4: Adjuncts to the secondary survey with resuscitation.

<ul><li>X-ray examinations</li><li>Extended focused assessment with sonography for trauma (eFAST)</li><li>CT scans</li><li>Bronchoscopy</li></ul>	<ul><li>Esophagoscopy</li><li>Contrast urography</li><li>Angiography</li><li>Transesophageal ultrasound</li></ul>

An *extended focused assessment with sonography for trauma (eFAST)* examination should be performed on all patients with multisystem trauma or isolated trauma to the torso and it is highly sensitive and specific assessment modality for torso injury. Additionally, eFAST gives the physician with an opportunity to evaluate bilateral thorax in terms of pneumothorax and hemothorax.

If bleeding sources cannot detect by bedside imaging (i.e. X-ray, FAST, eFAST) during primary and secondary survey for unstable trauma patient, if the patient needs further information for operation, the surgeon and emergency physician must decide whether or not the patient will take to the computed tomography (CT) scan or operating room. If the cervical spine injury is not cleared with *NEXUS criteria or Canadian Cervical Spine Rule*, cervical spine of CT should be obtained. Chest CT should be performed in those with significant chest pain, dyspnea, sternal tenderness, or abnormal thoracic ultrasound (US) or CXR findings.

SPECIFIC INJURY MANAGEMENT AND TREATMENT

Head Trauma

Traumatic brain injury (TBI) is a leading cause of morbidity and mortality worldwide and MVT accidents are the cause of death due to TBI in 55.8% of youth ages of 5–14 and 47.4% of young ages of 15–24. Today TBI is most frequently classified as mild, moderate, or severe using the GCS. A CT scan is the gold standard for detecting the pathologic findings for the TBI patient. Prevent hypovolemia and hypoxemia, maintain airway patency and avoid using hypotonic solution to prevent further brain damage. Many patients with moderate or severe head injuries are taken directly from the emergency room to the operating room. In many cases, surgery is performed to remove a large hematoma or contusion that is significantly compressing the brain or raising the pressure within the skull.

Neck Trauma

The neck is divided into three zones: zones 1, 2, and 3 (**Fig. 7**). Zone 2 injuries undergo surgical exploration; zone 1 and 3 wounds undergo further evaluation. Wounds that do not penetrate the platysma are not life threatening (**Fig. 8**).

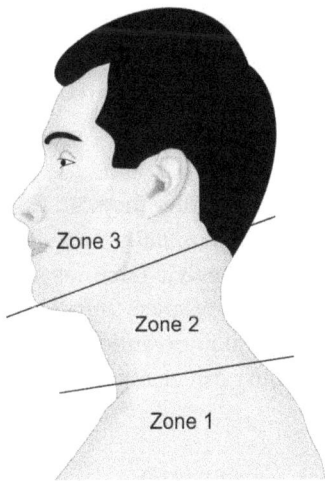

Fig. 7: Zones of the neck.
Source: Adapted with permission from David B Levy, 2017.

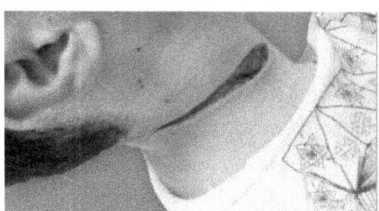

Fig. 8: Zone 2 wound that do not penetrate the platysma.
Source: Adapted with permission from Gaziantep University Faculty of Medicine Emergency Department archive.

A modern sensitive imaging technology, including computed tomographic angiography (CTA), is widely available. In a "no-zone" management approach, patients are divided into two groups as a stable and unstable and the unstable patient should be taken immediately to the operation room.

Thoracic Trauma

Thoracic trauma can cause serious organ injuries such as heart, the great vessels that can cause the death of the patient. Early intervention (i.e. chest tube insertion, emergency thoracotomy) of life-threatening injuries such as tension pneumothorax, open pneumothorax is crucial to reduce the morbidity and mortality.

Abdominal Trauma

Abdominal trauma can cause hemorrhagic shock due to exsanguinations in injured patients and is associated with high mortality and morbidity rates. If intra-abdominal injury is suspected, early surgical consultation is necessary after restored the patient's vital functions. If the patient hemodynamically unstable, the physician should assess possible intra-abdominal injury by using FAST or DPL. If the patient hemodynamically stable and physician could not evaluate abdomen with physical examination or in the presence of acute abdomen signs, should obtained further imaging information such as contrast-enhanced CT for identified abdominal injury.

Pelvic Injury

When pelvic fractures are not recognized earlier they can cause hemorrhagic shock and death due to severe bleeding. In the hemodynamically unstable patients, the physician should obtain portable pelvic X-ray to identified pelvic fractures such as open book fracture, vertical displacement of the posterior pelvis and if presence, the pelvic binder or a sheet should be placed and consulted for surgical or radiological intervention to control ongoing pelvic hemorrhage. Clinically stable patient with pelvic injury can be obtained CT scan if imaging is required.

Retroperitoneal Injuries

The retroperitoneum is the anatomical region with the highest mortality rates after the trauma; therefore, early diagnosis and treatment of these lesions are crucial and there may not be signs of peritoneal irritation at the initial physical examination. CT scan is a diagnostic tool to detecting retroperitoneal injuries. ACS is recommended that early outpatient follow-up is crucial after 24-hour observation to avoid possible occult injuries.

Genitourinary Injuries

Genitourinary trauma is common in males. *The kidney* is the most commonly injured organ in the genitourinary system. *Ureteral trauma* is rare and mainly due to iatrogenic injuries or penetrating gunshot wounds. *Bladder trauma* is usually due to blunt injuries such as motor vehicle accidents and associated pelvic fractures. *Genital trauma* is common in males due to anatomical considerations. *The anterior urethra* is commonly injured by blunt trauma. *The posterior urethra* is usually injured in pelvis fracture cases. A contrast-enhanced CT scan and delayed images are the best methods for the diagnosis and staging of renal injuries in hemodynamically stable patients. Delayed phase imaging identifies collecting system/ureteric injury.

Musculoskeletal Injuries

Musculoskeletal injuries can threat of life and cause loss of limb. Most extremity injuries are appropriately diagnosed and managed during the secondary survey. It is very important to recognize the open fractures and joint dislocations and to make the reduction and splinting in order to prevent the serious complications. In addition, crush injuries and compartment syndrome should be considered. If there are any signs of vascular injury and/or if the ankle-brachial index is less than 0.9, should obtained the imaging tests to evaluate for associated vascular injuries, or transfer to a hospital where vascular surgery can be done.

■ SUMMARY

- The emergency physician has to approach to the multiple trauma patients systematically to reduce morbidity and mortality.
- Rapid assessment and resuscitation are needed at the second peak period, which is defined as the *golden hour*.
- *The primary survey* should be performed when the patient is admitted to the emergency room. The physician should begin to provide quick diagnosis and treatment of the life-threatening injuries (i.e. tension pneumothorax) as soon as possible during the primary survey phase.
- Try to perform *eFAST examination* as soon as possible as a part of the primary survey.
- Aggressive fluid resuscitation is not recommended by ACS because of increased mortality and morbidity. If the patient needs, give *1 L warm normal saline*.
- If indicated, give the patient *1:1:1 (plasma, platelets, and red blood cells)* ratio of blood products.
- The patient can benefit from *tranexamic acid* (loading dose 1 g over 10 minutes then infusion of 1 g over 8 hours) when administrated within first 3 hours after injury, if the patient needs blood transfusion.
- Rapidly *correct the coagulopathy*, if presented.

CHAPTER 70

Oral Problems (Oral Candidiasis, Oral Herpes Simplex)

Aman Sharma

ORAL CANDIDIASIS

INTRODUCTION

Candida species are amongst the normal flora present in human body. When there is disturbance of this normal flora, it leads to overgrowth leading to candidiasis or thrush. The species most commonly causing infection in humans is *Candida albicans*. Oral thrush is one of the most common fungal infections and can be found in all age groups though mostly found in the early and late stages of life. It is more of a clinical diagnosis, proper history, and physical examination are enough to establish a diagnosis but confirmatory laboratory studies must be sent for confirmation. Prophylactic doses should not be given to all affected individuals, but to reduce the severity and incidence for patients falling in high-risk groups. The disease has a favorable prognosis in most of the cases.

ETIOLOGY/CAUSES

These harmless commensals are found in various parts of body as normal flora but opportunistic overgrowth may lead into disease. Other than *C. albicans* other species of oral *Candida* are: *C. glabrata, C. guilliermondii, C. krusei, C. parapsilosis, C. pseudotropicalis, C. stellatoidea,* and *C. tropicalis*.

Usually it is a self-limiting disease; however, certain local and systemic factors may favor overgrowth and lead to invasive candidiasis. Predisposing conditions leading to infections are mentioned in **Table 1**.

CLASSIFICATION

Classification of oral candidiasis has been shown in **Table 2**.

PATHOPHYSIOLOGY OF THE CONDITION

Candida albicans is one of the most common inhabitants of oral and gut flora, found in about 50% of individuals. Inadequate functioning of the immune system leads to disturbance of microflora thus causing overgrowth and pathogenicity (**Flowchart 1**).

Table 1: Predisposing conditions leading to infections.

Local factors	Systemic factors
Impaired local defense mechanisms	Systemic immunosuppression
Diminished saliva production	Acquired immunodeficiency syndrome
Tobacco chewing and smoking	Immunosuppressant medications
Atrophic oral mucosa	Diabetes and other endocrine disorders
Oral lichen planus	Malnourished state
Topical steroids	Malignancies
Altered or immature oral flora	Congenital conditions
Poor hygiene of oral cavity	Broad-spectrum antibiotics
Dental prosthesis/dentures	

Table 2: Classification of oral candidiasis.

Primary oral candidiasis	Secondary oral candidiasis

• *Acute forms*:
  – Pseudomembranous
  – Erythematous
• *Chronic forms*:
  – Hyperplastic (nodular or plaque like)
  – Erythematous
  – Pseudomembranous
• *Candida-associated lesions*:
  – Denture stomatitis
  – Angular cheilitis
  – Median rhomboid glossitis
• *Keratinized primary lesions with candidal superinfection*:
  – Leukoplakia
  – Lichen planus
  – Lupus erythematosus
	• Oral manifestations of systemic mucocutaneous candidiasis:
	  – Thymic aplasia
	  – Candidiasis endocrinopathy syndrome

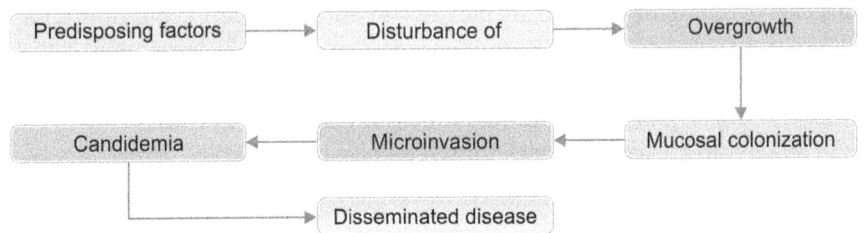

Flowchart 1: Pathophysiology of candidiasis.

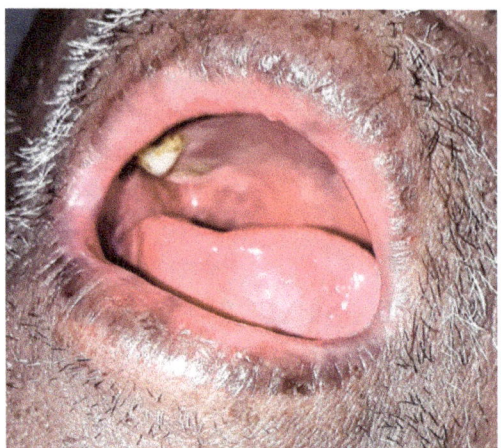

Fig. 1: Erythematous lesions over gingiva and hard palate.
Source: Courtesy by Dr Pandya Jignesh, DNB (Nephro).

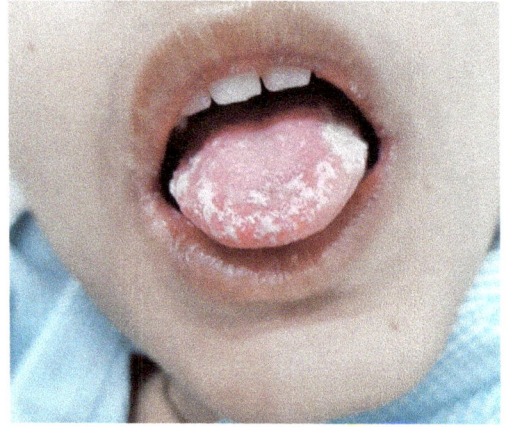

Fig. 2: Hyperplastic candidiasis.
Source: Courtesy by Dr Singh Devendra, DNB (Gastro).

CLINICAL PRESENTATION

Commonly called as oral thrush. Usually patients do not exhibit any symptoms. Most types of oral candidiasis are painless, but a burning sensation may occur in some cases.

It appears as patches of gray or white friable material covering an erythematous base on buccal mucosa, tongue, gingiva, palate, and tonsils (**Figs. 1 and 2**). Oral thrush is much more common in infants, and usually occurs within the first week of life.

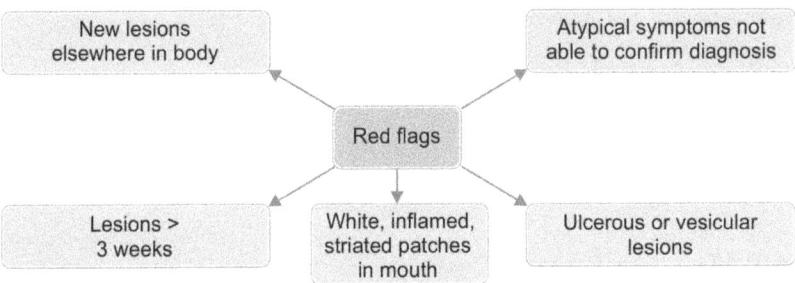

Flowchart 2: Red flags—oral candidiasis.

RED FLAGS

If the patient exhibits any of the red flag symptoms, they must be referred to a specialist/higher center for further evaluation and workup (**Flowchart 2**).

EVALUATION

History

- Infant—white coating present over tongue, difficulty in lactation
- Pediatric—whitish/gray coat over tongue usually asymptomatic
- Adults—intake of antibiotics or steroids.

Physical Examination

Physical examination reveals classical whitish lesions in oral cavity which are usually not easily removable and may cause pain and bleeding if scraped.

INTERPRETATION OF FINDINGS

In clinical practice such clinical findings give an idea of patient's current health status and enable the emergency physicians to make a differential diagnosis and not to miss immunodeficiency states and malignancies as well.

INVESTIGATIONS

Though diagnosing oral thrush is mostly clinical but samples should be obtained for identification of species causing the disease and its quantification. The following laboratory investigation techniques can be used as shown in **Box 1**.

Box 1: Laboratory investigation techniques.

- Culture of whole saliva
- Concentrated oral rinse
- Swab
- Smear
- Imprint culture
- Biopsy

TREATMENT

Conservative Measures

- Good Oral Hygeine
- Removal of dentures during night
- Oral rinses (chlorhexidine)

Pharmacological Treatment—Topical and Systemic

Antifungal agents that are available for the treatment of candidiasis fall into three main categories: (1) the polyenes (nystatin and amphotericin B); (2) the ergosterol biosynthesis inhibitors—the azoles (miconazole, clotrimazole, ketoconazole, itraconazole, and fluconazole), allylamines, thiocarbamates, and morpholines; and (3) DNA analog 5-fluorocytosine, and newer agents such as caspofungins (**Table 3**).

SUMMARY

Summary of candidal stomatitis (oral thrush) has been shown in **Flowchart 3**.

Table 3: Treatment of oropharyngeal candidiasis (OPC).

Severity	Antifungal drug	Dosage/Duration
First-line agents	• Fluconazole (PO/IV) • Clotrimazole troches • Nystatin suspension (100,000 U/mL) • Nystatin lozenges (200,000 U each)	• 100–200 mg/1–2 weeks • 10 mg five times/1–2 weeks • 4–6 mL four times/1–2 weeks • 1–2 lozenges four times/1–2 weeks
Second-line agents	• Itraconazole solution (PO) • Posaconazole (PO) • Voriconazole (PO/IV)	• 200 mg/4 weeks • 400 mg daily in divided doses • 200 mg twice daily
Agents used in refractory case of OPC	• Caspofungin (IV) • Micafungin (IV) • Anidulafungin (IV) • Amphotericin B (oral suspension) • Amphotericin B (IV)	• 70 mg loading dose followed by 50 mg daily • 100–150 mg daily • 100 mg loading dose followed by 50 mg daily • 500 mg every 6th hour • 0.3 mg/kg once daily

Chapter 70: Oral Problems (Oral Candidiasis, Oral Herpes Simplex)

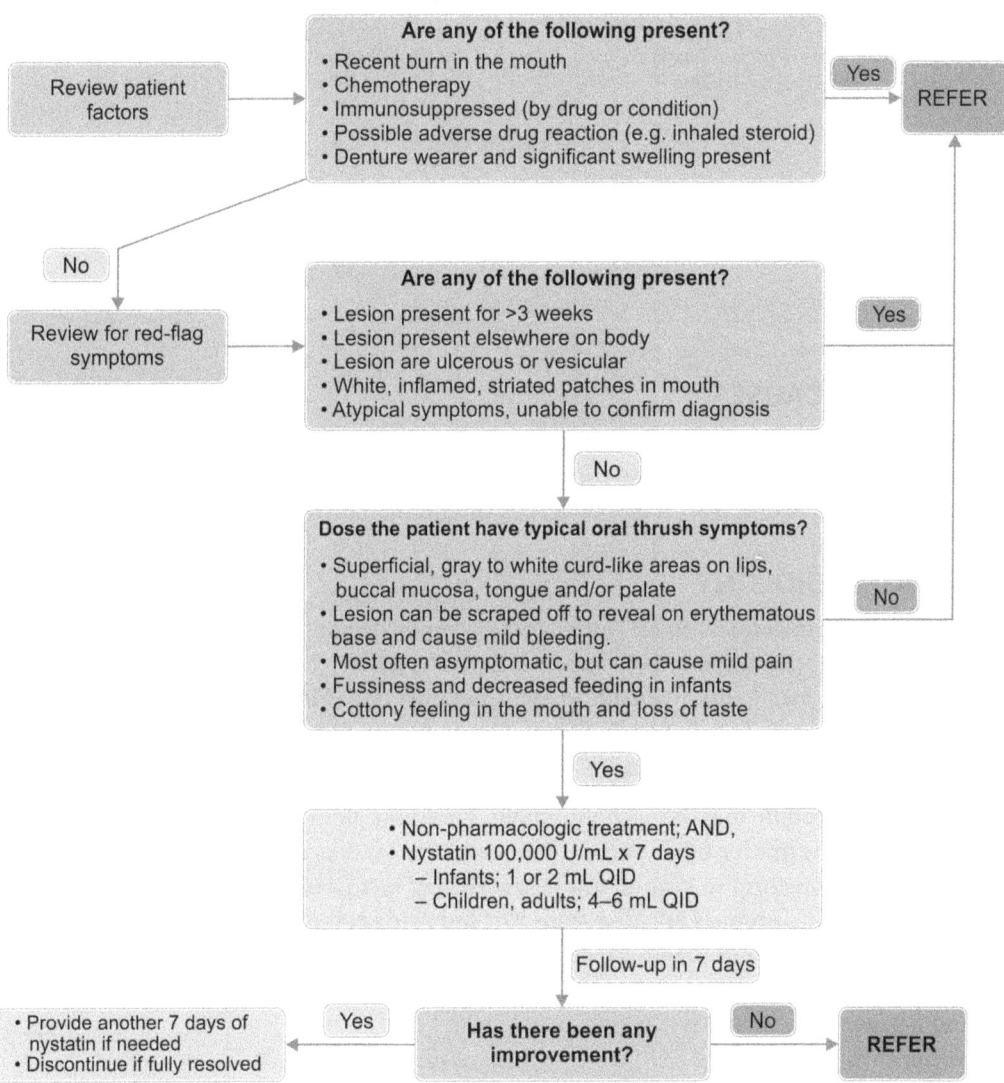

Flowchart 3: Summary of candidal stomatitis (oral thrush).

ORAL HERPES SIMPLEX

INTRODUCTION

Oral herpes simplex commonly known as herpes labialis is an infection commonly caused by herpes simplex virus (HSV). It is common in the young especially in the second decade of life and very contagious causing blisters over lips, mouth, tongue, or gums.

Flowchart 4: Common causes of herpes labialis.

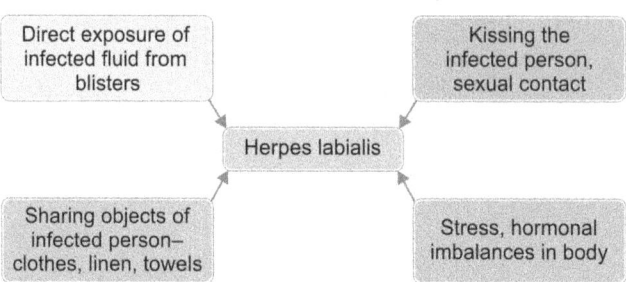

ETIOLOGY/CAUSES

Herpes simplex labialis is most commonly caused by HSV-1. The infection is typically spread between people by direct nonsexual contact, sharing the household objects of infected person leads to spreading of disease. Causes of herpes simplex labialis are shown in **Flowchart 4**.

PATHOPHYSIOLOGY

Once a person is infected with HSV, the virus becomes dormant after the primary infection and lays itself in facial nerve cells (trigeminal nerve ganglion). It reinfects when the person is exposed to triggering factors and leads to recurrent infection (**Flowchart 5**).

CLINICAL PRESENTATION

The primary infection may be asymptomatic. One may notice small fluid-filled vesicles/blisters around the lips or other parts of face within 1–3 weeks of initial contact. The blisters may burst and transform to scab in few cases. During recurrence of infection the severity is usually less than the primary infective state. The following common symptoms may be seen:
- Burning sensation and pain over the affected areas (lips, buccal mucosa, gingival, other parts of face)
- Itching over the blisters
- Fever
- Headache
- Malaise
- Running nose and cold.

RED FLAGS

Usually the disease is self-limiting but one must take precaution when any pregnant women or neonates are affected. If a patient has further progression of symptoms especially central nervous system (CNS) involvement or bacterial/fungal superinfection, the patient requires immediate hospitalization (**Flowchart 6**).

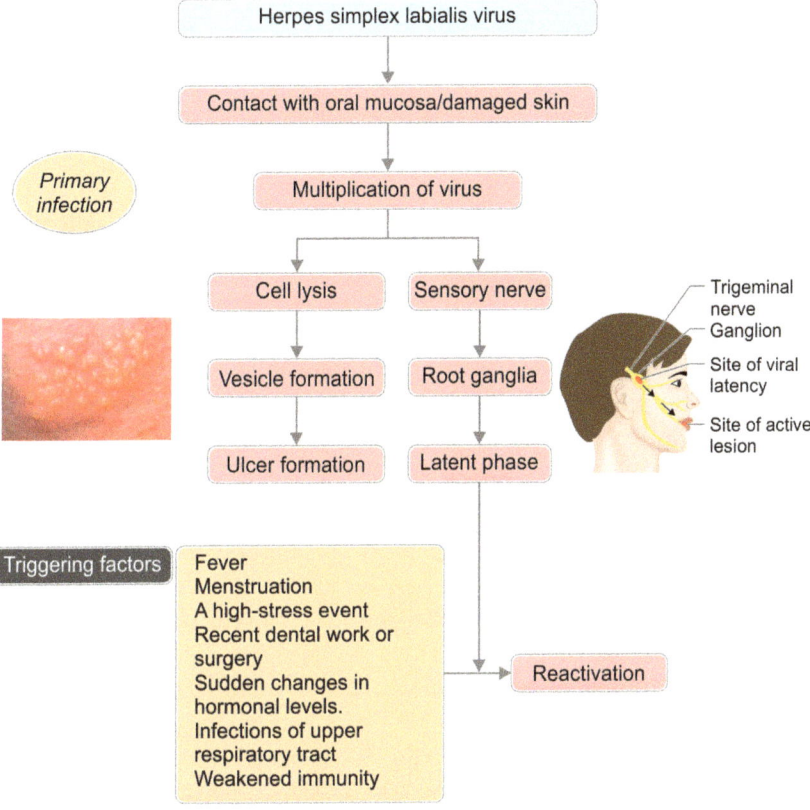

Flowchart 5: Pathophysiology of herpes labialis.

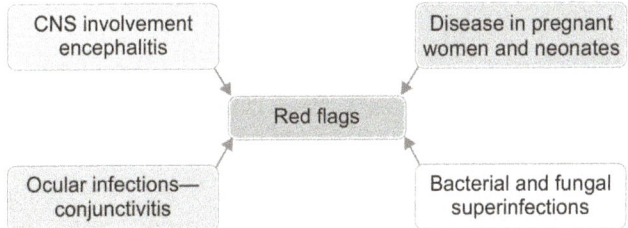

Flowchart 6: Red flags—herpes labialis.

EVALUATION

History

Contact with infected person, young individuals, history of cold, cough, or fever. It is usually a self-limiting condition and rarely requires hospitalization. It affects in early stages of life so one must not miss such earlier events during history taking and also the recurrence is associated with any stress.

Physical Examination

The physical examination of herpes infection reveals fluid-filled vesicles/blisters.
- Site—lips, oral cavity, tongue, gingival, hard, and soft palate
- Size—small (2–5 mm) usually in groups
- Shape—round/circular.

INTERPRETATION OF FINDING

Oral herpes simplex is diagnosed clinically with the classical presentation. In ED, one must always look for the red flags and differentiate it with similar lesions. Though it does not always require hospitalization, we should be precautious handling pregnant women and neonates.

INVESTIGATIONS

Various investigations can be utilized to identify the presence of HSV.
- *Cell culture*: It is the standard test for diagnosis, isolating HSV in the culture is the standard test for confirmation.
- *Polymerase chain reaction (PCR)*: It is more sensitive than cell culture, usually used in CNS involvement and eye infections.
- *Direct fluorescent antibody (DFA) method*: It differentiates between HSV-1 and HSV-2 infections.
- *Tzanck smear (also known as herpes skin test)*: Presence of Tzanck cells confirms infection by HSV.

  In case of superinfection with bacteria and fungi, punch biopsy may be taken for histological evaluation.

TREATMENT

Preventive Measures

Avoid contact with the infected person—touching, kissing, sexual contact. Do not use linens, clothes of infected person.

Pharmacological Therapy

Topical
- Acyclovir—5% cream, five times a day for 4 days
- Penciclovir—1% cream, every 2nd hourly (when awake) for 4 days.

Chapter 70: Oral Problems (Oral Candidiasis, Oral Herpes Simplex)

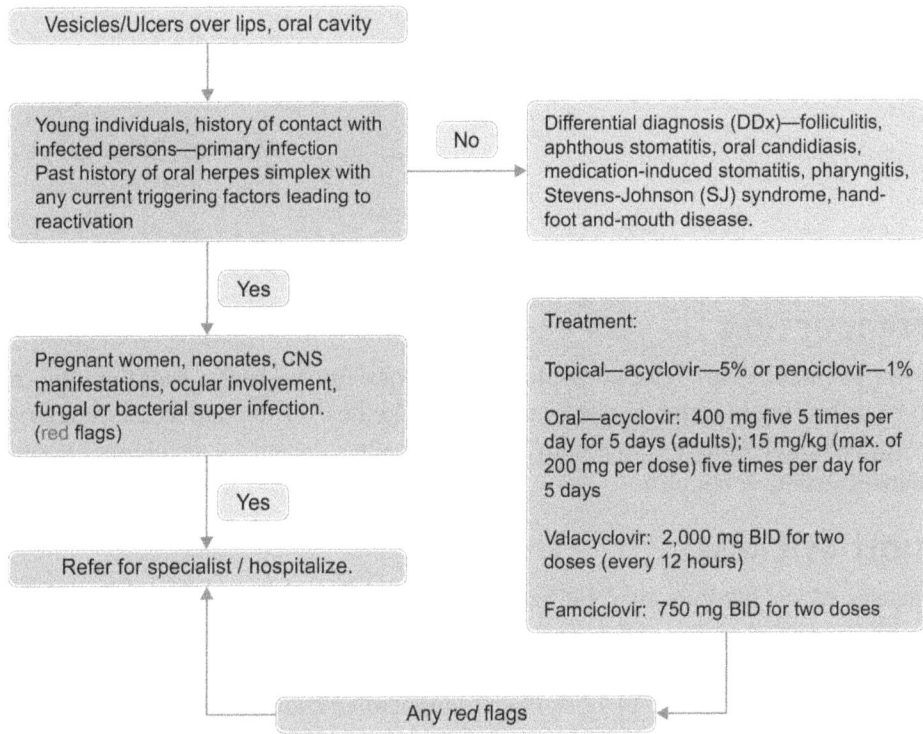

Flowchart 7: Summary of oral herpes simplex.

(ACE: angiotensin-converting enzyme; HRCT: high-resolution computed tomography)

Oral

- Acyclovir: 400 mg *five* times a day for 5 days (adults); 15 mg/kg (maximum of 200 mg per dose) *five* times a day for 5 days
- Valacyclovir: 2,000 mg *twice* daily for two doses
- Famciclovir: 750 mg *twice* daily for two doses or single dose of 1,500 mg stat.

SUMMARY

Summary of oral herpes simplex has been shown in **Flowchart 7**.

Palpitations

Aldo Tua, Roberta Petrino

INTRODUCTION

The term palpitations are referred by the patient when he/she feels a sense of abnormality of the heart beating in terms of rate or regularity. The heart is defined as skipping, frisking, fluttering, racing, or jumping. Frequently, the abnormality is lasting for a prolonged period and thus causes anxiety or anguish.

ETIOLOGY/CAUSES

The causes of palpitations may be several and different. Any situation that can cause acceleration or deceleration of the heart beating, or a change in the regularity can determine the unpleasant feeling referred as palpitation.

Causes of palpitations can be of cardiac or noncardiac etiology. About 40% of the causes are of cardiac origin, one-third are of psychiatric origin, while the remaining are of other or unknown origin. Most common causes of palpitation is summarized in **Table 1**.

Cardiac etiology is generally due to an impairment of the conduction system that causes brady- or tachyarrhythmias with the mechanisms like altered automatism, reentry of a premature beat, post-potential excitation due to cell membrane ion channels disturbances.

Psychiatric causes of palpitations may be:
- Anxious state
- Panic attack
- Conversion crisis.

Palpitations in these cases normally are more frequent, last longer than for cardiac causes and may be accompanied by different symptoms. In any case, it is necessary to rule out any cardiac cause before accepting the diagnosis of a psychiatric disorder, thus a 12-lead electrocardiogram (ECG) is mandatory and eventual other investigations.

Other etiologies include:
- *Physiological*: Exercise, pregnancy, excitement, emotional trauma
- *Hyperkinetic circulatory state*: Fever, hyperthyroidism, anemia, hypoglycemia
- Vasovagal syndrome
- *Drugs*: Aminophylline, atropine, antiarrhythmic, tricyclic antidepressants, calcium channel blockers

Table 1: Etiologies of palpitations.

Arrhythmic and arrhythmogenic causes of palpitations:
Supraventricular tachycardia
Ventricular tachycardia
Atrial flutter
Atrial fibrillation
Supraventricular and ventricular extrasystoles
Sick-sinus syndrome
Brady-arrhythmias
Brugada syndrome
Arrhythmogenic right ventricular dysplasia
Nonarrhythmic cardiac causes of palpitations:
Mitral valve prolapses
Aortic stenosis or insufficiency
Pulmonary embolism
Atrial mixoma
Congenital heart disease
Arterial hypertension
Pericarditis
Myocarditis
Pace maker mulfunction
Noncardiac causes of palpitations:
Exercise
Anxiety, fear, stress, panic attack
Emotional trauma
Fever
Hyperthyroidism
Hypoglycaemia
Anemia
Pregnancy
Poisoning and drug abuse with cocaine, amphetamines, other drugs
Alcohol and caffeine abuse
Shock

- *Toxic*: Cocaine, alcohol, amphetamines, tobacco
- Systemic mastocytosis
- Da Costa's syndrome or effort syndrome or neurocirculatory asthenia

PATHOPHYSIOLOGY

- *Palpitation intermittent*: Normally due to extrasystole (**Fig. 1**). The patient feels the beat after the extrasystole because the major end-diastolic filling after the pause and the increased strength of contraction.
- *Palpitations that appear only after exercise or excitement or emotional stress*: Normally the heart rate is not faster than 120 beats per minute (bpm) and regular. Palpitation is due to catecholaminergic stimulus and transitory hyperdynamic cardiovascular state.
- *Palpitation continuous and regular*: Generally due to supraventricular tachycardia (SVT) or atrial flutter or ventricular tachycardia (**Figs. 2 to 4**). The pathogenesis of the former is a reentry mechanism, around the atrioventricular node or through an atrioventricular accessory pathway. Atrial flutter is normally occurring in patient with a cardiac scar or cardiomyopathy and is sustained by reentry mechanism around the scar or around anatomic or functional atrial circuits. Ventricular tachycardia is the most threatening as it may evolve toward pulseless tachycardia or ventricular fibrillation. It is normally due to ischemia, dilative cardiomyopathy, hypokalemia or other arrhythmogenic congenital or acquired diseases.
- *Palpitation continuous irregular*: It may be due to atrial fibrillation (**Fig. 5**), but also to atrial flutter with variable ventricular conduction, multifocal atrial tachycardia (MAT), or frequent extrasystoles. Pathogenesis of atrial fibrillation is several mini reentry mechanism due generally to atrial walls distention and dilation. Very important to keep in mind the need for anticoagulation to prevent thrombus formation in the atria due to the absence of an efficacious atrial systole. MAT may be seen in chronic respiratory failure.
- Palpitation is associated with:
    - *Chest pain*: Possible myocardial infarction with arrhythmia (**Fig. 5**)
    - *Syncope*: Low cardiac output with arrhythmia, hypoglycemia
    - *Dyspnea*: Heart failure, chronic obstructive pulmonary disease (COPD) exacerbation
    - *Sweating*: Vasovagal syndrome, anxiety, hypoglycemia
    - *Polyuria*: SVT
    - *Diarrhea*: Thyrotoxicosis.
- *Positional palpitation*: It may be due to the presence of an intracardiac (atrial myxoma) or mediastinal mass that in certain positions triggers the arrhythmia.

CLINICAL PRESENTATION

As already described above, palpitation may be continuous or intermittent, may start and stop abruptly, and may be associated with other symptoms like chest pain, dyspnea, fever, sweating, syncope, polyuria, anxiety, or agitation. Very often when the patient comes to the emergency department (ED), palpitation is extinguished and is necessary to make a hypothesis according to the patient history and the associated symptoms. Whenever possible, it is important to ask the patient to tap on the table the rhythm and frequency of the palpitation. In **Table 2**, there is the correlation of the description of the palpitation and the possible causes are enumerated.

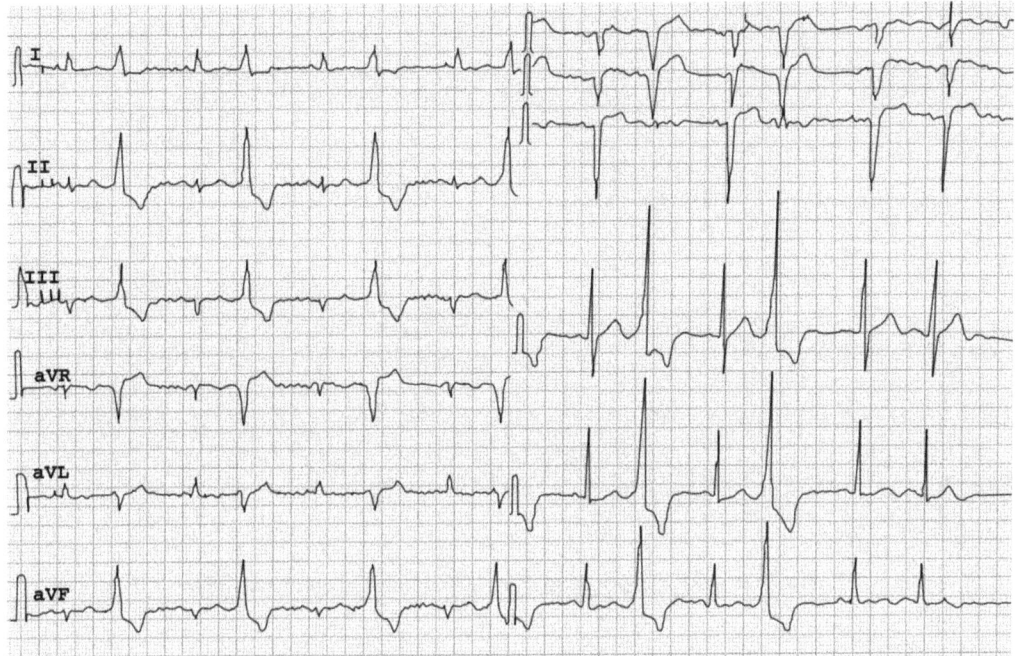

Fig. 1: 12 leads ECG showing a ventricular extrasytolic bigeminism.

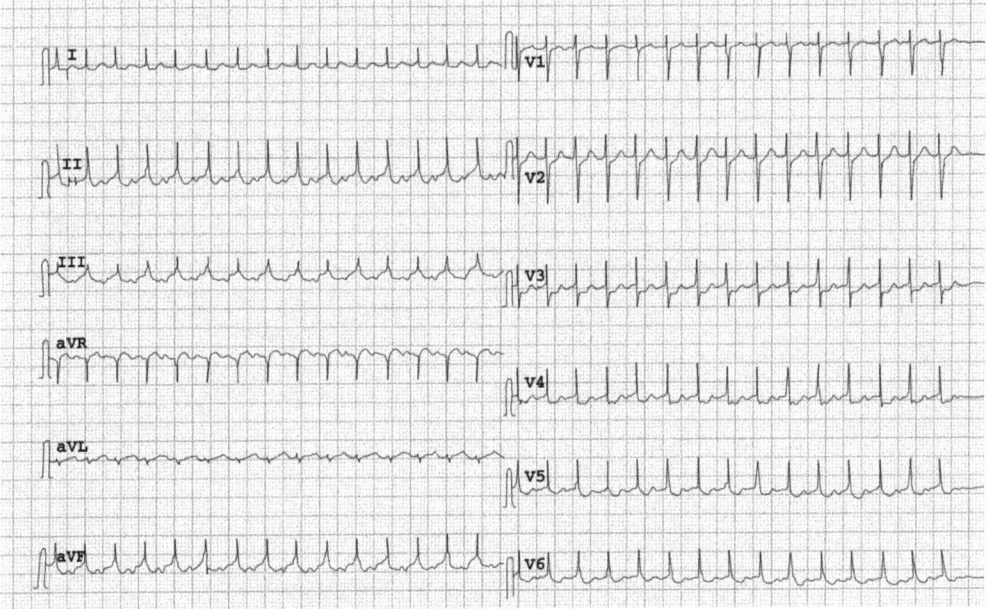

Fig. 2: 12 leads ECG showing a supraventricular tachycardia.

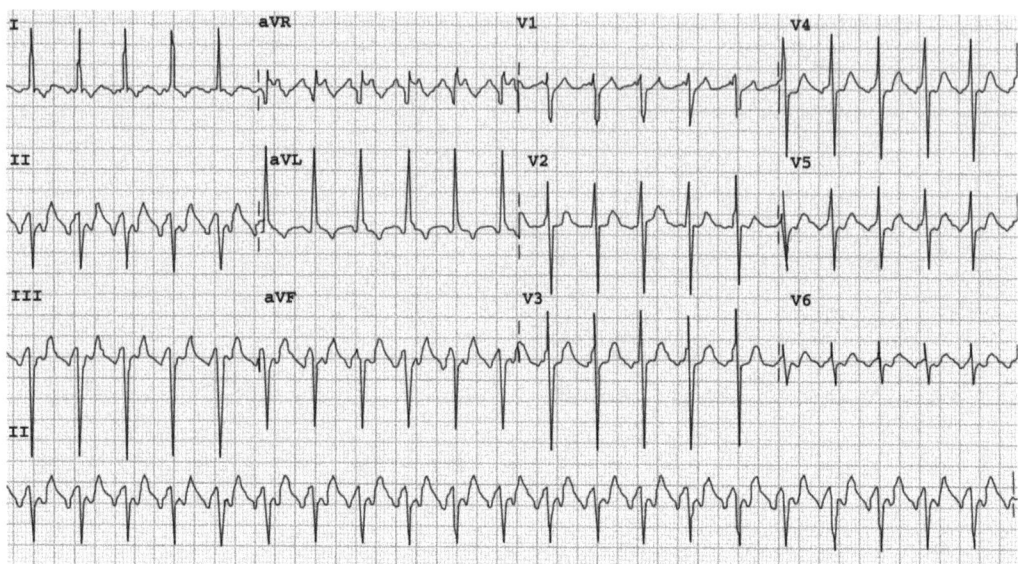

Fig. 3: 12 leads ECG showing an atrial flutter with conduction 2:1.

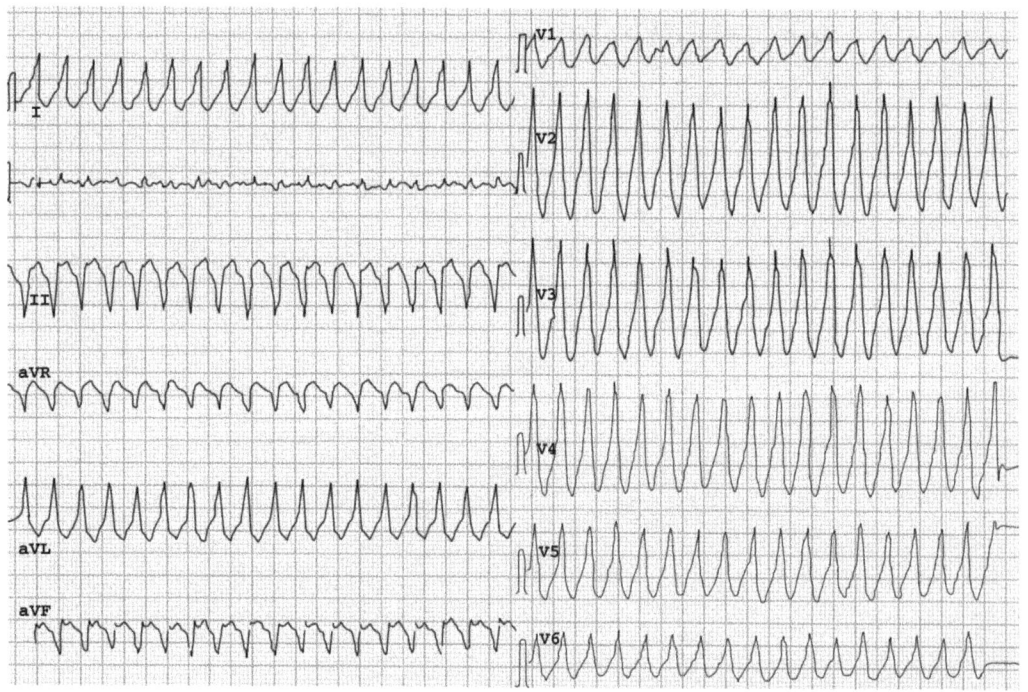

Fig. 4: 12 leads ECG showing a ventricular tachycardia.

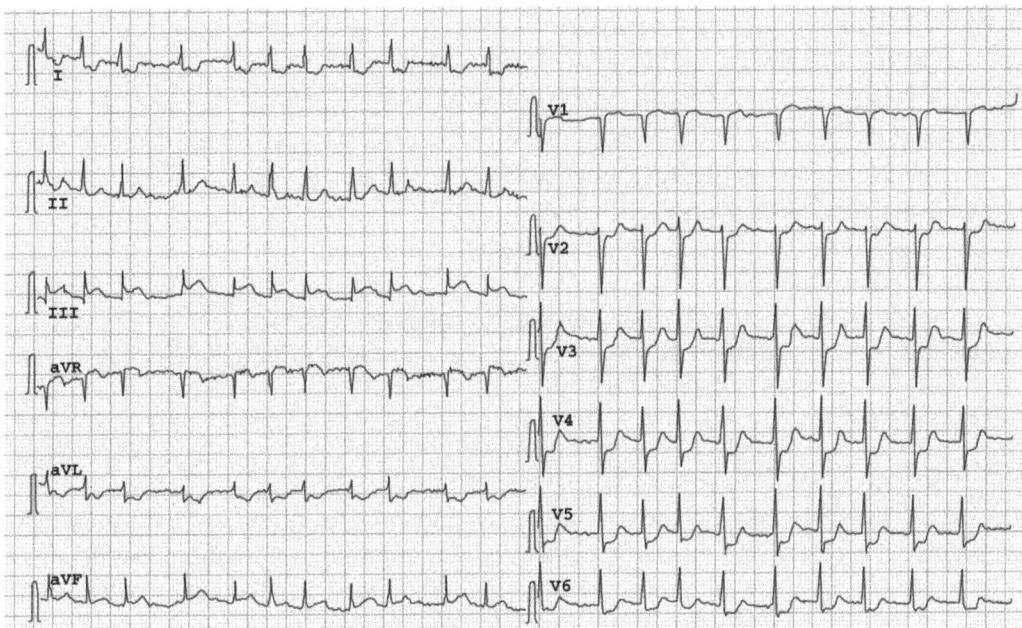

Fig. 5: 12 leads ECG showing an atrial fibrillation and an inferior STEMI.

Table 2: Description of palpitation and possible cause.

Description	Suggestion
Beat skipping and thumps	Extrasystole
Worsen at rest	Extrasystole
Fast and regular	Supraventricular or ventricular tachycardia
Sudden onset	Supraventricular or ventricular tachycardia
Ends with vagal maneuvers	Re-entry supraventricular tachycardia
Fast and irregular	Atrial fibrillation or flutter with varying block
Non-fast and irregular	II degree AV block or extrasystole
Hard and regular	Awareness of sinus rhythm (hypertension, anxiety, cocaine)
Dizziness, heart failure, syncope, shock	Ventricular tachycardia

The patient may be in shock or hemodynamically unstable or may present palpitation only in orthostatic or lying position.

Very often the patients are young and otherwise healthy so easily labeled as "anxious."

RED FLAGS

When palpitation is recurrent, persistent, and is provoked by *exertion*, or accompanied by *lightheadedness, syncope, chest pain, and dyspnea*, a careful workup is mandatory and if the diagnosis is not evident at the beginning a period of observation and monitoring is necessary.

Preceding episodes of syncope can be associated with long QT syndrome, idiopathic or acquired, that may develop torsade de pointes.

A syncope may also happen with the onset of an atrioventricular advanced block or a ventricular tachycardia.

The onset of chest pain and palpitation is always alarming as it can be due to a ventricular tachycardia or another arrhythmic complication of a coronary syndrome.

EVALUATION

History

The patient should be asked about the onset of palpitation, the duration, and the associated symptoms. The rate of heartbeat and regularity is an important information like the onset with a syncope, or other symptoms, and whether the patient was in activity or at rest. In particular, palpitation occurring during exertion or just after it is a warning sign for possible cardiomyopathy or conduction disturbance. Doctors should inquiry about the interruption of the palpitation: if it is sudden or Inturrepted by vagal maneuvers like Valsalva, a paroxysmal SVT is likely.

It is also important to know whether the patient is in a difficult or stressful period, is in sleep deprivation or with a fever.

Physical Examination

The patient should be evaluated according to airway, breathing, circulation, and disability (ABCD) approach.

Airway: If the patient is able to speak fluently, the airway is clear.

Breathing: Take respiratory rate and oxygen saturation, look for signs of cardiac decompensation, or respiratory failure, the presence of rales, wheezes, rhonchi on auscultation that may be the cause or the consequence of a tachyarrhythmia.

Circulation: Blood pressure and heart rate give immediately the idea of a cardiac arrhythmia and of the stability of the patient. In this phase, it is essential to make a 12-lead ECG directly at the triage, because it permits immediately to find the cause of palpitations in a wide majority of cases, or at least to disclose life-threatening situation like ventricular tachycardia or hemodynamically unstable tachyarrhythmia, myocardial infarction, or evident signs of electrolyte disorders like hyperkalemia.

Disability: Once excluded an obvious cardiac cause of palpitation, it is necessary to evaluate all the other signs and symptoms that may lead to the diagnosis like signs of hyperthyroidism, evidence of intoxication, psychosis, anxiety, panic attack, etc.

Flowchart 1: Approach to the patient presenting to the emergency department with palpitation.

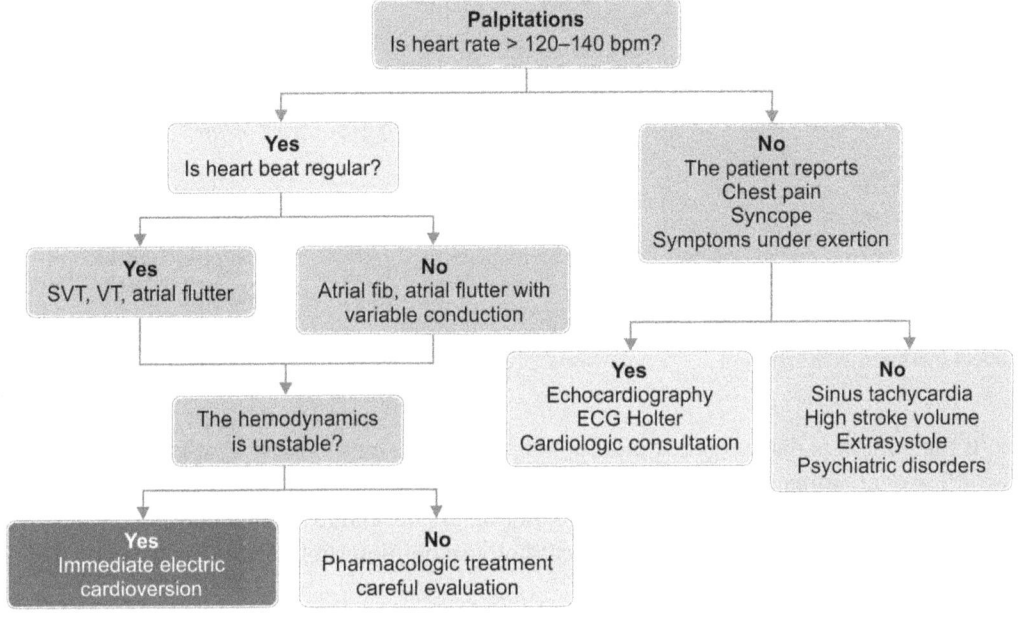

INTERPRETATION OF FINDINGS

If at the first clinical evaluation, an unstable cardiac or respiratory disease is evident, it will be necessary to start immediately the proper treatment and monitoring. An eventual arrhythmia that may be related to palpitation may need to be treated with the condition (e.g. high rate atrial fibrillation in pulmonary edema) or may be a consequence of the disease (e.g. MAT in COPD exacerbation with respiratory failure) and will resolve once the situation is getting better.

When at the ECG, it is clear that the pure cause of palpitation is an acute arrhythmia, the best option is to treat it immediately as described later in the text.

If the clinical examination excludes a cardiac or another medical problem, the probability of a psychiatric disorder is high, so a proper specialist consultation is recommended.

INVESTIGATIONS

As already reported, a 12-lead ECG is mandatory and needs to be available as soon as possible.

Laboratory test are recommended including complete blood count to exclude anemia, serum electrolytes, arterial blood gas analysis also required to evaluate respiratory failure hypercarbia, metabolic acidosis, carbon monoxide poisoning.

If the ECG is negative but the patient is describing episodes of syncope, dyspnea or chest pain, a period of observation or monitoring in the ED is recommended, and very often is possible to scavenge a new arrhythmic episode or another cardiac problem like ischemia.

Table 3: Indication to seek urgent or nonurgent expert opinion of a cardiologist according to the ECG finding.

ECG finding	Acute onset	Unknown
STEMI, coronary syndrome	Urgent	Urgent
Atrial fibrillation, atrial flutter	Urgent or deferred (if treated by the EP)	Nonurgent
Left ventricular hypertrophy, left bundle branch block	Urgent if acute cardiac decompensation	Nonurgent. Echocardiogram mandatory
Second degree atrioventricular block	Urgent for Mobitz II	Nonurgent for Mobitz I
Third degree atrioventricula block	Urgent	Urgent
Atrioventricular accessory pathway (Wolff-Parkinson-White pattern)	Urgent if associated with tachyarrhythmia	Nonurgent

If the patient is discharged should be referred to the cardiologist to apply a Holter ECG recording or an implantable loop recording.

An echocardiogram is recommended either before discharge or soon after.

As per ECG criteria shown in **Table 3** cardiologist opinion should be taken urgently.

TREATMENT

Arrhythmias

Extrasystoles are normally not treated unless really disturbing the patient. In this case, a beta-blocker or intravenous magnesium therapy is indicated.

Atrial fibrillation: According to the most recent guidelines, it is necessary to identify the time of onset because if it is less than 48 hours, it is possible to attempt a cardioversion, if not it is necessary to do a "rate control" approach and postpone the cardioversion after a period of anticoagulation. According to patient choice, it will be possible to do an electrical cardioversion that needs sedation, or a pharmacological cardioversion with flecainide, if the patient has not structural cardiac disease, or amiodarone if there is a cardiac disease or decompensation.

A hemodynamically unstable atrial fibrillation as any other unstable tachyarrhythmia requires an urgent electrical cardioversion.

In view of risk of thrombotic stroke oral anticoagulation therapy should be started.

The patient needs to be always referred to the cardiologist, in the ED or at discharge.

Supraventricular tachycardia: Reentry SVTs often are self-limited or may be interrupted by vagal maneuvers. If these are not efficacious, the drug of choice is adenosine, 6 mg intravenous flush, that can be repeated at 12 mg. A period of asystole after the drug is possible but the very short half-life of adenosine makes it a very safe option.

The third choice is a non-dihydropyridinic calcium channel blocker like verapamil, but it must be avoided in patients with a Wolff-Parkinson-White syndrome.

Ventricular tachycardia is generally treated with electrical cardioversion or, in a stable situation, can be treated with amiodarone or lidocaine.

Arrhythmias due to electrolyte alterations or drug poisoning need to be treated by treating the underlying cause.

Symptomatic bradycardias require the use of transthoracic or transvenous cardiac pacing, and a washout of the drugs that may have provoked the bradyarrhythmia.

Any other structural cardiac disease, or any noncardiac disease will be treated properly or referred to a specialist evaluation.

In a majority of cases, palpitation does not need pharmacological treatment but only reassurance of the patient and can be resolved by lifestyle modification.

SUMMARY

Palpitation is a common symptom that leads the patient to the emergency department. Approach to patient with palpitation is described in **Flowchart 1**. It is generally described as the sense of abnormality of the heart beating in terms of rate or regularity. About 40% of the cases or of cardiac origin, 30% have a psychiatric cause, and 30% of other medical causes.

Any acute arrhythmia may cause palpitation, for this reason a 12-lead ECG is mandatory every time a patient refers palpitation at the triage.

At the first evaluation, it is necessary to exclude all the possible life-threatening conditions that may cause or present with palpitation like unstable ventricular or supraventricular arrhythmia, cardiac ischemia, structural arrhythmogenic cardiac disease, poisoning, electrolyte disorders or advanced atrioventricular block. If not evident immediately, a proper period of monitoring and observation is mandatory.

Particular attention must be given when palpitation is provoked or followed by chest pain, dyspnea, lightheadedness, or syncope that may be the alarm sign of ischemia or a structural heart disease.

A careful evaluation of previous medical history, with recording of all the drugs and structural cardiac diseases, is of utmost importance, as well as the habit to consume alcohol or illegal drugs.

An acute arrhythmia or any other critical illness related to the symptom must be stabilized and addresses immediately, while in all the other cases it will be indicated a follow-up with some investigations like Holter ECG, or loop recording to scavenge eventual arrhythmic episodes. It is important to recognize the noncardiac causes of palpitations like thyrotoxicosis and hypoglycemia, and when all the organic causes have been excluded to address the patients toward a psychiatric evaluation.

CHAPTER 72

Pedal Edema

Ajay Singh Thapa

INTRODUCTION

The word is derived from the Greek word οἴδημα *oídēma* meaning "swelling." Previously this condition also known as "dropsy." This is an abnormal excessive accumulation fluid in the interstitium of the tissue of the lower leg. The condition is most of the time secondary to various systemic disease. A systemic approach to the edema requires for the diagnosis of the disease.

ETIOLOGY AND PATHOGENESIS

The accumulation of the fluid is due to these reasons:
- Increased hydrostatic pressure (heart failure)
- Decreased oncotic pressure (hypoalbuminemia)
- Increased blood vessel permeability (inflammation)
- Obstruction of the lymphatic system of the tissue (elephantiasis)
- Alteration of the water retaining properties of the tissue.

The mechanism of the edema is frequently overlapping one or more factors.

Usually causes of pedal edema are classified based on the mechanism and etiology of the condition (**Flowchart 1**).

RED FLAGS

Red flags of pedal edema have been shown in **Box 1**.

GRADING OF EDEMA

The grading of pedal edema has been shown in **Table 1**.

AN APPROACH TO THE PEDAL EDEMA

A detail history is a key component to distinguish the causes of the pedal edema.
- *Onset of edema*: If onset is less than 72 hours indicates, infection (e.g. cellulitis), deep venous thrombosis (DVT) and compartment syndrome.
- *Pitting or nonpitting*: The most of the time pitting edema points toward the systemic disease, venous insufficiency, DVT or infections; however, nonpitting edema indicates lymphatic system obstruction (lymphedema or pelvic malignancy).

Flowchart 1: Classification of causes of pedal edema based on the mechanism and etiology of the condition.

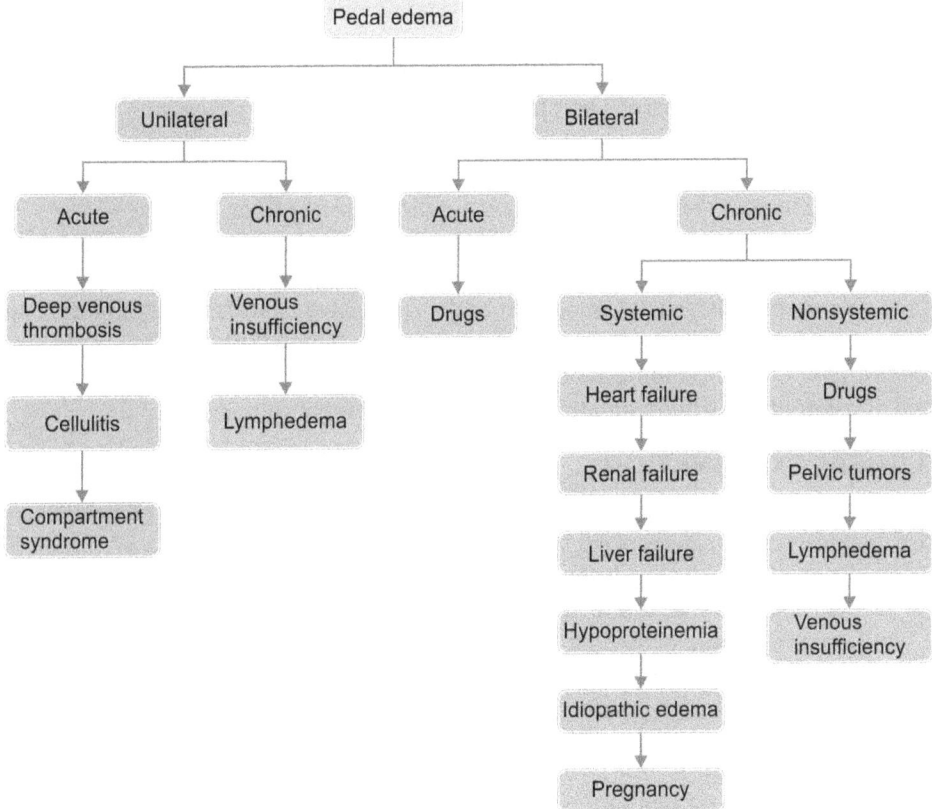

Box 1: Red flags of pedal edema.

- Unilateral painful swelling
- Fever
- Dyspnea
- Post-traumatic swelling
- Edema of rapid onset
- Rapid deterioration
- Unexplained weight loss
- Medications suggestive of heart failure, liver failure, renal failure, and endocrine diseases

Table 1: Grading of pedal edema.

Grade 1	Mild: both feet/ankle
Grade 2	Moderate: both feet plus lower legs or lower arms
Grade 3	Severe: generalized bilateral pitting edema, including both feet, legs, arms, and face

- *Site and distribution*: Is it unilateral or bilateral? The unilateral pedal edema causes generally secondary to DVT, cellulitis, lymphedema or venous insufficiency; however, bilateral pedal edema is primarily due to systemic disease: like liver failure, congestive cardiac failure, and kidney failure.
- *Aggravating factors*: The edema exacerbates by prolong standing in the venous insufficiency and congestive heart failure; however, it alleviates with leg elevation.
- *Past medical history*: The past medical history of chronic heart failure, liver disease, kidney disease, and endocrine disorder like hypothyroidism. The history of radiation and surgery for the malignancy should consider ruling out the cause of edema.
- *Associated symptoms*: The edema is associated with pain likely secondary to the infection, e.g. cellulitis, DVT or fracture. Painless edema with fatigue, breathlessness, paroxysmal nocturnal dyspnea is usually associated in the congestive heart failure but jaundice with abdominal distention and edema likely due to chronic liver failure.
- *Medications*: Calcium channel blockers like amlodipine cause bilateral edema and steroids and nonsteroidal anti-inflammatory drugs (NSAIDs) might cause it too.

CLINICAL EXAMINATION

The detail clinical examinations are required after meticulously obtaining clinical history to make a diagnosis of the causes of edema.
- *Technique to determine the edema*:
  - Press firmly with your thumb for at least 2 seconds on each extremity
    - Over the dorsum of the foot
    - Behind the medial malleolus
    - Lower calf above the medial malleolus
  - Record indention recovery time in seconds
    - Scoring system
      - No clinical edema = 0
      - ≤2 mm indentation = 1+ edema
        - Slight pitting
        - No visual distortion
        - Disappears rapidly
      - 2–4 mm indentation = 2+ edema
        - Somewhat deeper pitting
        - No readably detectable distortion
        - Disappears in 10–15 seconds
      - 4–6 mm indentation = 3+ edema
        - Pit is noticeably deep
        - May last >1 minute
        - Dependent extremity looks fuller and swollen
      - 6–8 mm indentation = 4+ edema
        - Pit is very deep
        - Last as long as 2–5 minutes
        - Dependent extremity is grossly distorted

- *Local inspections*: The redness skin changes over the edema suggest of infections and gray-brownish doughy skin suggests chronic venous insufficiency but dry, coarse, and brownish skin changes suggest the myxedema.
- *Local palpations*: Bilateral pitting edema gives a clue about systemic disease, rather unilateral tender pitting edema hints the local pathology like deep vein thrombosis (DVT) or cellulitis. Nonpitting unilateral edema suggests lymphedema.
- *General examinations*: It is important to look for jaundice, fever, pallor, lymphadenopathy, ascites, jugular vein pressure (JVP), and varicose veins to rule out systemic causes of edema.
- *Systemic examination*:
  - *Respiratory system:* Bilateral coarse crepitation over lower lobe or wheezes with bilateral pitting edema are suggestive of chronic heart failure.
  - *Cardiovascular system*: The third heart sound with raised JVP should consider the cause of congestive heart failure.
  - *Gastrointestinal system*: The jaundice, hepatomegaly, gynecomastia, spider naevi, ascites with bilateral pedal edema suggest the chronic decompensated liver failure.

INVESTIGATIONS

- *Complete blood count*: Anemia with edema suggests the kidney failure or congestive heart failure. Increased white blood cell (WBC) count indicates the inflammation.
- *Biochemistry*: Raised serum ALT, AST, bilirubin, altered prothrombin time (PT), hypoalbuminemia suggest the decompensated liver failure. Increased serum urea, creatinine, and raised potassium with edema notify the renal failure. Increased B-natriuretic peptide (BNP) with edema indicates the chronic heart failure.
- Raised D-Dimer is highly sensitive test for the DVT and should proceed further by venous Doppler to confirm the diagnosis.
- The dyslipidemia with hypoalbuminemia and proteinuria associated with bilateral edema indicates the nephrotic syndrome.
- *Chest X-ray*: Cardiomegaly with signs of pulmonary edema with bilateral edema gives a clue for the diagnosis of congestive heart failure.
- *Echocardiography*: It evaluates the functions of all ventricules and valves as well as measures the pressures of pulmonary arteries to diagnose the right and left heart failure.
- *Ultrasound Doppler of lower legs*: The most sensitive and specific image study for DVT and venous insufficiency.
- *Lymphoscintigraphy*: This is a radionuclide imaging study on Gamma Camera to look for the obstruction of lymphatic system to diagnose a lymphedema.

MANAGEMENT OF PEDAL EDEMA

The management is based on the likelihood diagnosis of the pedal edema.

Nonpharmacological

Fluid restriction: It is the initial management for the congestive heart failure, decompensated liver failure, and chronic kidney disease with bilateral pedal edema.

- *Diet*: Low salt diet is for congestive heart failure, low-protein diet for decompensated liver failure and renal failure. High-protein diet may advocate for the hypoproteinemia.
- *Exercise and weight reduction*: Elevations of lower limbs and limbs movement alleviates the symptoms in the venous insufficiency; however, high knee compressive stocking may require for the chronic venous insufficiency. The manual massaging, bandaging, and compressive stocking may use in the case of lymphedema. The weight reduction is the initial management for the obstructive sleep apnea.

Pharmacological

- *Diuretics*: The loop diuretics like furosemide or torsemides can be used in the congestive heart failure, chronic kidney disease, and liver failure, when patients fail to respond on nonpharmacological measures.
- *Antibiotics*: In the case of cellulitis, antibiotics are indicated as per local sensitivity to the microorganisms.
- *Anticoagulants*: Subcutaneous low molecular weight heparin followed by oral anticoagulants is advisable for the DVT.
- *Albumin*: Intravenous infusion of albumin may consider in the hypoalbuminemia state due to chronic liver failure for temporary relief.
- *Surgical treatment*: In the refractory cases of lymphedema, surgical bypass and debulking surgery may consider. Fasciotomy is indicated for the compartment syndrome.

CHAPTER 73

Penile Problems

Puneet Ahluwalia, Saurabh Patil

PHIMOSIS

Introduction

Phimosis is the condition in which a narrowed prepuce (foreskin of penis) cannot be retracted over the glans penis. It is derived from a Greek word *"phimos"* which means "muzzle."

At birth almost 96% of male newborns have phimosis which resolves over time, so that normal retractable prepuce is seen in around 50% by the end of 1st year, 90% by 3 years, and in 99% by 14 years of age.

Etiology/Causes

Phimosis can be divided into physiological and pathological (true) phimosis.

Physiological (primary) phimosis: During neonatal development, the inner epithelial lining of preputial skin is attached to the underneath glans. These naturally occurring adhesions and narrow prepuce inhibits retractability of prepuce over glans leading to physiological phimosis. As the child grows, epithelial debris get formed and accumulated under the prepuce causing its separation from glans. This along with intermittent erections of penis leads to normal retractable foreskin, over the variable period of time ranging from birth to 18 years of age or may rarely be even more. However, around 2% individuals may not achieve this normal retractability even throughout their lives.

Pathological (secondary) phimosis: The pathological or true phimosis is due to scarring of distal preputial skin. The various reasons for such scarring could be poor hygiene leading to recurrent balanitis (inflammation of glans penis) or posthitis (inflammation of preputial skin). Even overzealous attempts of forceful retraction of prepuce in physiological phimosis may lead to microtears, bleeding, inflammation, and healing with scarring.

The incidence of pathological phimosis is around 0.4/1,000 boys/year, much lesser compared to physiological.

Another causative factor for pathological phimosis is balanitis xerotica obliterans (BXO), a penile form of lichen sclerosus et atrophicus. BXO is a chronic inflammatory condition with unknown etiology affecting skin and mucous membrane, especially prepuce, glans penis, meatus, and distal urethra, accounting for the most common cause of secondary phimosis in children.

Clinical Presentation

It is important to differentiate between physiological and pathological phimosis as the treatments for both are different.

In physiological phimosis, the child is usually brought by anxious parents but the child himself may not be having any bothersome complaints, except for nonretractability of foreskin or ballooning of foreskin during voiding. The local symptoms like pain, swelling, redness are absent. Urinary flow is good.

This is contrary to pathological phimosis in which child may present with preputial pain and irritation, local infections leading to swelling and redness of skin, minor bleeding and sometimes dysuria, recurrent episodes of urinary tract infections (UTIs). The parents may notice poor urinary stream, especially in cases with associated BXO.

Few grading classifications according to the severity of phimosis have been proposed by various authors. Meuli et al. created the following scoring system:
Grade 1: Fully retractable prepuce and stenotic ring in the shaft
Grade 2: Partially retractable prepuce with partial exposure of the glans
Grade 3: Partially retractable prepuce with exposure of only meatus
Grade 4: No retractability.

Another grading of phimosis was proposed by Kikiros et al. according to severity of phimosis and appearance of foreskin.

Retractability of foreskin score:
Score 0: Full retractability, not tight behind glans, or easy retraction limited only by congenital adhesions to the glans
Score 1: Full retraction of foreskin, tight behind the glans
Score 2: Partial exposure of glans, prepuce (not congenital adhesions) limiting factor
Score 3: Partial retraction, meatus just visible
Score 4: Slight retraction, but some distance between tip and glans, i.e. neither meatus nor glans can be visible
Score 5: Absolutely no retraction.

Appearance of foreskin score:
Score 0: Normal
Score 1: Crack in prepuce, "skin-splitting" on gentle retraction
Score 2: Small white scar, partial circumferential
Score 3: Balanitis xerotica obliterans or severe scarring ± bleeding.

Evaluation

Phimosis is a fairly obvious clinical condition, requiring no specific laboratory tests or imaging modalities for diagnosis.

History

Though usual presenting complaint is ballooning of prepuce during voiding, a detailed history of all associated symptoms is vital in ruling out the likely complications.

History should also include episodes of recurrent fever, stream of micturition, and urinary problems.

Physical Examination

In physiological phimosis, the distal preputial skin is healthy, pliant with typical pink mucosa seen pouting or flowering on gentle traction. However in pathological phimosis, on gentle traction, there is abnormal scarring of prepuce and a cone-shaped structure is seen with a narrow white fibrotic ring at the tip. This clinical differentiation is very vital so as to avoid anxiety in parents and unnecessary surgical procedures.

Treatment

First and foremost thing in management of phimosis is to confirm whether it is physiological or pathological. Management depends on age of child, type and severity of phimosis, and associated complications. Once it is confirmed that the phimosis is physiological, the most important thing is to reassure parents about the normalcy of the condition. Parents should be taught about the care of foreskin.

Treatment of phimosis can be divided into nonsurgical or conservative and surgical treatment. Though traditionally circumcision is considered the standard treatment for phimosis, many topical ointments have been tried in recent years with a good success rate. In few recent trials, it was shown that only 8–14.4% of the total referrals had actual pathological phimosis requiring surgical intervention. Rest all could be managed conservatively and thus over-referrals could have been avoided.

Topical Preparations

Various topical preparations have been tried till date in form of steroids, estrogen, and nonsteroidal anti-inflammatory drugs (NSAIDs). Amongst these steroids have been most widely used and have shown more promising outcomes.

Topical steroids: Many studies in past few decades have shown a favorable success rate of topical steroid therapy, ranging from 70% to 95%. The mechanism of action of topical steroids is believed to be local anti-inflammation and immunosuppression. They also reduce the dermal synthesis of glycosaminoglycans, epidermal proliferation, and stratum corneum thickness thereby causing skin thinning.

Most commonly used preparation is betamethasone 0.05% twice daily for a period of 4 weeks. Other concentrations of betamethasone like 0.1%, 0.06% have also been tried with almost similar success rates. Other steroids like clobetasol propionate, triamcinolone, mometasone dipropionate, fluticasone showed comparable results.

Very few studies have mentioned the recurrence rates because of the short follow-ups in rest of the studies. The reported recurrence rate ranges from 2% to 14%, poor compliance being the most common reason. Almost all studies, who have reported the recurrence, have observed success after retreatment for few more months with same agent, and therefore reduction in need for circumcision.

Preputial Stretching

The nonsurgical adhesiolysis by frequent manual retractions of prepuce has found to be a safe and effective treatment option for phimosis regardless of the age of the boy. Combination of topical steroids along with stretching adds to the improvement of overall outcome.

Surgical Treatment

Circumcision: Male circumcision is one of the oldest surgical procedures known to humans. It is also one of the most commonly performed surgical procedures worldwide to the extent that approximately 37–39% of men are circumcised worldwide.

Though sometimes treatment of phimosis is as per the parent's preference, the absolute indication of circumcision is secondary phimosis. However, circumcision may be indicated in some cases of primary phimosis like recurrent balanoposthitis, recurrent UTIs especially in patients with urinary tract abnormalities. The contraindications for circumcision are an acute local infection and congenital anomalies of the penis like hypospadias, where the foreskin should be preserved as it may be helpful for a future reconstruction.

Techniques

1. *Circumcision using devices*
2. *Freehand circumcision*
    i. *Sleeve technique*
    ii. *Dorsal-ventral slit technique*
    iii. *Preputioplasties*

Complications of Circumcision

As complications can happen in any surgical procedure, circumcision is no exception. In one large systematic review of complications of circumcision, Weiss et al. found that the median frequency of any adverse event and any serious adverse event was 1.5% (range 0–16%) and 0% (range 0–2%), respectively. They also found that complications occurred more frequently in circumcision for older children than in neonates and infants.

Early complications: By and large the complications of circumcision procedure are usually minor and treatable like bleeding, surgical site infection or swelling, inadequate skin removal, etc. Other serious early complications include excessive bleeding, chordee, iatrogenic hypospadias, necrosis of glans, and amputation of glans. The excessive bleeding during or after circumcision, requiring blood transfusion, may occur in children with bleeding disorders like hemophilia. Therefore, it is very important to ask regarding any family history of such disorders before surgery.

Late complications: These include chordee, epidermal inclusion cysts, excess redundant foreskin, preputial adhesions or skin bridges, iatrogenic hypospadias recurrent phimosis, buried penis, suture sinus tracts, urethrocutaneous fistulae, and meatal stenosis. Most of these are treatable but require an additional surgical procedure, indicating the importance of proper operative technique.

Medical Benefits of Circumcision

Most of the studies in literature showed that uncircumcised males were more prone to sexually transmitted diseases like syphilis, chancroid, herpes simplex, and human papillomavirus (HPV), whereas circumcised men were more prone to urethritis. Few randomized controlled trials (RCTs) done in African patients have shown protective effects of circumcision against human immunodeficiency virus (HIV) with almost 50% risk reduction.

There is no direct causal association of phimosis with penile carcinoma. However, indirect benefit by reduction in HPV infection, which is a causative factor for penile carcinoma, may be expected. Still routine neonatal circumcision to prevent penile carcinoma is not indicated.

The protective effect of circumcision against UTIs may be seen only in cases of recurrent UTIs and children with congenital urinary tract abnormalities such as high-grade vesicoureteric reflux.

Summary

Phimosis is the nonretractability of prepuce over the glans penis. Most of the newborns have phimosis due to natural adhesions between prepuce and the glans, and this is physiological and as the child grows, he achieves normal retractability over a variable period of time. Secondary phimosis is a pathological condition, which must be differentiated clinically from primary phimosis. While primary phimosis can be managed conservatively or by manual stretching and topical steroids, secondary phimosis definitely requires some forms of treatment mostly surgical. There are various forms of treatment options available. The topical steroid application along with repeated manual stretching of prepuce is quite safe and has a good success rate. The absolute indication for circumcision is pathological phimosis (BXO) or sometimes primary phimosis with recurrent balanoposthitis or UTIs. Various devices are now available for circumcision with almost equal success rates as conventional freehand circumcision and with comparable complication rates. Complications associated with circumcision procedure are usually minor and treatable. Medical benefits offered by circumcision include protection against some sexually transmitted diseases including HPV, HIV, and against recurrent UTIs especially in cases of congenital urinary tract anomalies.

PARAPHIMOSIS

Introduction

Paraphimosis is a urological emergency in which foreskin is left retracted due to its entrapment behind the glans penis. This leads to strangulation of glans and lymphovascular compromise of the prepuce leading to venous engorgement, inflammation, pain, and even necrosis, further impending the reduction of foreskin.

Etiology/Causes

The cause is most often iatrogenic. It occurs when the foreskin is retracted for urethral catheterization, penile examination, or during per urethral procedure like cystoscopy or meatal dilatation. Failure to reposit the retracted foreskin back over glans results in paraphimosis. Less commonly it may be due to trauma during sexual intercourse or self-inflicted injuries.

Pathophysiology of the Condition

When retracted foreskin remains trapped behind glans penis prolonged time, the blood and lymphatic flow to and from prepuce and glans is obstructed. This leads to vascular engorgement and subsequent edema of prepuce. Paraphimosis is a urological emergency which, if left untreated, may ultimately result in glans necrosis and rarely autoamputation.

Clinical Presentation

Though paraphimosis can occur in any age group, its incidence is lesser in young children (0.2%) compared to other penile lesions like balanitis (5.9%), phimosis (2.6%), etc. Most common occurrence is in adolescent males with 1% incidence in all adult males above 16 years of age.

The preceding event in adults is usually a Foley catheter insertion and in children, a forceful retraction of foreskin for examination or for cleaning. Whatever may be the reason, failure to return the retracted foreskin to its normal position over the glans remains the main culprit.

Patient presents with a swelling in foreskin, usually with pain. The diagnosis is often confirmed on physical examination of prepuce and the glans, both of which are markedly edematous and congested. The proximal penile shaft usually remains unremarkable. The reduction of preputial skin becomes difficult and painful due to the swollen prepuce and constricted band of edematous tissues behind the glans.

Evaluation: History and Physical Examination

A detail history should be taken concerning foreskin retraction, urethral instrumentation or presence of urinary symptoms. The external genitalia should be examined in detail with a focus on the color and consistency of the glans and prepuce, the severity of constriction around the penile corona and condition of proximal penile shaft. Though glans remains pink healthy in most of the cases, long-standing cases may have dark red, dusky, or even black glans indicating its ischemic necrosis. The viability of glans can also be confirmed by its palpation, as normal healthy glans is soft and pliable and becomes firm and inelastic after necrosis.

Treatment

The main aim of treatment of paraphimosis is reduction of preputial and glans edema and restoration of prepuce to its original position. There are many different methods of reduction of phimosis as described here.

Manual Reduction

Manual reduction method may be tried in mild, early and uncomplicated cases. Because of the pain which gets further aggravated during manipulation, it may require some forms of anesthesia like topical lignocaine gel, oral narcotics, penile nerve block, or sedation.

Manual reduction is done by giving circumferential compression over edematous prepuce and glans with gloved fingers in order to disperse the edema fluid. The reduction can simply be achieved by pulling the foreskin upward toward the phallus, while maintaining the circumferential compression. Application of ice packs may also facilitate in reducing the edema; however, some surgeons discourage this method as it may further compromise arterial inflow to the already ischemic portion of the penis. Manual compression can also be achieved by tightly wrapping a compressive elastic dressing around edematous portion of the penis from the glans toward the base for 5–10 minutes.

Pharmacological Therapy

Another way of reducing the preputial edema is application of mannitol (20%)-soaked gauze around prepuce for a period of 30–45 minutes, with or without intermittent compression. This works on the principle of transfer of edema fluid from edematous prepuce down the osmotic gradient to hypertonic mannitol, reducing the edematous swelling.

In another reported technique, eutectic mixture of local anesthetic (EMLA) cream containing 2.5% lidocaine and 2.5% prilocaine is applied to the glans in a glove covering for around 30 minutes and trapped foreskin can then be reduced with gentle traction.

Injection of hyaluronidase (1 mL of 150 U/cc) also helps in reducing the edema. Hyaluronidase degrades the viscous hyaluronic acid and thereby increases the dispersion of edema fluid.

Minimally Invasive Therapy

This includes the most widely practiced method of multiple puncture technique, also known as Perth-Dundee technique. In this method, multiple (approximately 20) punctures with 26-gauge needle are made in edematous prepuce and the prepuce is then compressed to express out the edema fluid. As this is a painful method, it requires some forms of anesthesia usually topical or penile block.

Once the edema has subsided with the help of above described methods, paraphimosis can be reduced. For this, both the thumbs are placed on glans and rest all fingers are wrapped around the trapped prepuce. A gentle steady force is applied by thumb over glans along with countertraction achieved by constant pulling of prepuce outward back over the glans.

Surgical Treatment

Surgical intervention is required when above described methods have failed to reduce the paraphimosis. This involves longitudinal dorsal slit cutting of prepuce at 12 o'clock till constricting band site and reduction of trapped prepuce back over the glans. The cut edges are over sewn with absorbable suture without approximating them.

Circumcision is usually the last resort done reserved for recurrent episodes.

SUMMARY

Paraphimosis is a urological emergency in which foreskin is left retracted due to its entrapment behind the glans penis causing inflammation, strangulation of glans. It usually occurs after failure of prompt repositioning of foreskin after its retraction. Urgent medical attention is necessary to avoid further damage which may even cause ischemic necrosis of glans in long-standing cases. Paraphimosis can occur in any age group. The diagnosis is clinical, no tests are required. The treatment options include manual reduction, compression dressing, multiple puncture technique, dorsal slit, and lastly circumcision. Patients should be taught regarding the reduction of foreskin every time it is retracted.

■ PENILE FRACTURE

Introduction

Penile fracture is defined as disruption of the tunica albuginea with rupture of the corpus cavernosum secondary to trauma to penis in tumescent state. Penile fracture usually occurs during vigorous sexual intercourse or an aggressive manipulation of penis in an erect state. This is a urological malignancy and the rupture may extend to involve corpus spongiosum and urethra. The first case of penile fracture was reported by an Arab physician, Abu al-Qasim al-Zahrawi in Cordoba, more than 1,000 years ago.

Epidemiology

The incidence of penile fracture varies amongst different geographical areas, with higher incidence in Middle East and African regions compared to western countries or Asian continent. The incidence of penile fracture is under reported as patients avoid to seek medical attention due to embarrassment. The reported incidence is around 1 in 175,000. The age distribution also varies in different geographical areas with mean age in Africans 26.4 years, in Asians 33.7 years, in Europeans 38.7 years, and in North Americans 37.6 years with a range of 12–82 years.

Etiology/Causes

Overall, the most common cause of penile fracture is the blunt trauma during a vigorous sexual intercourse, when the erect penis slips out of the vagina and hits the perineum or pubic bone, giving rise to a buckling injury. Again, causative factors differ according to the region. Trauma during sexual intercourse is more common cause in western countries while in Middle East countries common causes include penile manipulations including kneading during masturbation, forceful bending of a tumescent penis during masturbation in order to achieve sudden detumescence—known as "Taghaandan maneuver," or even tucking the erect penis into underwear. Taghaandan maneuver alone is responsible for more than 50% of cases in Middle East countries, while it accounts for only 8% of cases in western population. Other reported causes are fall from bed during sleep on an erect penis, roll over injury during nocturnal tumescence, sudden change of position by female partner while an erect penis is still inside vagina causing its acute bend. "Woman on top" or reverse coitus is reported to be the riskiest position causing fracture penis.

Pathophysiology of the Condition

Tunica albuginea is a bilaminar structure covering both the corpora cavernosa. In flaccid state, the thickness of tunica albuginea is 2 mm, which decreases to 0.25–0.5 mm in tumescent state. It also has a high tensile strength which can resist extracavernous pressures up to 1,500 mm Hg. However, when erect penis is bent abnormally, there is sudden rise in intracavernosal pressure exceeding the tensile strength of the tunica albuginea. This leads to rupture of already thinned tunica, most commonly at ventrolateral aspect which is the thinnest part of tunica albuginea. The rupture of tunica albuginea is usually unilateral and transverse, involves overlying corpus cavernosum and may extend to corpus spongiosum and urethra. After penile fracture, penis becomes detumescent suddenly and a local hematoma develops over penile shaft confined by Buck's fascia. When Buck's fascia is disrupted, this hematoma may spread to the scrotum, perineum, and suprapubic region.

Clinical Presentation

Patient typically presents with a history of a cracking or popping sound in erect penis followed by immediate detumescence and development of pain and swelling in penis. Blood at tip of meatus, hematuria, and acute urinary retention give the hint of associated urethral rupture. Urethral injury incidence also varies region to region, with United States and Europe (20%) having higher incidence compared to Middle East and Asia (3%), may be related to the cause of trauma (intercourse related versus self-inflicted). Due to embarrassment, patients usually do not present to emergency room or present very late.

Evaluation: History and Physical Examination

Diagnosis of penile fracture is a clinical one with history and physical examination playing important role in establishing it. In history, one should ask regarding the time and type of trauma, presence of sudden detumescence and presence of blood at tip of meatus, hematuria, or any voiding disturbance.

On inspection, the most common finding is presence of penile swelling due to penile hematoma, bruising and deviation to one side, giving an "eggplant" appearance, also known as "aubergine sign." The deviation of swollen penis is opposite to the side of tear, because of the mass effect of hematoma. This defect can sometimes be palpable with a blood clot over it can be rolled under the fingers—known as "rolling sign." A butterfly hematoma in perineum suggests rupture of Buck's fascia or associated urethral injury. Rest physical examination remains unremarkable. Patients late after trauma usually have present with erectile dysfunction, penile curvature, palpable plaques like Peyronie's disease and rarely urethrocutaneous or urethrocavernous fistula. Differential diagnoses include rupture of penile vessels (superficial or deep dorsal vein, dorsal or deep cavernous artery), lymphangitis of penis and Mondor's disease.

Investigations

Though the diagnosis of penile fracture is made clinically, few radiological investigations help in confirmation of diagnosis, to locate the exact site of tear and to diagnose associated complications. Penile ultrasound is the preferred modality as it is readily available in emergency, cheap, noninvasive and useful in locating exact site of tear and in ruling out fracture in suspicious cases. In case of clinical suspicion of urethral injury, retrograde urethrography can be done before surgery. However, because of possibility of inaccuracy and its time-consuming nature, on table flexible cystoscopy just before catheter placement is preferable. Magnetic resonance imaging, cavernosography are not routinely used because of the high expenses, limited availability, and time-consuming nature.

Treatment

Treatment can be conservative or surgical. Conservative approach may be advocated in cases of intact tunica on imaging but strong clinical suspicion. It includes cold fomentation, anti-inflammatory agents, fibrinolytics (trypsin, streptokinase), and antiandrogens (like stilbestrol, to prevent erections). However, conservative approach is not recommended because of the long-term complications like corporeal fibrosis, delayed chordee with resultant shaft deformation (in up to 16% of cases), and plaque formation (in up to 50% of cases).

Many studies and reviews of literature have shown that prompt surgical is associated with fewer complications and better long-term results in terms of erectile function compared to conservative treatment.

Timing of Surgical Repair

It has been shown in some of the reports and reviews from the literature that prompt repair is associated with good functional results compared to delayed repairs. However, timing of repair does not significantly affect rates of erectile dysfunction and penile plaque formation. Therefore, cases presenting even after few days should not be denied for surgical repair as they can have a good functional results in long term.

The dressing should be loose so that glans can be checked for early ischemic color changes. Patient should be instructed to avoid sexual activity for a period of 4–6 weeks to allow complete healing of the repair.

A patient should be educated about the predisposing factors so to avoid recurrence. He should be instructed to avoid vigorous sexual intercourse, aggressive sudden penile manipulations, and unusual positions of intercourse like reverse coitus.

Long-term complication rates after a surgical repair are not very high. Reported complications include penile deviation due to fibrosis, skin necrosis, painful erections, and rarely erectile dysfunction.

Summary

Penile fracture is rupture of tunica albuginea due to trauma to penis in a tumescent state. Common causes vary geographically and include aggressive sexual intercourse, forceful penile manipulations, fall from bed, or roll over injury during nocturnal tumescence. Though the diagnosis is clinical imaging like ultrasound gives better idea on the number and site of tunica tear. Once diagnosis is confirmed, patient should be offered surgical repair at earliest and patients presenting even after few days should also be treated in same way. Surgical principles include evacuation of hematoma, identification and repair of tunica tear with running or interrupted absorbable sutures, repair of associated urethral injury. Long-term results are better in surgical repair group compared to conservative. However, no significant difference in erectile function could be found in early versus delayed treatment. So, all patients should be offered surgical management, irrespective of time between of fracture penis presentation to hospital. Reported long-term complications include penile curvature, skin necrosis, painful erections, and rarely erectile dysfunction.

CHAPTER 74

Procedural Sedation and Analgesia

Ronak Mankodi

INTRODUCTION

There is an ever increasing patient population including children and elderly, requiring sedation, and analgesia when being treated in the emergency department (ED).

Definition: Procedural sedation is a technique of administering sedatives or dissociative agents with or without analgesics to induce a state that allows the patient to tolerate unpleasant procedures.

On the basis of effect on various body functions, sedation levels are divided into minimal, moderate, deep sedation, and general anesthesia (**Table 1**).

Despite careful planning and performance, the depth of sedation needed or achieved cannot always be predicted. It is therefore important to prepare for managing deeper levels of sedation than anticipated. Most of the agents used can produce variable levels of sedation, so pay particular attention to dosing and to the patient's responses to the medications.

Dissociative sedation is a type of moderate sedation. Dissociation is a state in which the cortical centers are prevented from receiving sensory stimuli, but cardiopulmonary activity and responses are preserved.

Table 1: Different levels of sedation and their effects on bodily functions.

	Responsiveness	*Airway*	*Spontaneous ventilation*	*Cardiovascular function*
Minimal sedation/anxiolysis	Normal response to verbal stimulation	Unaffected	Unaffected	Unaffected
Moderate sedation/analgesia (conscious sedation)	Purposeful response to verbal or tactile stimulation	No intervention required	Adequate	Usually maintained
Deep sedation/analgesia	Purposeful response following repeated or painful stimulation	Intervention may be required	May be inadequate	Usually maintained
General anesthesia	Unarousable even with painful stimulus	Intervention often required	Frequently inadequate	May be impaired

Chapter 74: Procedural Sedation and Analgesia

Table 2: Types of sedation and their indications.

Type of sedation	Indications
Emergent	Cardioversion for life-threatening arrhythmias, neuroimaging for head trauma, reduction of fractures or dislocations with soft tissue or vascular compromise, care of contaminated wounds, or intractable pain.
Urgent	Stable fractures, abscess incision and drainage, care of clean wounds, foreign body removal, and laceration repair.
Nonemergent	Removal of a soft tissue foreign body, placing splints on fractures that require minimal manipulation, or changing splints on fractures that have already been reduced.

In emergency various types of sedation and their indications are described in **Table 2**. The need for sedation is sometimes more urgent than a full preprocedure evaluation.

RISK ASSESSMENT

Complications are primarily determined by the interaction of the depth of sedation and the patient's current medical condition. One of the most common tools to assess patient's underlying clinical condition is American Society of Anesthesiologists' physical status classification system.

Patient Assessment

Focused history is important to establish fasting state, prior experiences with sedation or anesthesia, current medications, and allergies. Focused physical examination reveals any potential difficult airway or cardiopulmonary compromise. A potentially difficult airway should be anticipated when the following findings or conditions are present: short neck, micrognathia, large tongue, trismus, morbid obesity, a history of difficult intubation, or anatomic anomalies of the airway and neck. At a minimum, difficult airway equipment should be present and available.

Airway Assessment Procedures for Sedation and Analgesia

Positive pressure ventilation, with or without tracheal intubation, may be necessary if respiratory compromise develops during sedation/analgesia. This may be more difficult in patients with atypical airway anatomy. Also, some airway abnormalities may increase the likelihood of airway obstruction during spontaneous ventilation. Some factors that may be associated with difficulty in airway management are listed below.

- *History*:
    - Previous problems with anesthesia or sedation
    - Stridor, snoring, or sleep apnea
    - Advanced rheumatoid arthritis
    - Chromosomal abnormality (e.g. trisomy 21)

- *Physical examination*:
  - *Habitus*: Significant obesity (especially involving the neck and facial structures)
  - *Head and neck*: Short neck, limited neck extension, decreased hyoid-mental distance (<3 cm in an adult), neck mass, cervical spine disease or trauma, tracheal deviation, dysmorphic facial features (e.g. Pierre-Robin syndrome)
  - *Mouth*: Small opening (<3 cm in an adult); edentulous; protruding incisors; loose or capped teeth; dental appliances; high, arched palate; macroglossia; tonsillar hypertrophy; nonvisible uvula
  - *Jaw*: Micrognathia, retrognathia, trismus, and significant malocclusion.

Cardiorespiratory conditions increase the complication rate. Most agents can cause vasodilation and hypotension, particularly in patients with preexisting hypovolemia. Drug or alcohol intoxication or reduced level of consciousness increases the risk of hypoxemia and hypoventilation. If possible, delay procedural sedation in intoxicated patients until mental status improve.

CURRENT PRACTICE GUIDELINES

Preprocedure Fasting

In urgent or emergent situations where complete gastric emptying is not possible, do not delay moderate procedural sedation based on fasting time alone.

Routine Capnography

Capnography* may be used as an adjunct to pulse oximetry and clinical assessment to detect hypoventilation and apnea earlier than pulse oximetry and/or clinical assessment alone in patients undergoing procedural sedation and analgesia in the ED.

Number of Personnel Required

For minimal and moderate levels of sedation, one emergency physician simultaneously administering sedation and performing the procedure with a nurse monitoring the patient appears to be an appropriate practice. However for deep sedation, two physician, one to perform sedation and monitor the patient and the other to perform the procedure.

EQUIPMENT

Sedation area must have all size-appropriate equipment for airway management and resuscitation. An ideal list is provided in **Box 1.**

---

*Capnography includes all forms of quantitative exhaled carbon dioxide analysis.

Box 1: Emergency equipment for sedation and analgesia.

Intravenous equipment (age- and size-appropriate):
- Gloves
- Tourniquets
- Alcohol wipes
- Sterile gauze pads
- Intravenous catheters
- Intravenous tubing
- Intravenous fluid
- Assorted needles for drug aspiration, intramuscular injection
- Intraosseous access kit
- Appropriately sized syringes
- Tape

Basic airway management equipment (age- and size-appropriate):
- Sources of compressed O_2 (tank with regulator or pipeline supply with flow meter)
- Source of suction
- Suction catheters
- Yankauer-type suction
- Face masks
- Self-inflating breathing bag valve set
- Oral and nasal airways
- Lubricant

Advanced airway management equipment:
- Supraglottic airway devices
- Laryngoscope handles (tested)
- Laryngoscope blades
- Endotracheal tubes
- Stylet
- Gum-elastic bougie

Pharmacologic antagonists:
- Naloxone
- Flumazenil

Emergency medications:
- Epinephrine
- Ephedrine
- Vasopressin
- Atropine
- Nitroglycerine (tablets or spray)
- Amiodarone
- Lidocaine
- Glucose (intravenous or oral)
- Diphenhydramine
- Hydrocortisone, methylprednisolone, or dexamethasone
- Benzodiazepines
- Beta blocker
- Adenosine

MONITORING

There are two types of monitoring: Interactive and electronic. *Interactive monitoring* is the direct observation of the patient to assess the depth of sedation and observe for hypoventilation or apnea, upper airway obstruction, laryngospasm, vomiting, or aspiration. Thus interactive monitoring requires an unobstructed view of the patient's face, mouth, and chest wall. *Electronic monitoring* uses equipment to assess arterial oxygenation, ventilation, blood pressure, and cardiac rate and rhythm. Moderate and deep sedation requires constant observation and continuous monitoring.

Pulse oximetry is not a substitute for monitoring ventilation. Quantitative capnography may be used as an adjunct to pulse oximetry and clinical assessment to detect hypoventilation and apnea earlier than pulse oximetry and/or clinical assessment alone in patients undergoing procedural sedation and analgesia in the ED. Capnography during procedural sedation allows the early recognition of adverse events.

Monitoring of vitals including heart rate, blood pressure, and pulse oximetry must be taken and recorded legibly before beginning sedation and after each dose of medication, upon completion of procedure, beginning of recovery period, and upon discharge. For mild sedation, intermittent measurements are sufficient. For moderate and deep sedation, it is recommended that blood pressure be assessed every 5 minutes and heart rate and pulse oximetry be continuously monitored. Patients are at the highest risk of hypoxia and hypoventilation during the period immediately after intravenous (IV) medication administration (until the peak effect of the medication has been reached) and during the immediate postprocedure period (when external stimuli are discontinued and the stimulating pain of the procedure has subsided).

TECHNIQUE

Preprocedure Analgesia

Preprocedure administration of analgesics like opioids makes the patient more comfortable during painful procedures. Sedatives should be administered after time of peak action of analgesics in nonurgent to semi-urgent procedures as it decreases postprocedure analgesic requirement and oversedation may result if analgesic medications are given after sedation. Shorter-acting agents are preferred to drugs with a longer duration of action to minimize postprocedure respiratory depression.

Oxygen Supplementation

The use of supplemental oxygen throughout procedural sedation is a common ED practice. The benefit is that enhanced oxygen reserves permit a longer period of normal oxygenation in the event of apnea or respiratory depression. The disadvantage is that supplemental oxygen therefore negates oximetry as an early warning device.

Two studies of ED propofol sedation without supplemental oxygen have reported desaturation rates of 11.6% and 31%. These rates are higher than the 5–7% similarly observed in studies with supplemental oxygen.

A randomized, controlled trial showed no apparent benefit to supplemental oxygen during ED moderate sedation; however, this question has not been similarly studied for deep sedation. In the case of apnea, a preoxygenated patient will tolerate a longer period of apnea without requiring assisted ventilation, with the associated risk of gastric insufflation. Thus, although unproven, the administration of supplemental oxygen with propofol seems prudent, particularly when the patient's respiratory status can be monitored with capnography, in addition to pulse oximetry.

Sedation Management

Observe and monitor the patient until the peak effect of the initial sedative dose has been reached. If necessary, titrate with additional medications to the desired sedation level. Once the patient has achieved the target sedation level, the actual procedure may begin. If the patient begins to regain alertness before completion of the procedure, additional sedative doses may be required. However, additional sedative doses given to extend procedural sedation are associated with an increased risk of respiratory depression. As larger cumulative doses of the drug are given, the half-life of each bolus will increase. After the patient recovers from sedation, analgesics are administered as needed for patient comfort.

Pharmacologic Agents for Sedation

Pharmacologic agents for sedation are given in **Table 3.**

COMPLICATIONS

Reported rates of complication during procedural sedation in ED vary from 0.1% to 4%. Factors associated with an increased rate of complications include age more than 65 years, level of sedation, premedication with fentanyl, use of short-acting agents and procedural sedation and analgesia performed at night, when procedural sedation and analgesia could be administered by physicians with varying levels of training and experience and when consultant-level supervision is not always physically present.

Serious adverse events include the need for assisted ventilation, endotracheal intubation, or treatment of hypotension or cardiac dysrhythmias. Minor adverse events resolve spontaneously and include sedation to a deeper level than intended, transient hypoxia, or emesis. Complications can occur unexpectedly, so careful preparation, appropriate procedural monitoring, and careful selection of the target sedation level will minimize the rate of occurrence and severity of adverse events.

FOLLOW-UP AND PATIENT INSTRUCTIONS

At the completion of sedation and the procedure, patients should be monitored until they return to baseline mental status and cardiopulmonary function. A structured assessment, such as the Aldrete Score©, can be used to assess the patient's recovery and safety for discharge (**Table 4**).

Table 3: Pharmacologic agents for sedation.

Agent (references)	Role	Route	Initial dose—Adult Elderly	Repeat dose	Initial dose—Adult	Repeat dose	Initial onset time (min)	Peak effect time (min)
Propofol	Sedation/ Amnesia	IV	10–20 mg (given slowly)	10–20 mg (given slowly)	0.5–1.0 mg/kg	0.5 mg/kg every 3–5 mins	½–1	1–2
Midazolam	Sedation/ Amnesia	IV (over 1–2 mins)	0.5 mg	0.5 mg	1–2 mg (max single dose 2.5 mg)	After 2–5 mins	1–2	3–4
Ketamine	Sedation/ Amnesia/ Analgesia	IV (give over 30–60 secs)	10–30 mg		1 mg/kg	0.25–0.5 mg/kg every 5–10 mins	½–1	1–2
Ketamine	Sedation/ Amnesia/ Analgesia	IM			4–5 mg/kg	2–2.5 mg/kg every 5–10 mins	½–1	1–2
Ketamine	Analgesia (sub-dissociative)	IV			0.3 mg/kg		½–1	1–2
Fentanyl	Analgesia with other sedatives	IV			Up to 0.5 µg/kg	Up to 0.5 µg/kg every 2 mins	1–2	3–5
Fentanyl	Sedation/ Analgesia	IV			Up to 0.5 to 1 µg/kg	0.5–1.0 µg/kg every 2 mins	1–2	3–5
Ketofol (ketamine and propofol)	Sedation/ Amnesia/ Analgesia	IV			0.5 mg/kg–0.75 mg/kg of both agents		½–1	1–2

Contd...

Contd...

Agent (reference)	Role	Route	Age	Initial dose—Pediatric	Maximum dose	Repeat dose	Maximum dose	Initial onset time (min)	Peak effect time (min)
Propofol	Sedation Amnesia	IV	6 months–2 years	1 mg/kg–2 mg/kg*		0.5 mg/kg every 3–5 mins*	3 mg/kg*	½–1	1–2
			> 2 years	0.5–1.0 mg/kg*					
Midazolam	Sedation/Amnesia	IV	6 months–5 years	0.05–0.1 mg/kg	2 mg (single dose)	Up to 0.2 mg/kg after 2–5 mins	Total 6 mg		
			6–12 years	0.025–0.05 mg/kg	2 mg (single dose)	0.1 mg/kg	Total 10 mg	1–2	3–4
IM Ketamine	Sedation/Amnesia/Analgesia	IM	>3 months only	4–5 mg/kg		2–2.5 mg/kg IM after 5–10 mins		½–1	1–2
IV Ketamine	Sedation/Amnesia/Analgesia	IV (Over 30–60 secs)	>3 months only	1.5–2 mg/kg		0.5–1.0 mg/kg IV after 5–10 mins		½–1	1–2
Ketofol (ketamine and propofol)	Sedation/Amnesia/Analgesia	IV	>3 months only	0.5 mg/kg propofol and ketamine				½–1	1–2

(IM: intramuscular; IV: intravenous)
* Reduce dose significantly in patients who are debilitated or have decreased cardiac function.

Table 4: Aldrete Score*— For the safe discharge of the patient after procedural sedation.

Activity	Respiration	Circulation	Consciousness	Oxygen saturation
2: Moves all extremities voluntarily/on command	2: Breathes deeply and coughs freely	2: BP + 20 mm Hg of preanesthetic level	2: Fully awake	2: SpO_2 > 92% on room air
1: Moves 2 extremities	1: Dyspneic, shallow or limited breathing	1: BP + 20–50 mm Hg of preanesthetic levels	1: Arousable on calling	1: Supplemental O_2 required to maintain SpO_2 > 92%
0: Unable to move extremities	0: Apneic	0: BP + 50 mm Hg of preanesthetic levels	0: Not responding	0: SpO_2 < 92% with supplemental O_2

*A score of more than and equal to 9 is required for safe discharge after procedural sedation.

The duration of observation before discharge is variable. It depends on the quantity of sedatives given, the patient's response, the duration of the procedure, and the occurrence of any adverse events. Most adverse events occur during procedural sedation itself, typically within a few minutes of sedative administration. The occurrence of adverse events more than 5 minutes after completion of the procedure is rare (<1%). Patients should be instructed to return if they develop respiratory complaints or nausea or vomiting. The follow-up interval required for patients who undergo ED procedural sedation is usually related to the procedure rather than the sedation itself.

CHAPTER 75

Rabies Prophylaxis

Pooja Kataria, Seema Sharma

INTRODUCTION

"Rabies" has been derived from the Sanskrit word *"Rabhas"* which means "to do violence" or from Latin word *"Rebere,"* which means "to rave," meaning talking irrelevantly. Another name of rabies is hydrophobia. Rabies is a disease of carnivores and zoonotic diseases of warm blooded animals like dogs, cats, jackals, and wolves. Rabies is suspected in any human being by sudden onset neurological disorder, e.g. encephalitis which is characterized by hyperactivity, or paralysis and progressive to coma and death within 7 days of onset.

ETIOLOGY

Rabies is caused by Rhabdoviridae family virus which is ribonucleic acid (RNA) containing *Lyssavirus* type I virus. In the neurons, these viral particles are seen as inclusion bodies, called "Negri bodies" which is pathognomonic of rabies, but their absence does not rule out the disease. Virus is found in various body fluids like saliva, milk, urine, and lymph of rabid animals and in saliva (highly infectious), semen, sweat, and tears among affected persons. The cornea of human cases also constitutes an infective material.

HOST FACTORS

Main concern is that human being (warm blooded) is susceptible to rabies. Dogs are responsible for most of the cases in India. In few cases cats, jackals, and monkeys are also causing rabies.

MODE OF TRANSMISSION

Disease is transmitted by lick, scratch, or deep bite (saliva) by an infected animal. From the wild animals (sylvatic cycle) it is transmitted to domestic animals (urban cycle) and accidently to human beings. However, the disease is not transmitted from person-to-person as they do not have biting tendency and saliva also does not contain virus in optimum number. Man-to-man transmission is possible through corneal grafting as rabies antigen has been detected in the corneal cells of a case of hydrophobia. Virus never enters the circulation, so there is no hematogenous route of transmission. Route of entry of virus is via percutaneous route.

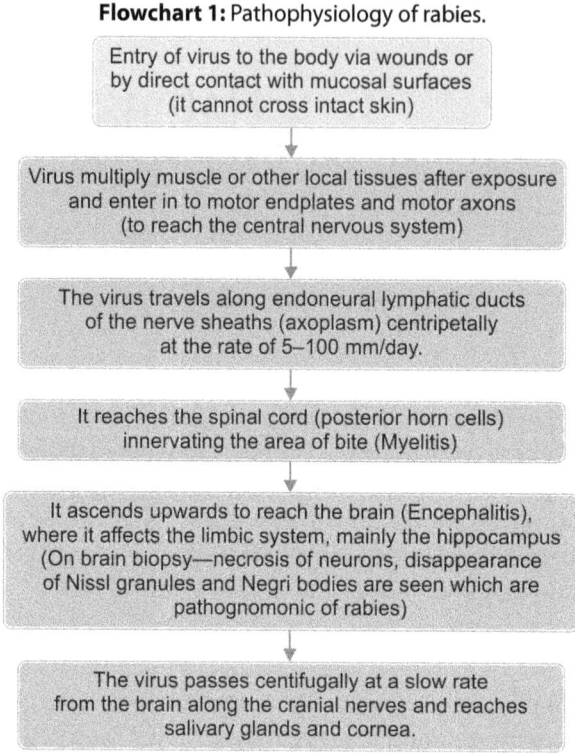

Flowchart 1: Pathophysiology of rabies.

Note: Throughout the passage of rabies virus (RABV) to the brain tissue, the virus never enters the circulation. Hence there is no production of antibodies or viremia. However, during its centrifugal passage from CNS to salivary glands, cornea and other organs antibodies are produced. Though the production of antibodies is too late, they are not beneficial.

PATHOPHYSIOLOGY

Pathophysiology of rabies is described in **Flowchart 1**.

CLINICAL FEATURES

Furious Rabies (80–90% Cases)

Stages of furious rabies along with their signs and symptoms are given in **Table 1**.

Paralytic Rabies (10–20% Cases)

- It is seen mostly in partially immunized individuals
- Gradual ascending paralysis
- Urinary retention and constipation
- Hydrophobia is usually absent
- Stupor, coma, and death (1-2 weeks).

Table 1: Signs and symptoms of furious rabies.

Stage		Signs and symptoms
A	Prodromal stage	• Tingling, numbness, and pain at the site of bite (first specific symptom due to virus replication in dorsal root ganglia and inflammation induced by cellular immunity. • Itching at the site of bite. • Headache, malaise, and fever.
B	Stage of excitement	Sensory system: • Aerophobia (fear of air) can be elicited by fanning a current of air across the face, which causes violent spasms of the pharyngeal and neck muscles. • Photophobia • Sensitive to sensory stimuli like touch, pain, cold, and hot.
		Motor system: • Increased tone and spasticity of muscles. • Exaggerated deep tendon reflexes.
		Sympathetic system: • Increased lacrimation • Increased salivation • Increased perspiration • Increased libido • Dilatation of pupils.
C	Stage of paralysis	• Paralysis of muscles of deglutition—an attempt to swallow food and water reflexly results in painful spasms. • Later, even the sight or sound of water results in severe painful spasms of the muscles of deglutition *"hydrophobia"* (pathognomonic).
D	Death	• Death is the rule in hydrophobia. • It occurs within 8–10 days.

LABORATORY DIAGNOSIS

Various samples and test can be used for diagnosis of rabies in human beings. Some of them are as follows:
- *Antigen detection*: By direct fluorescent antibody test; sample used are skin and hair follicle.
- *Ribonucleic acid detection*: By reverse transcriptase polymerase chain reaction; samples used are skin, hair follicle, saliva, and tears.
- *Virus isolation:* By rabies cell culture inoculation test and mouse inoculation (MI) test; samples used are saliva, tears, and cerebrospinal fluid (CSF).
- *Antibodies detection*: By indirect immunofluorescence and enzyme-linked immunosorbent assay (ELISA); sample used are serum and CSF.
- Postmortem detection of antigen, antibodies RNA detection, and virus isolation by various methods in brain tissue.

PREVENTION OF RABIES

Prevention of rabies can be done by two ways; first by vaccination of dogs so that human transmission is interrupted and second by vaccination of humans both pre- and postexposure.
- *Postexposure prophylaxis (PEP)*: Prevention of disease in an infected person
- *Pre-exposure immunization*: To prevent infection in healthy person.

Postexposure Prophylaxis

The World Health Organization (WHO) rabies exposure categories are listed in **Table 2**.

Steps involved in Management of Wound and Postexposure Prophylaxis
- Priorities should be given to all bite wounds and scratches. All bite wounds and scratches should be washed thoroughly with soap and plenty of water. Wash the wound with running water for 15 minutes.
- Rabies immunoglobulin (RIG) indicated for severe category III exposures. If suturing of wound is indicated it should be done only after RIG infiltration into the wound.
- After that rabies vaccination schedule is indicated.
- Vaccine can be given intradermal (ID) or intramuscular (IM), in deltoid area of the arm in adult and for aged less than 2 years the anterolateral area of the thigh is recommended.
- WHO-recommended IM PEP regimens are vaccine administration on days 0, 3, and 7 intramuscularly and the fourth dose between days 14 and 28.

Category III Exposures and where Rabies Immunoglobulin is indicated

After giving the first dose of vaccine as PEP administer RIG (passive immunization) as soon as possible (not beyond 7 days of first dose of vaccine). RIG neutralizes the virus within few hours at wound site there are two varieties of RIG; human RIG (hRIG) and equine RIG (eRIG) both have efficacy and later one is less costly. Nowadays, eRIG highly purified, skin testing before administration is unnecessary. WHO recommends—the maximum dose is 20 IU (hRIG) and 40 IU (eRIG) per kg body weight. There is no minimum dose. Calculated RIG should be infiltrated in maximum amount into and around wound, and not required to inject remaining dose as IM away from wound.

If RIG is not available, thorough, prompt wound washing, together with immediate administration of the first vaccine dose, followed by a complete course of rabies vaccine, is highly effective in preventing rabies.

Table 2: The World Health Organization (WHO) rabies exposure categories.

Category I	Touching or feeding animals and licks on intact skin
Category II	Nibbling of uncovered skin, minor scratches, or abrasions without bleeding
Category III	Single or multiple transdermal bites or scratches, contamination of mucous membrane or broken skin with saliva from animal licks, and exposure due to direct contact with bats

Note: Individuals with WHO category II or III exposures should receive postexposure prophylaxis (PEP) without delay.

PEP for Rabies-exposed Individuals who can Document Previous Pre-exposure Prophylaxis or PEP

- No indication for RIG
- Any one of the vaccination schedule can be applied as PEP regimens:
  - *On days 0 and 3*: 1-site ID vaccination
  - *On day 0 only*: 4-site ID vaccination (equally distributed on four areas left and right deltoids, thigh or suprascapular areas)
  - *On days 0 and 3*: 1-site IM vaccine administrations.
- Only wound treatment is required (no vaccine no RIG) if re-exposure within 3 months of completion of PEP).

Pre-exposure Prophylaxis

Pre-exposure prophylaxis (PrEP) is indicated in people who are at higher risk due to their occupation. The "at risk" groups are veterinarians, travel to rabies affected countries and areas, forest staff and hunters, zoo employees, slaughter house workers, taxidermists, dogs/animal handlers, laboratory personnel working with rabies virus (RABV), and pet owners.

Note

- Pre-exposure prophylaxis makes administration of RIG unnecessary after a bite.
- Rabies vaccination likely provides lifetime protection, with vaccine booster in case of an exposure.
- A routine PrEP booster or serology for neutralizing antibody titers would be recommended. PrEP regimens for individuals of all ages are on days 0 and 7 IM/ID vaccine administrations are recommended. But if person is immunodeficiency third dose should also be given on 21 or 28 days. A complete PEP course, including RIG, is indicated to immunocompromised individual after exposure even after PrEP.

CHAPTER 76

Rashes in Newborn and Infants

Nadeem Uddin Qureshi, Irene Oriaifo, Mohammed Moizuddin Qureshi, Rekha Gadiparthi

■ HIGH-YIELD FACTS

- *Nevus flammeus*, or *port-wine stain*, when present in the area innervated by the ophthalmic branch of the facial nerve, is associated with Sturge-Weber syndrome, a neurocutaneous disorder with vascular malformations of the brain and intractable seizures.
- Multiple or clustered capillary hemangiomas may be associated with deep tissue and parenchymal involvement, and further evaluation is necessary.
- Dermal melanoses, or *Mongolian spots*, are dark blue-gray patches of melanocytes located in the dermis. Mongolian spots should not be confused with bruising.
- Seborrheic dermatitis can be recognized clinically by the presence of greasy scales and erythematous plaques.
- Diaper dermatitis is usually caused by irritation of the skin from prolonged contact with feces and urine. Sparing of the skin folds is diagnostic.
- Atopic dermatitis is usually caused by dry skin, can be recognized by distribution.
- Candida skin or oral infections may be secondary to excessive use of oral antibiotics. Treatment includes antifungal agents such as nystatin, ketoconazole, or clotrimazole as well as consideration of probiotics and hygiene.
- Multiple café au lait spots of neurofibromatosis increase the risk for auditory and central nervous system (CNS) tumors.
- Vascular malformations in a "beard distribution" on the face are associated with airway hemangiomas.

■ TERMINOLOGY OF PRIMARY LESIONS

- Macules are nonpalpable lesions less than or equal to 1 cm.
- Patches are nonpalpable lesions greater than 1 cm.
- Papules are palpable lesions less than or equal to 5 mm.
- Plaques are palpable lesions greater than 5 mm.
- Nodules are palpable lesions greater than 5 mm in both width and depth.
- Telangiectasias are dilated superficial blood vessels.
- Vesicles are clear fluid-filled lesions less than or equal to 5 mm.
- Bullae are clear fluid-filled lesions greater than 5 mm.
- Pustules are pus-filled lesions less than or equal to 5 mm.

With the urgent need for adjustment to the extrauterine environment that the newborn faces, many different adaptive changes occur across all organ systems, including the skin. Skin lesions, or rashes, commonly occur, many of which are benign, but which usually are a cause of considerable concern for parents.

BENIGN NEONATAL SKIN LESIONS

Miliaria crystallina are lesions caused by obstruction of eccrine sweat gland ducts located high in the outer layer of epidermis. Multiple thin-walled vesicles form over head, neck, and upper trunk.

Miliaria rubra, or prickly heat, caused by sweat duct obstruction deeper in the epidermal or dermal layers. Erythematous small papules noted over face, neck, upper trunk. Common in infants and children during hot, humid weather (**Fig. 1**).

Neonatal acne is characterized by presence of open or closed comedones, papulopustules over cheeks and forehead. Thought to be due to placental transfer of maternal androgens, hyperactive neonatal adrenal glands or due to inflammatory response of skin to *Malassezia furfur* in severe cases. Treatment is not required as it is self-limiting; however, topical ketoconazole or hydrocortisone can be used in severe cases (**Fig. 2**).

Milia are tiny white-yellow discrete pearly papules, 1–2 mm, frequently occurring on the face and scalp. They are superficial inclusion cysts of the pilosebaceous units that contain laminated keratinized material of sebaceous origin. They are firm and unlike pustules are not easily denuded by pressure. Cause is unknown. The lesions resolve spontaneously and no treatment is necessary.

Transient pustular melanosis is a transient benign eruption seen in newborns at birth (**Fig. 3**). More common in black infants. Presents as pustules which rupture to form fine scales and hyperpigmented macules. May have all stages of lesions present anywhere on body but predominantly seen over forehead, neck, and lower back. A Wright stain of the contents will show a predominance of neutrophils, and absence of microorganisms.

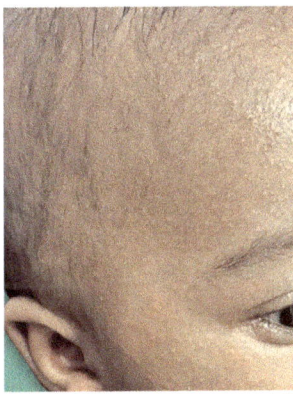

Fig. 1: Miliaria rubra.

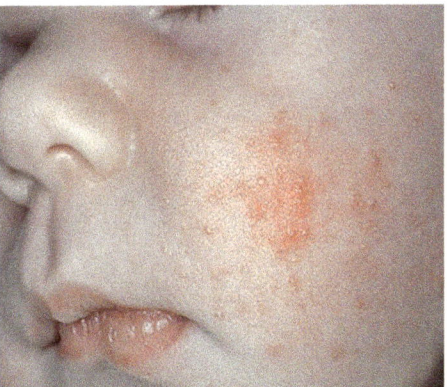

Fig. 2: Neonatal acne.

Infantile acropustulosis is a recurrent condition characterized by groups of pruritic vesiculopustular lesions on palms and soles (**Fig. 4**). Lesions can occur on the dorsa of the feet, hand, fingers, ankles, and forearms. Can present from birth to 2 months of age. Resolves spontaneously by 2–3 years of age. Cause is unknown. Lesions start as tiny, red papules which evolve into vesicles and then pustules. Lesions appear similar to scabies. High potency topical steroids and antihistamines may help relieve itching.

Erythema toxicum is a transient rash characterized by papules and pustules on an erythematous base. Usually evident within first 48 hours of life and resolves spontaneously in 1–2 weeks without any sequelae. It can present as clumps of lesions in different areas or more diffuse, except palms and soles. Cause of this condition is unknown, thought to be secondary to an inflammatory reaction to microbial colonization at birth. Wright staining of the lesion contents will show collections of eosinophils with absence of infectious organisms (**Fig. 5**).

Seborrheic dermatitis is common within the first 4 weeks of life. It is characterized by red scaling eruption predominantly over hair bearing areas and intertriginous areas like scalp, eyebrows. eyelashes, perinasal, postauricular areas, neck, axilla, and groin. Scalp lesions consist of thick tenacious, salmon-colored scaly dermatitis, commonly known as "cradle cap" (**Fig. 6**). Pathogenesis is unknown although *Pityrosporum* and *Candida* are implicated as causative agents. Seborrheic dermatitis is usually nonpruritic and responds well to low-potency

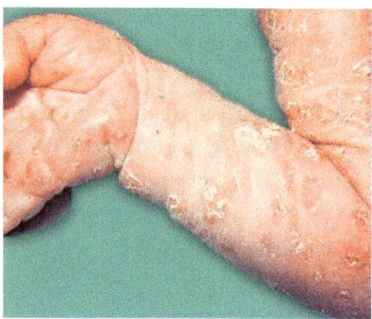

Fig. 3: Transient pustular melanosis.

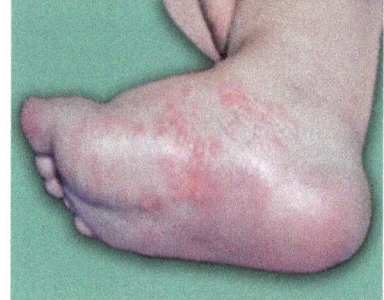

Fig. 4: Infantile acropustulosis.

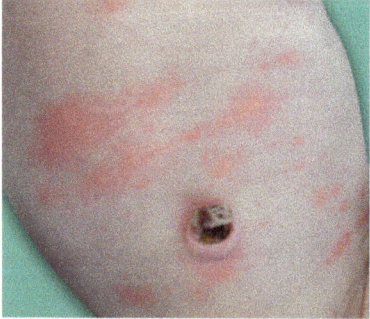

Fig. 5: Erythema toxicum.

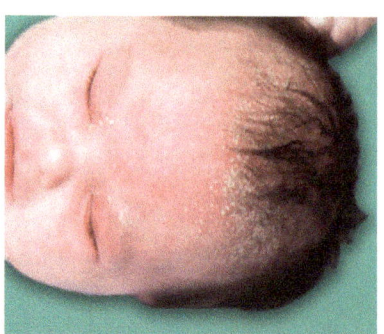

Fig. 6: Seborrheic dermatitis.

topical corticosteroids, topical antifungal cream. Antiseborrheic shampoo and oatmeal baths often help.

Oral candidiasis also known as oral thrush or moniliasis. It is a superficial mucous membrane infection more common in premature infants. It can be seen in immunocompromised children or in those with underlying systemic diseases. *Candida albicans* is the most common cause. It is characterized by soft, creamy white plaques seen on tongue, palate, and buccal mucosa. Scraping of these lesions is difficult, and this differentiates from milk deposits. Scraping of these lesions reveals erythematous base or punctate bleeding (**Fig. 7**). Oral thrush can be asymptomatic but can cause pain, fussiness, decreased feeding leading to dehydration and inadequate nutritional intake. Treatment includes topical application of nystatin over the affected sites. Recurrent infections can be treated with oral fluconazole for 10–14 days.

Diaper dermatitis encompasses all causes of skin irritation localized to the diaper area. Irritant dermatitis is the most common cause characterized by erythema, scaling, and excoriation sparing the intertriginous areas. Failure to change diapers frequently and prolonged skin contact with urine and feces or from soaps and chemicals present in the diaper contribute to the rash (**Fig. 8**). Absorbable disposable diapers have decreased the incidence of this problem. Secondary infection with *Candida* should be suspected when intertriginous areas are involved with the appearance of satellite lesions or diaper rash fails to respond to symptomatic treatment (**Fig. 9**). Candida skin or oral infections may also be secondary to excessive use of oral antibiotics. Treatment includes topical antifungal agents such as nystatin, ketoconazole, or clotrimazole as well as frequent change of diapers.

Drooling or spit-up rash is common in newborn and infancy. Erythematous rash seen on chin, cheeks, and neck creases (**Fig. 10**). Usually caused due to prolonged contact with food or stomach acid that has been spit up. This rash comes and goes. It can be prevented by rinsing the face with water after all feedings or spit ups.

Infantile Scabies

Scabies is highly contagious infestation caused by the mite *Acarus scabiei (Sarcoptes scabiei),* which burrows under the skin. The burrow which is produced by the female mite is

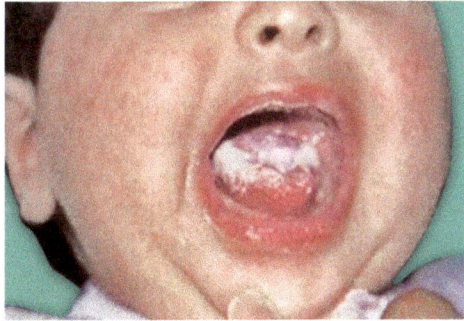

Fig. 7: Oral candidiasis.

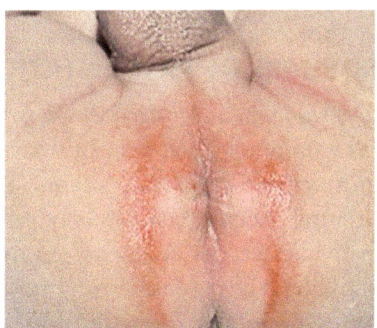

Fig. 8: Irritant diaper dermatitis.

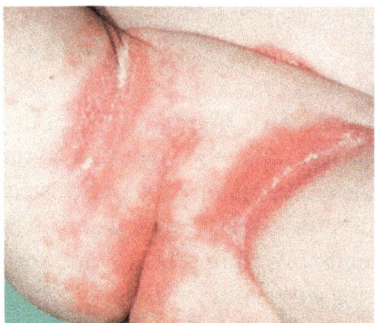
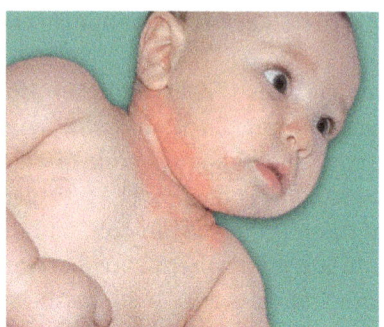

Fig. 9: Candidal diaper rash.   **Fig. 10:** Drool rash.

pathognomonic sign for scabies. It consists of small scaly linear papule with pinpoint vesicles at the end. Infants are more likely to develop an intense and persistent nodular reaction to the mite. Lesions are characterized by pruritic papules, pustules, and vesicles over the head, neck, trunk, palms, soles, lateral and instep portions of the feet, lateral aspect of wrist (**Figs. 11A to E**). Eradication of scabies requires topical application of 5% permethrin cream to the patient, all household members and close contacts. Thorough cleaning of all dirty clothing, towels, bedding, car seat covers is essential.

Two courses of treatment 1 week apart are necessary to kill the live mites and second to eliminate mites that had not hatched at the time of first application.

Infantile eczema also known as atopic dermatitis. Usually begins between birth and 6 months of age and lasts about 2–3 years. Erythematous itchy papules and plaques that ooze and crust can occur over the cheeks, forehead, scalp, trunk, and extensor surfaces of the extremities (**Fig. 12**). These patches are often symmetrical. Cause of atopic dermatitis remains elusive. Thought to be due to chronic elevation of immunoglobulin E (IgE) or aberrant cutaneous response to histamine and other mediators of inflammation. Atopic dermatitis can occur in families and in association with other atopic conditions like asthma, allergic rhinitis, and food allergies. Children with eczema should be closely monitored for secondary bacterial and viral infections. Treatment includes adequate hydration and lubrication of skin, antipruritic agents to break itch-scratch cycle, topical steroids to relieve itching, and reduce inflammation.

■ DISORDERS OF PIGMENTATION

Dermal melanosis, or *Mongolian spots*, single or multiple slate gray or bluish black irregular macules commonly seen over buttocks and lumbosacral area (**Fig. 13**). More common in African-American and Asian infants. These are due to accumulation of melanocytes deep within dermis. Usually self-resolve over years. Special variants of Mongolian spots, nevus of Ota (involving face, periocular area), nevus of Ito (involving shoulder) may persist. Mongolian spots should not be confused with bruising.

Neurofibromatosis is an autosomal dominant disorder characterized by multiple café au lait spots. Presence of six or more lesions measuring greater than 5 mm in an infant, the

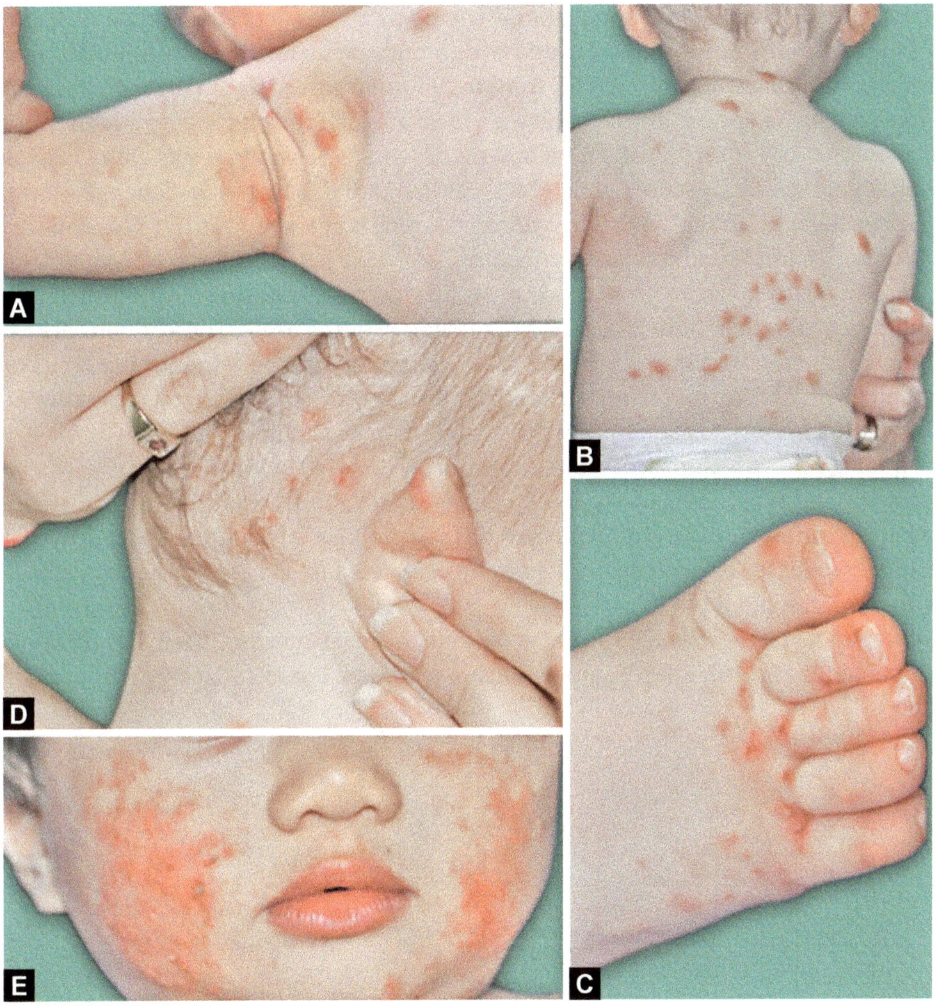

Figs. 11A to E: Infantile scabies.

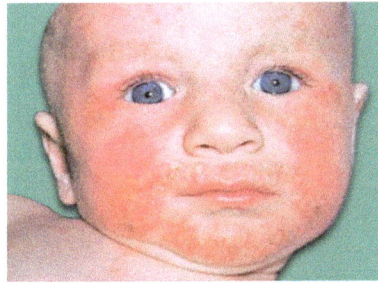

Fig. 12: Infantile eczema.

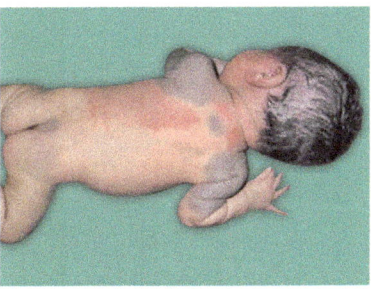

Fig. 13: Mongolian spot.

presence of axillary freckling, optic glioma, iris hamartomas, or Lisch nodule is diagnostic (**Fig. 14**). These disorders are associated with a high incidence of optic gliomas, acoustic neuromas, and a variety of other CNS tumors. Neurofibromas are small, rubbery, purplish lesions that usually appear during adolescence or pregnancy, but plexiform neurofibromas may be present at birth. The patient with neurofibromatosis who presents with headache or focal neurologic signs must be evaluated for an intracranial mass lesion. Other causes of café au lait spots include McCune-Albright syndrome, which is characterized by polyostotic fibrous dysplasia and multiple endocrine abnormalities.

Urticaria pigmentosa can present at birth or first few months of life. They are characterized by multiple small reddish-brown papules or plaques over the trunk. These lesions are caused by vascular effects of histamine released from infiltrating mast cells in the cutaneous tissue. Development of a wheal and flare reaction after firm stroking of the lesion is a positive Darier sign (**Fig. 15**). Lesions are usually self-limited and resolve in adolescence.

In infancy, these lesions can sometimes blister and widespread erosions can result in dehydration and sepsis. With temperature changes, metabolic insults, such as fever or viral illnesses, large numbers of degranulating lesions can produce flushing and systemic symptoms of histamine release. These patients should be counseled to avoid certain medications and iodinated contrast media.

Incontinentia pigmenti is an X-linked dominant disorder occurring in females and is usually present at birth (**Fig. 16**). It is a neurocutaneous syndrome characterized by four overlapping

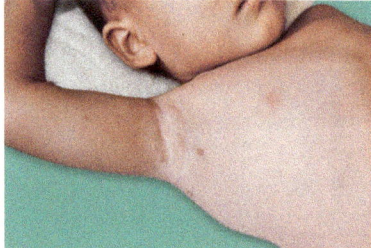

Fig. 14: Neurofibromatosis with axillary freckling (Crowe sign).

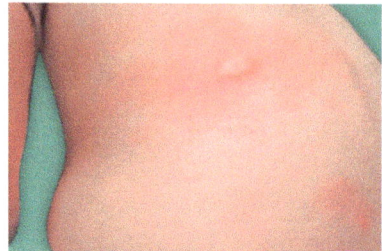

Fig. 15: Darier sign for urticaria pigmentosa.

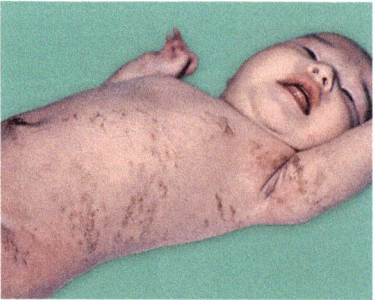

Fig. 16: Incontinentia pigmenti.

phases of skin presentation. The first stage usually within first 2 weeks of life manifested by inflammatory vesicles or bullae. The second stage presents usually before 6 months of age as the blisters evolve into warty plaques. As the plaques disappear, hyperpigmented whorls appear during stage 3. The final stage occurs later in adulthood with hypopigmentation and loss of hair and sweat glands. Approximately 30% of patients will have seizures, CNS abnormalities, and mental retardation.

VASCULAR LESIONS OF INFANCY

Cutis marmorata is a vascular phenomenon, characterized by reticulate reddish-blue mottling of the skin caused by transient vascular constriction and dilation. It occurs symmetrically over trunk and extremities (**Fig. 17**). It is a physiological response to cold temperature, and disappears on rewarming. When cutis marmorata is fixed, asymmetrical and does not disappear with rewarming consider vascular malformation called cutis marmorata telangiectatica congenita.

Harlequin color change is a benign transient color change, seen in approximately 10% of newborns. Usually presents as well-demarcated color change with dependent half displaying erythema and the other half appears pale. Thought to be due to temporary imbalance in the cutaneous blood vessel tone secondary to autonomic nervous system immaturity. It resolves spontaneously (**Fig. 18**).

Vascular malformations are common skin presentations at birth or in the first few months of life. They can be secondary to abnormalities of the capillary, venous, arterial, or lymphatic systems. Most are benign and self-limited, but a few may herald serious systemic consequences. The *salmon patch (nevus simplex or stork bite)* is a common capillary malformation may represent persistent fetal vessels, usually located on the forehead, upper eyelids, glabella, and posterior neck, and is present at birth. They become more apparent when baby cries or strains and usually resolve within 1-2 years, but if present on the back of the neck may persist for life.

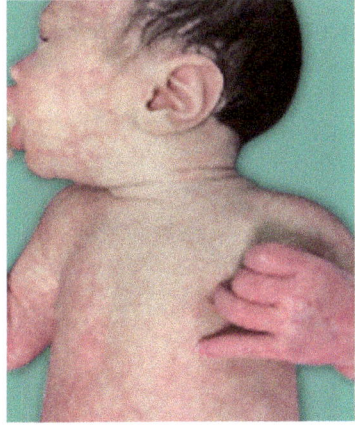

Fig. 17: Cutis marmorata.

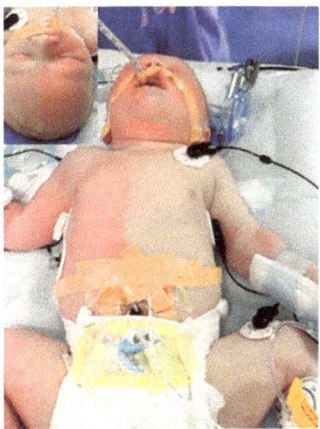

Fig. 18: Harlequin color change.

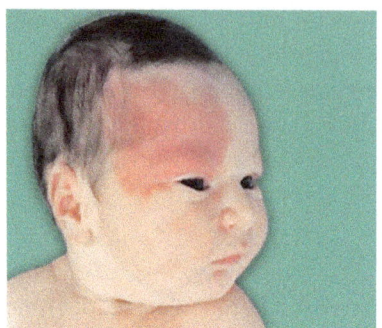 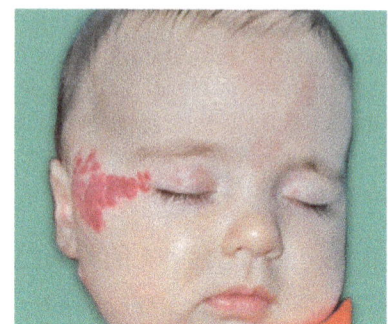

Fig. 19: Nevus flammeus.   **Fig. 20:** Strawberry hemangioma.

Nevus flammeus, or *port-wine stains*, are persistent vascular malformations of deep dermal capillaries and postcapillary venules. Mature capillaries infiltrate the deeper dermis and subcutaneous tissues causing purple-red macules in newborn. They neither enlarge nor regress but become more hyperpigmented as the child grows. Most common over head and neck, when present in the distribution of ophthalmic branch of trigeminal nerve can be associated with Sturge-Weber syndrome, a neurocutaneous disorder with vascular malformations of the brain and intractable seizures (**Fig. 19**).

Simple capillary hemangiomas are the most common vascular tumors in infancy. They are caused by proliferation of vascular endothelium and appear as small red telangiectasias that rapidly proliferate and protrude above skin to become the characteristic strawberry hemangiomas over the first year (**Fig. 20**), then become stable and involute by 5–9 years. Multiple or clustered capillary hemangiomas may be associated with deep tissue and parenchymal involvement, and further evaluation is necessary. Hemangiomas over the lower face, in an infant presenting with stridor or upper airway involvement suggest airway hemangiomas. Most of them will eventually involute; however, large lesions causing functional impairment may require steroids, and pulsed dye laser or surgery.

There are a number of hereditary and congenital conditions with vascular, hyper- and hypopigmented lesions, bulla, or ichthyotic scales that are beyond the scope of this text.

CHAPTER 77

Rib Fractures

Sandeep Jain

INTRODUCTION

Rib fractures are the most common injuries following blunt chest trauma in patients presenting to the emergency department (ED). It can present as single or multiple rib fractures; simple or flail fracture segment. Rib fractures themselves are not a life-threatening injury but can be an indirect indicator of an underlying thoracic or abdominal injury. Treatment is aimed at pain control, maintenance of oxygenation and pulmonary toileting. Most of these injuries can be managed by the Emergency Physicians themselves. Decision relating to discharge from ED or admission requires careful evaluation.

APPLIED ANATOMY

There is twelve pair of ribs. All ribs articulate with vertebral column posteriorly. Anteriorly only ribs 1-7 directly articulate with sternum (vertebrosternal) and thus are called true ribs. Ribs 8-10 articulate anteriorly with costal cartilage (vertebrocostal) and are called false ribs. 10 and 11 ribs do not attach anteriorly and are called floating ribs. Upper ribs 1-3 are protected by the bones of shoulder girdle with their muscular attachment providing a barrier to rib fractures.

CAUSES

- Majority of the rib fractures in adults are due to motor vehicle injuries.
- In older patients, falls are the primary causes of rib fractures.
- Assaults
- Recreational injury in contact sports such as football, rugby, etc.
- Pathological fractures due to metastasis from carcinoma of prostate, breast, and thyroid.

PATHOPHYSIOLOGY

Rib cage protects the underlying visceral structures due to its osseous content. Maintenance of its integrity is required for normal respiration. Following trauma ribs are commonly fractured at its weakest part—posterolateral angle. Fracture of multiple ribs indicates a higher energy transfer. Fracture of first rib is associated with higher mortality and morbidity due to higher energy required to cause fracture. It is usually associated with injury to underlying thoracic aorta or subclavian vessels. Lower rib fractures (9-11 ribs) have a higher incidence of associated liver or splenic injury. In children, due to pliable bones a higher energy is required to cause fracture, thereby indicating potential serious underlying visceral injury.

Rib fractures can impair ventilation and oxygenation by:
- Splinting of the chest wall due to severe pain associated with it causing atelectasis, pneumonia and respiratory insufficiency.
- Flail segment (fracture of two or more ribs at two or more places), leading to loss of skeletal integrity, impaired costovertebral and diaphragmatic excursions, causing ventilator insufficiency.
- Fractured segment causing laceration of the underlying lung parenchyma leading to pneumothorax and/or hemothorax.
- Associated lung contusions impairing oxygenation leading to hypoxemia and respiratory distress syndrome.

CLINICAL PRESENTATION

Following trauma patients may present with:
- Pain in chest especially with inspiration
- Difficulty in breathing
- Anxiety and agitation due to hypoxemia
- Cyanosis and somnolence are late signs of impending respiratory arrest
- Palpable crepitus.

RED FLAG SIGNS

- Severe breathing difficulty
- Hemodynamic compromise
- Cyanosis
- Altered mental state
- Flail chest
- Associated pneumothorax or hemothorax
- First rib fracture.

EVALUATION OF THE PATIENT

All patients of trauma are evaluated as per the Airway, Breathing, Circulation, Disability, Exposure (ABCDE) approach of advanced trauma life support (ATLS).
- History of trauma can be taken from the patient or the attendants. Details of scene at the site-deformed vehicle/steering wheel, deployment of airbags, can indicate rib fractures.
- On examination, contusions or abrasion over chest wall, tenderness and palpable crepitus suggests rib fractures.
- Deformity or paradoxical chest wall movement indicates flail chest. During inspiration, the flail segment is pulled in and pushed out during expiration leading to increased work of breathing and respiratory insufficiency.

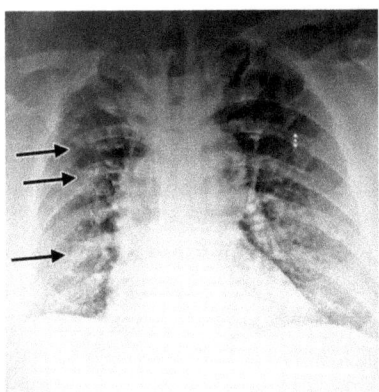

Fig. 1: Chest X-ray showing multiple right-sided rib fractures.

- Tachypnea, reduced air entry, low oxygen saturation, and subcutaneous emphysema are suggestive of underlying hemothorax or pneumothorax.

INVESTIGATIONS

- Anteroposterior view on chest X-ray is the first line of investigation. It is useful in diagnosing life-threatening condition such as pneumothorax or hemothorax (**Fig. 1**). Only 50% of the rib fractures are picked up on a routine chest X-ray. Presence of gas in subcutaneous space is highly suggestive of pneumothorax. Presence of widened mediastinum (>8 cm) is an indicator of blunt aortic arch injury.
- A plain computed tomography (CT) scan of chest is immensely useful in diagnosing rib fractures. Additionally it can pick up occult pneumothorax, hemothorax, and lung contusions. If widened mediastinum is suspected, a contrast-enhanced CT is advised.
- Bedside ultrasonography in hands of a trained Emergency Physician helps in diagnosing rib fractures and associated life-threatening visceral injuries.
- Bone scan is the preferred modality of investigation in suspected pathological fractures.
- In presence of tachypnea or hypoxia, a baseline arterial blood gas is advised.

MANAGEMENT

Treatment of rib fractures include:
- Prehospital care includes maintenance of airway and supplemental oxygen.
- Treatment of associated hemothorax/pneumothorax/aortic arch injury takes precedence over treatment of rib fracture itself.
- Adequate pain control is the mainstay of treatment of rib fractures. It prevents splinting of fractured segment, thus allowing the patient to maintain good ventilation. It also prevents atelectasis and subsequent pneumonia. Various modalities of pain control are recommended—oral/parenteral analgesics, intercostal or paravertebral nerve blocks and epidural analgesia.

- Single rib fractures in patients who can cough and clear secretions can be managed on outpatient basis with oral analgesics. More than 2 rib fractures need parenteral analgesics in the form of nonsteroidal anti-inflammatory drugs (NSAIDs) ± opioids. These patients need to be admitted for observation in the hospital. High-risk patients with isolated rib fracture, such as age older than 70 years, associated cardiac or lung disease should be admitted for observation.
- Incentive spirometry prevents atelectasis and allows pulmonary toileting and should be started early in the treatment.
- Judicious use of intravenous fluids avoids lung congestion and hypoxemia.
- Routine follow-up chest X-rays are not recommended in the absence of clinical findings such as decreased air entry or persistent pain.
- Surgical management includes open reduction and internal fixation (ORIF). This is usually done when thoracotomy is performed for other injuries, failure to maintain oxygenation and difficulty in weaning off the ventilator.

COMPLICATIONS

- *Hypoventilation and hypercarbia*: Pain associated with multiple rib fractures and splinting of chest wall segment leads to inadequate ventilation.

Flowchart 1: Summary of rib fracture evaluation and management.

```
Pain, tenderness, subcutaneous
emphysema, contusion in chest
     Difficulty in breathing
              │
              ▼
     Suspect fracture ribs
              │
              ▼
   Support airway, breathing,
   circulation-supplementary
   oxygen, intravenous fluids
              │
              ▼
Check for associated chest injuries—   Yes   Immediate surgeon reference for
pneumothorax/hemothorax/flail         ───►   management
      chest/lung contusion                   Intercostal drain insertion
              │                              Intravenous analgesics
              No
              ▼
     Intravenous analgesics         ───►    Isolated one/two rib
      Chest radiograph                      fractures with no other injury
              │                                       │
              ▼                                       ▼
   Multiple rib fractures, flail              Discharge from ED on
   chest, associated injuries                   oral analgesics
              │
              ▼
       Admit in hospital
```

- *Pneumonia*: Atelectasis due to inadequate coughing and pulmonary toileting leads to pooling of secretions and secondary bacterial infection.
- *Respiratory failure*: It can occur due to altered chest wall mechanics leading to increased work of breathing and fatigue. More commonly it occurs due to underlying lung contusion or pneumonia.
- *Associated injuries*: Underlying hemothorax, pneumothorax or lung contusion is the major cause of mortality and morbidity in patients with rib fractures and their treatment takes precedence.
- *Intra-abdominal injuries*: Injuries to abdominal organs such as liver, spleen, and kidney are associated with lower rib fractures.
- *Nonunion*: Small number of rib fractures does not unite leading to persistent pain.

SUMMARY

The summary of rib fracture evaluation and management are shown in **flowchart 1**.

CHAPTER 78

Scrotum (Acute)

Rakesh Khera, Prafull Mishra

INTRODUCTION

The acute scrotum is defined as "the constellation of new onset pain, swelling, and/or tenderness of the intrascrotal contents". Patients may describe the onset of symptoms as rapidly as occurring within minutes or up to 24-48 hours depending on the etiology. The acute scrotum is generally an umbrella term that includes a wide variety of unique disease processes. Rapid evaluation and investigations are necessary due to the time dependency of certain morbid but reversible conditions, such as acute testicular torsion.

Knowledge of the relevant anatomy (**Fig. 1**) is important to understand the differential diagnosis and subsequent steps in the evaluation. The testes are ovoid-shaped organs roughly 3-5 cm by 3 cm by 3 cm and vertically-oriented. The tunica albuginea covers them with continuous internal septations which acts as the structural support for the organ. This, in turn, is enveloped by the tunica vaginalis. Posterolateral to the testis is the epididymis, a curved structure roughly 6-7 cm in its longest dimension. The efferent ductules converge to form the ductus epididymis and eventually the vas deferens.

The vascular anatomy of the scrotal contents is also important to know. The testes receive a supply of blood from the testicular artery, deferential artery, and the cremasteric artery. Deferential artery and the cremasteric artery are branches of the inferior vesical and inferior epigastric artery, the testicular artery branches directly from the abdominal aorta. The testes are drained via small branching veins forming the pampiniform plexus and ultimately the testicular vein. The testicular vein drains directly into the inferior vena cava on the right while it drains into the left renal vein on left.

The vascular structures, vas deferens, and nerves are all encased within the spermatic cord, a conduit allowing passage from the peritoneum to the scrotum through the inguinal canal. The cremaster muscle is also found within the spermatic cord. The tunica vaginalis usually surrounds only part of the testis and epididymis and then attaches posteriorly to the scrotal wall. However, when the tunica vaginally surrounds the testis and part of the spermatic cord, the testicle is no longer fixed to the scrotal wall and able to twist freely. This is known as the bell-clapper deformity and has an incidence of up to 12%.

ETIOLOGY

The causative etiologies of an acute scrotum are broad and include those who are infectious, inflammatory, ischemic, traumatic or idiopathic. Given the nature of these, an acute scrotum

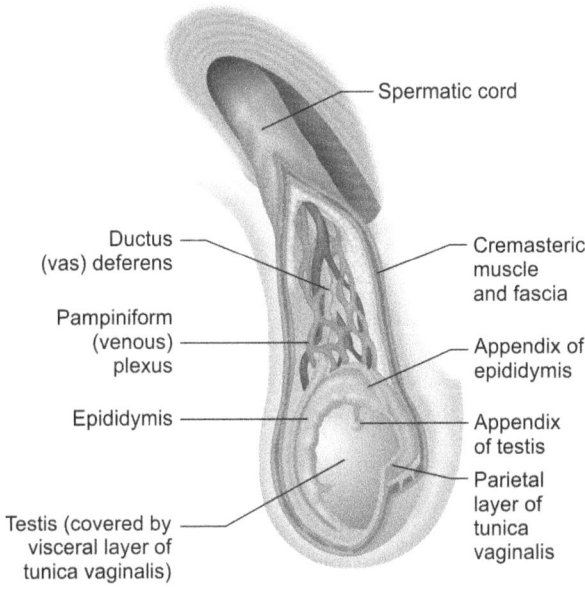

Fig. 1: Anatomy of the scrotum.

should be considered similar to patients presenting with an acute abdomen. By far the most common causes are epididymo-orchitis, spermatic cord torsion (commonly referred to as testicular torsion), varicoceles, testicular appendage torsion and inguinal hernias. The incidence and frequency of these etiologies are variable by age groups. Acute scrotal pain in children is much more likely to represent torsion of the spermatic cord or testicular appendages whereas patients older than 30 years are much more likely to have epididymitis. A complete differential diagnosis is discussed later.

EPIDEMIOLOGY

There is little data which specifically reports the incidence of the acute scrotum as a presenting complaint, but male genitourinary complaints are estimated at between 0.5% and 2.5% of all emergency department visits. The annual incidence of testicular torsion, however, is estimated 1 in 4,000. This means however that an estimated 1 in every 160 men will experience spermatic cord torsion within their first 25 years of life. Although it is possible to occur at any age, the incidence drops off dramatically in the adult years. Even among children, however, the most common cause of acute scrotal pain is torsion of the appendix testis rather than that of the spermatic cord.

Epididymitis is the most common cause of acute scrotal pain in adults. It is estimated that over 600,000 cases are diagnosed in the United States (US) emergency departments each year, and this condition was responsible for 1 out of every 144 outpatient visits for men between 18 years and 50 years of age. The condition tends to have a bimodal age incidence due to differing microbiological etiologies and risk factors.

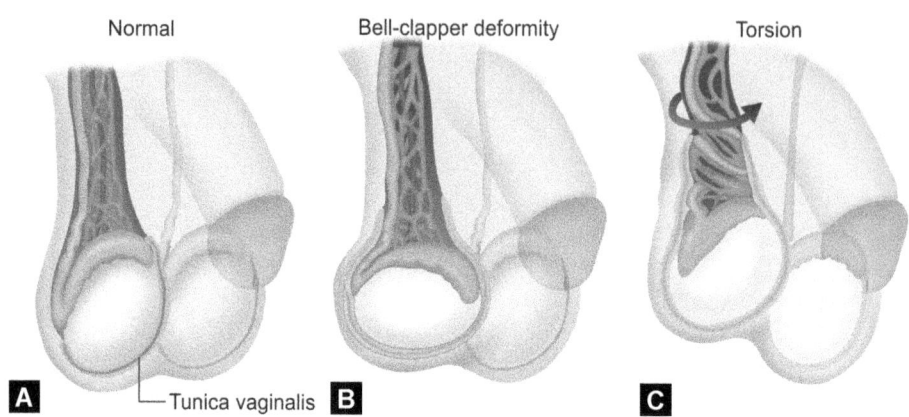

Figs. 2A to C: Pathophysiology of testicular torsion.

PATHOPHYSIOLOGY

Spermatic cord torsion may be intravaginal or extravaginal. Extravaginal torsion is seen almost exclusively in neonates and occurs to the increased mobility of the testicle before the descent into the scrotum when attached to the scrotal wall via the tunica vaginalis occurs. During intravaginal torsion, frequently associated with the bell-clapper deformity, the spermatic cord twists on itself ultimately pinching off arterial blood supply to the testicle leading to ischemia and infarction. The degree of torsion may be variable, usually causing venous occlusion and congestion first. Most cases of spermatic cord torsion leading to infarction are twisted at least 720° (**Figs. 2A to C**).

Epididymitis is a genitourinary tract infection which is usually due to continuous spread of infections from pathogens affecting the bladder of the urethra. In men less than 35 years old, this is most commonly associated with sexually transmitted organisms such as *Chlamydia trachomatis* and, less commonly, *Neisseria gonorrhoeae*. Men older than 35 years or those without sexual partners usually present with gram-negative urinary pathogens which are also responsible for cystitis and prostatitis, predominantly *Escherichia coli*. Other urinary pathogens such as *Klebsiella pneumoniae*, *Proteus mirabilis*, and *Ureaplasma urealyticum* may be seen. Rare organisms can occur such as cytomegalovirus, *Mycobacterium*, and other fungal causes may be seen in immunocompromised hosts such as those with human immunodeficiency virus (HIV).

DIAGNOSTIC EVALUATION

The diagnostic evaluation begins with proper history taking. History taking should include exact temporal course of events, the intensity of pain, and, in particular, when the pain started. If the patient is a small child, this history can only be obtained from parents. History should also include any new systemic symptoms or diseases already present particularly local problems, such as an inguinal hernia. Symptoms of hematologic disease and any newly arisen hematomata or petechiae, bleeding should be asked about specifically. On physical examination, the scrotum should be inspected, and a general physical examination should be performed. The involved testis should be palpated, and its position, size, and tenderness (if present) should be noted in scrotum and the abdomen is palpated, and the cremasteric reflex is tested. The Ger (is retraction of the scrotal skin that comparison to the other side) and Prehn (improvement of pain when the affected testicle is supported against gravity) signs are no longer relevant in everyday practice. The testis and epididymis should be evaluated separately.

History Taking in the Acute Scrotum
- Age
- Past medical history
- General symptoms
- Local symptom: pain, swelling?
- Pain: site? intensity? duration of onset?
- History of trauma
- Any prior surgery
- Nausea and vomiting
- Fever
- Dysuria
- Petechia, hematoma or bleeding.

Physical Examination of the Acute Scrotum
- Position, tenderness and orientation of the testes (Brunzel sign = secondary high position of a testis)
- Dimension of the testes
- Cremasteric reflexes
- Site of maximal tenderness
- Color of the overlying scrotum
- "Blue dot sign"
- Inguinal and abdominal examination.

Ultrasound and Scrotal Doppler

In recent years, ultrasonography (USG) has emerged as the excellent radiological study for diseases of the scrotum and testes, although there is no consensus on its reliability for the exclusion of testicular torsion. Some authors consider it reliable for this purpose as long as the ultrasonographic technique meets certain specified criteria. Two essential factors are the expertise of the radiologist performing the ultrasonographic study and the high quality of the USG apparatus used, which must have a 7-13 MHz linear transducer with Doppler and power-Doppler functions. Morphologically, an ultrasonographic study yields an estimate of testicular volume and an assessment of the echogenicity and any pathological features of the right and left testes in comparison to each other. For differential diagnosis, the study should include a search for an enlarged epididymis, a hydatid, a hematoma, or a tumor.

The USG evaluation of testicular perfusion includes both the arterial and the venous flow. The demonstration of central vessels in the testicular parenchyma is important, as perfusion may be preserved in the periphery and the outer coverings of the testis even in the presence of testicular torsion.

For accurate flow measurements in the testicular parenchyma, the wall filter and the pulse repetition frequency should be adapted to the flow velocity (1-5 cm/s). The wall filter permits a choice of especially low frequency ranges, so that low flow velocities can be measured. The pulse repetition frequency corresponds to the impulse-generator frequency and should be low for low flow velocities. The gain should be set optimally to keep artifacts to a minimum. The resistance index (RI) of the testicular vessels should be determined as well. An RI above 0.7 (mean: 0.43-0.75) with reversal of diastolic flow may indicate partial torsion. This cutoff value is appropriate from puberty onward; for prepubertal children, RI values up to 1.0 are considered normal (mean: 0.39-1.0). Diastolic flow and the venous flow curve may be hard to demonstrate in infants and small children. The examiner can also try to demonstrate the testicular vessels in the area of the funiculus. Here, the finding of a spiral course is highly sensitive (96%) for testicular torsion. A comparison of the two sides is obligatory. Aside from the performance of the individual tests mentioned, it is medicolegally very important for the findings and their interpretation to be thoroughly documented in the medical record.

Other Tests

Testicular perfusion could also be evaluated with magnetic resonance imaging or scintigraphy, but these tests are of little value for the diagnostic workup of the acute scrotum in routine clinical practice because they are time-consuming, expensive, and not available at all places.

There is no single test that can exclude testicular torsion. A reasonable blood profile to obtain in cases of suspected torsion consists of a complete blood count (with differential, if indicated). A urine routine and culture sensitivity test is needed to rule out urinary tract infection.

■ DIFFERENTIAL DIAGNOSIS OF THE ACUTE SCROTUM

The differential diagnosis of the acute scrotum (torsion, infection, trauma, systemic disease, and other causes) in childhood and adolescence has been shown in **Table 1**.

Table 1: Differential diagnosis of the acute scrotum in childhood and adolescence.

Torsion	Infection	Trauma	Systemic disease	Other causes
• Testicular torsion • Hydatid torsion	• Epididymitis • Orchitis	• Hematoma • Hematocele • Testicular rupture	• Henoch-Schönlein purpura • Lymphoma/leukemia	• Scrotal edema • Scrotal emphysema • Appendicitis • testicular tumor • incarcated inguinal hernia

Torsion

Testicular Torsion

Testicular torsion is a sudden rotation of a testis about its axis, resulting in twisting of the spermatic cord. The venous drainage of the testis is blocked and arterial perfusion is reduced, resulting in infarction of the testicular parenchyma. Following which perfusion of the testis reduces and rapidly is totally lost. Complete testicular torsion, by definition, involves a full 360° rotation. Irreversible damage of the testicular parenchyma can occur after 4 hours of ischemia. Studies have shown that only 50% of children who have had testicular ischemia for 4 hours or more go on to have normal sperm analysis in adulthood. The cause of testicular torsion is thought to be an abnormal degree of mobility of the suspension of the entire testis, or of the testis within its coverings, so that the testis rotates about its own axis during physical activity, or a suddenly occurring cremasteric reflex. Anatomical variants such as the bell-clapper anomaly, in which the gubernaculum, testis, and epididymis are not anchored as they normally are, predispose to testicular torsion. Supravaginal torsion (i.e. torsion occurring above the tunica vaginalis) is more common in infants, while intravaginal torsion of the spermatic cord is the usual occurrence in adolescence and is more common overall.

The pain is acute and severe and may be accompanied by nausea and vomiting; shock-like symptoms though may be present generally are rare. The involved testis is often fixed in position near the body, or else it may lie obliquely instead of vertically, because of shortening of the twisted spermatic cord. Absence of the cremasteric reflex is a sign of testicular torsion.

The morphological appearance of the testis on USG and Doppler study depends on the duration of testicular parenchymal ischemia. In the initial phase, there is usually a progressive increase in volume of the testis and a rather diffuse hypoechogenicity. Later on, inhomogeneities arise that are taken to represent irreversible testicular parenchymal damage. There is a lack of consensus in the literature about the reliability of Doppler USG for assessing testicular parenchymal perfusion. Overall, its sensitivity and specificity are generally estimated at 89–100%, though different publications on this question use different ultrasonographic criteria for establishing the diagnosis, so that the comparability of findings across studies is limited. The decisive criterion for adequate testicular perfusion is the unambiguous demonstration of central arterial and venous flow. The demonstration of an arterial flow signal alone cannot exclude partial torsion. Spectral analysis (triplex mode) should be performed, and the RI should be determined. The finding that the vessels of the spermatic cord are twisted into a spiral can be helpful in the differential diagnosis. A comparison with the contralateral testis is obligatory in every case. In complete testicular torsion, no central perfusion can be seen.

Whenever Doppler USG arouses suspicion of testicular torsion, emergency surgical exploration of the testis is indicated. The surgical approach can be either inguinal or scrotal. Infants nearly always have supravaginal torsion and should thus be operated on by an inguinal approach.

After detorsion of the vessels, the degree of ischemic damage of the testicular parenchyma should be assessed. Orchiectomy should be performed only if the testis is necrotic and gangrenous; in all other cases, the testis should be anchored to the scrotum with two sutures after derotation, the testis can later be reassessed ultrasonographically for reperfusion and potential secondary parenchymal changes. Contralateral orchiopexy is mandatory as well, because the second testis is also at increased risk of torsion.

Intermittent testicular torsion is a special case in which the initially severe acute pain rapidly improves. Doppler USG reveals a hyperperfused testis. The differential diagnosis must include orchitis, although the pain of orchitis is normally continuous. Perfusion must be reassessed with Doppler USG at close intervals, so that further episodes of torsion will not be missed and treated accordingly.

Neonatal Testicular Torsion

Neonatal testicular torsion is another special case. The testicular torsion often occurs before birth, making the diagnosis of torsion difficult. The percentage of severe testicular damage is 100%, according to some studies, although there have been reports of testicular preservation by direct surgical intervention. Accordingly, there are conflicting opinions about the need of intervention in neonatal testicular torsion, ranging from the view that this is an acute emergency demanding immediate testicular exploration all the way to diagnostic and therapeutic conservative management. USG can yield additional information about the current extent of testicular parenchymal damage. Doppler USG of the testis can be difficult to perform in a neonate. Whenever perfusion cannot be demonstrated with certainty, immediate exploration of the testis must be done. Marked atrophy of the parenchyma on USG may be an exceptional reason to consider delayed testicular exploration.

Pathophysiologically, the processes of ischemia and reperfusion lead to a cascade of immunological reactions in which leukocytes are activated and inflammatory cytokines [tumor necrosis factor-alpha (TNF-α) and interleukin-1β (IL-1β)] and adhesion molecules are released. N-acetylcysteine (NAC) has been found to have a protective effect on testicular tissue in animal models; thus, in the future, there may well be a form of drug therapy that will be given to patients with testicular torsion in addition to surgery.

Hydatid Torsion

In hydatid torsion, small appendages of the testis and epididymis undergo torsion and become ischemic. These appendages are embryologic remnants of the Müllerian and Wolffian ducts (appendix testicularis and appendix epididymidis). The clinical manifestations resemble those of testicular torsion. An important point for differential diagnosis is that the point of maximal tenderness is often directly above the testis, not on the testis. On transillumination, a bluish shimmering structure (the "blue dot sign") is often visible. USG often reveals a twisted hydatid as a hyper- or hypoechogenic structure between the testis and the epididymis, but demonstration of a hydatid alone is not diagnostic for torsion, as nontwisted hydatids can be seen as well. Doppler USG also often reveals accompanying hyperemia of the epididymis.

Hydatid torsion is generally treated conservatively, with bed rest, local cooling, and, in some cases, anti-inflammatory drugs. For severe and persistent symptoms, surgical removal of the hydatid can be considered in some cases not responding to conservative management.

Infection

Epididymitis and Orchitis

Epididymitis and orchitis are bacterial or viral or infections of the epididymis and testis. Bacterial infections are very rare in children, unlike in adults. The symptoms of both conditions generally arise more slowly than those of testicular torsion; unlike in testicular torsion, the testis is neither fixed nor in a higher position. The cremasteric reflex is usually preserved. There may be lower urinary tract symptoms (LUTS) indicating a concomitant urinary tract infection.

In these disease entities, scrotal USG reveals hyperemia with increased vascularity, along with enlargement of the epididymis or testis. Low RI values may be seen. Further findings may include thickening of the tunica albuginea or an accompanying secondary hydrocele.

Urinalysis is a part of the workup of these infectious conditions. In cases of recurrent infection, more diagnostic evaluation is indicated to exclude structural anomalies [the evaluation might include, USG kidney, ureter, and bladder (KUB), uroflowmetry, cystoscopy, and retrograde urethrogram (RGU), micturating cystourethrogram (MCU)].

Epididymitis and orchitis are managed conservatively. The need for antibiotic treatment in the absence of a demonstrated urinary tract infection is currently debated.

Trauma

Blunt trauma can cause a hematocele or swelling of the testis or scrotum. Ultrasonographic imaging is needed to rule out post-traumatic torsion or capsule rupture. The treatment is then decided upon individually in each case.

Systemic Disease

The acute scrotum as the initial manifestation of a systemic disease is a challenge for differential diagnosis. When the scrotum is involved in Henoch-Schönlein purpura, the epididymis and testis are often enlarged. Physical examination reveals the pathognomonic petechiae on the calves. Both leukemia and lymphoma also can present with scrotal involvement as their initial manifestation. In such cases, the ultrasonographic findings are generally not definitive, but laboratory tests reveal the diagnosis.

Other Diseases

Irreducible/incarcerated large inguinal hernia can cause testicular ischemia, sometimes presenting acutely. A swelling in the area of the inguinal canal points to the diagnosis. Here, too, USG is a useful in differential diagnosis along with the physical examination. If complete reposition is not possible, immediate surgery is indicated.

Acute idiopathic scrotal edema and emphysema is an entity in which the scrotum becomes swollen for unknown reasons. The testes are not involved. The marked swelling makes diagnosis by palpation impossible; the condition can only be diagnosed with ultrasonographic imaging.

Acute abdominal inflammation or infection (e.g., appendicitis) can also present with the clinical picture of an acute scrotum. In such cases, the physical examination, laboratory tests, and USG usually suffice to establish the diagnosis.

Testicular tumors are generally painless. Intratumoral hemorrhage can, however, present with an acute scrotum. USG reveals the tumor mass. Germ-cell tumor markers should be determined [alpha-fetoprotein, beta-human chorionic gonadotropin (β-HCG)].

SUMMARY

The acute scrotum is a medical emergency because any delay can bring about irreversible damage to the testicular parenchyma. The percentage of patients with an acute scrotum who need emergency scrotal exploration because of testicular torsion is probably less than 20%. It is, therefore, of vital importance to identify the patients who do not need surgery by use of the appropriate diagnostic procedures. The treatment is decided upon on the basis of the findings of the physical examination and Doppler USG, as soon as these have been performed. Whenever there are unequivocal findings in Doppler and physical examination, immediate scrotal exploration should be done. When in doubt, explore!

CHAPTER 79

Shoulder Dislocation

Praveen Saraogi

INTRODUCTION

Shoulder joint also known as glenohumeral joint. It is flexible ball-and-socket joint. It is most mobile joint of the body. Shoulder joint capsule is very loose, this allows the shoulder to dislocate easily. It is muscle-dependent joint as it lacks strong ligament. Primary stabilizers of the shoulder include the biceps brachii and tendons of rotator cuff which fuse to all side of the capsules except the inferior margin.

TYPES OF SHOULDER DISLOCATION

- *Anterior dislocation*: It is most common type of dislocation when head of humerus is displaced forward, toward the front of the body. It accounts for 95% cases in young people as it is sports related injury and in older people, it is usually by a fall on an outstretched arm.
- *Posterior dislocation*: The proximal end of the humerus is displaced toward the back. It accounts for 2–4% of all shoulder dislocations and is the type most likely to be related to seizures and electric shock.
- *Inferior dislocation*: Proximal end of the humerus is displaced inferior. It is the rarest and can be caused by various types of trauma in which the arm is pushed violently downward.

MECHANISM OF INJURY

Normal shoulder can become unstable (dislocated) as a result of trauma, shoulder can be dislocated by direct trauma such as blow directed at the proximal humerus. Indirect force is the most common cause of shoulder sprain, subluxation, or dislocation.

The combination of abduction, extension, and external rotation forces applied to arm can result in an anterior dislocation. Axial loading of the adducted internally rotated arm may produce a posterior dislocation.

In convulsive disorder, violent muscles contraction usually causes posterior dislocation.

SIGNS AND SYMPTOMS

Acutely dislocated shoulder is very painful. Humeral head may be palpable anteriorly, while posterior shoulder shows a hollow beneath the acromion. Attitude of arm is in slight abduction and external rotation. Because of frequent association of axillary nerve injury and, to a lesser extent, vascular injury, essential part of examination is neurovascular status of upper extremity.

Checking the skin sensation just above the deltoid insertion on the lateral shoulder is completely unreliable. Nerve injury is presented as a delayed recovery of active shoulder motion.

Asymmetry of shoulder contours can be visualized.

Recognition of posterior dislocation include:
- Limited external rotation of the shoulder
- Limited elevation of the arm
- Posterior prominence
- Flattening of anterior aspect of the shoulder
- Prominence of coracoid process.

This injury may be misdiagnosed as "frozen shoulder" for which vigorous physiotherapy may be mistakenly instituted.

RADIOLOGIC STUDIES

Anteroposterior X-ray View

Plain radiography with anteroposterior view (AP) is obtained. However, this is not true AP view of glenohumeral joint. To take true AP radiograph of the shoulder joint, X-ray must be perpendicular to the plane of scapula.

Lateral X-ray View

The view at right angle to the AP view in plane of scapula is the scapular lateral view. Presence of head compression fracture is demonstrated in axillary view and Stryker notch.

Computed Tomography

This scan is helpful in revealing the extent of fracture of the glenoid or humeral head compression fracture. CT offers a method for determination of size and location of glenoid rim defect.

NONOPERATIVE TREATMENT

Acute traumatic dislocation of the glenohumeral joint should be reduced as quickly and gently as possible. Early relocation promptly eliminates stretch and compression of neurovascular structure.

Kocher's Leverage Technique

In this maneuver, affected limb is flexed at elbow at 90°, arm is adducted against the body, slowly arm is externally rotated at 70°C, now lift the externally rotated arm in sagittal plane as far as possible and then internally rotate to bring patients hand toward the opposite shoulder. This brings head in position.

Milch Technique

Patient lies supine, surgeon stand on the same side and places his fingers over the affected shoulder. To steady the displaced humeral head, the thumb is braced against it. Next, the surgeon's other hand gently abduct and externally rotates the patients arm into an overhead position while fixing the humeral head so that it does not move from its dislocated position. Surgeon now gently pushes the humeral head back in to glenoid fossa with their thumb.

POST REDUCTION CARE

After reduction repeat AP and lateral radiograph to verify adequacy of reduction, check patient's neurological status.

Shoulder is immobilized by adhesive tapping for 2–5 weeks. Shorter period is indicated for patient older from 30 years, owing to their lower prediction for recurrence and greater tendency for should stiffness.

Position of immobilization should be one of the comfortable adductions and internal rotation, tight bandaging is not required.

After reduction of traumatic posterior dislocation of shoulder, shoulder is immobilized in a sling and swathe position. However, if the shoulder tends to subluxate in sling and swathe position, a shoulder spica (handshake cast) is applied.

SUMMARY

We conclude that the shoulder has a hierarchy of supporting mechanism. Minimal loads, such as gravitational pull on the arm, are resisted by passive mechanism such as the concavity of the joint surface provided by the glenoid and its labrum and adhesion cohesion of joint fluid. Larger loads are resisted by the action of the cuff muscles.

Finally, the ability of the shoulder to resist massive loads depends on the ligaments, the capsule, and bony support of the joint. Severe abduction and external rotation forces challenge the anteroinferior glenohumeral ligaments, if these ligaments do not hold, a subluxation or dislocation occurs.

CHAPTER 80

Skin Problems

Ramanjit Singh, Neha Dubey

ALLERGIC CONTACT DERMATITIS

■ INTRODUCTION

Allergic contact dermatitis (ACD) is an adverse allergic reaction, which is inflammatory in nature caused by contact with a specific exogenous allergen to which the patient has developed allergic sensitization earlier. The clinical response of the skin to the allergen is seen as eczematous inflammation of the skin.

■ ETIOPATHOGENESIS

Allergic contact dermatitis is a classic cell-mediated delayed-type hypersensitivity reaction. It results from exposure and sensitization of a genetically susceptible individual to an environmental allergen. This allergen upon re-exposure triggers an inflammatory reaction.

■ CLINICAL APPROACH

History
- Take medical and environmental exposure history
- History of use of topical agents
- History of use of personal care products (soap, shampoo, creams, deodorant, styling products, etc.)
- *Occupational history*: Occupations requiring frequent hand washing, chemical exposure, and use of gloves.

Clinical Features
- *Classic presentation*: Erythema, edema, papules and/or vesicles in the acute phase associated with pruritus
- Scaling, fissuring, and lichenification in chronic phase
- Pruritus is key symptom.

Commonly Implicated Allergens
- *Nickel*: A metal found in artificial jewelry, belt buckles, keys, eye glasses frames, etc.
- Fragrances
- Neomycin
- Formaldehyde
- *Bacitracin*: Topical antibiotic in general wound care
- *Paraphenylenediamine*: Used as a permanent hair dye.

INVESTIGATIONS
Patch Testing
The commercially available patch testing kit (Indian standard series) is optimal in situations where causative allergen cannot be ascertained clinically.

TREATMENT
- Identification and removal of inciting agent(s)
- Moderate to potent topical corticosteroids
- Antihistamines

STEVENS-JOHNSON SYNDROME

INTRODUCTION
Stevens-Johnson syndrome (SJS) is a life-threatening adverse mucocutaneous drug reaction characterized by necrosis and detachment of the epidermis that is of extensive nature. It can occur at any age, with an increasing incidence after the fourth decade and affects women more frequently.

ETIOPATHOGENESIS
- Drugs (**Table 1**)
- *Infections*: Mycoplasma pneumoniae, immunization, and viral diseases
- Post-bone marrow transplant
- Lupus erythematosus.
  In response to an inciting drug/causative agent, there is a cell-mediated cytotoxic reaction against keratinocytes which leads to massive apoptosis.

CLINICAL APPROACH
History
- After the first exposure, epidermal necrolysis usually begins within 8 weeks
- With a history of prior reaction it can begin within hours
- Fever, headache, malaise, and rhinitis 1-3 days prior to mucocutaneous lesions.

Table 1: Medications and risk of Stevens-Johnson syndrome.

High risk	Low risk
Allopurinol	Acetic acid nonsteroidal anti-inflammatory drugs (NSAIDs)
Carbamazepine	Aminopenicillins
Lamotrigine	Cyclines
Nevirapine	Cephalosporins
Oxicam NSAIDs	Quinolones
Phenytoin	Macrolides
Phenobarbital	
Phenylbutazone	
Sulfasalazine	
Sulfadiazine	
Thiacetazone	

Clinical Features

Cutaneous

- Initial lesions erythematous, dusky red, and purpuric macules
- Diffuse, extensive erythema sets in after confluence of necrotic lesions
- Initial eruptions are symmetrically distributed, involving face, trunk, and proximal limbs and these spread rapidly to become generalized
- They further evolve into flaccid blisters, which break easily leaving behind raw areas
- Patients can be classified into three categories based upon the extend of involvement of body surface area(BSA):
  1. *Stevens-Johnson syndrome*: Less than 10% of BSA involved
  2. *Stevens-Johnson syndrome/toxic epidermal necrolysis (TEN) overlap*: 10-30% BSA involved
  3. *Toxic epidermal necrolysis*: More than 30% BSA involved.

Mucous Membrane

- Seen in approximately 90% cases
- At least two sites are involved
- Can either precede or follow skin eruption
- Initial erythema is followed by painful erosions of ocular, oral or genital mucosa
- Leads to photophobia, conjunctivitis, dysphagia, and painful micturition
- The oral cavity and vermilion border of the lips show painful hemorrhagic erosions, coated with greyish white pseudomembranes and crusts on lips
- Severe forms result in cornel ulceration, anterior uveitis, purulent conjunctivitis, and synechiae formation between eyelids and conjunctiva.

General Symptoms
- High fever
- Pain
- Weakness
- Respiratory distress
- Proteinuria
- Hematuria
- Microalbuminuria.

MANAGEMENT
- *Diagnosis*:
  - Hemogram
  - Liver function test (LFT) and kidney function test (KFT)
  - Blood sugar
  - Blood culture
  - Electrolytes.

PROGNOSIS
- Prognostic scoring system for patients with Stevens-Johnson syndrome and epidermal toxic necrolysis (**Table 2 and 3**).

TREATMENT
- Withdrawal of offending drug(s)
- *Symptomatic treatment*:
  - Maintain hemodynamic equilibrium—fluid replacement, intake and output (I/O) charting
  - Ambient temperature maintained at 28–30°C
  - Use air fluidized bed

Table 2: Prognostic factors of Stevens-Johnson syndrome.

Prognostic factors	Points
Age > 40 years	1
Heart rate > 120 beats/min	1
Malignancy	1
BSA involved > 10%	1
Serum urea level > 10 mm	1
Serum bicarbonate levels > 20 mm	1
Serum glucose level > 14 mm	1

(BSA: body surface area)

Table 3: Prognostic scoring system for patients with epidermal necrolysis.

Scorten	Mortality rate (%)
0–1	3.2
2	12.1
3	35.8
4	58.3
5	90

- Barrier nursing
- Start antibiotics if clinical infection is suspected
- Nutritional support
- Daily ophthalmologic evaluation
- *Specific treatment*:
    - Systemic corticosteroids—although their use here is controversial, but they tend to prevent the rapid progression of the disease when used in the early phase
    - Intravenous immunoglobulins (Ig)—IgG in a dose of 0.5–1.0g/kg for 4–5 days
    - Cyclosporine A—an immunosuppressant, used in a dose of 3–5 mg/kg body weight in tapering doses over 14–30 days have proved beneficial
    - Plasmapheresis
    - Anti-tumor necrosis factor (TNF) agents

FOLLICULITIS

INTRODUCTION
Bacterial infection involving the hair follicle is known as folliculitis.

ETIOLOGY
- Coagulase positive Staphylococcus organism (commonest)
- Commensals of the skin (e.g. demodex, micrococcus, and pityrosporum) may become pathogenic in immunocompromised patient.
- *Klebsiella*, *Proteus*, and *Enterobacter* cause gram-negative folliculitis with long-term antibiotic use.

CLINICAL FEATURES
- *Superficial folliculitis*:
    - Acute superficial folliculitis
        - *Staphylococcus aureus* infects the follicular ostium

- Affecting mostly the scalp and extremities
- Follicular pustules with surrounding erythema
- Heal without scarring within 7–10 days
  - Chronic folliculitis of leg
    - Chronic, recurrent infection by *S. aureus*
    - Commonly in young adult males
    - Symmetrical follicular pustules on shins and sometimes thighs
- *Deep folliculitis*:
  - Sycosis barbae
    - Seen in young males
    - Erythematous follicular papule or pustule over beard region
  - Furuncle (boil)
    - Deep infection of hair follicle involving the perifollicular region, caused by *S. aureus*
    - Deep seated, tender, small, and inflammatory follicular nodules affecting the hair bearing areas
    - Associated with pain and fever
  - Carbuncle
    - Deep infection of a group of hair follicles with *S. aureus*
    - Coalescence of furuncles
    - Common in diabetics and immunocompromised
    - Tender, hard indurated swelling to start with, followed by pus discharge from multiple points after 7–10 days.

TREATMENT

- Appropriate topical and systemic antibiotics.

DIAPER DERMATITIS

INTRODUCTION

Diaper dermatitis or diaper rash is an acute inflammatory dermatosis occurring due to prolong use of diaper. It is one of the most common dermatosis reported in children.

ETIOPATHOGENESIS

The causes of diaper dermatitis are multifactorial.
- *Age*: Incidence is highest at 9–12 months of age
- *Diet*: Lower incidence has been reported in infants who are partially or totally breastfed. This is attributed to the difference in the intestinal microflora and urine components in these infants

- *Intestinal Candida albicans*: There is a direct correlation between the severity of diaper dermatitis and the presence of fecal *Candida*. It secondarily invades an already damaged skin
- *Contact between skin and excreta*: The incidence of diaper dermatitis increases with the increase in frequency of bowel movements
- *Type of diaper*: Disposable diapers with gel absorbent material are better and are associated with less chances of diaper rash.

Increased hydration of the skin due to prolong wearing of moist diapers increases the probability of skin surface damage because of friction. This in addition to a high skin pH of 6–7 creates an optimal environment for diaper dermatitis.

MANAGEMENT

- Frequent change of diapers
- Cleaning with warm water and allowing to dry after each diaper change
- Diaper free period for at least 30 minutes to 1 hour after every change
- Use of good quality disposable diapers
- Topical preparations containing zinc, Lassar's paste, and soft paraffin can be applied before putting a diaper on as it protects the skin
- Low potency nonfluorinated topical steroids(e.g. hydrocortisone) may be used to control inflammation and eczematization
- Topical and oral antibiotics are required in case of secondary bacterial infection.

ERYSIPELAS

INTRODUCTION

Erysipelas is an acute bacterial skin infection involving the upper dermis and superficial cutaneous lymphatics. It presents as a well-demarcated tender intensely erythematous indurated plaque and this helps in differentiating it from cellulitis.

ETIOPATHOGENESIS

- Primarily caused by streptococci
- Once inoculated into the skin from a potential portal of entry, the infection invades and spreads through the lymphatics.

CLINICAL APPROACH

- *History of*:
    - Recent trauma
    - Pharyngitis—in case of facial involvement
    - Prodromal symptoms—fever, chills, and malaise.

Clinical Features
- In 80% cases, lower extremities are involved and next common site is the face
- Begins as an erythematous patch, which progresses to a fiery red, indurated well-demarcated tender shiny plaque
- In some cases associated with lymphadenopathy
- Severe cases may present with vesicles and bullae.

MANAGEMENT
- *Diagnosis*:
  - Mostly clinical
  - Elevated erythrocyte sedimentation rate (ESR) and C-reactive protein (CRP).

TREATMENT
- Limb elevation
- Increase hydration
- Warm saline compresses twice a day for 10–15 minutes
- *Oral antibiotic therapy*:
  - Penicillins
  - First-generation cephalosporins.

CELLULITIS

INTRODUCTION
Cellulitis is an acute skin infection involving the subcutaneous tissue and commonly affects the lower extremities.

ETIOLOGY
- *S. aureus*
- Group A streptococci
- Hemophilus influenza type B—facial cellulitis in children
- May occur secondary to eczemas, trauma, burns, malnutrition, diabetes mellitus, and tinea pedis.

CLINICAL FEATURES
- Involved site shows erythema, induration and tenderness
- Associated with fever, malaise and lymphadenopathy

MANAGEMENT

- *Diagnosis*:
  - Clinical
  - In case of open wound with discharge a swab for culture sensitivity should be taken
  - Hemogram, ESR, and CRP

TREATMENT

- Foot end elevation
- Nonsteroidal anti-inflammatory drugs (NSAIDs)
- Penicillinase inhibitors
- Cephalosporins

LYMPHANGITIS

INTRODUCTION

Lymphangitis is defined as inflammation of a lymphatic channel secondary to an infection occurring at a distant site. It manifests as red streak on the skin extending proximally towards regional lymph nodes.

ETIOLOGY

- Group A beta hemolytic streptococci are the most common cause
- *S. aureus*
- *Pseudomonas* species
- *Wuchereria bancrofti*.

CLINICAL APPROACH

- *History of*:
  - Minor trauma to the skin at a site distal to the affected area
  - Fever, chills, malaise, and muscle aches.

Clinical Features

- Irregular erythematous tender streaks extend from primary site of infection towards the draining lymph nodes
- Primary site of infection may show a wound or abscess or area of cellulitis
- Associated lymph nodes are tender and swollen.

MANAGEMENT

- *Diagnosis*:
  - Clinical and based upon the history
  - Complete blood count (CBC) shows leukocytosis
  - Blood culture
  - Incision and drainage of abscess areas followed by culture and Gram staining.

TREATMENT

- Elevate and immobilize the affected area to reduce swelling and pain
- Appropriate oral antibiotics in patients who appear nontoxic
- Parenteral antibiotics in patients with signs of systemic illness.

FROSTBITE

INTRODUCTION

Localized damage to skin and tissues due to freezing by extreme cold environment is known as frostbite.

PATHOPHYSIOLOGY

- Characterized by four overlapping pathologic phases
- *Prefreeze*: A considerable decrease in blood flow as a result of skin cooling and vasoconstriction
- *Freeze thaw*: Ice crystals form intra- or extracellularly, causing protein and lipid derangement, cellular shifts of electrolytes, dehydration, cell membrane lysis, and death
- *Vascular stasis*: Vessels constrict and dilate or blood may leak from vessels
- *Ischemic phase*: The later phase is characterized by tissue ischemia and infarction.

RISK FACTORS

- Cold exposure
- Neuroleptic and sedative drugs
- Old age and immobility
- Diabetes, malnutrition, peripheral neuropathy, and cardiac disease
- Constricting clothing and footwear
- Exposed areas like nose, cheeks, toes, and fingers are frequently affected.

CLINICAL FEATURES

- First-degree injury is seen as erythema and mild edema.
- Second-degree injury—substantial edema and formation of clear blisters, which heal by forming an eschar.

- Third-degree injury—hemorrhagic blisters, blue-grey discoloration of the skin, thick gangrenous eschar formation, trophic ulceration, and severe cold sensitivity.
- Fourth-degree injury—muscle, bone, and tendons are involved.

TREATMENT
- Rapid rewarming is done by immersing the affected area in warm water for 15–20 minutes.
- If the wound is contaminated, tetanus prophylaxis and antibiotics might be required.
- Ibuprofen, thrombolytic therapy, heparin, vasodilators, and hyperbaric oxygen.

HERPES ZOSTER

INTRODUCTION
Herpes zoster, also known as shingles, occurs due to reactivation of varicella-zoster virus (VZV). Population at risk are adults above the age of 50 years, although it can occur at any age, especially in individuals with depressed cell mediated immunity.

ETIOPATHOGENESIS
The VZV causes a primary infection in children known as chicken pox. After the primary infection, the virus lies dormant in the dorsal root ganglion cells. There is formation of VZV specific memory T cells. Over a period of time this immunity declines and increases the risk of herpes zoster.

After reactivation, the virus reaches the designated dermatome causing neuronal damage on the way and forms vesicular rash.

CLINICAL APPROACH
History
Prodromal symptoms consisting of fever, malaise, itching, and paresthesias preceding the rash by few hours to several days.

Clinical Features
- Active phase sets in with the development of erythematous macules and papules progressing to form vesicles within 24 hours
- Progress to become pustules in a week
- Resolution phase results in formation of crust over the lesion within 14–21 days
- In the chronic phase there is postherpetic neuralgia
- *Herpes zoster ophthalmicus*: Vesicles are present over lid margins and sides and tip of the nose
- *Herpes zoster oticus*: Erythematous vesicular rash in the external auditory canal and pinna associated with vertigo, tinnitus, nausea, vomiting hearing loss, and severe otalgia.

MANAGEMENT
- *Diagnosis*:
  - Diagnosis is mostly clinical once the rash appears
  - For atypical cases—polymerase chain reaction (PCR), skin biopsy, and viral culture.

TREATMENT
Beneficial if started 72 hours within the onset of rash.
- *Antivirals*:
  - Acyclovir (800 mg thrice a day for 7 days)
  - Valaciclovir (1 gm thrice a day for 7 days)
- *Systemic corticosteroids*:
  - Recommended for conditions like Ramsay Hunt syndrome and ocular complications
  - Beneficial when combined with antivirals.

IMPETIGO

INTRODUCTION
It is a superficial infection of the skin that is highly communicable. It is generally seen in preschool aged children, although it can sometimes affect adults, especially playing close contact sports.

ETIOLOGY
- *S. aureus*
- *Streptococcus pyogenes*.

CLINICAL FEATURES
Clinical features of impetigo are described in **Table 4**.

TREATMENT
- Treat the *S. aureus* carrier sites to like the anterior nares with topical mupirocin to prevent recurrence.
- *Topical therapy*:
  - Mupirocin 2% ointment and fusidic acid 2% ointment three times a day for 10 days.
  - Silver sulfadiazine, retapamulin, and indolmycin.
- *Systemic therapy*:
  - Penicillinase inhibitors—gram-negative organism and polymicrobial infections.
  - Cephalosporins—effective against *S. aureus* and Streptococcus pyogenes and many other gram-positive organisms.

Table 4: Clinical features of bullous impetigo and nonbullous impetigo.

Clinical features	Bullous impetigo	Nonbullous impetigo
Causative organism	Staphylococcus aureus	Staphylococcus aureus/Streptococcus pyogenes
Age	Neonates and infants	Pre and primary school children
Clinically	Painless flaccid bullae with erosions and surrounding erythema	Small vesicle or pustule evolving into a honey colored crusted plaque
Extension	Extends peripherally with central clearing	Extends peripherally without central clearing
Complications	Cellulitis, pneumonia, and SSSS	Poststreptococcal glomerulonephritis

(SSSS: Staphylococcal scalded skin syndrome)

SCABIES

INTRODUCTION

Scabies is a contagious infestation of skin caused by a mite *Sarcoptes scabiei*. With an estimated 300 cases annually, it is the cause of significant global morbidity.

It generally affects people living in overcrowded conditions, although it can affect individual from any socioeconomic status. Other high risk population includes elderly, immunocompromised, and developmentally delayed individuals.

ETIOPATHOGENESIS

Scabies is the result of infestation with *Sarcoptes scabiei* mite. It is transmitted by direct skin to skin contact and fomite transmission (bed linen and clothes) is limited. Once in contact with the skin, the adult female mite burrows its way into the epidermis and lays eggs over several days. Within 2–4 days the larvae hatch and develop into adult mites within 10–14 days. Approximately 3 weeks after the first exposure, the affected individual develops a hypersensitivity reaction to the mite, its eggs and feces.

CLINICAL APPROACH

History

- History of recent travel
- History of nocturnal aggravation of pruritus
- History of similar complains in family members/room mate
- History of living in overcrowded conditions.

Clinical Features
- Generalized pruritus typically worse at night
- Classic presentation includes burrows, typically over finger web spaces, flexure aspect of wrist, elbows, axillae, breast, and genitals. In few cases they are difficult to find.
- Erythematous papules
- Norwegian scabies also known as crusted scabies is a rare form that results in hyperinfestation, inflammation, and hyperkeratosis. It is commonly seen in people suffering from malnutrition, immunodeficiency states like human immunodeficiency virus (HIV), leukemia, and T cell lymphoma.

DIAGNOSIS
- Diagnosed mostly on the basis of history and characteristic skin lesions at classical sites
- Presence of burrows, although seen infrequently
- Skin scrapping examined under microscope
- Burrow ink test (covering a lesion with ink and then removing it with alcohol leaves ink tracking on the burrow)
- Dermatoscopy.

TREATMENT
- In order to prevent reinfestation and transmission, it is important that all household contacts be treated simultaneously, even those without any symptoms (**Table 5**).

Table 5: Drugs and their applications used in the treatment of scabies.

Drug	Application	Age	Caution	Comments
Permethrin 5% cream	To be applied on whole body for 12–14 hours, preferably at night, preceded and followed by bathing. Repeat after 7 days	>3 months		First-line treatment
10% crotamiton lotion/cream	24 hours, may be repeated in 24 hours; wash off 48 hours after last application		Contact dermatitis	Second-line treatment
1% lindane cream	8–12 hours in adults; 6–8 hours in children, followed by a bath. Repeat after 7 days	To be used with caution in children	Ataxia, tremors, neurotoxicity, bone marrow suppression	Second-line treatment
Benzyl benzoate 28% in adults, 10–12.5% in children	Applied for 24 hours, can be repeated after 1 day gap			

Contd...

Contd...

Drug	Application	Age	Caution	Comments
Sulfur (8–10%) precipitated in petroleum jelly (compounded)	Daily for 3 consecutive days	Safe in pregnancy		Effective but not commonly used due to messy application and bad odor
Oral ivermectin adults—12 mg; children—6mg	Generally stat dose, may be repeated in 2 weeks	Safety not established in infants < 15 kg, pregnant or lactating women		

WARTS

INTRODUCTION

Infection of the keratinizing and nonkeratinizing epithelium with human papillomavirus (HPV), producing cutaneous, oral, and genital lesions is known as warts. Can occur in any age group, but particularly common in adults and those handling poultry, meat, and fish. They are also commonly seen in immunocompromised and those on immunosuppressives.

ETIOLOGY

- Common warts (verruca vulgaris)—mainly by HPV 2, other associated types are HPV 1, 4, 7, 27, and 57.
- Plantar warts—HPVs 1, 2, 4, 27, and 57.

Warts are mostly transmitted directly through skin-to-skin contact and autoinoculation. Transmission via clothing, swimming pool surfaces, and contaminated articles accounts for indirect transmission.

CLINICAL APPROACH

- *Common warts*:
    - Also known as verruca vulgaris
    - Present as skin colored dome shaped sessile papules, nodules with finger like projection
    - Solitary or in group sometimes leading to plaque formation
    - Commonly involved sites—hands, around nails, knees, and face
    - Usually asymptomatic, but painful when present over palmar aspect
    - New lesions can appear at sites of trauma.
- *Plantar warts*:
    - Initially appear as a shiny "sago-grain" like papules, and gradually enlarges to form a well demarcated lesion with a hyperkeratotic surface

- As opposed to corns and calluses, plantar warts do not interrupt the dermographic line, reveal bleeding points on pairing, and are more painful on lateral pressure (corns are more painful on direct pressure).

MANAGEMENT

- *Diagnosis*:
  - Clinical
  - Paring
  - Biopsy
- *Treatment*:
  - Topical therapy
    - Topical trichloroacetic acid (TCA) 50% applied under supervision twice a week until clearance
    - Salicylic acid (12–26%) with lactic acid as colloid ion
    - Tretinoin 0.05% cream at night
    - Formalin (37% formaldehyde in water) for plantar warts
    - Cantharidin 0.7%
  - Interventional therapy
    - Electrosurgery
    - Cryotherapy
    - CO_2 laser
    - Intralesional bleomycin
  - Systemic therapy
    - Oral zinc sulfate 10 mg/kg/day for 2 months
    - Oral cimetidine 30–40 mg/kg/day for 3–4 divided doses for 6 weeks.

TINEA CORPORIS

INTRODUCTION

It is defined as dermatophytosis (superficial fungal infection) of the glabrous skin, excluding the skin of palms, soles, and groin. It is highly prevalent in tropical and subtropical regions. Poor personal hygiene, malnutrition, and debilitating conditions like diabetes mellitus are some of the predisposing factors.

ETIOPATHOGENESIS

- *Trichophyton rubrum* (majorly)
- *Trichophyton mentagrophytes*
- *Microsporum canis*.

Aided by the moist and warm conditions, the causative organisms invade and reside in the stratum corneum.

After an incubation period of 1-3 weeks, it starts spreading centrifugally. The border is active and advancing whereas the center is clear.

CLINICAL FEATURES

- Characteristic morphology is an annular or polycyclic scaly lesion
- Erythematous advancing border with clear center
- Vesicles and pustules are commonly seen in inflammatory lesions.

MANAGEMENT

- Clinical
- KOH examination of skin scrapings for fungal elements.

TREATMENT

- *Topical antifungals*:
  - Miconazole 2% cream bid for 7-14 days
  - Sertaconazole 2% cream bid for 7-14 days
  - Clotrimazole 1% cream
  - Terbinafine 1% cream bid for 7 days
- *Oral antifungals*:
  - Fluconazole 150-300 mg od twice a week for 3-4 weeks
  - Itraconazole 200-400 mg od for a week
  - Terbinafine 250 mg od for 14 days.

TINEA CRURIS

INTRODUCTION

Dermatophyte infection involving the groins is known as tinea cruris. Predominantly affecting the males, it is also known as *jock's itch or dhobi's itch*. Fairly common in tropical areas, it is frequently associated with tinea pedis. Excessive sweating, high environmental temperature, wearing sweat absorbent athletic clothing, and constant mechanical irritation of the apposed skin surface in obese are some of the factors responsible for its recurrence.

ETIOLOGY

- *T. rubrum*
- *T. mentagrophytes*
- *Epidermophyton floccosum*.
  Transmission may occur both by direct contact and fomites.

CLINICAL FEATURES
- Characteristic lesion is a well demarcated, raised margin composed of papules and vesicles with a clear center
- Seen on the medial aspect of upper thighs and genitocrural region
- Bilateral
- Spread to involve the abdomen, buttocks and lower back, and perianal region
- Predominant feature is itching.

TREATMENT
- Same as in Tinea corporis.

TINEA PEDIS

INTRODUCTION
Also known as athlete's foot, it is the dermatophyte infection of the feet. It is believed to be the most common fungal infection in the world. It is more common in men and is being increasingly reported in children. More common in the summer months, especially in the tropical and semitropical countries, the incidence of this infection is more during the summer months.

ETIOPATHOGENESIS
- *T. rubrum*
- *T. mentagrophytes*
- *E. floccosum.*

Increased sweating washes off the lipids on skin surface that inhibit the growth of the fungus. Common site is the web space between the fourth and fifth toes. Some of the factors favoring the tinea pedis are as follows:
- Use of community pools or bath increases the chances of infection
- Use of occlusive footwear
- Immune deficiency states like diabetes mellitus and HIV
- Atopic dermatitis.

CLINICAL FEATURES
Clinical features of tinea pedis are described in **Table 6**.

MANAGEMENT
- *Diagnosis*:
  - KOH mount of scale

Table 6: Clinical variant and features of tinea pedis.

Clinical variant	Clinical features
Chronic intertriginous type	• Fissuring, scaling, and maceration in interdigital space • May spread to the soles or instep of foot
Chronic papulosquamous type	• Inflammation • Patch of moccasin like scaling over sole
Vesicular or vesiculobullous type	• Small vesicles or pustules • Scaling
Acute ulcerative type	• Maceration, denudation, and ulceration • White hyperkeratosis • Pungent odor

- *Treatment*:
    - Avoid known predisposing factors
    - Maintain a dry environment on the feet
    - Shoes to be air dried regularly
    - In the presence of severe infection with the presence of secondary bacterial infection a systemic antibiotic has to be added
    - Topical and oral antifungal treatment remains the same as mentioned earlier
    - In presence of vesicles, adjunctive treatment with Burrow's solution compresses is given.

URTICARIA

INTRODUCTION

Urticaria is a cutaneous disorder characterized by the presence of transient, pruritic, erythematous, and slightly edematous plaques. May presents with wheals, angioedema or both. It is a worldwide disease, in the general population ranges from 1% to 5%. It is more common in women and female:male ratio of approximately 2:1 for chronic urticaria. But ratio varies with different physical urticarias—dermographism occurs more in women and delayed pressure urticaria is more common in men.

CLASSIFICATION

- *Ordinary spontaneous urticaria*:
    - Acute urticaria
    - Chronic urticaria
    - Contact urticaria
- *Physical urticaria*:
    - Dermatographism
    - Delayed pressure urticaria

- Vibratory angioedema
- Cholinergic urticaria
- Exercise induced urticaria
- Solar urticaria
- Heat urticaria
- Cold urticaria
- Aquagenic urticaria
- Adrenergic urticarial

CAUSES OF URTICARIA

Causes of urticaria are shown in **Table 7**.

CLINICAL FEATURES

- Itchy erythematous macules develop into wheals consisting of pale to pink, edematous, and raised areas of skin with a surrounding red flare.
- *Sites*: Anywhere on the body including scalp, palms, and soles, variable in numbers and size.
- Urticaria can be differentiated in to 2 group, acute and chronic urticaria (**Table 8**).

PHYSICAL URTICARIA

- Characterized by the development of wheals and pruritus promptly after application of the appropriate physical stimulus.

Table 7: Causes of urticaria.

Immunologic	Physical

• IgE mediated
  – Food
  – Drugs
  – Aeroallergens
  – Insect venom
• Complement mediated
  – Transfusions
  – Systemic disorders
  – Vasculitis
  – Paraneoplastic
	• Dermographism
	• Heat urticaria
	• Cold urticaria
	• UV-induced
	• Pressure induced
	• Aquagenic
	• Vibratory

Infections	**Hereditary disorder**
• Bacterial, viral, and parasitic	• Hereditary angioneurotic edema • CI deficiency • Hereditary cold urticaria
Nonimmunologic factors	**Chronic idiopathic urticaria**
• Alcohol and DAO deficiency	

(CI: complex I; IgE: immunoglobulin E; UV: ultraviolet; DAO: diamine Oxidase)

Table 8: Types of acute urticaria and chronic urticaria.

Type	Acute urticaria	Chronic urticaria
Time of onset	<6 week	>6 week
Causes	Immunological reactions to medications, foods, contact allergens, insect venoms, viral infections, and idiopathic	Idiopathic, autoimmune, drug-induced, complement-mediated, secondary to a systemic disorder, and rarely caused by foods, etc.
Natural history	Typically self-limited	Chronic with episodic exacerbations

- Wheals typically fade within 30-60 minutes.
- In delayed pressure urticaria wheals lasts for several hours, may be up to 48 hours.

URTICARIAL VASCULITIS
- Clinically indistinguishable from that of chronic urticaria.
- In contrast to chronic urticaria, lesions of urticarial vasculitis last for longer than 24 hours.
- Associated with burning and pain in addition to itching.

INVESTIGATIONS
- *Acute urticaria*:
    - Complete blood count with differential, ESR, LFT, and urinalysis
    - The history and physical examination provides clue to additional tests—hepatitis A, B, and C; infectious mononucleosis; thyroid antibodies; thyroid function tests; and antinuclear antibodies
    - Skin tests
    - Radioallergosorbent test (RAST)
    - Food testing
    - Oral challenge tests
    - Serum IgE
- *Chronic urticaria*:
    - Complete blood count with differential count
    - Stool for ova and parasites
    - ESR, CRP, antinuclear antibody (ANA), rheumatoid factor (RF) testing (for rheumatologic disorder)
    - Hepatitis B and C
    - Serum cryoglobulins and complement assays
    - Thyroid profile and thyroid antibodies
    - Autologous serum skin test (ASST)
    - C4 and C1—esterase assays

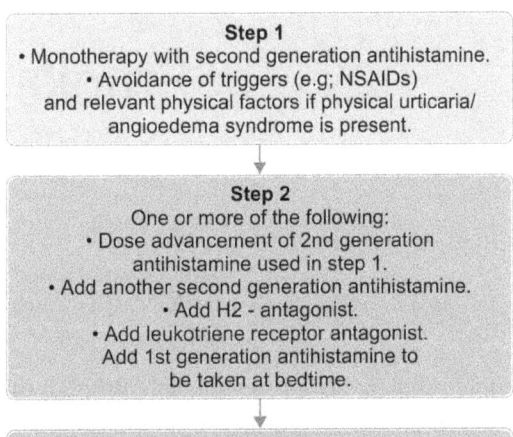

Flowchart 1: Treatment of urticaria.

Step 1
- Monotherapy with second generation antihistamine.
- Avoidance of triggers (e.g; NSAIDs) and relevant physical factors if physical urticaria/angioedema syndrome is present.

Step 2
One or more of the following:
- Dose advancement of 2nd generation antihistamine used in step 1.
- Add another second generation antihistamine.
- Add H2 - antagonist.
- Add leukotriene receptor antagonist.
Add 1st generation antihistamine to be taken at bedtime.

Step 3
- Dose advancement of potent antihistamine (e.g; hydroxyzine or doxepin) as tolerated

Step 4
Add an alternative agent:
- Other anti-inflammatory agents, immunosuppresants. Omalizumab or cyclosporine.

(NSAIDs: nonsteroidal anti-inflammatory drugs)

- *Contact urticaria*:
  – Prick test
  – Scratch test
  – Radioallergosorbent test
- *Physical urticaria*:
  – By stroking the skin—dermographism
  – Provocation test—cholinergic urticaria
  – Ice cube test—for cold urticaria
  – Phototesting—solar urticaria
  – Application of heated cylinder—heat urticaria
  – Inducing wheals after bath or shower—aquagenic urticaria
- *Urticarial vasculitis*:
  – Complete blood count, ESR, blood urea nitrogen (BUN), creatinine, ANA, anti-deoxyribonucleic acid (DNA), anti-Smith (anti-Sm), complement assay, anti-C1q antibodies, cryoglobulins, Schirmer's test, and pulmonary function tests
  – Skin biopsy
  – Direct immunofluorescence.

TREATMENT

Treatment of urticaria has been described in various steps as is shown in **Flowchart 1.**

CHAPTER 81

Smoke Inhalation

Eric Revue

INTRODUCTION

Inhalation of smoke, frequent during fires, is responsible for high initial mortality related to the systemic effects of two asphyxiant components found in inhaled gases: carbon monoxide (CO) and cyanide (CN).

Inhalation of fire smoke is a complex that combines a gas phase, a soot phase and water vapor.

The anoxic attack is linked to an oxygen deprivation (decrease in the partial pressure of oxygen), and of the toxic pulmonary and systemic action of asphyxiating gases. Hemoglobin is loaded into CO decreasing the amount of hemoglobin available for the transport of oxygen, and the toxicity of CN prohibits the cellular use of oxygen contributes to hypoxia.

Respiratory lesion induced by inhalation of fumes is a negative prognostic factor significantly aggravates morbidity/mortality in the presence of skin burns.

Management of victims of inhalation of fire fumes requires a rigorous diagnostic procedure to detect and start an urgent treatment on the scene.

During the past 50 years, synthetic polymers contain nitrogen or halogens, have been introduced in buildings. Resulting in the release of hydrogen cyanide (HCN) and inorganic acids in fire smoke but CO is still the major toxicant.

For example, the first 48 hours after the 9/11 World Trade Center (WTC) attack in New York in 2001, 50% of victims had inhalation lesions and two-thirds of patients who had skin burns.

Mortality ranges from 20% to 80% depending on authors. In 77% of cases, deaths are, in these patients, secondary to respiratory failure.

ASPHYXIATING GASES

They are products of degradation of polysulfones and other polymers—sulfur.

The main lethal agents are:
- Cyanide
- Carbon monoxide
- Carbon dioxide (CO_2)
- Hydrogen sulfide (H_2S)
- Sulfur dioxide (SO_2).

These gases are depressants of the central nervous system and are responsible of hyperventilation, which increases the absorption and distribution of all toxic dissolved in the blood.

IRRITATING GASES

These gases are:
- Volatile organic components (benzene, nitromethane, ethyl acetate)
- Aldehydes, carbon components (acrolein, formaldehyde, butyraldehyde) from plant degradation (wood, cotton, papers)
- Chlorine derivatives (hydrochloric acid, hydrofluoric acid, hydrobromic acid and carbon oxyhalides) from the degradation of materials containing chlorine (polyvinyl chloride or PVC)
- Nitrogen derivatives (nitrogen monoxide, ammonia, isocyanates, amines) from polymer degradation of nitrogen and polyurethanes.

Benzene is depressor of the central nervous system. Patients may complain of headache, nausea, drowsiness, dizziness, or coma. Acute exposure (5-10 minutes) at a high concentration (about 20,000 ppm) can cause death, attributed to respiratory arrest, central nervous system depression or cardiovascular collapse.
- Nitromethane causes methemoglobinemia, a hemolysis, acute renal failure, acute respiratory distress syndrome (ARDS)
- Ethyl acetate causes irritation of mucous membranes, neurological symptoms, convulsions and coma
- Aldehydes (formaldehyde, butyraldehyde) are 5-50 times more toxic than acid hydrochloric acid, and are responsible for eye irritation and high pulmonary toxicity
- Chlorine derivatives (hydrochloric acid, hydrofluoric acid, hydrobromic acid, and carbon oxyhalides) are very irritating for the eye and the upper airways. All these derivatives have a marked toxicity for the lungs and sometimes systemic toxicity.

TOXICITY OF FIRE SMOKE

The mechanism of toxicity of fire fumes is twofold, pulmonary and systemic.

Pulmonary toxicity is linked to a triple effect: thermal, chemical and mechanical.

Inhalation of fire smokes exposes three main risks: superior *airway burns* (oral cavity, oropharynx and larynx); *physical obstruction* by divisional particles bronchial and pulmonary parenchyma (associated with inflammatory mucosal reaction) altering gas exchange.

By able to reach high temperatures, smoke is responsible of burns of the tracheobronchial tree, mainly through liquid droplets but also by the irritating gases and the soaked, burning soot.

Particle size determines their level penetration into the bronchoalveolar tree. They penetrate even further into the tracheobronchial tree than their diameter is small. They then cause a mechanical obstruction.

Deposition of soot on the mucous membranes can induce chemical burns.

The exact number and nature of the components present in the smoke are generally unknown, as are their respective toxicity. So while a victim of a smoke inhalation fire has been exposed to multiple toxic components, two toxic, CO and CN, intervene in urgent antidote therapeutic.

Soot deposits on the face, nasal and oral cavities and on the tracheobronchial tree account for penetration fumes and the risk of systemic toxicity of CN.

In addition to these asphyxiating gases, the irritating gases may have clinical expression of their essentially systemic toxicity:

Systemic toxicity of inhaled gases: The symptoms include hyperpnea, due to direct stimulation of the chemoreceptors of the carotid and aortic bodies by CN. CN also stimulates the nociceptors, leading to a brief sensation of dryness and burning in the nose and throat. In milder cases of CN poisoning, the symptoms are headache, nausea, vertigo, anxiety, altered mental status, tachypnea, and hypertension and there may be an odor of bitter almonds in the patient's expiration. In more severe cases, the patient will have dyspnea, bradycardia, hypotension and arrhythmia. In most severe cases, symptoms are unconsciousness, convulsions, cardiovascular collapse followed by shock, pulmonary edema and death due to respiratory arrest 3-4 minutes after the last gasp.

CARBON MONOXIDE POISONING

Carbon monoxide is an odorless and colorless gas resulting from incomplete combustion of components containing carbon. After inhalation, CO diffuses rapidly through the alveolocapillary membrane, dissolves in the plasma, enters the red blood cells where it links to hemoglobin to carboxyhemoglobin (HbCO) form, unfit for oxygen transport and responsible for tissue hypoxia. CO has 200 times higher affinity than oxygen for hemoglobin. A gas containing 0.1% of CO can result in the formation of 50% HbCO.

For situations of pregnant women, the passive passage of CO between mother and fetus is increased by the HbCO pressure gradient.

The affinity of CO for fetal hemoglobin is still 2.5 times greater than that for maternal hemoglobin. Reaching fetus appears correlated with the importance and severity of symptoms maternal. Fetal HbCO concentration increases more slowly in the fetus than in the mother.

In addition, the half-life of HbCO in the fetus is longer than in the mother (7 hours vs 4 hours).

Clinical Presentation

In case of fire, any patient who has been burned or has inhaled fumes disorders of consciousness is suspected of intoxication of CO. Nonspecific symptoms may appear headache, nausea, vomiting, confusion, disorientation, visual disturbances.

In severe intoxications, patients may present: a polypnea, a tachycardia, seizure, and coma. Cardiovascular disorders have been described: tachycardias, rhythm disorders, atrioventricular blocks, hypotension, and ischemic injury/infarction. Cardiocirculatory arrest is the leading cause of toxic death.

Cyanosis may be lacking in the early days of CO poisoning—correct pulsed saturation oxygen (SpO_2)—a does not exclude CO poisoning. Severity is often evaluated by measuring the HbCO.

Noninvasive measurement methods estimate in prehospital the level of CO: measurement of CO exhaled by measurement of saturation venous HbCO by Rad 57®. The value exhaled CO, expressed in parts per million (ppm) CO, is reliable in cooperating subjects capable of apnea 20 seconds in order to balance the blood levels and alveolar CO. The Rad 57®, meanwhile, has a sensitivity of 48% and a specificity of 99%. Values greater than 9% in the smoker and 6% in the nonsmoker as suspicious. These measures must be confirmed by the blood test.

Electrocardiogram (ECG) may show conduction disturbances and repolarization. Electrocardiographic abnormalities seem correlated to the intensity and duration of the CO exposure.

Subtraction from the toxic environment is the first step to be taken, then the patient must be placed under high-concentration oxygen therapy.

Extraction of the toxic exposure and normobaric oxygenation are the first-line treatments.

Intoxication with asphyxiating gases associated with early injection of hydroxocobalamin (OHCob) in case of suspicion of severe CN poisoning. The treatment of respiratory lesions is mainly symptomatic.

Hydroxocobalamin is currently the antidote for the most effective CN poisoning with the least side effects. Its use must be early, so prehospital to the 5-g dose intravenously in adults and 70 mg/kg in children, renewable once in case of failure. In case of poisoning with severe CO, hyperbaric oxygen therapy (HBOT) must be realized, with two goals: (1) to increase the quantity dissolved oxygen in the plasma and immediately available to the cells, and (2) restore the levels of intramitochondrial energy.

The inhalation of smoke is responsible of acute illness life-threatening, but also of chronic disease with neurological or respiratory sequelae. Among the survivors, inhalation with intoxication to fumes is a cause of post-intervallary syndrome. This syndrome appears to be due to initial hypoxia and ischemia infusion targeting the less vascularized brain areas (pallidum, periventricular, and hippocampus) and resulting in multifocal necrotic lesions, extensive demyelination. It results in the appearance in 10–30% of cases of neuropsychiatric signs, at a distance from acute intoxication (from 7 days to 21 days) and after apparent recovery. Patients who suffer from this syndrome recover in 50–75% of cases in less than a year.

Treatment

The treatment intoxication (whatever they are) combines treatment symptomatic, treatment purifier/evacuator and treatment-specific, antidotic.

Normobaric Oxygen Therapy

First treatment to be undertaken urgently, normobaric oxygen therapy with a high-concentration mask to treat hypoxia, reverse the CO binding with hemoglobin and palliate the related lung failure thermal and chemical burn. Invasive ventilation may sometimes be necessary if the patient is unconscious or case of obstruction of the upper airways. In this case, ventilation will be performed with a fraction of inspired oxygen (FiO_2) at 100%. The duration of normobaric oxygen therapy up to symptoms disappears or until the HbCO level is less than 10%.

Hyperbaric Oxygen Therapy

In cases of severe CO poisoning, HBOT must be proposed to increase the amount of dissolved oxygen in the plasma and to restore energy levels of intramitochondrial by raising the inhibition of cytochrome a3. Recommended by the European Committee for hyperbaric medicine for intoxicated patients at high risk of immediate- or long-term complications term, This committee recommends HBOT for patients with unconsciousness (grade B), with neurological involvement (Babinski's sign, cerebellar syndrome, osteotendinous hyperreflexia), cardiac, respiratory or psychiatric (grade B) and for pregnant women.

Treatment should be done as soon as possible. Beyond 24 hours and in the absence of symptoms, an HBOT is no longer recommended (grade C).

For children, close to those of the adult: severe neurological symptoms, syncope, persistence of symptoms after several hours normobaric oxygen therapy, myocardial ischemia, arrhythmias, psychiatric symptoms, particularly HbCO high, children less than 6 months lethargic or irritable.

Finally, concerning pregnant women, Koren et al. suggest a beneficial action of HBOT on the fetal outcome. The half-life of HbCO goes from approximately 1 hour 30 minutes for normobaric oxygen therapy at 20 minutes for HBOT at 3 atmospheres absolute (ATA).

The main contraindication for HBOT is pneumothorax without drainage. HBOT does not appear to aggravate hydrocyanic intoxication in case of cointoxication CO-CN.

CYANIDE TOXICITY MECHANISM

The determining role of CN in the toxicity of fumes has been demonstrated by the CN assays taken in prehospital settings. Cell anoxia, which results from CN intoxication, aggravated by other inhaled toxins (including CO) is responsible for multiple and nonspecific disorders.

Cyanide has a high affinity for sulfur components. In cells, it binds to the ferric iron of the heme of cytochrome oxidase a3 thus incapacitating the Krebs cycle of mitochondria.

It interrupts the formation of adenosine triphosphate (ATP) and diverts aerobic metabolism to the benefit of a metabolism anaerobic lactic acid producer.

Clinical Presentation

Diagnosis

Cyanide poisoning seems to be an overlooked diagnosis in fire victims. In 1991, Baud showed that persons from fire accidents were poisoned by both CN and CO. The diagnosis of CN poisoning presents a dilemma for first-responders. Clinicians are often able to diagnose CO poisoning by either arterial or venous blood sampling measuring HbCO or by oximetry although the latter may be unreliable.

The neurological system and the cardiovascular system are the first affected. Neurological symptoms are headache, dizziness, agitation, confusion, psychomotor retardation, convulsions, loss of consciousness. Symptoms range from collapse to cardiac arrest.

Respiratory symptoms are hyperventilation, then a respiratory arrhythmia (appearing in 20 minutes for 90 ppm exposure and appearance instantaneous exposure to 200 ppm). The presence of soot in the mouth or sputum, dysphonia and conjunctival hyperemia is predictive of a significant exposure to fumes and therefore to CN.

Metabolically, there is metabolic acidosis with hyperlactatemia and confirms, indirectly, the diagnosis.

Diagnosing CN poisoning, however, remains a challenge in the emergency setting as methods to detect and measure CN in blood are usually not readily available and that patients may often be exposed to both CO and CN. In patients with a history of fire accident, combined with severe neurological symptoms with a Glasgow Coma Scale (GCS) scoring less than 8 and either soot particles in the mouth or tracheal expectoration is likely to be an indicator of concomitant CN poisoning.

Baud et al. found a relationship of proportionality between the dosage of CN and the determination of lactates. They determined that lactate level greater than 8 mmol/L (72 mg/dL) had a sensitivity of 94% and a specificity of 70% in the diagnosis CN intoxication greater than 1 mg/L. The rate of lactic acid is inversely correlated with pH, Systolic blood pressure and respiratory rate. There is also an increase of the anionic hole. CN poisoning must be strongly suspected in presence of at least two of the following three criteria:

1. Signs of neurological involvement, convulsions, coma
2. Soot in the mouth or in the sputum
3. Metabolic acidosis with lactates greater than 10 mmol/L.

Treatment

The treatment of CN poisoning is aiming at basic life support including 100% oxygen, assisted ventilation if the patient is unconscious (GCS <8) or the airway seems compromised, decontamination, correction of acidosis and blood pressure support combined with the use of an antidote. Currently there are four types of antidotes: (1) OHCob, (2) sodium thiosulfate, (3) dicobalt edetate and (4) methemoglobin forming antidotes. Initial evaluation of antidotal efficacy is based on correction of hypotension and lactic acidosis.

Mechanism of Detoxification of Cyanides

Knowledge of CN detoxification mechanisms allows to envisage therapeutic tracks. The complex cytochrome oxidase-CN, unstable, detoxifies naturally in several ways
- A very small part is eliminated in unchanged form by the urine and respiration
- The fixation of the CN ion on aldehyde functions or ketone gives nontoxic components
- The fixation of the CN ion on the iron or on the cobalt of molecules organic compounds (such as methemoglobin and cobalamin, vitamin B_{12}) gives cyanmethemoglobin and cyanocobalamin, stable and nontoxic

- In 80-90% of cases, the CN ion is converted into thiocyanate. The thiocyanate ion toxic is eliminated by the urinary tract. OHCob works by combining with CN forming cyanocobalamin (vitamin B_{12}). It acts quickly and dissolves in all compartments immediately after its administration. It broadcasts in 30 minutes in cerebrospinal fluid (CSF). It is then excreted by the kidneys and eliminated by the urinary tract. This is the main antidote for CN used in Europe due to toxicity CN intoxication, absence of contraindication or significant side effects.

An intravenous injection of 5-10 g per adult and 70 mg/kg per child is recommended. The effectiveness of therapy is judged in the field by the improvement of hemodynamic conditions.

The earlier the treatment is administered, the more is effective. Its availability in all mobile hospital units and resuscitation ambulances are recommended for many years. Victims must receive the appropriate treatment at the scene of the fire.

CONCLUSION

Immediate treatment includes 100% oxygen, assisted ventilation if the patient is unconscious (GCS <8), decontamination, correction of acidosis and blood pressure support. Antidotes include OHCob, sodium thiosulfate, dicobalt EDTA and methemoglobin-inducers.

Fire smoke poisoning is responsible for half of these deaths. Of the hundreds of components contained in these fumes, CO and CN are the two most toxic. The presence of soot in the upper airways, associated with a lactate level greater than 10 mmol/L, is very suggestive of CN poisoning. Subtraction to the toxic environment is the first measurement to perform, then the patient should be placed under oxygen therapy.

Hydroxocobalamin is currently the antidote the most effective CN poisoning with the least side effects. HBOT is indicated in case clinically severe intoxication with CO, and at the pregnant woman. Act on fire prevention and the equipment in smoke detectors of dwellings has significantly decreased in the United States through the introduction of these devices among individuals.

CHAPTER 82

Sore Throat (Pharyngitis)

Akanksha Rastogi, Amit Mittal

INTRODUCTION

Pharyngitis or "sore throat" means the inflammation of the pharynx (i.e. back of the throat). It is one of the most common symptoms seen by the physician on an outpatient department (OPD) basis. Acute pharyngitis (AP) is more commonly seen than chronic pharyngitis (seen in syphilis, tuberculosis and leprosy). Systematic approach and management is needed to curtail over prescription of antibiotics and also early identification of the complications to reduce morbidity. This chapter will focus on AP.

ETIOLOGY/CAUSES

It is broadly classified into infectious and noninfectious causes.
1. Infectious (Differentiating features of viral and bacterial pharyngitis are described in **Fig. 1**)
   a. *Viral (most common)*: Respiratory viruses account for approximately 25-45% of the cases. Rhinovirus (20%), coronavirus (5%) and adenovirus (2-5%), influenza virus are more common. Other viruses include coxsackievirus, Epstein-Barr virus (EBV) (infectious mononucleosis **Fig. 2**), enterovirus, respiratory syncytial virus, etc.
   b. *Bacterial*:
      - Group A streptococcus (GAS) (15-30%), most common bacteria **Figure 3**
      - Others, e.g. group C and G streptococci, *Mycoplasma, Chlamydia, Fusobacterium, Arcanobacterium haemolyticum.*
   c. Human immunodeficiency virus (HIV) and others sexually transmitted infections, e.g. *Neisseria gonorrhoeae, Treponema pallidum*, etc.—less common in general population, however prevalence rises among those with high-risk behavior.
2. Noninfectious
   a. Allergic rhinitis, sinusitis, gastroesophageal reflux disease (GERD), active or passive smoking, exposure to dry air especially in winter season, iatrogenic (trauma caused by endotracheal intubation), drugs [angiotensin-converting enzyme (ACE) inhibitors, chemotherapeutic drugs].

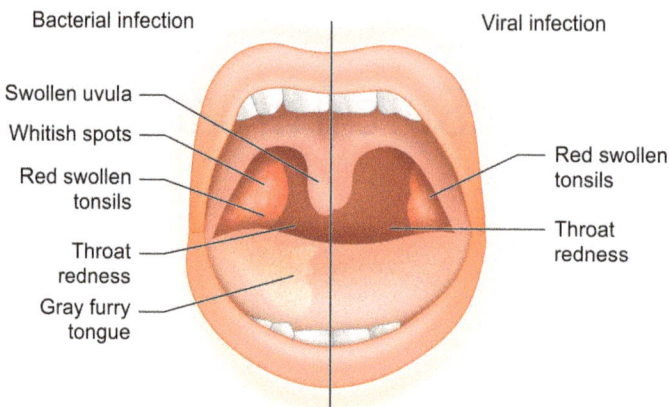

Fig. 1: Differentiation between viral and bacterial infection.

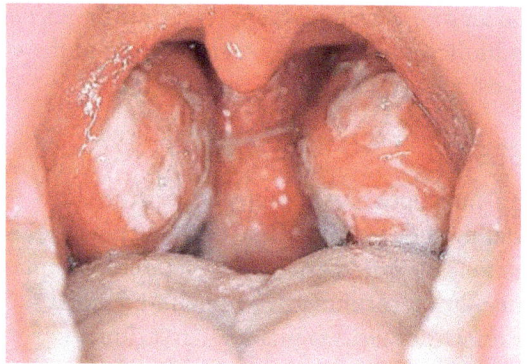

Fig. 2: Infectious mononucleosis.

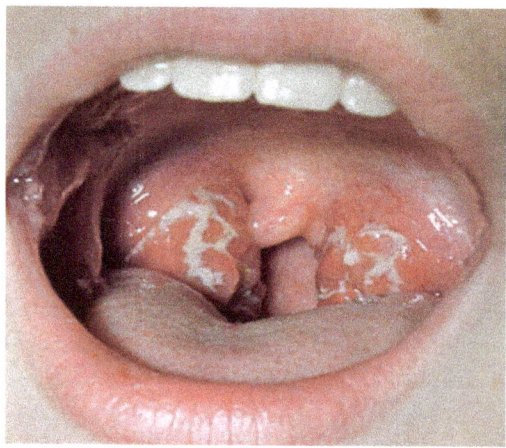

Fig. 3: Streptococcal pharyngitis.

PATHOPHYSIOLOGY OF THE CONDITION

Approximately half of the cases of pharyngitis are seen in childhood and young adults (<18 years of age). It affects all age groups (incidence declines after 40 years of age) with no gender preponderance. Highest incidence of pharyngitis is usually noted in winter and spring season. It is transmitted usually through respiratory route by droplets of saliva expelled through sneezing, coughing by the infected individual. Other mode of spread is hand contact with infected person. The risk of transmission depends upon the virulence of the infecting strain and inoculum size.

Pathological strains of *Streptococcus pyogenes* can be differentiated by Lancefield antigens and by blood agar hemolysis. Streptococcal infections are characterized by local invasion and release of proteases and extracellular toxins. The M protein resembles the myocardial sarcolemma and is responsible for virulence and antigens causing rheumatic heart disease in few individuals. However, some streptococcus strains produce erythrogenic toxins resulting into scarlet fever. Acute glomerulonephritis results from immune complex deposition in glomeruli.

CLINICAL PRESENTATION

Pharyngitis may present as throat pain, fever, cough, nasal congestion, headache, oral ulcers, viral exanthems, scarlet fever (fine, popular, bright red rash on neck), and strawberry tongue.

RED FLAGS

Alarming symptoms and signs that require urgent management:
- Dysphagia (difficulty in swallowing) for solids and eventually liquids
- Odynophagia (painful swallowing)
- Weight loss
- Features of upper airway obstruction, e.g. hoarseness of voice (hot potato voice), pooling of saliva, stridor, respiratory distress
- Deep neck space infections manifesting as trismus (reflex spasm of the internal pterygoid muscle) along with intense unilateral throat pain, toxic look, high-grade fever with rigors
- Bulging of pharyngeal wall/soft palate/floor of the oropharynx
- Ipsilateral otalgia.

EVALUATION

History
- Onset—sudden (bacterial cause) or gradual (viral cause)
- Duration and progression—viral recovers in 5–7 days without any specific treatment. GAS pharyngitis recovers sooner within 1–3 days of antibiotic use
- Seasonal history—viral (variable) and bacterial (winter-spring)
- Past history—dental problems, GERD
- Drugs—ACE inhibitors, tricyclic antidepressants, recent multiple courses of antibiotics cause oral candidiasis

- Social history—piercings and sexually transmitted infections, smoking, excess alcohol intake
- How are the symptoms now? —progression or improvement.

Physical Examination
- Ask the patient to remove any dentures, open full mouth, deviate tongue to one side, examine palate, oropharynx, tonsils, posterior pharyngeal wall, cervical lymph nodes
- Throat examination: Look for pustular exudates on tonsils
- Voice change
- General examination: Fever, cervical lymphadenopathy.

INTERPRETATION OF FINDING
- Age: *Viral* (<4 and >45 years of age), *bacterial* (5-15 years of age)
- Viral infections have cough, nasal congestion, rhinitis, conjunctivitis, myalgia, mild odynophagia and mild fever. On examination—small nontender cervical lymphadenitis and erythematous exudates on pharynx *(= red AP)*.
- Bacterial pharyngitis has acute onset and presents with high fever with chills, vomiting and severe odynophagia. On examination—large tender cervical lymphadenitis, scarlatiniform skin rash, severe inflammation and patchy white exudates on tonsils *(= white AP)*.
- Sometimes, clinical examination cannot distinguish viral from bacterial etiology clinically.

INVESTIGATIONS
They have a limited practical value.
- *Throat culture* is the gold standard diagnostic test for GAS.
- *Rapid antigen detection testing (RADT)* performed by throat swab (done only in bacterial infections by GAS) with sensitivity of 75-90% and specificity of 88-100%. It has a shorter turnaround time.
- *Complete blood count*—neutrophilic leukocytosis in bacterial infections, atypical lymphocytosis in infectious mononucleosis.
- *Monospot test*—in EBV (95% sensitivity).
- *Serum biochemical tests*—kidney function test (KFT), liver function test (LFT) to look for multiorgan dysfunction in suppurative infections.
- *Serologic testing*—HIV, sexually transmitted diseases (STDs).
- *X-rays cervical spine*: Plain lateral films in extension and flexion show loss of normal curvature with a soft tissue bulge in front of it.
- *Computed tomography (CT) scan/magnetic resonance imaging (MRI) neck and CT chest*—to look for suppurative complications in detail.

COMPLICATIONS
- *Suppurative (1-2%)*: It occurs in untreated bacterial infections, when infection spreads to the drainage areas resulting in peritonsillar abscess, retropharyngeal abscess, acute

otitis media, cervical adenitis, and rarely thrombophlebitis of the internal jugular vein (Lemierre's syndrome) and meningitis.
- *Nonsuppurative*: Acute rheumatic fever, poststreptococcal glomerulonephritis seen after few weeks of pharyngitis.

TREATMENT
Aim of the Treatment
- Symptomatic relief to the patient.
- Reducing the contagious time span.
- Preventing local suppurative and nonsuppurative complications.

Management depends upon the etiology. Evaluation and management of pharyngitis have been shown in **Flowchart 1**.

Nonpharmacological
- Refrain from smoking, tobacco chewing
- Hydration with frozen ice or popsicles or hot beverages (soups, tea).

Flowchart 1: Evaluation and management of pharyngitis.

```
Red flag symptoms and signs
    +                    −
    ↓                    ↓
Refer to            Suspicion of viral pharyngitis
emergency for       (cough, coryza, conjunctivitis, oral
hospitalization     ulcers, rhinorrhea, viral exanthem)
                    +                    −
                    ↓                    ↓
            Symptomatic and supportive   Suspicion of GAS pharyngitis
            care (recovery in 7 days)    (high fever, sudden onset sore
                                         throat, tonsillopharyngeal edema/
                                         exudates, scarlatiniform rash)
                        +                    Uncertain            −
                        ↓                       ↓             Rule out acute
                Perform RADT                                  HIV/gonorrhea/
                                        CENTOR Criteria       non-infectious
            +           −               (1 point for each)    causes
            ↓           ↓               • Fever > 38°C,
        Treat with    Any of the        • Tonsillar or pharyngeal exudates,
        antibiotics   following, e.g.   • Tender cervical lymphadenitis,
        for GAS       Immunosuppression,• Absence of cough
                      ARF, High GAS     (Total points ≥ 3 is diagnostic)
                      prevalence area, close
                      contact with ARF
            +                       +           −
                            Throat culture → Supportive care
```

Pharmacological
- *Topical therapy*: Lozenges and throat sprays which contain menthol, dyclonine, benzocaine, lidocaine, ambroxol
- *Drugs*:
    - Analgesics with titrated dosages, e.g. paracetamol, nonsteroidal anti-inflammatory drugs (NSAIDs) (ibuprofen 200-400 mg, aspirin 325 mg, acetaminophen 325 mg) help to relieve pain
    - Antibiotics—(in adults with GAS pharyngitis or its complication)
        Drug of choice: Penicillin (since it is studied in detail and found to reduce development of acute rheumatic fever)
        Options:
        - *Adults*:
            - Oral penicillin V (500 mg) two to three times daily for 7-10 days
            - Amoxicillin oral 50 mg/kg once daily (maximum = 1,000 mg) or 25 mg/kg twice a day × 8-10 days.

        Intramuscular long-acting penicillin G is more effective
        - <27 kg: 600,000 units single dose IM
        - >27 kg: 1,200,000 units single dose IM

        If penicillin allergy, options are:
- Cephalosporin—cefuroxime 250 mg twice daily/cephalexin 500 mg twice a day for 10 days
Or
- Macrolides—azithromycin 500 mg once daily × 5 days or
- Clarithromycin 250 mg twice a day × 10 days
Or
- Lincosamides—clindamycin 300 mg three times a day for 10 days.
Children:
- Penicillin V, oral 250 mg two to three times daily × 10 days
- Amoxicillin 50 mg/kg/day orally.

SUMMARY
- Acute pharyngitis is very common and mostly of viral origin.
- Detailed history and examination is must to distinguish the etiology.
- Identify the patient who needs investigation by throat swab c/s or RADT (i.e. GAS pharyngitis and specific inv for treatable pathogens—HIV/syphilis).
- Antistreptococcal Ab testing is not routinely recommended.
- In nonspecific chronic pharyngitis—exclusion of malignancy is an important aspect which requires a detailed history along with careful physical examination.
- Avoid overprescribing of antibiotics.
- Glucocorticoids have a limited role.

CHAPTER 83

Stridor

Yatin Mehta, Kamal Lashkari, Prashant Kumar

INTRODUCTION

Stridor is a harsh, vibratory sound of variable pitch produced by turbulent airflow during respiration through a partially obstructed airway. The term stridor originated from the Latin word *stridere*, which means to make a shrill sound or harsh noise as to creak.

Stridor is usually inspiratory sound but also can occur on expiration or can be biphasic. Inspiratory stridor usually points to an obstruction at or above the larynx, while expiratory and biphasic respiratory stridor generally indicate an obstruction below the larynx. In biphasic stridor, there is fixed airway obstruction at the level of the glottis, subglottis, or upper trachea. Loud stridor points toward significant narrowing of the airway. The characteristics of the voice provide additional important information. While hoarseness may suggest vocal cords dysfunction, a muffled voice with a low-pitched stridor indicates supraglottic pathology such as epiglottitis.

Stridor is an important physical finding that requires prompt evaluation and often emergency intervention. Further workup may be necessary to establish a definite diagnosis, among all modalities flexible airway endoscopy is the procedure of choice in most circumstances.

Characteristics of stridor in sound analysis are regular, sinusoidal oscillations with a fundamental frequency of approximately 500 Hz, frequently accompanied by several harmonics.

PATHOPHYSIOLOGY

A complete understanding of the normal airway anatomy and airflow dynamics is important for the evaluation of the upper airway obstruction. Anatomically, the large airways can be divided into the extrathoracic and intrathoracic regions. On inspiration, intrathoracic pressure becomes lower than atmospheric pressure, drawing air into lungs through the airways. The trachea has some compliance, allowing the intrathoracic portion to increase in diameter during inspiration and decrease during expiration. These changes in diameter are normally limited by support from cartilaginous rings and tone provided by contraction of smooth muscle. All of this prevents the trachea from collapsing with expiration, even though the tracheal air column in healthy patients is wider on inspiration than it is on expiration. Airway narrowing in the nasal, nasopharyngeal, or oropharyngeal areas (i.e. adenoid hypertrophy, micrognathia,

Table 1: Types of stridor.

Stridor	Features
Inspiratory stridor	Obstruction is in the extrathoracic region, during inspiration the pressure inside the airway falls below atmospheric pressure resulting in airway collapse
Expiratory stridor	Obstruction exists in intrathoracic region. Intrathoracic pressure rises due obstruction during expiration, resulting in airway collapse
Biphasic (inspiratory and expiratory) stridor	In biphasic stridor obstruction is fixed rather than dynamic, resulting in sound production on both inspiration and expiration. Fixed airway obstruction may be caused by external compression, intraluminal airway masses, e.g. hemangioma or foreign body, and mural changes in the airway, such as subglottic stenosis

macroglossia, and tonsil hypertrophy) can generate typically low-pitched sound. It is called as snoring if it is produced during sleep and stridor when patient is awake. Different types of stridor and their features are described in **Table 1**.

CAUSES

Stridor can be due to congenital or acquired causes and are described in **Table 2**.

CLINICAL PRESENTATION

They are divided into acute, subacute, and chronic onset and are described in **Table 3**.

EVALUATION

History

The initial evaluation of children with stridor must begin with a rapid assessment of airway, breathing, and circulation (ABC) and immediate intervention should be done on case-to-case basis. Key steps are to evaluate upper airway patency, work of breathing, evidence of hypoxemia and exhaustion, and to closely monitor for the possibility of rapid deterioration. Time of onset is important determinant for diagnosis. Rapidly progressive symptoms with fever indicate epiglottitis or bacterial tracheitis while symptoms without fever suggest foreign body aspiration or anaphylaxis. Laryngotracheitis (croup) and peritonsillar and retropharyngeal abscesses tend to have a subacute or intermittent course. Chronic or recurrent episodes of stridor may be congenital or acquired. History taking should also include the previous admissions secondary to respiratory diseases, allergy, necessity of intubation, mechanical ventilation, surgery, prenatal and perinatal events like infections, prematurity, and complicated delivery.

Physical Examination

Initial assessment starts with ABC of resuscitation. Once the patient is stabilized then a detailed physical examination and diagnostic testing should be conducted. Breathing should

Table 2: Congenital and acquired causes of stridor.

I. Congenital stridor	
A. Craniofacial dysmorphology (with micrognathia and glossoptosis)	• Pierre-Robin syndrome • Treacher-Collins syndrome (mandibulofacial dysostosis) • Hallermann-Streiff syndrome (oculomandibular) • Möbius syndrome • de Lange syndrome • Freeman-Sheldon (whistling face)
B. Macroglossia	• Beckwith's syndrome • Congenital hypothyroidism • Glycogen storage diseases • Down's syndrome • Diffuse muscular hypertrophy of the tongue • Localized lingual tumors
C. Laryngomalacia D. Congenital subglottic stenosis E. Congenital laryngeal webs F. Laryngotracheoesophageal cleft G. Congenital vocal cord paralysis H. Vascular rings and slings I. Congenital tracheal anomalies J. Congenital calcification of tracheal cartilage	
K. Congenital tumors and cysts	• Congenital subglottic hemangioma • Laryngeal lymphangioma and cystic hygroma • Cysts and laryngoceles • Miscellaneous congenital tumors
L. Birth trauma—edema M. Metabolic stridor—laryngysmus stridulosa N. Immunologic stridor—hereditary angioneurotic edema O. Neurogenic stridor—reflex laryngospasm	
II. Acquired stridor	
A. Infectious stridor	• Epiglottitis • Croup • Acute spasmodic laryngitis • Diphtheria • Retropharyngeal abscess
B. Immunologic stridor—juvenile rheumatoid arthritis	
C. Trauma	• Foreign bodies • Iatrogenic stridor: – Postintubation, i.e. after extubation – Postinstrumentation – Postoperative • External trauma • Thermal and chemical trauma
D. Neoplasia	• Laryngeal papillomatosis • Miscellaneous tumors and nodes

Table 3: Clinical presentation.

Onset	Causes	Symptoms
Acute (symptoms develop within minutes or a few hours, and may progress rapidly)	a. Foreign body aspiration	Sudden respiratory distress
	b. Anaphylaxis—commonly be caused by food allergens (e.g. egg, peanuts, seafood, and milk) or medications. It is a common cause of acute-onset stridor, which is sometimes severe and life threatening, especially when edema involves the retropharynx or larynx	Barking cough, swallowing difficulty, dyspnea, wheezing along with rash, and rapidly developing respiratory arrest
	c. Bacterial tracheitis—also known as pseudomembranous croup or bacterial laryngotracheobronchitis. Most common causative organism is *Staphylococcus aureus*, other etiologies include *Haemophilus influenzae* type b and *Moraxella catarrhalis*	Initial symptoms and signs are generally suggestive of viral respiratory tract infection for first 1–3 days, afterward serious signs of illness including stridor and respiratory distress may develop
	d. Epiglottitis—it is severe inflammation of the epiglottis with adjacent supraglottic structures	The classic presentation for epiglottitis is high fever, irritability, and the "4Ds"—dyspnea, drooling, dysphonia and dysphasia
	e. Airway burns—smoke or steam inhalation and ingestion of caustic materials can also cause thermal injury to the upper respiratory tract	
Subacute onset—typically presents with respiratory symptoms that progress gradually over the course of a few days to stridor	a. Laryngotracheitis (croup) characterized by varying degrees of inspiratory stridor, cough, seal-like barking, and hoarseness. Croup mainly affects children between ages 6 months and 4 years with a peak incidence at 12–24 months	Symptoms usually start gradually, beginning with nasal irritation, coryza, and congestion and progressing to inspiratory and sometimes expiratory stridor. Furthermore, it progresses over 12–48 hours to include fever, barking cough, hoarseness, and stridor. Mostly croup is self-limiting disease, but occasionally causes significant respiratory distress and can be life-threatening
	b. Retropharyngeal abscess and peritonsillar abscess—it can develop as a complication of tonsillitis or pharyngitis Common causative organisms include *S. aureus*, *Haemophilus* species, group A beta-hemolytic streptococcus, *Bacteroides* species, *Peptostreptococcus* species and *Fusobacterium* species	Physical signs of retropharyngeal abscess include fever, cervical adenopathy, stridor, torticollis, drooling, and neck stiffness. As the disease progresses, symptoms include dysphagia, muffled or "hot potato" voice, and inspiratory stridor

Contd...

Contd...

Onset	Causes	Symptoms
Chronic or recurrent—chronic stridor is commonly caused by a structural abnormality that may be congenital or acquired, leading to intrinsic or extrinsic obstruction of the upper airway	a. Laryngomalacia—it is the most common cause of chronic extrathoracic airway obstruction causing stridor in newborns	Stridor is usually inspiratory and tends to be worse during lying down position, feeding, and sleeping. In laryngomalacia, stridor is produced due to weak and immature laryngeal and supralaryngeal structures which collapse during inspiration. As these structures strengthen with age, stridor disappears gradually
	b. Tracheomalacia—develops due to weakening of the supporting cartilage and muscle of the trachea. Tracheomalacia can be primary or secondary. Primary tracheomalacia is found in association with congenital anomalies Acquired or secondary forms may develop as a result of prolonged intubation, mechanical ventilation, tracheostomy, or severe tracheobronchitis	During expiration trachea collapses, producing expiratory stridor and wheeze. Usually most lesions are intrathoracic, causing stridor during expiration, which is accompanied often with a croup like cough
	c. Vocal cord paralysis and vocal cord dysfunction—after laryngomalacia, vocal cord paralysis is the second most common laryngeal abnormality in the newborn and young infant. The onset may be acute, subacute, or intermittent, depending on the etiology	Vocal cord dysfunction typically presents with recurrent acute episodes of dyspnea and stridor, often misdiagnosed as asthma. The stridor is exaggerated with exercise and resolves during sleep

be observed both during rest and activity. The patient's work of breathing should be assessed, including the presence of nasal flaring, cyanosis, retractions, and the patient's preferred body position. Patient should be examined for craniofacial malformation, size of the tongue, presence of surgical scars and hemangiomas. Presence of lymphadenopathy suggests an intrathoracic process and clubbing may indicate an underlying congenital heart disease or bronchiectasis.

INVESTIGATIONS

Airway management is priority over diagnostic investigations. Complete blood count (CBC) with inflammatory markers can help identify infectious etiology. Radiography is necessary for evaluating a child with severe or atypical features, suspected of radiopaque foreign body, epiglottitis, retropharyngeal abscess, and laryngotracheitis. A normal chest X-ray does not rule out a foreign body aspiration. Plain chest radiograph can also help identifying intrathoracic etiology like mediastinal lymphadenopathy, masses, or vascular rings. Ultrasonography of the neck or computed tomography (CT) with contrast can potentially show the anatomical extension of the lesion and help differentiating a true abscess from cellulitis. CT is also used to look for enlarged lymph nodes, tumors, aberrant arteries, and vascular rings, but intraluminal lesions may be missed. Magnetic resonance imaging (MRI) is valuable for evaluation of children with suspected tracheal stenosis or obstruction because it is able to image the trachea across the long axis. MRI also provides a good evaluation of the mediastinum. Direct visualization of the larynx is important diagnostic tool for chronic or recurrent stridor. Visualization of the airways with nasopharyngoscopy, laryngoscopy, and bronchoscopy allows definitive diagnosis of the cause of stridor in children.

■ TREATMENT

Treatment of all cases of stridor starts with appropriate management of airway involving specialist skilled in securing difficult airways (e.g. anesthesiologist, intensivist, and otolaryngologist). Options may include temporary or definitive airway including emergency tracheotomy. Specific management of each condition is discussed in **Table 4**.

Table 4: Specific conditions and treatment.

Foreign body	The removal of foreign body from the respiratory tract by team of surgeon and the anesthesiologist. CT or bronchoscopy can be considered in more stable patients
Anaphylaxis	Immediate adrenaline is the treatment of choice. Intramuscular (IM) injection is the preferred route for epinephrine administration for anaphylaxis in most settings and in patients of all ages
Tracheitis and epiglottitis	Antibiotic treatment against causative organisms should be started
Croup	Corticosteroid therapy is routinely recommended by all experts
Laryngomalacia	The management of laryngomalacia depends on the severity of symptoms. In the majority of otherwise normal children, laryngomalacia is not dangerous and resolves spontaneously. Surgical treatment includes supraglottoplasty, accessory routes for feeding and sometimes, in extreme cases, tracheostomy
Vocal cord paralysis	Those with unilateral paralysis tend to present with hoarseness and are at risk for aspiration. Bilateral vocal cord paralysis typically presents with concomitant airway disease and progressive airway obstruction which may require urgent airway intervention including endotracheal intubation and tracheostomy

Contd...

Contd...

Vocal cord dysfunction	In children, disorder often spontaneously resolves with time. The benign nature of the dysfunction should be explained to the patients. In the adults, excellent response to speech therapy has been reported
Retropharyngeal and peritonsillar abscess	Treatment includes surgical drainage and intravenous antibiotics
Postextubation stridor	A cuff leak test can be performed if risk factors for postextubation stridor from laryngeal edema are present like prolonged duration of intubation, traumatic intubation, and large endotracheal tube, and aspiration, presence of an orogastric or nasogastric tube. For those who have a reduced cuff leak, administering a short course of glucocorticoid therapy at least 4 hours prior to extubation is recommended

SUMMARY

Stridor may result from a variety of conditions that can be either congenital or acquired. The timing, acuity of onset, and associated symptoms help to narrow the differential diagnosis. The initial evaluation of patient with stridor must begin with a rapid assessment to identify patients who need immediate intervention and stabilization. Management of many cases of stridor may need teamwork and close coordination among various skilled specialist including anesthetist, intensivist, and otolaryngologist. Once the focused clinical history and physical examination narrows the diagnostic possibilities, radiographic studies and direct examination of the airway are considered for further evaluation. Approach to patient with stridor is summarized in **Flowchart 1**.

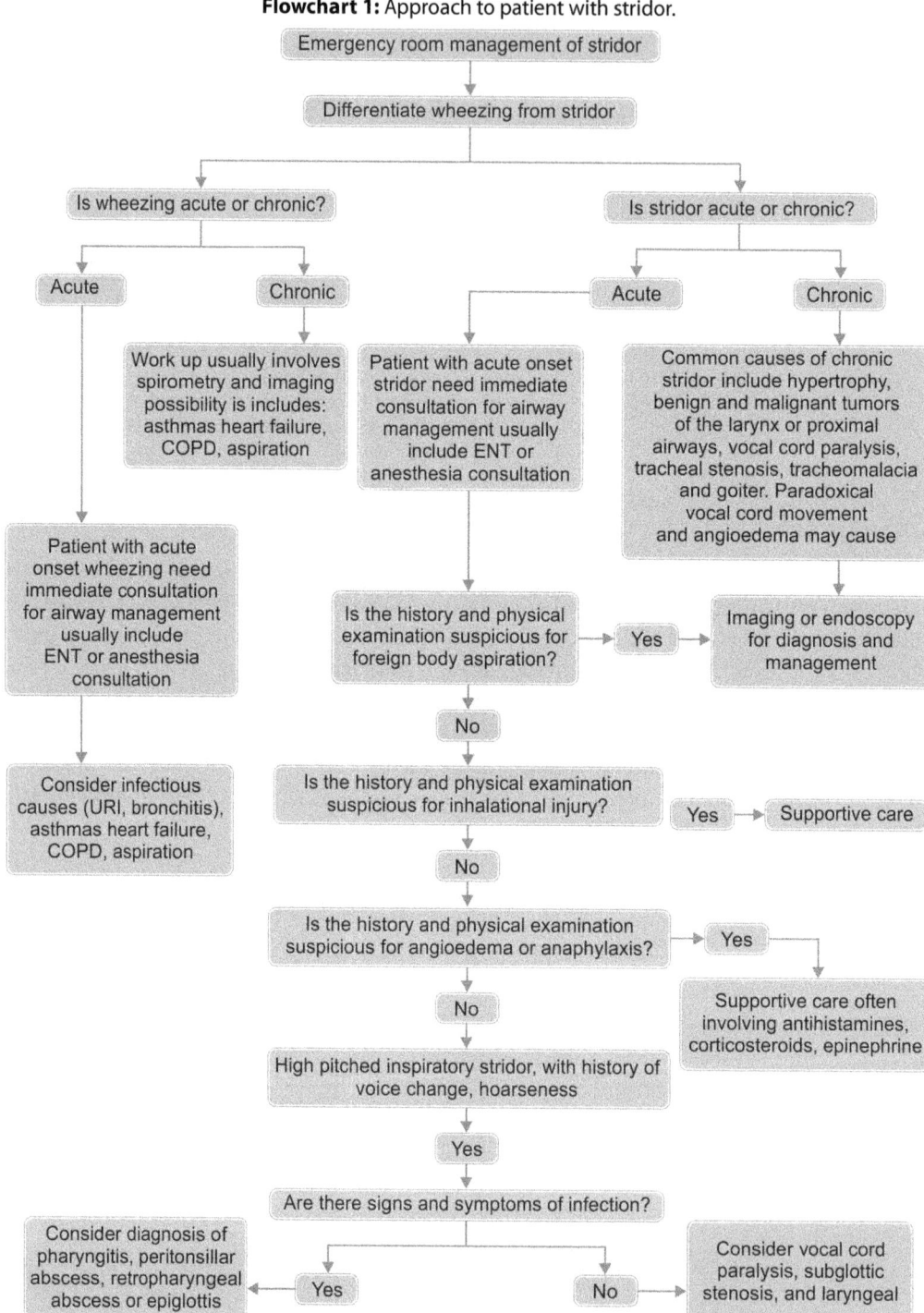

Flowchart 1: Approach to patient with stridor.

Tetanus Prophylaxis

M Sai Surendar

INTRODUCTION

Tetanus is caused by a neurotoxin (tetanospasmin) produced by *Clostridium tetani*, an anaerobic spore-forming bacillus. Tetanus spores are widespread in the environment, including soil and manure. They can survive in hostile conditions for long periods of time. Transmission occurs when the spores are introduced into the body most often is due to a puncture wound but also through unnoticed wounds, through injecting drugs and sometimes due to an abdominal surgery. Tetanus is a notifiable disease in certain countries.

All wounds in emergency department (ED) should be cleaned thoroughly and should be considered for tetanus risk.

TETANUS-PRONE WOUNDS

They include:
- Wounds or burns that require surgical intervention that is delayed for more than 6 hours.
- Wounds or burns that show a significant degree of devitalized tissue or a puncture type injury particularly where there has been contact with soil or manure.
- Wounds containing foreign bodies.
- Compound fractures.
- Wounds or burns in patients who have systemic sepsis.

High-risk tetanus: Prone wounds are those with heavy contamination with material likely contain tetanus spores like soil, manure, or extensive devitalized tissue.

TETANUS PROPHYLAXIS IN TETANUS PRONE WOUND

- If the wound, burn or injury meets the above criteria and is considered to be high risk, human immunoglobulin should be given for immediate protection, irrespective of the tetanus immunization history of the patient (**Table 1**).
- The dose of human tetanus immunoglobulin is normally 250 IU by intramuscular injection or 500 IU if more than 24 hours have elapsed since injury or there is a risk of heavy contamination or following burns.
- Tetanus vaccination should be injected at different site from immunoglobulin so that it does not get neutralized by the passive immunization.

Table 1: Tetanus prophylaxis in different types of wound.

Immunization status	Clean wound	Tetanus-prone wound	High-risk wound
Fully immunized (i.e. five dose of vaccine at appropriate intervals)	Nil	Nil	Human tetanus immunoglobulin
Primary immunizations complete, boosters incomplete but up to date	Nil	Nil	Human tetanus immunoglobulin
Primary immunization incomplete or boosters not up to date	Tetanus vaccine in ED and completion of schedule by GP	Human tetanus immunoglobulin, tetanus vaccine in ED, and completion of schedule by GP	Human tetanus immunoglobulin, tetanus vaccine in ED, and completion of schedule by GP
Not immunized, immunocompromised, or immunization status uncertain	Tetanus vaccine in ED and completion of schedule by GP	Human tetanus immunoglobulin, tetanus vaccine in ED, and completion of schedule by GP	Human tetanus immunoglobulin, tetanus vaccine in ED, and completion of schedule by GP

- Patient who are immunosuppressed may not be adequately protected against tetanus, despite having been fully immunized and should treated as if they are incompletely immunized.
- In patients where the tetanus boosters are incomplete but up to date, tetanus booster is not needed but may be given if booster is due and it is convenient to grow now.
- Where an immediate tetanus vaccine is given, further doses should be arranged as per recommended schedule.

CHAPTER 85

Torticollis (Wryneck)

Harshil Mehta

INTRODUCTION

Torticollis is also known as cervical dystonia or wryneck. Torticollis is a combination of two Latin words, i.e. *tortus*—twisted and *collum*—neck.

Head and neck is turned into fixed or dynamic posturing (due to tonic component), flexion, and rotation.

It occurs due to more prominent spasm of neck muscles [sternocleidomastoid (SCM), trapezius, and other neck muscles], on one side than the other resulting into turning or tipping of the head.

Spasmodic torticollis is an adult onset segmental or focal dystonia in which variable combination of neck extension, flexion, tilting, and rotation is seen. Such posture can present at any time even at rest. It may worsen with some activity (action or stress) and may resolve completely.

Depending upon tonicity of different segmental muscles, four types of presentations are noticed including (**Fig. 1**):
1. Rotational—rotation of chin toward opposite shoulder.
2. Laterocollis—head is displaced with the ear moved toward the shoulder from increased tone in the ipsilateral cervical muscles.
3. Anterocollis—forward deviation of the head in the sagittal plane with the chin moving toward the chest.
4. Retrocollis—backward deviation of the head in the sagittal plane.

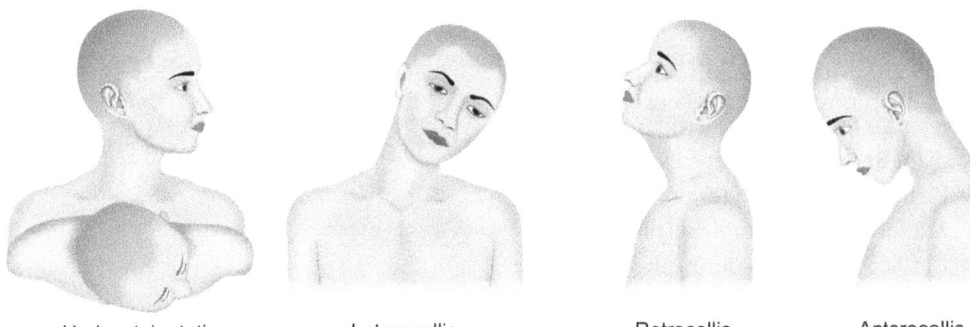

Fig. 1: Four types of presentations of torticollis.

Onset of idiopathic cervical dystonia is typically seen between 30 years and 50 years of age. Females are affected twice as frequently as males. Congenital muscular torticollis occurs in not more than 0.4% of neonates.

ETIOLOGY/CAUSES

Torticollis is mainly classified in dystonic and nondystonic torticollis.

Dystonic Torticollis

It manifests as contractions of neck muscles that are sustained and involuntary leading to abnormal postures and movements of the head.

It is observed mainly due to following reasons:
- *Primary/idiopathic*: It is a painful chronic progressive neurological movement disorder causing the neck to turn any side involuntarily. Studies have shown neurochemical changes in basal ganglia. Initial symptoms are mild which may progress with frequency and severity. During any activity like walking or during periods of increased stress symptoms may worsen. Studies suggest that 33-40% of the patients may experience head tremors and over 75% of patients report neck pain.
- *Secondary torticollis*: It is very uncommonly seen. It results from:
    - Perinatal cerebral injury
    - Kernicterus
    - Cerebrovascular diseases
    - Segmental brain lesions of various etiologies, e.g. skull base tumors
    - Peripheral/central trauma
    - Paraneoplastic syndromes
    - Neurodegenerative disorder
    - Metabolic disorder
    - Drugs like antipsychotics/neuroleptic antiemetics and chemicals that affect brain structures like thalamus, basal ganglia, and brainstem.

Nondystonic Torticollis

It may occur as a result of abnormal positions of head due to various etiologies. In such patients, palpable muscular hypertonus/hypertrophy and sensory tricks should be absent. It can be divided into:
- *Congenital torticollis*: It is the most common type of torticollis at birth. The incidence is 0.3-2.0%. It occurs due to:
    - Birth trauma or in-utero malposition
    - Malformation of cervical spine
    - Cervical muscle hypertrophy
    - Arnold-Chiari malformation

- *Acquired torticollis*: Various etiologies are given below for noncongenital muscular torticollis:
    - Neurological causes like syringomyelia or tumors
    - Abnormalities of cervical spine, e.g. fracture clavicle or scapula
    - Infections like cervical spine osteomyelitis or in the posterior pharynx.

PATHOPHYSIOLOGY

- *Congenital torticollis*: It results from soft tissue neck trauma during or just before delivery. The common explanation involves unilateral shortening of SCM muscle due to birth trauma and fibrosis of the same muscle.
- *Acquired torticollis*: The mechanism of acquired torticollis varies according to underlying disease process. Acute torticollis may be self-limiting on cessation of certain etiology.

CLINICAL PRESENTATION

Early in the morning, symptoms are basically absent. It increases with fatigue gets worsened as day passes. It is also aggravated by stress, anxiety and with some specific tasks like watching television, reading or writing.

Primary Torticollis

Involuntary jerking or twisting associated with abnormal head posture without any other neurological signs:
- Mild neck stiffness
- Pulling sensations in the neck
- Subtle head posture deviation
- Hypertrophy of neck muscles
- Headache
- Shoulder or neck pain
- Sensory tricks—known as "Geste Antagoniste"or "Gegendruck phenomenon". Its presence is a diagnostic clue to this disease. It also temporarily deceases dystonic posturing.

Secondary Torticollis

Any neurologic, medical disorders or any drug exposure, orthopedic or history of trauma may give rise to secondary torticollis.

Factors differentiating Primary from Secondary

Following are the factors seen in secondary torticollis:
- Sudden onset
- Severe pain
- Onset early during pediatric age group
- Fixed posture

- Absence of sensory tricks
- Rapid progression
- Presence during sleep.

PHYSICAL EXAMINATION

The objective of examination is to locate evidence for torticollis as the obvious finding of primary process with associated features elsewhere.
- The presence of craniofacial asymmetry suggests congenital or long-standing dystonia.
- Patients with traumatic torticollis should be immobilized and evaluated for range of motion (ROM).
- Posterior pharynx should be examined for any sign of infection of inflammation.
- Neck should be palpated for any mass, adenopathy or tenderness.
- A complete neurological examination should be done.
- Characterization of head/neck movements includes tonic and phasic components.
    - *Phasic component* includes:
        - *Spasmodic jerks*: Rapid, irregular clonic jerks with slower recovery
        - *High-frequency oscillation*: Regular or irregular tremors.
    - *Tonic component*: Head is turned to any one direction according to pathology. Only with simple torticollis, no head tilt is present.

Congenital Torticollis

A firm, palpable, nontender soft tissue mass in the SCM must often felt in congenital torticollis shortly after birth. The mass usually enlarges in size by 4–6 weeks and then decreases.

INVESTIGATIONS

After taking detailed history including perinatal history (mainly in congenital torticollis) and physical examination, some test may help to determine accurate pathology.

Rarely any laboratory test is required for torticollis diagnosis except DNA test in cases of a positive family history.

In radiological workup, following modalities can be used:
- *Plain cervical X-ray*: Useful in distinguishing any bony changes like spondylosis or scoliosis or any other structural changes in spine due to chronic dystonia.
- *Magnetic resonance imaging (MRI)*: Cervical cord MRI is useful to document pathologies for multiple radiculopathy like cord impingement.
- *Cranial computed tomography (CT)/MRI*: It indicated when the physical examination shows signs of pyramidal tract abnormality, ophthalmoplegia or dementia.
- *Contrast swallowing studies*: It may be performed before botulinum toxin injections in consultation with speech pathologist.
- *Electromyography*: useful in distinguishing myopathic from neuropathic pathology.

DIFFERENTIAL DIAGNOSIS
- Cranial nerve VI palsy
- Spasmus nutans
- Sandifer syndrome
- Myasthenia gravis
- Essential tremor
- Multiple sclerosis
- Parkinson's disease
- Tardive dyskinesia.

TREATMENT

Different modalities are available to treat the condition. Medical therapy includes various medications, physiotherapy and when conservative therapy goes fail, surgical intervention is required.

Medications

The goal of medical therapy is to reduce morbidity and prevention of complications. There are two categories of medicines:
1. *Dystonia reducing*: Pramipexole, trihexyphenidyl, glutamate release inhibitors, botulinum toxin.
2. *Selective adjunctive*: Clonazepam, baclofen, propranolol.
    - Botulinum toxin is the most recommended treatment for spasmodic torticollis. It paralyzes dystonic muscle by preventing release of acetylcholine presynaptic axon of motor end-plate. The agonist muscle is allowed to move freely by disabling the movement of antagonist muscle. With this injection, for approximately 12–16 weeks patients experience relief from torticollis. Commonly seen side effects with botulinum toxin are pain at injection site, dysphagia, dry mouth, fatigue, and weakness of injected muscles.

Deep Brain Stimulation

For all types of dystonia, Postventral globus pallidus internus (GPi) deep brain stimulation (DBS) is commonly utilized stereotactic target. Effects of this therapy are not immediate. Improvement in pain is the first effect then motor disability and later severity.

PHYSICAL THERAPY

Physical therapy is a noninvasive and cost-effective manner to treat torticollis. In infants and small children, passive stretching and proper head positioning is used. Applying heat, traction to the neck and massage are helpful to relieve head and neck pain. For neck spasms, stretching exercises and neck braces are helpful.

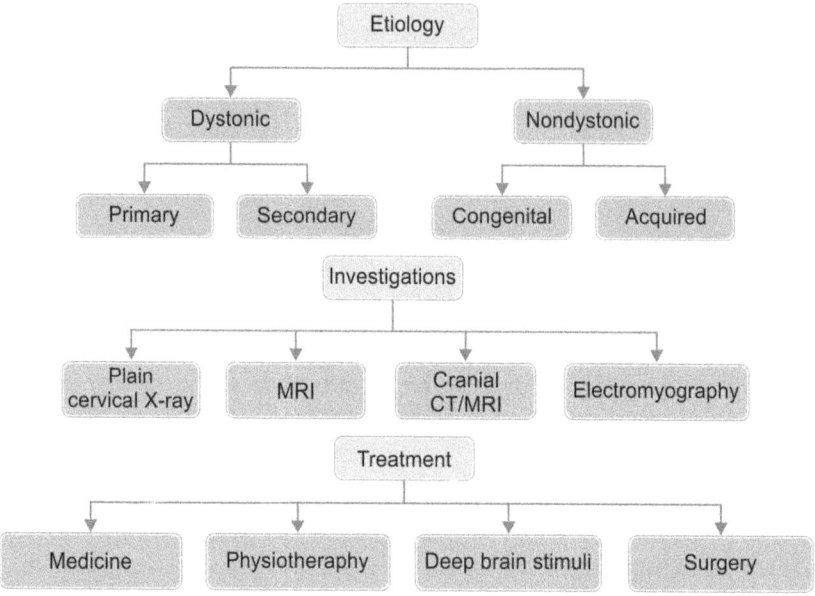

Flowchart 1: Etiology, investigations, and treatment of torticollis.

Surgical Intervention

Those patients who do not respond to physical therapy or medical therapy are the candidates for surgical modality.

SUMMARY

Torticollis is the presentation of abnormal muscular spasms. Studies have shown that with conservative treatment 85–90% of cases of congenital torticollis are resolved. Torticollis may resolve spontaneously. Chance of relapse is always there.

Etiology, investigations, and treatment of torticollis have been shown in **Flowchart 1**.

CHAPTER 86

Tremor

Devendra Richhariya

INTRODUCTION

Tremor is one of the most common movement disorders in neurology outpatient and also in general practice. Tremor is rhythmical oscillatory movement disorder and due to contraction of reciprocally innervated muscles. Tremors are may be due to normal physiological response or may be due to severe neurological response like Parkinson's disease or stroke. So the sound knowledge about the tremor is necessary for appropriate tremor evaluation and treatment to improve the quality of life of patient suffering from the tremors.

EPIDEMIOLOGY AND CLINICAL FEATURES

The tremor most commonly treated in general practice is "essential tremor" of which the cause is not known. The prevalence of essential tremor more than the Parkinson's tremor and increases with age. Essential tremors are generally benign and started with shaky feeling inside followed by the intermittent tremors during anxiety and fatigue and ultimately progress to permanent phenomenon but disappear during sleep. Hands are most commonly affected.

CLASSIFICATION

Phenomenological Classification

1. *Resting tremor*: Present during sitting lying down when body is relaxed and increased during activities.
2. *Postural tremor*: Present in body part maintained in a particular position, e.g. outstretched hand.
3. *Kinetic tremor*: Present during activities like eating, writing and can affect the daily routine. Seen in cerebellar tremor, dystonic tremor, and primary writing tremor.
4. *Intention tremor*: It is cerebellar tremor and occurs when someone try to touch the target.

Etiological Classification

1. *Essential tremor*: Bilateral symmetrical postural or kinetic tremor involving hand and forearm aggravated by stress and alcohol. Usually have family history, progression is slow but severity increases with time. Most of patients do not have neurological symptoms.

2. *Parkinson's tremor*: During course of Parkinson's disease, about 70% of patients have tremor, asymmetrical and gradually progressive in onset, special characteristic of pill rolling type of tremor and associated with tremor of lips jaw and lower limbs.
3. *Drug-induced tremor*: Symmetrical occurs due to initiation of drugs and decrease with the withdrawal of the medication. Multiple medications, advance age, brain disease, renal disease are the common risk factors. Beta-adrenergic agonists, antidepressants, neuroleptics, anticonvulsants, dopamine agonist and antagonists, heavy metals antiarrhythmic, thyroxine corticosteroids are the common drugs that can induce tremor.
4. *Neuropathic tremor*: It is associated with chronic inflammatory demyelinating neuropathy, other signs of peripheral neuropathy are also present on examination.
5. *Dystonic tremor*: It is commonly associated with primary dystonia. Tremors are irregular and variable. Tremor that occurs while writing (primary writing tremor), mild blepharospasm, slight torticollis indicates dystonic tremor and botulinum toxin injection is the treatment of choice.
6. *Orthostatic tremor*: Mostly in the legs when person is erect, unsteadiness on standing and causes postural instability. A very strong urge to sit or to move that often person avoid the situation of long standing such as queuing. Women are affected more. Clonazepam, primidone, gabapentin, and benzodiazepine are beneficial.
7. *Psychogenic tremor*: Abrupt onset generalized shaking mostly in stress full life conditions. Coactivation signs and entrainment sign are diagnostic of psychogenic tremor.
8. *Wilson tremor*: Tremor in Wilson disease and treatable. Wilson disease is characterized by clinical feature of ascites, jaundice, chronic liver disease in nonalcoholic young patients with KF ring dystonia, dysarthria and diagnosis is confirmed by serum ceruloplasmin and 24-hour urinary copper excretion.

■ EVALUATION OF TREMOR

- *History*: As tremors are visible, history about onset of tremor sudden or gradual any precipitating aggravating or relieving factors should be noted. Family history and medication history are also important.
- *Examination*: Tremor should be observed right from the history taking. Observe the tremor in every position of patient like sitting supine and walking. Horizontal or vertical head tremor is usually feature of essential tremor. In Parkinsonism localized face lip and jaw tremor are common. Detail examination of cranial nerves gait balance and muscle tone is essential to find out neurological cause of tremor. Ocular examination for nystagmus (cerebellar disease) KF ring (Wilson disease) is helpful.
- *Laboratory test*: Consider complete hemogram, liver function test, renal function test, thyroid function test, serum ceruloplasmin, screening for heavy metals such as mercury and arsenic may be helpful. Brain imaging can be helpful to rule out any neurological disorder.
- *Electromyography*: Detail information about tremor can be acquired by simple test called electromyography. Tremor activity is recorded by applying needle, wire surface electrode

Table 1: Drugs useful in essential tremor.

Primidone	Start with 12.5/25 mg at night, and increase up to 250 mg/day
Beta-blockers	Propranolol start with 40 mg/day increase to 120 mg/day
Benzodiazepines	Alprazolam 0.25–3 mg/day, clonazepam 0.5–4 mg/day
Clozapine	6–75 mg/day
Gabapentin	Up to 1,200 mg/day
Flunarizine	Up to 10 mg/day clonidine or mirtazapine up to 30 mg/day

over the involved muscle. Electromyography is also helpful in differentiating the essential tremor and tremor due to Parkinsonism.
- *Accelerometer*: It is considered a gold standard for evaluation of tremor. This is also helpful in differentiating Parkinson's tremor from the essential tremor.
- *Others*: Other methods for evaluation of tremor are Tremor rating scale, Archimedes spiral drawing and handwriting assessment, volumetry, nine-hole pegboard test, Gibson maze test.

TREATMENT

Treatment of tremor depends upon evaluation and underlying cause. Dopamine agonist levodopa in Parkinson's disease and propranolol and primidone are effective in essential tremor. Clonazepam, gabapentin topiramate can be tried for refectory essential tremor.

Drugs Useful in Essential Tremor

Drugs useful in essential tremor have been shown in **Table 1**.

For medically refractory essential tremor, deep brain stimulation, and unilateral thalamotomy are effective.

CONCLUSION

Essential tremor is most common movement disorder in general practice. History taking, detail neurological examination is essential to ascertain the cause of tremor. Medical treatment is preferred but surgery is advisable in tremor refractory to medical management.

CHAPTER 87

Vertigo (Dizziness)

Kishalay Datta, Rigenjyoti Kalita

INTRODUCTION

Vertigo is the perception of movement, where no movement exists. The Latin word *vertō* stands for "a whirling or spinning movement."

Vertiginous symptoms in patients are often linked to several explanations like giddiness, anxiety, weakness, syncope, presyncope, and disturbances in balance.

Vertigo with nausea and vomiting, gait disturbances, spontaneous nystagmus, and postural instability can also be caused by injury to peripheral or central vestibular structures.

ETIOLOGY

Vertigo or dizziness may be associated with metabolic, neurological, cardiovascular, and psychiatric causes. **Table 1** highlights the causes of vertigo.

PATHOPHYSIOLOGY

Vertigo arises due to mismatch of information arising from three systems:
1. Visual
2. Vestibular
3. Proprioception.

These three systems are responsible for maintenance of body's equilibrium and orientation with respect to gravity.

Table 1: Causes of vertigo.

Peripheral causes	Central causes
Acute otitis media	Vertebral basilar artery insufficiency
Cerumen or hair in external auditory canal (EAC)	Subclavian steal syndrome
Benign positional vertigo	Cerebellar hemorrhage/infarction
Labyrinthitis	Infection in brain
Vestibular neuronitis	Trauma/tumor
Ménière's disease	Multiple sclerosis
Trauma	Cervical spine muscle and ligamentous injury
Acoustic neuroma	Migraine

Visual inputs provide additional information about body's position in space.

Proprioceptive organs located in muscles and joints (joint sensation) send information about relative positions of the parts of the body.

Vestibular apparatus in ear consist of utricle, saccule, and three semicircular canals. The semicircular canals contain fluid called endolymph which provides information about movement and angular momentum and the otoliths present there provide information about the orientation of the body with respect to gravity.

Vertigo is caused by freely moving debris within the semicircular canal under the influence of gravity. The movement of fluid in the canals causes specialized hair cells inside the canals to move, causing afferent vestibular impulses to fire. Sensory inputs are then transmitted by eighth cranial nerve, which enter the brainstem and proceed to the four vestibular nuclei in the brainstem and to cerebellum. From there impulses travel along two pathways: (1) the medial longitudinal fasciculus and (2) the vestibulospinal tract. Connections between these structures and the oculomotor nuclei [vestibulo-ocular reflex (VOR)] complete the entire system.

Healthy vestibular systems allow the eyes to compensate for body movements in different directions and to maintain a visual axis that is stable with respect to the environment.

A periodic rhythmic eye movement called nystagmus sometimes accompanies with vertigo. Nystagmus has a *slow* and a *fast* component.

Slow component is due to the VOR and is generated by excitation of the semicircular canal, producing eye movement away from that canal.

The fast component of nystagmus is caused by the cortex, which exerts a quick corrective movement in the opposite direction. Direction is always named after the fast phase.

Finally to conclude, peripheral vertigo is caused by disorders affecting the vestibular apparatus and the eighth cranial nerve; whereas central vertigo is caused by disorders affecting central structures, such as the brainstem and the cerebellum.

CLINICAL PRESENTATION

Patient usually presents with spinning of head while stationary. Other presenting features may be nausea, vomiting, unsteadiness, jerking eye movements, headache and hearing loss, frequent falls, neurological or muscular issues.

Characteristic features of types of vertigo are listed in **Table 2**.

RED FLAGS

Red flags have been shown in **Box 1**.

EVALUATION

History

Evaluation of the patient with dizziness begins with careful history taking, complete neurological examination, which also must include vestibular examination.

The history should focus on the nature of the symptoms, the duration, and aggravating and relieving factors.

Table 2: Characteristics between central and peripheral vertigo.

	Peripheral	*Central*
Onset	Sudden	Gradual or sudden
Intensity	Severe	Mild
Duration	Usually seconds to minutes	Usually weeks, but can be minutes with vascular causes
Associated nausea/diaphoresis	Frequent	Variable
Auditory symptoms	May be present including tinnitus	None
Headache/neck pain		
Nystagmus	Usually horizontal	Horizontal, rotatory, or vertical
Central nervous system (CNS) symptoms	Absent	Usually present
Horizontal head impulse, nystagmus, and test of skew	Normal	At least one abnormal

Box 1: Red flags—look for "DANISH."

- Dysdiadokokinesia
- Ataxia
- Nystagmus
- Intention tremor
- Slurring of speech
- Hypotonia

It is also important to ask the patient if they have experienced any abnormal eye movements during a dizzy spell or when sudden change in the position of the head occurs.

Time of onset and duration of vertigo symptoms also carefully evaluated in history.

Acute onset of vertigo which lasts for minutes can be due to migraine or brain or vascular disease especially in elderly population. Cardiovascular and drug history should be elicited.

Patient and family members should be inquired about any history of anxiety and depression.

Physical Examination

Physical examination begins with complete ear, neurologic, and otological examinations in patients presenting with vertigo.

Patient's pulses and blood pressure should be checked in both arms.

Any significant difference may give suspicion about subclavian steal syndrome, which also can cause vertebrobasilar artery insufficiency.

Head and Neck Examination

External auditory canal and tympanic membrane should be examined for evidence of otitis media, cholesteatoma, and other pathology.

Test for hearing like Weber and Rinne testing should also be done.

Detailed otoscopic examination is necessary to rule out causes in ear. Also cerumen or a foreign object impaction in the ear canal has to be checked for.

The neck should be auscultated along the course of the carotid artery for carotid or vertebral artery bruits suggesting atherosclerosis.

Eyes should be examined for abnormalities of pupils and extraocular movements. Special attention should be given for cranial nerve 3 and 6 and for descending sympathetic tract involvement.

Nystagmus characteristics are one of the most valuable tools for distinguishing peripheral from central causes of vertigo.

The abnormal jerky nystagmus of inner ear disease consists of slow and quick components. The eyes slowly "drift" in the direction of the diseased, hypoactive ear, then quickly jerk back to the intended direction of gaze.

Positional nystagmus, induced by rapidly changing the position of the head, strongly suggests an organic vestibular disorder.

Dix-Hallpike maneuver (**Figs. 1A to C**): It is a diagnostic maneuver used to identify benign paroxysmal positional vertigo (BPPV).

Patient's eyes must be open, while being seated upright during performing this test after premedicating with dimenhydrinate.

To test the right posterior semicircular canal, rotate the head 30–45° to the right. Keeping the head in this position, rapidly bring the patient supine until the head is 20° below the level of the examining table. This is called Dix-Hallpike position.

Rotatory nystagmus following a latency of no more than 30 seconds is considered a positive test.

Return the patient to the upright sitting position, and repeat the test on the other side. The side exhibiting the positive test is the side of the lesion.

Patients with spinal injury, carotid bruits, vertebrobasilar insufficiency, or cerebrovascular accidents (CVAs) should take precautions while performing this test.

Epley's maneuver (**Figs. 1D and E**): It is used to treat BPPV by keeping the patient in Dix-Hallpike position for 1–2 minutes.

The patient's head is then rotated 90° in the opposite direction, keeping the head and neck in a fixed position, the individual rolls on their shoulder rotating the head another 90° in the direction they are facing. The eye should be observed for nystagmus.

Finally the patient is brought up in a sitting position, maintain 45° rotation of head and holding this position for 30 seconds.

HINTS testing: HINTS testing is an important advancement in the assessment of acute vestibular syndrome.

HINTS stands for three bed side tests namely (1) horizontal head impulse test, (2) nystagmus, and (3) test of skew. These tests when taken together reliably help to distinguish central (usually stroke) from peripheral acute vestibular syndrome.

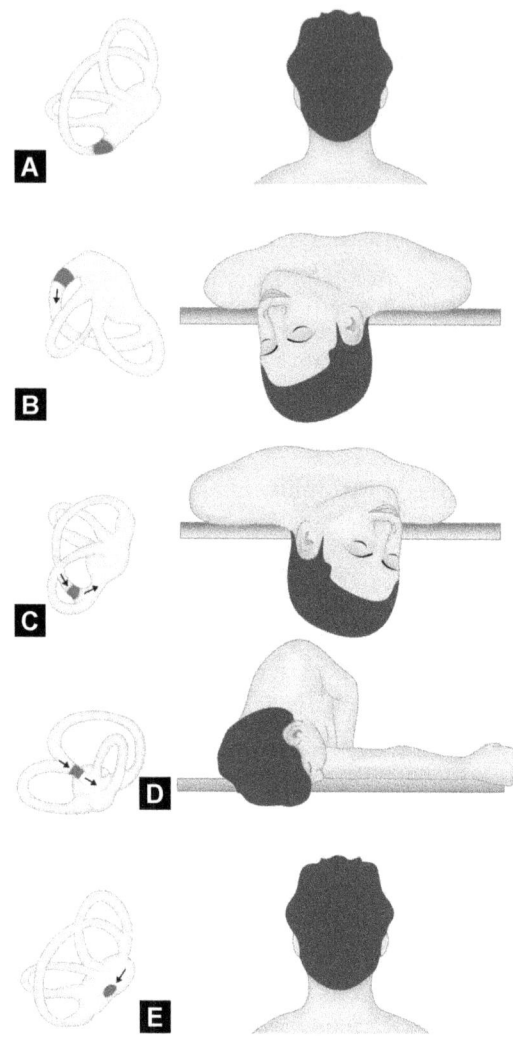

Figs. 1A to E: (A to C) Dix-Hallpike position test; (D and E) Epley maneuver.

INVESTIGATIONS

Imaging and Ancillary Tests

Most patients with vertigo do not require extensive diagnostic testing.

Hypoglycemia can present as vertigo, so finger stick blood glucose test is must.

Patients of infectious pathology should undergo routine blood tests.

Tests for blood counts, thyroid function test, electrolytes, and electrocardiogram (ECG) may be helpful to establish the cause of vertigo.

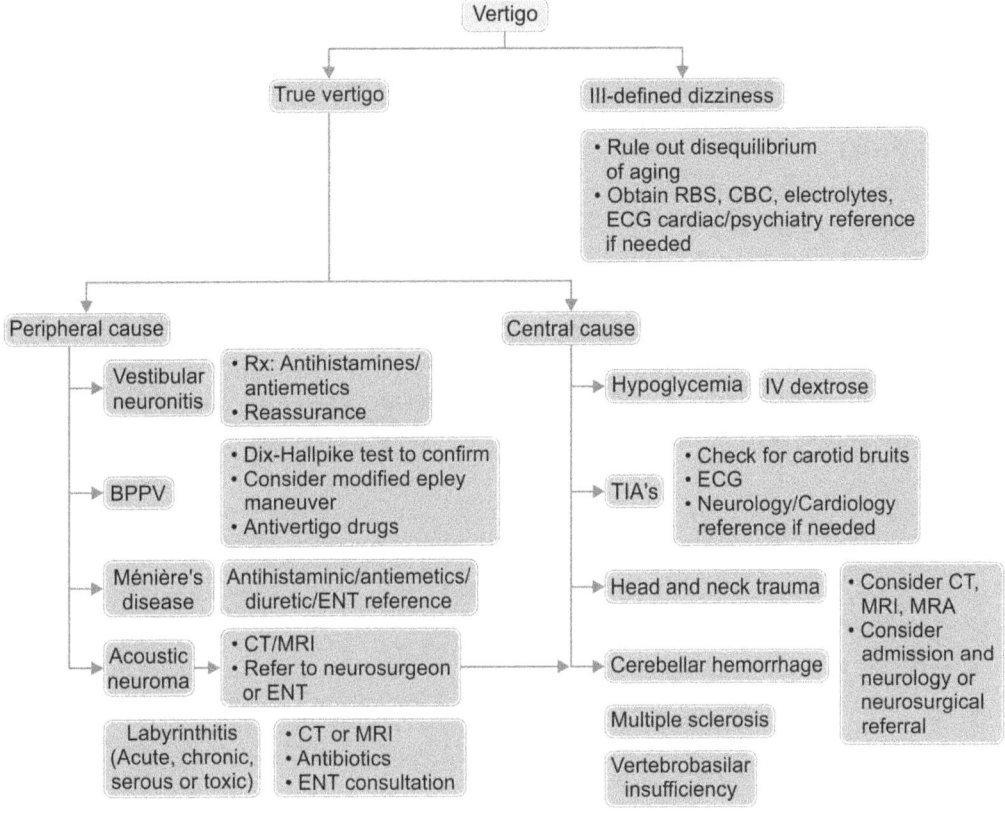

Flowchart 1: Clinical and diagnostic approach to vertigo.

Radiologic Imaging

Computed tomography (CT) and magnetic resonance imaging (MRI) are the best modality to evaluate if there is suspicion of intracranial pathology.

Magnetic resonance imaging with angiography or diffusion-weighted imaging (DWI) is particularly useful for the diagnosis of stroke, tumors, sclerotic, and demyelinating lesions.

MANAGEMENT

Treatment plan has to be started after making a final diagnosis of a specific diseases causing vertigo.

Diazepam in 2–5 mg intravenous (IV) doses is effective in stopping vertigo.

Anticholinergic or antihistamines with anticholinergic activity are extremely useful in treating peripheral vertigo, e.g. meclizine (25 mg tid), diphenhydramine hydrochloride (25–50 mg tid) and dimenhydrinate IV, promethazine hydrochloride (25 mg orally).

Acute bacterial labyrinthitis requires IV antibiotics and vestibular rehabilitation exercise. Surgical drainage and debridement might be needed.

Ménière's disease is often treated successfully by vasodilation and diuretic therapy.

Cerebellar hemorrhage causing vertigo should undergo CT or MRI and neurosurgery consultations.

In addition, BPPV generally improves with canalith repositioning procedures.

SUMMARY

In general practice, it is important to determine whether the patient has true vertigo or not, and if yes whether it has a central or peripheral cause.

In elderly patient's vertigo might be the sole manifestation of a life-threatening underlying pathology.

Most vertigo having peripheral cause can be discharged from ED.

Patients with central vertigo may require neuroimaging and other diagnostic tests to establish the life-threatening causes of vertigo. Clinical and diagnostic approach to vertigo is described in **Flowchart 1**.

CHAPTER 88

Voice Disorders

Deepak Dalmia

INTRODUCTION

Voice disorders are medical conditions involving abnormal pitch, loudness, or quality of the sound produced by the larynx and thereby affecting speech production.

ETIOLOGY

The larynx contains the vocal cords and serves as the production of voice and opening to the tracheobronchial tree.

Laryngeal disorders that affect the vocal cord mobility lead to voice disorders.
- Professional voice
- Puberphonia
- Laryngitis (chorditis)
- Benign vocal cord lesion (vocal cord nodule, vocal cord cyst, vocal cord hemangioma)
- Contact granuloma or ulcer (postintubation)
- Vocal cord paralysis (iatrogenic o viral)
- Spasmodic dysphonia
- Neurologic disease (multiple sclerosis, amyotrophic lateral sclerosis, myasthenia gravis, parkinsonism)
- Benign laryngeal tumor—leukoplakia of vocal cord, papilloma, hemangioma, neurofibroma
- Vocal cord carcinoma.

PATHOPHYSIOLOGY

Professional Voice

People who use their voice professionally in public for a prolonged period (singers, politician, teachers) often develop voice disorder due to vocal cord nodule, vocal cord granuloma.

Puberphonia
- A type of voice disorder occurs due to habitual use of a high-pitched voice after puberty.
- Generally it is psychogenic or may be occasionally associated with laryngeal muscle tension, vocal cord asymmetry, nonfusion of thyroid lamina.

Laryngitis

Excessive use of voice, laryngopharyngeal reflux, allergic reaction, inhalation of irritating substance (smoke).

Benign Vocal Cord Lesion (Figs. 1 and 2)

- Polyps and nodules result from injury to the lamina propria of the true vocal cords.
- Granulomas result from injury to the perichondrium overlying the vocal processes of the arytenoid cartilages either due to intubation or laryngopharyngeal reflux.

Vocal Cord Paralysis

- Unilateral vocal cord paralysis is most common. About one-third of unilateral paralyses are neoplastic in origin, one-third are traumatic, and one-third are idiopathic.
- Recurrent laryngeal nerve paralysis is caused by neck or thoracic lesions (aneurysm, thyroid carcinoma, tumor of lung, esophagus, and mediastinum).
- Following thyroidectomy.

Spasmodic Dysphonia

Intermittent spasm of laryngeal muscles causing abnormal voice leading to dysphonia.

Benign Laryngeal Tumor (Fig. 3)

- Papilloma, hemangioma, neurofibroma can affect any part of larynx.
- Papilloma may be associated with human papillomavirus 6, 11, 16, 18.

Vocal Cord Carcinoma (Fig. 4)

- Associated with chronic smokers, premalignant lesion of vocal cord like leukoplakia and papilloma has increased propensity to develop vocal cord carcinoma.

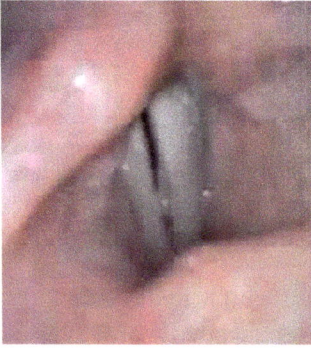

Fig. 1: Vocal cord polyp.

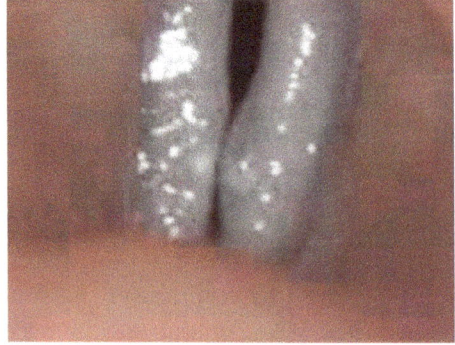

Fig. 2: Vocal cord cyst.

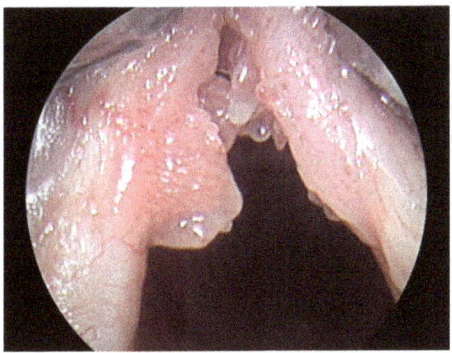

Fig. 3: Vocal cord papilloma.

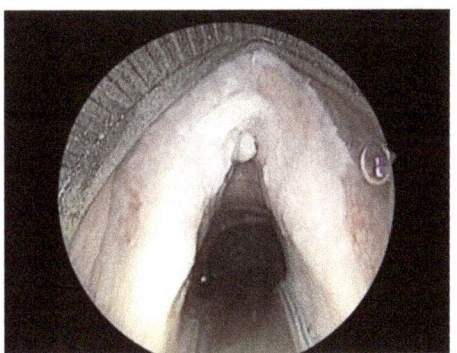

Fig. 4: Vocal cord leukoplakia.

CLINICAL PRESENTATION

Professional Voice
The voice becomes breathy and hoarse which is gradual onset.

Puberphonia
- Puberphonia is characterized by the failure to transition into the lower pitched voice of adulthood in male.
- In conjunction with an atypically high pitch, common symptoms include a weak, breathy, or hoarse voice as well as a low vocal intensity, pitch breaks, and shallow breathing.

Laryngitis
- Fever, malaise, dysphagia, and throat pain.
- Sudden change of voice.
- Constant urge to clear throat.
- Volume is typically greatly decreased; some patients have aphonia. Hoarseness, a sensation of tickling, rawness.

Benign Vocal Cord Lesion
Vocal cord nodule, polyp, and granuloma all develop slowly developing breathy voice and hoarseness.

Vocal Cord Paralysis
In unilateral paralysis, the voice may be hoarse and breathy.

Spasmodic Dysphonia
- In adductor spasmodic dysphonia, patients attempt to speak through the spasmodic closure with a voice that sounds squeezed, effortful, or strained.

- In abductor spasmodic dysphonia, sudden interruption of sound caused by momentary abduction of vocal cord.

Benign Laryngeal Tumor

Hoarseness, breathy voice, dyspnea, aspiration, dysphagia, and hemoptysis.

Vocal Cord Carcinoma

- Hoarseness is the first symptom with pain.
- Occasional lymphadenopathy.

RED FLAGS

If voice changes or disorder associated with stridor, urgent specialist opinion should be taken.

EVALUATION

Puberphonia

History

Adolescent or adult male.

Clinical Examination

- To examine the larynx if it is high in position.
- Palpation of laryngeal area if high in muscular tension.
- Presence of breathy voice, an indication of speech in the Falsetto register, and other distortions of vocal quality.

Laryngitis

History

Unusual change of voice following fever or upper respiratory tract infection (URTI).

Clinical Examination

- Febrile
- Both indirect laryngoscopy and direct laryngoscopy show erythema and edematous larynx.

Benign Vocal Cord Lesion

History

Slowly developing hoarseness of voice with vocal abuse.

Clinical Examination

- Laryngoscopy (vocal cord polyp is usually unilateral, vocal cord nodule is bilateral that occurs at membranous cord, granuloma often bilateral).
- Stroboscopy.

Vocal Cord Paralysis
History
History of chronic heavy metal exposure, connective tissue disorder, diabetes, alcoholism, thyroid surgery.

Clinical Examination
Laryngoscopy.

Spasmodic Dysphonia
History
History of squeezed, effortful, and strained voice.

Clinical Examination
Laryngoscopy.

Benign Laryngeal Lesion
- Direct laryngoscopy
- Contrast-enhanced computed tomography (CECT) of larynx.

Vocal Cord Carcinoma
- Direct laryngoscopy
- CECT of larynx to know the extent of disease and cervical adenopathy.

INVESTIGATIONS
- Indirect laryngoscopy
- Direct laryngoscopy
- Flexible fiberoptic laryngoscopy
- Endoscopy
- Spectrograph
- Videostroboscopy
- Electroglottography (EGG)
- Electromyography (EMG)
- Aerodynamic measurements
- Pitch measurements
- Perceptual assessment of voice (pitch, loudness, resonance, respiration, phonation).

TREATMENT

Puberphonia

Direct Voice Therapy

- Cough
- Glottal attack before a vowel
- Speech range masking
- Laryngeal musculature relaxation technique
- Lowering of larynx to appropriate position
- Humming while sliding down the scale.

Indirect Voice Therapy

Creating an environment where direct treatment options will be more effective like counseling by psychologist.

Surgery

- Indication is when traditional voice therapy is ineffective.
- Relaxation thyroplasty or window relaxation thyroplasty.

Laryngitis

- Symptomatic treatment.
- Cough suppressants, voice rest, and steam inhalations relieve symptoms and promote resolution of acute laryngitis.
- Specific treatments to control gastroesophageal reflux.
- Steroid has a supportive role in case of edematous larynx.

Benign Vocal Cord Lesion

- Correction of voice abuse
- Speech therapy
- Treatment of reflux.

Microlaryngeal Surgery

- An operating microscope is used to examine, biopsy, and operate on the larynx. Images can be recorded on video as well. The patient is anesthetized, and the airway is secured by high-pressure jet ventilation through the laryngoscope, endotracheal intubation, or, for an inadequate upper airway, tracheotomy.
- Tissue can be removed precisely and accurately either by cold instruments or LASER minimizing damage (possibly permanent) to the vocal mechanism.

Vocal Cord Paralysis
- In unilateral paralysis, treatment is directed at improving voice quality through augmentation, medialization, or reinnervation.
- Augmentation involves injecting collagen, micronized dermis, or autologous fat into the paralyzed cord, bringing the cords closer together to improve the voice and prevent aspiration.
- Medialization is shifting the vocal cord toward the midline by inserting an adjustable spacer laterally to the affected cord by a procedure called thyroplasty.
- Reinnervation has only rarely been successful.
- In bilateral vocal cord paralysis, airway is to be maintained first by tracheostomy.

Spasmodic Dysphonia
- For adductor spasmodic dysphonia, surgery has been more successful than other approaches. Injection of botulinum toxin into vocal adductors has restored a normal voice in up to 3 months. Because the effect is temporary, injections may be repeated.

Benign Laryngeal Lesion
- Smaller lesions may be excised endoscopically by using a CO_2 laser.
- Larger lesions extending beyond the laryngeal framework often require pharyngotomy or laryngofissure.

Vocal Cord Carcinoma
- CO_2 laser-assisted cordectomy with neck dissection if required.

SUMMARY
- Proper evaluation of cause of voice disorder is essential for the treatment.
- Most of the vocal cord lesions can be dealt with microlaryngeal surgeries.
- Puberphonia and professional voice require a good speech therapy along with the surgery.

CHAPTER 89

Vomiting in Adults

Ravindra Kale

INTRODUCTION

Vomiting refers to expulsions of gastric contents due to strong abdominothoracic muscle and gut contractions. It may occur as a protective response to certain ingested toxins or may be an indicator of serious organ system dysfunction. Vomiting is usually associated with nausea (subjective feeling to vomit) and retching (abdominal contraction without oral expulsion). Vomiting should be differentiated from regurgitation and rumination which are effortless expulsion of food.

ETIOLOGY

Vomiting and nausea are associated with a variety of gastrointestinal (GI) and non-GI disorders (**Table 1**). In tropical countries, acute onset vomiting most commonly is due to gastroenteritis or systemic infections and usually associated with diarrhea. Food borne infections can be due to contaminated water or food material. *Staphylococcus aureus* and

Table 1: Etiology of vomiting

GI causes	Other organ systems	Miscellaneous
Gastric—gastritis GERD Peptic ulcer Malignancy Gastric outlet obstruction Gastroparesis	Endocrine metabolic Uremia Diabetic ketoacidosis Pregnancy Addison's disease Hypercalcemia	Drug induced NSAIDs Antimalarials Chemotherapeutic agents Oral contraceptive Alternative medicine
Hepatobiliary Hepatitis Cholecystitis Biliary colic Pancreatitis	*Cardiac* Acute MI *Cerebral lesions* Brain tumor Hemorrhage Brain abscess	Toxins Alcohol Food borne Poisoning
Bowel obstruction Ischemic bowel	Psychiatric Bulimia Anorexia nervosa	Radiation Motion sickness
Food poisoning		Cyclic vomiting syndrome

Bacillus cereus produce toxins which cause emesis. Viral infection by rotavirus, adenovirus, etc. can also cause gastroenteritis. Systemic infections like meningitis, hepatitis, upper respiratory infections can also cause nausea and vomiting.

Other most frequent cause is medication. Drugs act on vomiting center as well as on GI tract to cause nausea and vomiting. Nonsteroidal anti-inflammatory agents commonly cause gastritis and peptic ulcers sometimes resulting in stricture and resultant obstruction. They also can cause acute kidney injury. Nonsteroidal anti-inflammatory drug (NSAID) analgesic like tramadol frequently causes nausea and emesis. Aspirin and cardiac antiarrhythmic, antihypertensive can induce emesis. Other common agents are anticancer treatment, metronidazole, antidiabetic (metformin, exenatide), antidepressants [selective serotonin reuptake inhibitor (SSRI), tricyclic antidepressants (TCAs)], oral contraceptives, diuretics, and nicotine. Consumption of bottle gourd (known as *lauki* or *dudhi* in India) juice is a treatment advocated by alternative medicine practitioners. Bitter juice contains toxin cucurbitacin and can lead to nausea, vomiting, GI bleeding, and death.

Mechanical gut obstruction due to various causes is associated with abdominal distention, pain and nausea which may get partial relief on vomiting. Obstruction could be due to strictures, volvulus or adhesions or due to extrinsic compression by superior mesenteric artery. Gastroparesis due to diabetes; neurological conditions like Parkinsonism and malignancy can cause nausea and vomiting in 70-80% patients. Other abdominal conditions like acute cholecystitis, appendicitis, and pancreatitis may also induce nausea, vomiting.

Cyclic vomiting syndrome is an idiopathic disorder characterized by intermittent episodes of nausea and vomiting with intervening normal periods. Each episode lasts for 4-6 days with exacerbation due to emotional stress, food allergy, menses, or pregnancy. Patients of diabetic gastroparesis and marijuana addicts can also have cyclic pattern of vomiting.

PATHOPHYSIOLOGY

Vomiting primarily appears to be a protective reflex; may occur in response to various types of stimuli. Unpleasant, strong thoughts, pain, smell or sight can produce vomiting. Area postrema also known as chemoreceptor trigger zone is located outside blood–brain barrier and is sensitive to various toxins including food borne as well as endogenous like in uremia and ketoacidosis and drugs. Labyrinth in inner ear is sensitive to movements. Muscarinic MI and histaminic H1 receptors get stimulated in motion sickness, morning sickness, and ear infection. Cannabinoid CB1 receptors located in dorsal vagal nuclei in brain stem inhibit vomiting reflex. Neurokinin NK-1 receptors in area postrema are activated by substance P and are responsible for chemotherapeutic agents induced vomiting. Serotonergic 5HT3 receptors on vagal afferents are stimulated by serotonin release by enteroendocrine cells in response to toxins and drugs. Coordination of vomiting is done at vomiting center in medulla. Stimulation of brain 5HT3 receptors release dopamine which acts on D2 receptors in vomiting center. This starts emesis by induction of nausea, gastric contraction, and inhibition of gut peristaltic slow waves. Thoracic muscles contract with closed glottis leads to retching. Reverse peristalsis in small intestine in combination of thoracoabdominal muscle contraction leads to expulsion of food contents through mouth.

CLINICAL PRESENTATION

Vomiting must be differentiated from regurgitation which is effortless expulsion of gastric contents. Acute onset vomiting usually is result of strong painful stimuli in abdomen, gut obstruction, toxins, metabolic causes (uremia, diabetic ketoacidosis) or food borne infections. Early morning vomiting is seen in pregnancy, alcohol, and metabolic disorders. Vomiting after meals occurs in gastroparesis, gastric outlet obstruction, and achalasia cardia. Achalasia patients may also reports regurgitation of food at night and nasal regurgitation. Bilious vomiting with obstipation and abdominal distention suggest intestinal obstruction. Sudden onset vomiting without nausea or retching (projectile vomiting) may indicate raised intracranial pressure usually due to intracerebral space occupying lesions. It may be associated with headache and visual symptoms.

RED FLAGS

- Abdominal pain
- Jaundice
- Weight loss
- Hematemesis
- Presence of lump
- Severe headache
- Postural symptoms.

EVALUATION

History

Evaluation of patient with acute onset vomiting (<1-week duration) requires detailed history of recent travel, food habits, associated abdominal pain or diarrhea. Vomiting and diarrhea of acute onset suggest acute gastroenteritis. History of amenorrhea is important in woman of childbearing age. Careful interrogation about any poisoning or drug overdose is required. History of associated abdominal pain, distention, and obstipation may suggest peritonitis due to perforation, pancreatitis or obstruction. Vomiting relieves abdominal pain due to obstruction but not in other conditions like pancreatitis and cholecystitis. Presence of anorexia, nausea, vomiting before onset of jaundice suggests acute hepatitis. History of postural giddiness, excessive thirst, and oliguria suggest significant volume depletion. History of fever and headache with or without altered sensorium points toward meningeal irritation or raised intracranial pressure. Vomiting due to gastric outlet obstruction or gastroparesis occurs within an hour after meals and may contain food ingested hours before. It may be associated with postprandial fullness. Cough and fever may be indicative of aspiration. Dyspnea and chest pain after vomiting should alert for possible esophageal perforation.

Physical Examination

Assessment should be made for hydration and nutritional insufficiency. Tachycardia, orthostatic hypotension, and dehydration suggest significant volume loss. Lymphadenopathy may be due to tuberculosis or disseminated malignancy. Jaundice and epigastric lump with excoriation marks on skin may suggest obstructive jaundice due to malignancy. Distended abdomen with high pitch bowel sounds suggests intestinal obstruction while absent bowel sound and tender abdomen with guarding suggests peritonitis. Per rectal examination may reveal impacted fecal matter, growth, rectal shelf (pelvic metastatic deposits) or empty rectum (intestinal obstruction). Presence of blood on examining finger could be due to rectal growth, ulceration or ischemic bowel. Epigastric lump with visible peristalsis and presence of succussion splash suggest gastric outlet obstruction.

INVESTIGATIONS

Complete blood counts, creatinine, electrolytes, arterial blood gas (ABG), serum calcium, serum glutamic pyruvic transaminase (SGPT), random blood sugar, and ketones to be sent and chest and abdominal radiographs to be ordered to look for obstruction, bowel perforation and esophageal perforation (Boerhaave's syndrome). Further evaluation with cross-sectional imaging [computed tomography (CT)/magnetic resonance imaging (MRI)] may be required. ABGs to be sent for acid–base imbalance.

TREATMENT

Management of acute vomiting requires assessment for etiology, dehydration, electrolyte imbalance, and possible complications. Patients with mild symptoms can be managed with oral prokinetics and antiemetics. Poisoning and drug overdose are to be treated by nasogastric aspiration and lavage, activated charcoal and specific antidote. Start antiemetics. Fluid resuscitation should be started according to degree of dehydration. Endoscopy can be done, if required, after initial resuscitation. Patient with gastric outlet obstruction may require nasogastric aspiration and lavage to empty stomach before endoscopy.

Patients with chronic vomiting should be assessed for malnutrition. Replacement of fluid, electrolytes, and vitamins is done wherever indicated. Chronic vomiting should be treated with prokinetics and antiemetic agents. Most commonly used antiemetics are substituted benzamides, which acts as D2 receptor antagonist. D2 receptor antagonism at area postrema reduces nausea and vomiting while effect on gastric D2 receptors improves gastric emptying. Metoclopramide and levosulpiride are available in oral and intravenous (IV) preparation. Rapid IV metoclopramide injection may produce restlessness. Metoclopramide crosses blood–brain barrier and causes dystonia, extrapyramidal symptoms, tardive dyskinesia, QT prolongation, and hyperprolactinemia. It also acts on peripheral 5-HT4 receptor causing acetylcholine release leading to increased antroduodenal motility. Domperidone is much safer as it does not cross blood–brain barrier although it can cause hyperprolactinemia and galactorrhea. It can be used in levodopa induce vomiting in Parkinson's diseases. Itopride acts as antagonist of D2 receptor and acetylcholine esterase inhibitor. Motilin agonist erythromycin enhances gastric emptying.

The 5-HT3 antagonist ondansetron and granisetron are useful in postsurgical and chemotherapeutic agents induced vomiting. They block 5-HT3 receptors in stomach and vomiting center. Side effects are raised liver enzymes, QT prolongation, and headache. Ondansetron can be used safely in pregnancy. Palonosetron is very effective in chemotherapeutic drugs induced nausea and vomiting.

Ginger and doxylamine-pyridoxine combination is also used in pregnancy.

Phenothiazines like prochlorperazine block D2 receptors and muscarinic M1 receptors. They are potent antiemetic but with extrapyramidal side effects. Olanzapine does not have extrapyramidal side effect and is a good alternative.

Antihistaminic agents—cyclizine and dimenhydrinate block central H1 receptors and are useful for motion sickness.

Combination of glucocorticoids, NK1 receptor antagonist (aprepitant), and cannabinoids (tetrahydrocannabinol) is used for chemotherapeutic-induced vomiting.

SUMMARY

Vomiting is expulsion of GI food contents due to abdominothoracic muscle contractions and occurs in a wide variety of conditions. It can be treated by various antiemetic and prokinetics. Presence of significant adverse effects poses difficulty in prolong treatment with these agents.

CHAPTER 90

Weight Gain (Obesity)

Jasvinder Singh Anand

INTRODUCTION

Obesity affects at least nine organs systems and is one of the most prevalent and expensive medical problems seen in daily practice. Several chronic diseases can be impacted by preventing and treating obesity. Despite of knowing the importance of screening and evaluation of obesity, detection, and counseling rates among physicians remain low. The primary reason for the same is that the physicians find it time consuming and nonrewarding. Obesity is a global epidemic and its momentum is not going to slow down in near future. Obesity is a risk factor for many disorders like hypertension, dyslipidemia, heart disease, diabetes mellitus, stroke, obstructive sleep apnea, and cancer. One of the major worries is that many of these conditions like hypertension, dyslipidemia, and diabetes mellitus can be silent killers. Even small gains in weight are associated with increased health risks.

ETIOLOGY AND PATHOPHYSIOLOGY

An excess of body fat mass attributable to a greater number and/or size of fat cells (adipocytes) relative to other cell types is the defining characteristic of obesity.

"One need not be a rocket scientist to understand that increased food intake tends to be associated with obesity." Consuming an extra candy bar (~220 kcal) as a snack every day will result in a gain of approximately 11 lb (5 kg) in 1 year and approximately 22 lb (10 kg) in 3 years.

Lifestyle plays a major role in the development of obesity. Those having an urbanized and sedentary life are definitely more predisposed to obesity compared to the ones having a rural and active lifestyle. In rural Japan, the prevalence of type 2 diabetes was approximately 4%, whereas among Japanese who have immigrated to the United States, the prevalence rises to more than 21%.

It used to be said that the only exercise effective in combating obesity was pushing one's chair back from the dining table. It is now recognized that physical activity—i.e. increased energy expenditure—has a much more positive role in reducing fat storage and adjusting energy balance in the obese, particularly if associated with modification of the diet.

The biggest risk factor amongst the sedentary behaviors for obesity and diabetes is prolonged TV watching. In the Nurses' Health Study, after adjustment for age, smoking, exercise level, and dietary factors, every 2-hour increment spent watching TV was associated with a 23% increase in obesity and a 14% increase in the risk of diabetes.

Sleep deprivation also significantly increases the risk of obesity as it results in excessive eating especially of energy dense and carbohydrate-rich foods.

Smoking cessation can lead to an average weight gain of 4-5 kg. Nicotine withdrawal is the main culprit as it leads to an increase in food consumption.

Several drugs like antipsychotics, antidepressants, and antidiabetics can lead to weight gain. Hence, taking the drug history becomes extremely important to rule out the causes of obesity.

The hormonal causes of obesity like Cushing's syndrome, hypothyroidism and polycystic ovary syndrome (PCOS) should also be thought of while evaluating a patient of obesity.

■ CLINICAL PRESENTATION AND COMPLICATIONS

Body mass index (BMI) is recommended, because it provides an estimate of body fat and is related to risk of disease. A desirable or healthy BMI is 18.5-24.9 kg/m^2; overweight is 25-29.9 kg/m^2, and obesity is at least 30 kg/m^2. Obesity is further subdefined into class I (30.0-34.9 kg/m^2), class II (35.0-39.9 kg/m^2), and class III (at least 40 kg/m^2).

Obese persons with excess abdominal fat are at higher risk for diabetes, hypertension, dyslipidemia, and ischemic heart disease than obese persons whose fat is located predominantly in the lower body (**Fig. 1**).

Waist circumference is highly correlated with abdominal fat mass and is often used as a surrogate marker for abdominal (upper body) obesity.

The World Health Organization (WHO) has indicated that waist circumference thresholds denoting increased risk in the Asian population should be 90 cm for men and 80 cm for women.

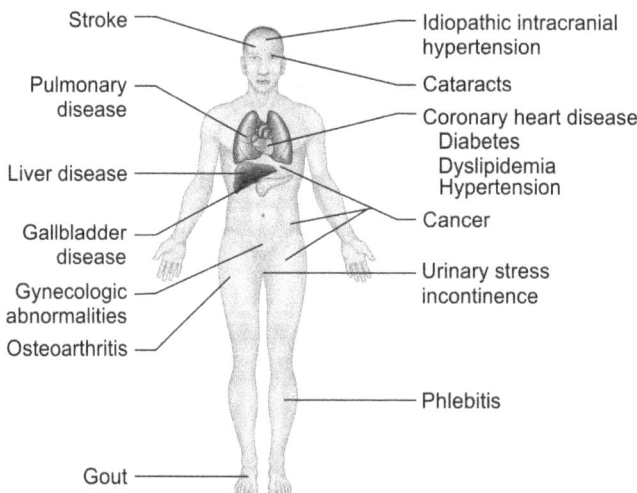

Fig. 1: Obese persons with higher risk for diseases.

RED FLAGS

Morbid obesity is a term used to define patients who meet criteria for bariatric surgery (BMI ≥40 kg/m², or BMI 35.0–39.9 kg/m² and one or more severe obesity-related medical complications, such as hypertension, type 2 diabetes mellitus (T2DM), heart failure, or sleep apnea).

According to the National Heart, Lung, and Blood Institute (NHLBI)/the North American Association for the Study of Obesity (NAASO) guide, patients at very high absolute risk, in need of intense risk factor modification and management, include people with established coronary heart disease; patients with other atherosclerotic diseases such as peripheral arterial disease, abdominal aortic aneurysm, or symptomatic carotid artery disease; and people with type 2 diabetes or sleep apnea. Patients with metabolic syndrome and those most likely to be insulin-resistant also require urgent treatment

EVALUATION: HISTORY AND PHYSICAL EXAMINATION

While evaluating a patient of obesity, there are several questions whose answers can guide us in managing the patient.
- What factors contribute to the patient's obesity?
- How is obesity affecting the patient's health?
- What is the patient's level of risk regarding obesity?
- What are the patient's goals and expectations?
- Is the patient motivated to enter a weight management program?
- What kind of help does the patient need?

A useful and convenient technique is to ask the patient to describe a typical day. "I want to learn more about your diet. Can you take me through a typical day or an example of a day, starting first thing in the morning and continuing into the evening?" This open-ended and nonjudgmental approach allows patients to reveal their dietary pattern without guilt or embarrassment.

An informative open-ended question is, "What is the most physically active thing you do over the course of a week?"

A thorough medication history should be taken to uncover possible drug-induced weight gain or medications interfering with weight loss.

The threshold for excessive abdominal fat is defined as a waist circumference of at least 90 cm in men and at least 80 cm in women amongst Asians. According to the NHLBI/NAASO guide, "To measure waist circumference, locate the upper hip bone and the top of the right iliac crest. Place a measuring tape in a horizontal plane around the abdomen at the level of the iliac crest. Before reading the tape measure, ensure that the tape is snug, but does not compress the skin, and is parallel to the floor. The measurement is made at the end of a normal expiration."

INVESTIGATIONS

There is no single laboratory test or diagnostic evaluation that is indicated for all patients with obesity. The specific evaluation performed should be based on presentation of symptoms, risk factors, and index of suspicion. Based on several other screening guideline recommendations, however, most if not all patients should have a fasting lipid panel (total, low-density lipoprotein (LDL) and high-density lipoprotein (HDL) cholesterol and triglyceride levels) and blood glucose measured at presentation, along with blood pressure (BP) determination.

TREATMENT

Three factors are necessary for physicians to intervene: (1) adequate recognition of obesity as a medical problem, (2) willingness to provide intervention, and (3) adequate skills or resources to do so. Even a modest weight loss, in the range of 5–10% from the patient's presentation weight, can result in significant initial improvement in the comorbidities of obesity. The initial management of individuals who would benefit from weight loss is a comprehensive lifestyle intervention: a combination of diet, exercise, and behavioral modification. The two major goals of the Diabetes Prevention Program lifestyle intervention were a minimum of 7% weight loss and a minimum of 150 minutes of exercise per week (such as brisk walking).

Dietary therapy: We suggest tailoring a diet that reduces energy intake below energy expenditure to individual patient preferences, rather than focusing on the macronutrient composition of the diet. Metabolic studies using state-of-the-art techniques have shown all adults will lose weight when fed less than 1,000 kcal/day. Thus, even subjects who are concerned that they are "metabolically resistant" to weight loss will lose weight if they comply with a diet of 800–1,200 kcal/day.

Exercise: Physical activity should be performed for approximately 30 minutes or more, 5–7 days a week, to prevent weight gain and to improve cardiovascular health.

Behavior modification: Behavior modification or behavior therapy is one cornerstone in the treatment for obesity. The goal of behavioral therapy is to help patients make long-term changes in their eating behavior by modifying and monitoring their food intake, modifying their physical activity, and controlling cues and stimuli in the environment that trigger eating. The key features of typical behavioral programs include self-monitoring, goal setting, nutrition and exercise education, stimulus control, problem solving, cognitive restructuring, and relapse prevention.

Drug therapy: Drug therapy may be an important constituent of the treatment regimen for obese individuals; it can be considered for those with a BMI greater than 30 kg/m^2, or a BMI of 27–29.9 kg/m^2 with comorbidities, who have not met weight loss goals (loss of at least 5% of total body weight at 3–6 months) with a comprehensive lifestyle intervention. In current practice, only two categories of weight loss drugs (appetite suppressants and lipase inhibitors) have been approved, and only two drugs are currently available for the specific indication of weight loss—phentermine and orlistat. Phentermine, an adrenergic reuptake inhibitor, augments adrenergic signaling within the central nervous system and peripheral tissues. Phentermine decreases appetite and food intake and increases resting metabolic rate to promote weight loss. Its side effects include tachycardia and hypertension. Orlistat, a lipase inhibitor, reversibly binds to lipase and prevents both absorption and digestion and absorption of certain dietary fats. Because orlistat also interferes with the absorption of fat-soluble vitamins, patients using this drug need to supplement fat-soluble vitamins A, D, E, and K. Orlistat has significant gastrointestinal side effects including diarrhea, steatorrhea, flatulence, fecal incontinence, and oily rectal discharge.

Surgery: Candidates for bariatric surgery include adults with a BMI greater than or equal to 40 kg/m², or a BMI of 35–39.9 kg/m² with at least one serious comorbidity, who have not met weight loss goals with diet, exercise, and drug therapy. Most patients in whom the surgery is a success achieve weight losses of 25–35% of body weight. The two most significant outcome measures of bariatric surgical success are weight loss and resolution of comorbidities. Larger weight loss goals are more appropriate for more profoundly obese individuals who are contemplating surgical interventions. Even with surgery, ideal weight is hardly ever achieved, and after a number of years at a plateau, weight gain often recurs. Contraindications to surgery include active substance abuse, defined noncompliance or inability to comply with medical care, schizophrenia, borderline personality disorder, or uncontrolled depression. The long-term follow-up of patients who have undergone gastric bypass surgery is needed to ensure adequate protein, calorie, vitamin, and mineral nutrition. Supplemental vitamin B_{12}, iron, and calcium are routinely added to standard multivitamins.

SUMMARY

Obesity will likely be the most significant medical problem that health care providers will face over the coming decades. This chronic disease has to be addressed aggressively by the physicians, providing preventive and therapeutic care. Because this topic traditionally has not been taught in medical school or residency training, physicians will need to acquire the knowledge, skills, and attitudes necessary to be effective obesity care providers.

CHAPTER 91

Weight Loss

Sharad Bedi

INTRODUCTION

Weight loss is one of the common complaints noted in a physician's clinic and is especially worrisome in the elderly. It may be voluntary or involuntary. Voluntary weight loss is generally not harmful and does not require any intervention. Involuntary weight loss is the condition which generally pushes an individual to see a doctor.

It is defined as a condition in which patient looses weight which does not have a reason or is not done purposefully. It also excludes weight loss which has happened following treatment of some known disease. It is also known as unintended or unintentional weight loss. Some other terminologies used categories of weight loss include:
- *Unexplained weight loss also known as isolated involuntary weight loss*: It is defined as weight loss which has not been done purposefully and the workup has failed to find a cause.
- *Sarcopenia geriatric syndrome*: It is defined by low muscle mass as per the reference charts and poor physical performance. Low muscle mass is defined as values less than two standard deviations below reference range.
- *Cachexia metabolic syndrome*: In this syndrome an underlying illness is the cause of low muscle mass. Other characteristics include fatigue and anorexia, decreased muscle strength, low fat-free mass index, and abnormal laboratory test. The weight loss should be more than or equal to 5% in less than a year.

ETIOLOGY

There are a large number of causes which can cause involuntary weight loss. Some of the common causes include:
- *Infections*: Tuberculosis, human immunodeficiency virus (HIV), hepatitis B, hepatitis C, worm infestations, abscess, empyema.
- *Chronic diseases*: Chronic kidney disease, chronic liver disease, congestive heart failure.
- *Malignancy*: Gastrointestinal (GI) cancers, prostate, renal, lung cancer, lymphomas.
- *Collagen vascular diseases*: Systemic lupus erythematosus, rheumatoid arthritis, sarcoidosis.
- *Gastrointestinal diseases*: Inflammatory bowel disease, celiac disease.

Box 1: List of medications leading to weight loss.

- Nonsteroidal anti-inflammatory drugs
- Opioids
- Antibiotics like metronidazole
- Angiotensin-converting enzyme (ACE) inhibitors
- Chemotherapy drugs
- Antiretroviral drugs
- Antihistaminics
- Metformin
- Antiepileptics like topiramate
- Bisphosphonates
- Alcohol, tobacco
- Ephedra
- Diuretics
- Selective serotonin reuptake inhibitors

Table 1: Etiological classification of causes of weight loss based on appetite.

Involuntary weight loss with preserved/increased appetite	Involuntary weight loss with loss of appetite
Uncontrolled diabetes mellitus	Malignancy
Hyperthyroidism	Severe cardiac or respiratory failure
Malabsorption	Advanced renal disease
Pheochromocytoma	Esophageal disease
Vigorous physical activity	Gastroduodenal disease
	Depression
	Human immunodeficiency virus (HIV)
	Chronic inflammatory disease of any cause

- *Psychiatry diseases and neurologic illnesses*: Bulimia nervosa, depression, anxiety disorder, bipolar disorder, Parkinson's disease.
- *Endocrinology disorders*: Diabetes mellitus, hyperthyroidism, Addison's disease.
- *Drugs*: A lot of drugs are implicated in weight loss by different mechanisms like decreasing appetite, inducing nausea, altered taste, etc. selective serotonin reuptake inhibitors (SSRIs), levodopa, metformin, theophylline by suppressing the appetite. Nonsteroidal anti-inflammatory drugs (NSAIDs), metformin, iron, antibiotics lead to nausea. Azathioprine and antiretrovirals can cause pancreatitis leading to nausea, pain abdomen, and poor appetite. A list of common drugs causing weight loss is depicted in **Box 1**.

Etiological classification of weight loss which is based on appetite is described in **Table 1**.

PATHOPHYSIOLOGY

Weight loss has a complex pathophysiology and is not just the reverse of weight gain. When body uses more calories as compared to intake it results in weight loss. Certain diseases not only increase the calorie expenditure but also decrease the appetite most commonly by cytokine-mediated mechanisms. For example, in cancers, cytokines such as tumor necrosis factor-alpha (TNF-alpha) and interleukin-6 (IL-6) decrease the appetite and simultaneously increase the muscle and fat breakdown. In acute illnesses, weight loss is once again mediated by cytokines. Weight loss which has normal leptin signals is reversible. This phenomenon is not seen in carcinomas. By contrast, the weight loss attributable to inadequate food intake alone has normal leptin signaling and is reversible with nutritional repletion.

■ CLINICAL FEATURE AND INTERPRETATION

A detailed history, general physical and systemic examination is must to find an underlying cause in any case of weight loss. Before proceeding further, whether weight loss is the only complaint or are there associated symptoms should be established.

History

A detailed history is very helpful in finding the cause of weight loss. The salient points to be noted include:
- Whether the weight loss is voluntary or involuntary; whether it coincides with change in diet, exercise or lifestyle.
- Amount of weight loss—more than 5% as compared to baseline body weight is considered significant. But patients generally tend to under or overestimate the weight loss. Change in cloth size can help in quantifying the weight loss. Opinion of family members can be taken to quantify further.
- Pattern of weight loss—any progressive or sudden weight loss is more worrisome.
- Duration in which weight loss happened—more than 5% over 6–12 months demands a detailed workup.
- Patients should be assessed regarding appetite, food intake, and bowel habits. Assessment of patients' nutritional intake should be done by asking the number of meals and snacks in a day, other nutritional and vitamin intake.
- Symptoms regarding chronic infections and chronic diseases should be asked.
- Patients should be assessed for their living situation and any causes of anxiety and depression should also be assessed.

Physical Examination

A detailed general physical and systemic examination must be a part of the workup. The salient points to be noted in physical examination are:
- General physical examination include vital signs, body weight, body mass index (BMI), skinfold thickness, midarm circumference, weight hip ratio.
- Ideal body weight is calculated as 22.5 multiplied by height in meters. The interpretation of BMI and skinfold thickness should be as shown in **Tables 2 and 3**.
- Further examination should be done focused on the system most expected after a detailed history.

Table 2: Interpretation of body mass index (BMI).

BMI <18.5	Below normal weight
BMI 18.5–25	Normal weight
BMI 25–30	Overweight
BMI 30–35	Class I obesity
BMI 35–40	Class II obesity
BMI >40	Class III obesity

Table 3: Interpretation of skinfold thickness.

Skinfold thickness measurement	Standard	80%	60%
Adult male	12.5	10	7.5
Adult female	16.5	13	10
Nutritional status	Normal	Moderate	Poor

- *Assessment of weight loss*: The most common method for assessment of weight loss is documented weight loss, or at least two of the following three criteria:
  1. Change in size of clothes
  2. Near ones corroborating the weight loss
  3. Patient himself estimates the amount of weight lost.

Too short a time frame may select for only the most acute illnesses; too long a time frame may reflect other long-term physiologic changes rather than an underlying serious illness. After analyzing multiple studies, weight loss as 5% or more of usual body weight within the preceding 6–12 months is being accepted as the most appropriate duration.

APPROACH TO WEIGHT LOSS IN ELDERLY

Elderly patients may develop weight loss due to certain social factors as loss of independence, feeling of loneliness, retired status. They should be specifically observed for eating habits, daily activities and any signs and symptoms suggestive of depression or age-related memory loss. Elderly patients often tend to lose weight in the range of 0.1–0.2 kg/year to 0.5% per year which is considered to be physiologic and does not increase the risk of morbidity and mortality. Any weight loss beyond this range and found to be involuntary should be appropriately worked up. The most common cause of weight loss in old people, especially those living alone are isolation, poor financial status, and forced food which may not be as per their preference.

RED FLAG SIGNS
- Early satiety
- Dysphagia

- Abdominal pain
- Change in bowel habit
- Melena/Hematochezia
- Respiratory symptoms
- Bone pain.

INVESTIGATIONS

Once the underlying cause of weight loss is diagnosed clinically, investigations should be focused on confirming the same. In cases where no cause could be found in spite of detailed history and examination, some preliminary test should be done to look for the underlying cause. These include:
- Complete blood count and peripheral smear
- C-reactive protein and erythrocyte sedimentation rate, serum ferritin levels, vitamin D_3 levels
- Kidney function and liver function test
- Blood sugar fasting and postprandial and hemoglobin A1c (HbA1c)
- Thyroid function test, fasting lipid profile
- Stool for occult blood, fecal Sudan stain for fat malabsorption, fecal elastase (chronic pancreatitis)
- Viral markers—hepatitis B and C, HIV
- Electrocardiogram, Chest X-ray—PA, sonography—whole abdomen
- Mantoux test
- Antinuclear antibody and tissue transglutaminase IgA testing
- Carcinoma screening based on the probabilities like carcinoembryonic antigen (CEA), cancer antigen 19-9 (Ca19-9), Ca-125, alpha-fetoprotein (AFP), prostate-specific antigen (PSA).

TREATMENT

Treatment of this entity is based on management on the underlying cause. Patient in whom no cause is found needs a close follow-up over next 6 months to ensure that no such cause is missed which can be treated. Serial follow-up of lean body mass should be done in all patients.

The aim of the treatment should be to identify the underlying cause and treat them. Sometimes causes of weight loss may be very subtle like unavailability of vegetarian food for some people who avoid nonvegetarian food due to cultural reasons. Presence of social stigma leading to depression, avoidance of social contact due to personality disorders, spiritual disturbances, and dental problems are other causes which can cause weight loss.

Suitable substitution of pharmacological management should be done if found to be the reason for weight loss. In certain cases, patients may need psychological and behavioral support including diet counseling and nutritional support. Patients who fail to accept well orally in spite of all measures should be tried enteral tube feed. Diet should be adequately supplemented with micronutrients and vitamins.

Flowchart 1: Approach to a patient with weight loss.

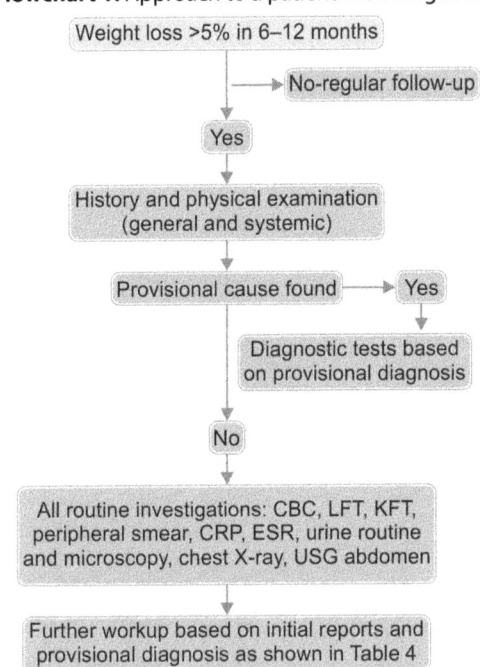

Table 4: Summary of common causes of weight loss, their signs and symptoms, investigations, and treatment.

Clinical condition	Signs and symptoms	Lab investigations	Treatment
Pulmonary tuberculosis	Evening rise of temperature, night sweats, cough	Sputum acid-fast bacillus (AFB), chest X-ray (CXR)-posteroanterior (PA)	Anti-tubercular treatment (ATT)
Hyperthyroidism	Increased appetite, loss of weight, anxiety, tremor, sweating, diarrhea	Triiodothyronine (T3), thyroxine (T4), thyroid stimulating hormone (TSH)	Antithyroid drugs like propylthiouracil, carbimazole, or methimazole
Bacterial endocarditis	Fever, joint pains, night sweats, shortness of breath (SOB), fatigue, valvular heart disease, murmur	Echo and blood cultures	Treated with appropriate intravenous antibiotics for 4–6 weeks
Sarcoidosis	Fever, fatigue, cough	CXR, biopsy from appropriate tissue	Corticosteroids
HIV/AIDS	Fever, night sweats, generalized lymphadenopathy	Western blot	Treated with highly active antiretroviral treatment (HAART)

Contd...

Contd...

Clinical condition	Signs and symptoms	Lab investigations	Treatment
Malabsorption syndrome	Steatorrhea, watery diarrhea, nausea, dyspepsia	Fecal Sudan stain for fat malabsorption, fecal elastase (chronic pancreatitis)	Treated with gluten-free diet if necessary, avoidance of milk and milk products, corticosteroids, low-fat diet
Worm infestation	Pain abdomen, increased frequency of stools, decreased appetite	History, stool routine microscopy	Albendazole/mebendazole
Depression	Depressed mood, lack of sleep, fatigue	History	Antidepressants and behavioral therapy
Carcinomas	Fever, night sweats, generalized lymphadenopathy	Appropriate cancer markers, imaging studies	Appropriate chemotherapy/surgery/radiotherapy
Alcoholism	Poor appetite, drowsiness, lethargy	History, liver function test (LFT), USG-WA, FibroScan	Appropriate behavioral counseling/deaddiction therapy
Diabetes mellitus	Polyuria, polyphagia, polydipsia	Blood sugar (BS)—fasting and postprandial, HbA1c	Antidiabetic therapy
Treatment related	Fatigue, drowsiness	History, treatment charts	Withdrawal/substitution of the offending agent

■ CONCLUSION

Weight loss particularly involuntary or unintentional weight loss can become a major cause of morbidity and mortality if left unrecognized or untreated. A stepwise algorithmic approach as summarized in **Flowchart 1** and **Table 4** can help in early and easy diagnosis and timely treatment.

Index

Page numbers followed by *b* refer to box, *f* refer to figure, *fc* refer to flowchart, and *t* refer to table.

A

Abdomen 177
  acute 4, 16*t*
  computed tomography of 15
  red flags of acute 15*t*
  surgical causes of acute 13
  ultrasonography of 15
  ultrasound 16, 297
Abdominal anatomy 1, 11
Abdominal examination 444
  ultrasound 10
Abdominal pain, 1, 8, 9*t*, 12*fc*, 13, 14, 18, 86, 138
  acute 13, 17*t*
  causes of acute 13*t*
  chronic 18
  diffuse 2
  localized 20
  lower 14
  mild-moderate 11
  pathophysiology of 13
  presence of 86
  recurrent 18
  signs in 3*t*
  symptoms in 3*t*
Abdominal surgery 86
  previous 9
Abdominal symptoms 355
Abdominal X-ray, role of 10
Abetalipoproteinemia 28
ABG analysis 187
Abortions, recurrent 58
Abscess 280
  brain 375
  deep 117
  dental 203
  intra-abdominal 3
  lactation 80
  lung 112, 117, 357

  pain to 193, 196
  parotid 74
  perirectal 9
  peritoneal 19
  peritonsillar 177, 628, 637
  retropharyngeal 628, 637
  spinal epidural 483
  subphrenic 375
Absorptive function, loss of 85
Acarus scabiei 573
Acetaminophen 372
Acetyl choline, release of 26
Achalasia 234
  cardia 233
Achilles tendon 38
  injury 41
Acid
  injuries 271
  reflux 22
  suppression 497
Acid-fast bacilli 360, 394, 462
Acidosis 183
Acne, neonatal 571, 571*f*
Acoustic neuroma 242
Acquired asplenia 412
Acquired bleeding disorders 56, 61, 64, 71
Acquired genetic defects 28
Acquired immunodeficiency syndrome 231
Acropustulosis, infantile 572, 572*f*
Acute coronary syndrome 105, 236, 238
Acute scrotum 584, 592
  diagnostic evaluation 586
  differential diagnosis of 588
  epidemiology 585
  etiology 584
  history taking in 587
  pathophysiology 586
  physical examination of 587

  sifferential diagnosis of 588*t*
  ultrasound 587
Acyclovir 529
ADAMTS13 enzyme 69
Adenoid hypertrophy 631
Adenoma, bronchial 357, 363
Adenosine triphosphate 128, 441
Adequate hydration, maintenance of 172
Adequate renal function 89
Adrenal crisis 19
Advanced airway management equipment 559
Advanced trauma life support 120
  guidelines 133
Aedes aegypti 437
Aerobic culture 360
Afebrile seizures 154
Agranulocytosis 332
Air fluid levels, multiple 17
Airway 161, 235, 241
  breathing and circulation 338, 359, 450
  maintain 158
  management 496
  equipment, basic 559
  reflex, protective 169
  resistance, level of 162
  secretions, presence of 169
  secure 158
Albumin 544
Alcohol 104, 129, 143
  withdrawal 143
  seizure 151
Alcoholic hepatitis 49
Alcoholism 318, 444, 680
Aldehydes 619
Aldolase 505
Alendronate 231
Aleukemic leukemia 295
Alkali burns 271

Allergen
 exposure 170
 implicated 597
Allergic contact dermatitis 596
 clinical features 596
 etiopathogenesis 596
 treatment 597
Allergic disorders, suspected 171
Allergic reaction 68
Allergic rhinitis 172, 626
Allergic vasculitis 295
Allergy 155, 245, 247
Allopurinol 598
Alpha-adrenergic agonists 340
Alpha-methyldopa 375
Aluminum 414
 containing antacids 137
 phosphate 414
Alveolar-arterial oxygen gradient, elevated 240
Amantadine 378
Amebiasis 295
American National Athletic Trainers 41
American Society of Anesthesiologists 557
Aminoglycosides 388
Aminotransferases 505
Amiodarone 181-183
Amnesia 95, 124
Amniotic fluid embolism 236
Amoxicillin 475, 630
 clavulanate combination 475
Amphotericin B 524
Ampicillin 475
 sulbactam combination 475
Amylase 88
Amyloidosis 138, 442
Amyotrophic lateral sclerosis 657
Anal fissure 24
 chronic 24
 differential diagnosis of 9
 management of chronic 26
Anal injury 24
Anal rectal muscle function, evaluation of 139
Analgesia 461
 airway assessment procedures for 557
 procedural 556
Anaphylactic shock, history of 11
Anaphylaxis 236, 282, 636
Anasarca 281
Ancillary tests 654

Androgen receptor molecules, selective 507
Anemia 20, 27, 27t, 69, 237, 282, 433
 approach to 31
 causes of 33fc
 classification of 27
 differential diagnosis of 32t
 of chronic
  disease 29, 32
  disorder 29
 pathophysiology of 31
 signs of 57
 to blood loss, treatment of 33fc
 types of 29t
Anesthesia, general 310
Aneurysms, diagnosis of 479
Angina 100, 102
 abdominis 5
 unstable 100
Angioedema 279
Angiotensin-converting enzyme 164, 166, 276, 626
 inhibitors 170
Angle closure glaucoma 273
Anhidrotic ectodermal dysplasia 300
Anidulafungin 524
Ankle anterior drawer test 38
Ankle joint, level of 38
 movements of 43
Ankle sprain 36, 37, 43, 44fc
 diagnosis of 38, 40
 isolated simple 43
 management of 42
 recurrent 43
 symptoms of 37
 treatment of chronic 41
Ankylosing spondylitis 295
Anomalous 141
Anorectal manometry 139
Anorexia 19
Antalgic gait 321, 322
Anterior drawer test 38, 39f
Antiaggregants 126
Antiallergic drugs 279
Antiarrhythmic agent 183
Antibiotic therapy 5, 475
Antibody 54
 detection 567
 mediated destruction 28
Anticancer treatment 665
Anticoagulant 261
 therapy 56
 use of 515

Anti-cyclic citrullinated peptide 460
Anti-D antibody 68
Antidepressant 137, 378, 380, 665
 tricyclic 151, 665
Antidiuretic hormone 361
Antiepileptic drug 147, 148, 160
 noncompliance with 144
Antigen detection 567
 testing, rapid 628
Anti-hepatitis A virus, detection of 397
Antihistamine agents 287, 437, 445, 668
Antihistaminic therapy 172
Antihypertensive drug ACE inhibitors 164
Anti-inflammatory drugs 343
Antineutrophil cytoplasmic antibody 505
Antinuclear antibody 276, 297, 460, 505
Antiphospholipid syndrome 295
Antiplatelet 126
 agents 474
 therapy 261
Antipyresis, pharmacological 306
Antipyretics 172
Antirheumatic drugs, disease-modifying 298
Anti-rheumatic drugs
 modifying 413
 start disease-modifying 462
Antitetanus 437
Antithrombin III deficiency 477
Antithrombotic agents 474
Antithyroid drugs 328
Antitussives 173
 role of 172
Antiviral drugs 75
Anxiety 238
 cause of 442
 history of 652
Anxious state 530
Aortic aneurysm 2, 9
 abdominal 1, 9
 leaking 363
Aortic dissection 9, 102, 109, 110, 237
 acute 101
Aortic stenosis 144
Aortic syndrome, diagnosis of 11
Aplastic anemia 29, 32
Appendicitis 16, 17, 592
 acute 1, 4, 13

Index

diagnostic of 16
harbinger of acute 13
Appendix
  epididymidis 590
  testicularis 590
Appetite, loss of 396
Arcanobacterium haemolyticum 626
Arch support 343
Arcus senilis 105
Argatroban 61
Argemone alkaloid-contaminated cooking 358
Argon plasma coagulation 361
Arnold-Chiari malformation 642
Arrhythmia 134, 183, 184, 236, 237, 538, 539
  acute 539
  cardiac 177, 382
  respiratory 623
Arrhythmogenic causes of palpitations 531
Arterial blood
  gas 88, 120, 133, 135, 185, 239, 241, 360, 380, 667
  analysis 239
  pressure 31, 470
  specimen, heparinized 185
Arterial embolism, peripheral 470
Arterial hypertension 73
Arterial hypoxemia 185
  detecting 184
Arterial oxygenation, decreased 182
Arterial ulcers 478
  treatment of 479
Arteriovenous malformation 33, 183, 360
Artery disease, peripheral 469, 478
Arthritic cause 342
Arthritis
  in women 395
  infective 455
  inflammatory 463
  post-traumatic 122
Arthropod 423
  types of 423*f*
Asbestosis 112
Ascites 45
  cardiac 45
  causes of 46*t*
  etiology of 46*t*
  evaluation of 50*fc*
  fluid
    analysis 48
    cell count of 48

malignant 46
nonhepatic 51
pathophysiology of 47
Ascorbic acid 231
Asperger's syndrome 75
Aspergillus niger 245
Asphyxiating gases 618
Aspiration
  acute 236
  recurrent 164
Aspirin 474
Asplenia, anatomic 412
Asterixis 132
Asthma 163, 238
  acute 236
  bronchial 104, 237
Ataxia 133
  telangiectasia 318
Ataxic dysarthria 318
Ataxic gait 318, 322
Atelectasis 162
Atmospheric pressure 382
Atonia 153
Atopic dermatitis 570
Atresia, congenital 84
Atrial fibrillation 535*f*, 538
Atrial myxoma 112, 117
Atrial natriuretic peptide 46
Aubergine sign 553
Auditory canal, external 243, 252, 253
Aura 142
Autism 75
Autoimmune 282, 324
  conditions 295
  disease 68, 73, 455
  disorders 28
  thrombocytopenia 56
Autonomic cephalalgias, trigeminal 370
Autonomic dysfunction 132
Autonomic function 141, 153
Avil 279
Axillary nerve injury 593
Axillary node 80
Axonal injury, diffuse 129
Azithromycin 389, 630

B

Babesiosis 28
Bacillus anthracis 405
Bacillus calmette-guérin vaccine 394, 409, 413, 417

Bacillus cereus 665
Back pain 20
  management of simple 483
  nonpharmacological modalities simple 483
  pharmacological therapy simple 483
Bacteremia 388
Bacterial cultures 171
Bacterial endocarditis 679
Bacterial fermentation, translocation of 85
Bacterial hydrolysis 441
Bacterial infection 184, 625*f*
  secondary 168
  suspected 171
Bacterial labyrinthitis, acute 655
Bacteroides 4
Baker's cyst 471
Balance error scoring system 125
Balanitis xerotica obliterans 545
Ball and socket joint 593
Barbiturates 318
  short-acting 375
Bariatric surgery 673
Barium swallow 232
Barotrauma 242
Barr virus 297
Barrett's esophagus 234
Bartonella quintana 437
Basal cell cancer 436
Basal ganglia diseases 321
Baylor bleeding score 345
Becker's muscular dystrophy 320
Bedside glucose
  measurement 133
  testing 176
Bedside testing 231
Behçet's disease 300
Bell's disease 76
  clinical suspicion of 76
Bell's palsy 72, 73, 75
  cause of 72
  diagnosis 75
    confirmation of 76
  differential diagnosis for 74*b*
  pathogenesis of 73
Bell-Clapper deformity 586
Benzocaine 182
Benzodiazepine 147, 148, 151, 287, 380
Benzyl benzoate 609
Beriberi 282
Berlin edema 270

Bernard-Soulier syndrome 54, 56
Beta-haemolytic streptococci, group A 247
Bethesda system 327t
Bevacizumab treatment 358
Bicuspid aortic valve 101
Biliary cirrhosis 112, 114
Biliary obstruction 442
Bilirubin, metabolism of 442f
Biopsy
　image-guided 79
　vacuum-assisted 79
Biphasic fever 300
Birmingham eye trauma terminology 262, 265b
Birth injury 74
Bisacodyl 22
Bitot spots 443
Bivalirudin 61
Bladder obstruction, presence of 11
Bladder trauma 519
Bleeding
　history of 55
　managing active 63
　mild-to-moderate 70
　noninjury-related 56
　sources of 345b
Bleeding disorders 52, 54, 56, 57, 59t, 62, 63, 70, 71
　classification of 52t, 55fc
　congenital 61
　diagnosed 55
　etiology of 52
　inherited 56, 71
　laboratory investigation of 60fc
　mucocutaneous manifestation of 57
　screening 60b
Blood
　alcohol content 284
　and urine tests 133
　counts, differential 491
　cultures 88, 297
　gases 283
　glucose 158
　investigations 171
　malignancies 282
　massive transfusion of stored 52
　stained discharge 79
　sugar regulation 479
　tests 139, 353
　traces of 79
　urea nitrogen 88, 347, 496

Blood loss 28
　acute 28, 31t
　chronic 28
Blood pressure 259
　low 183
Blood products
　administration of 61
　components derivation 64fc
　transfusion
　　complications of 68
　　pitfalls 66
　　principles of 63
Blood smear 62
　peripheral 31, 491
Blood transfusion 35, 443, 496
　guidelines 34
　effect of 34
Blood-brain barrier 667
Blumberg's sign 4, 8
Blunt injuries 264, 276
Blunt trauma 591
　chest 358
Body mass index 670
　interpretation of 677t
Body's equilibrium, maintenance of 650
Boerhaave syndrome 101
Bone
　deformity of 37
　fracture 202, 470
　lesions, malignant 473
　marrow transplantation 358
　pains 326
　tissues 474
　trauma, evidence of 133
Bony crepitus, presence of 177
Bony tenderness, absence of 40
Bordetella pertussis 388
Borrelia recurrentis 437
Borrelia vincentii 332
Bothersome symptoms 167
Botulinum toxin 26, 645
　use of 76
Bowel gangrene 15
Bowel gas, paucity of 17
Bowel obstruction 5, 14, 49, 83, 91fc, 92, 175
　causes
　　of large 84b
　　of small 84b
Bowel perforation 17
Brachial plexus injury 119
Bradycardia 132, 283

relative 295
symptomatic 539
Bradycardic heart rate 8
Bradykinin 18
Brain
　computed tomography of 157
　development, disorders of 152
　functions, maintain core 128
　infarcts, bilateral 317
　injury, traumatic 123, 517
　malformations 156
　natriuretic peptide 48, 107
　stimulation, deep 645
　tumor 129, 156, 296, 317
Brainstem
　infarct, upper 129
　neoplasms 375
　reflexes 132
　　absent 134
Breast
　biopsy 81
　cancer 45
　　varies, frequency of 77
　contralateral 80
　disease 77
　disorders 77
　fatty enlargement of 82
　inspection of 80
　lesions, vast majority of 77
　lump, feeling of 79
　mass 79
　　evaluation of 80
　　management of 81
　mild tenderness in 278
　pain 77
　　evaluation of 77
　problems 77
　skin, redness of 77
　tissue, examination of 177
　ultrasonography 78
　ultrasound 79
Breathing 134, 158, 161
　and circulation, assess 158
　exercise 381
　holding spells 156
　rapid 380
　shortness of 380
　sounds, bronchial 105
Breathlessness 382
Brincidofovir 404
Bronchial artery 362
　embolization 362
Bronchial hyper-reactivity 168

Bronchiectasis 112, 164, 165, 168, 170, 357
Bronchoalveolar lavage 360
Bronchodilator
   role of 172
   therapy 172
Bronchogenic carcinoma 165, 357
Bronchopneumonia 165
Bronchoscopy
   diagnostic 168
   flexible 172
Bronchospasm 162
Brucella serology 297
Brucellosis 286, 295, 303
Buck's fascia 553
Budd-Chiari syndrome 48, 441
Bullous emphysema 357
Bullous impetigo, clinical features of 608f
Bupivacaine 314
Burns 175
Burrow's solution 614
Butyraldehyde 619
Bystander 143

C

Cachexia 282
   metabolic syndrome 674
Caffeine, avoidance of 78
Calcaneofibular ligament injury 37
Calcium 500
   channel blockers 25, 137, 340, 469
Calcium-binding protein B antibody 125
Caliber esophagus, small 233
Canadian C-spine rule 96
Cancer, diagnosis of 77, 79
Candida 572, 573
   albicans 520, 573
   skin 570
Candidal diaper rash 574f
Candidal stomatitis 525fc
Candidiasis, pathophysiology of 521fc
Cannulas, common 514t
Capillary hemangiomas, simple 578
Carbamazepine 318, 598
Carbon dioxide, pressure of 134
Carbon monoxide 129, 371
   poisoning 236, 237, 537, 620
Carboxyhemoglobin 185, 620
Carboxyhemoglobinemia 181

Cardiac abnormalities 168
Cardiac arrest 134, 382
Cardiac disease, structural 539
Cardiac disorders 282
Cardiac examination 144
Cardiac failure 501
Cardiac output 31
Cardiac tamponade 236
Cardiac traumatic hemolysis 28
Cardiac troponin 106
Cardiac valves, defective 28
Cardiocirculatory arrest 620
Cardiopulmonary compromise 557
Cardiopulmonary diseases 162, 182
Cardiopulmonary illness 184
Cardiorespiratory arrest 132
Cardiovascular abnormalities 234
Cardiovascular collapse 149
Cardiovascular diseases, chronic 412
Cardiovascular disorders 620
Cardiovascular system 543
Carnett sign 21
Carotene 181
Caspofungin 524
Catamenial hemoptysis 358
Catheter thrombolytic therapy 474
Cat-scratch disease 486
Causes of death, injury-related 508f
Cefazolin 476
Cefuroxime 476
Celiac disease 18, 20, 22, 112
Cell
   area of network of 142
   culture 528
Cellulitis 424, 470, 475, 540, 542, 603
   clinical features 603
   etiology 603
   management 604
   treatment 604
Central nervous system 69, 128, 129, 135, 152, 154, 164, 177, 283, 295, 374, 384
   infection of 176
   pathology, history of 143
Central retinal
   artery occlusion 274, 276
   vein occlusion 274, 276
Central venous pressure 31
Cephalexin 476, 630
Cephalosporins 475, 607, 630
Cerebellar ataxia 318
Cerebellar disease

bilateral 318
unilateral 318
Cerebellopontine angle tumors 74
   removal of 74
Cerebral cortex 170
Cerebral hemispheres 128
Cerebral lacerations 129
Cerebral palsy 317, 321
Cerebral pathologies 141
Cerebral perfusion pressure 130
Cerebral vein thrombosis 371
Cerebrospinal fluid 130, 135, 252, 253, 297, 305, 372, 391, 401
   analysis 157
Cervical
   disk disease 101, 103
   spine 628
   sprain 93, 98fc
Cetirizine 279
Charcot-Marie-Tooth disease 319, 320
Chest
   computed tomography of 185
   injuries 363
   tightness 380
   trauma 236
   tube insertion 518
   wall 235
   X-ray 75, 110, 335, 360
Chest pain 99, 108fc, 109fc, 231, 362, 382
   approach to 110
   causes of 99, 100fc, 102t
   evaluation of 103
   life-threatning causes of 99f
Cheyne-Stokes respirations 132
Chickenpox 396
Chikungunya 437
Child abuse 93
Chlamydia 626
   trachomatis 586
Chloride channel activators 140
Chlorpromazine 181, 182, 377
   oxidation products of 183
Cholangitis 10, 442
   ascending 442
Cholecystitis 10, 16, 442
Cholera
   DTP 422
   vaccine 420
Cholestasis 443
Cholesteatoma 248

Cholesterol 672
Chorda tympani 73
Choreiform gait 321
Chronic illness, signs of 57
Churg-Strauss syndrome 295
Cidofovir 404
Ciliary neurotrophic factor 300
Ciprofloxacin 246
Circadian rhythm 300
Cirrhosis 49
   chronic complication of 51
Cirrhosis-portal hypertension 45, 282
Clarithromycin 389, 630
Clavicle fracture 118, 121*fc*
Clay-colored stools 442, 443
Clindamycin 231, 476
Clomiphene 82
Clopidogrel 474
Clostridial sepsis 28
Clostridium
   botulinum 26
   perfringens sepsis 442
   tetani 390, 410
Clotrimazole 246, 612
   troches 524
Clotting disorder 52
Coagulopathy, correct 69
Cobalamin 623
Cochlear implants 412
Cognitive behavioral therapy 380
Cold
   compresses 279
   feeling of 326
Coleoptera 423
Colitis 18
Collagen vascular diseases 674
Collateral ligaments 465
   lateral 464
   medial 464
Colloid cyst 324
Colon, diseases of 137
Colorectal cancer 84, 137
Colorectal resection 86
Coma 128
   diagnostic algorithm for 135*fc*
   etiology of 129*t*
   medically induced 128
Combined pill 278
Common bile duct 443
Communicable disease symptom 162
Compartment syndrome 470, 540

Complete blood count 21, 32*fc*, 60, 88, 96, 120, 145, 259, 276, 335, 371, 460, 543, 628, 667
Concussion 123, 129, 202
   standardized assessment of 124
Condylar fracture 449
Congenital disorders 176
Congestive heart failure 163, 175, 183, 184, 237, 357, 444, 469
Conjunctiva 184
Conjunctival tears 265
Conjunctivitis 272, 395, 598
Connective tissue
   diseases 38, 455
   disorders 487
Consciousness
   impaired level of 136
   level of 128
   loss of 382
   state of 128
Constipation 8, 13, 16, 18, 86, 87, 137, 139*fc*, 175
   chronic 22, 137
   experience occasional 137
   in adult, management of 138*fc*
   risk of 137
Constrictive pericarditis 282
Contraceptive, use of emergency 278*fc*
Contusion 265
   injuries 267
Convulsive status epilepticus, generalized 150
Core biopsy, advanced form of 81
Core needle biopsy 79, 81
Corneal abrasion 268, 268*f*
Corneal injury, penetrating 266
Corneal reflexes 131
Coronary angiogram 185
Coronary artery disease 104, 237
Coronary heart disease 100
Corpus spongiosum 552
Cortical sensory testing 144
Corticospinal tracts 503
Corticosteroids 69, 494
   use of 136
Corynebacterium diphtheriae 389
Costal cartilage 579
Costochondritis 103
Cough 162, 167
   acute 167
   characteristics of 163, 165*t*
   chronic 168, 173
   complications of 163

   consequences of ineffective 162
   development of 164*fc*
   dry 163, 169
   effectiveness of 162
   etiologies of 163, 167, 169*t*
      acute 172
   evaluation
      of chronic 164, 164*b*, 166*fc*
      of pediatric 171*t*
   management of 172
      pediatric 167
   mechanism of 163, 164*fc*
   nonspecific 168
   normal 168
   pathophysiology of 169
   productive 163
   recurrent 168
   sound of 169
      traditional recognizable 169*t*
   subacute 168, 173
   treatment of acute 173
   type of 168
   variant asthma 168
   wet 169
Cowpox 404
Cramp
   severe 500
   symptoms for 500
Craniotomy, decompressive 136
C-reactive protein 4, 21, 171, 304, 457, 472, 482, 491
Creatine kinase 335, 505
   muscle-brain 107, 240
Creatinine 10, 88, 96, 667
Cresylate acetate 246
Crigler-Najjar syndrome 441
Crimean-Congo hemorrhagic fever 58
Crohn's disease 6, 21, 22, 24, 84, 230, 286
Crotamiton lotion 609
Croup 636
Cruciate ligament
   anterior 464
   posterior 464, 465
Crush injury 74
Crush trauma 471
Crying episodes, intensity of 176
Crying infant, management of excessively 179*fc*
Cryoprecipitate 63, 64, 74
Cushing's reflex 132
Cushing's syndrome 320, 670
Cushingoid 281

Cutaneous disease 389
Cutis marmorata 577, 577f
Cyanide toxicity mechanism 622
Cyanosis 105, 114, 181, 186fc, 621
   causes of 182t, 187
   central 183, 183
   deep 183
   detection of 184
   diffuse 114
   etiology of 185
   peripheral 183
   presence of 183
   threshold of 182
   treatment of 187
Cyanotic heart diseases, congenital 114
Cyclooxygenase 97, 112, 306
Cyclosporine A 600
Cystic fibrosis 112, 164, 168, 170, 357, 364
   suspected 171
Cystic masses 80
Cytomegalovirus 295, 303, 487

D

Da Costa's syndrome 531
Dabigatran 61
Danazol 82
Dapsone 182
Darier sign 576f
Decongestants 172, 279
Deep vein thrombosis 385, 470, 474
Defecography 139
Dehydration 175, 334, 374
Demyelination 317
Dengue 295
Dense adhesions 90
Dental problems 193
Dental surgery, bleeding after 204
Dental trauma 201
   types of 201
Deoxyhemoglobin 181, 182, 185, 186
   levels of 184
Depression 680
   history of 652
Dermal melanosis 574
Dermatitis 486
Dermatomyositis 320, 455
Desmopressin 66
Detoxification of cyanides, mechanism of 623
Dexamethasone 375
Dexogenation, clinical signs of 183

Dextromethorphan 172
Diabetes
   mellitus 471, 475, 478, 669, 680
   risk for 670
Diabetic foot ulcers 477, 478
   treatment of 479
Diabetic ketoacidosis 19, 130, 666
Diaper dermatitis 570, 573, 601
   etiopathogenesis 601
   management 602
Diaper, type of 602
Diarrhea 20
   chronic 19
Diazepam 149, 375, 500
Dicloxacillin 476
Dieulafoy's disease 357
Dieulafoy's lesion 347, 495
Dimorphic anemia 31
Diphenhydramine hydrochloride 655
Diphtheria toxoid 410, 414
Diphtheria-tetanus-pertussis 407, 417
Diplegic gait 317
Diptera 423
Direct fluorescent antibody 402
   method 528
   testing 402
Disimpaction 22
Disk herniation 95
   central 483
Dislocation without fracture, treatment of 309fc
Disseminated intravascular coagulation 28, 53, 54, 56, 69, 358
   score 70t
Diuretic therapy 49
   high doses of 49
   intolerance to 49
Diverticular disease 5, 84
   clinical suspicion of 5
Diverticulitis, acute 1, 5
Diverticulosis 5, 137
Dix-Hallpike maneuver 653
Dix-Hallpike position test 654f
Dizziness 58, 382, 650
Dolichocolon 5
Dorsal dislocation, treatment of 309fc
Dorsiflexion 36
Doxycycline 231
Drool rash 574f
Dropped head syndrome 502

Drug
   abuse 128
   antifungal 524
   class of 11
   fever 296
   intoxication 130
   overdose 130
   reaction 236
   toxicity 132
Drug-resistant *Streptococcus pneumoniae* 391
Dubin-Johnson syndrome 441
Duchenne muscular dystrophy 320
Duct
   ectasia 78
   inflammatory lesion of 78
   localization of affected 79
Dysarthria 318
Dysdiadokokinesia 318
Dysfibrinogenemia 61
Dyslipidemia 104, 669
Dysmetria 318
Dysmnesic symptoms 145
Dysmorphic erythrocytes 349
Dyspepsia 22, 99
   functional 19
Dysphagia 19, 229, 598
   specific disorders causing 233
   symptoms, evaluation of 232fc
   transfer 230
Dyspnea 58, 183, 235, 282, 380
   acute 241fc
   causes
      of acute onset 236b
      of chronic 237b
   etiologies of acute 238t
   evaluation of 236
   profile, multidimensional 235
Dysrhythmias 175
Dystonia 449
   causes 667
   reducing 645
Dystonic reaction 449
Dystonic torticollis 642

E

Ear
   complete examination of 244
   discharge 252, 254
      causes of 253t
   dry 246
   fullness of 243
      symptoms of 251

infection
  external 242
  middle 242
  itching of 254
  pain 243
  plugs 245
  pulling of 176
  wax 242
Earache 242
Ecchymoses, location of 38
Ecchymosis 470, 471
Echocardiogram 185
Echocardiography 107
Ecstasy 129
Ectopic pregnancy 10
Eczema 245
  infantile 574, 575*f*
Effort syndrome 531
Ehler-Danlos syndrome 54, 101, 456
Electrolyte 88, 96, 160, 335, 667
  imbalance 12, 90
  rich fluid, loss of 85
Elephantiasis 540
Emergency contraception 277
Emergency department, seizure in 147, 148*fc*
Emergency medical service 339, 510
Emergency medications 559
Emergency thoracotomy 518
Emotional stress 77
Emphysema 162
Empyema 112, 117, 388
Encephalitis 129, 152, 177, 296, 395, 565
Endemic fungi 164
Endocarditis, infective 112, 117
Endocrine
  abnormalities, multiple 576
  disorders 29, 137
Endocrinology disorders 675
Endogenous 53
Endolymph 651
Endometriosis 19, 84
Endoscopic retrograde cholangiopancreatography 445, 446
Endoscopic ultrasound 446
Endoscopy 497
Endothelial injury 53
Endothelin 46
Endotracheal tube 359
Enemas 22
Enteric fever 303
Enteric nervous system 19

Enteritis, regional 2
Enterocolitis, necrotizing 17
Enteroendocrine cells 665
Enzyme
  deficiency 28
  linked immunosorbent assay 460
Eosinophil 171
Eosinophilia 169
Eosinophilic esophagitis 18
Ephemeroptera 423
Epidermal necrolysis 600*t*
Epididymis 584
Epididymitis 351, 585, 591
Epidural hematoma 129
Epigastric artery, inferior 584
Epiglottitis 236, 388, 636
Epilepsy 141
  recurrence 154
  subsequent 154
Epistaxis 256, 355
  management of 258, 258*fc*, 261
Epithelial cells, desquamated 246
Epitrochlear area, right 489
Epitrochlear lymphadenopathy 489
Epley's maneuver 653, 654*f*
Epstein-Barr virus 295
Erectile dysfunction 555
Erosive esophagitis 18
Erosive gastritis 495
Erysipelas 602
  clinical features 603
  etiopathogenesis 602
  management 603
  treatment 603
Erythema toxicum 572, 572*f*
Erythematous
  itchy papules 574
  lesions over gingiva 522*f*
  swelling 245
Erythroblast maturation, defects affecting 28
Erythrocyte sedimentation rate 21, 96, 276, 290, 297, 372, 457, 482, 491
Erythromycin 497
  deficiency 29
Escherichia coli 4, 245, 247, 462
Esophageal cancer 233, 234
Esophageal dysphagia 230
Esophageal motility, ineffective 232
Esophageal reflux 103
Esophageal varices 495
Esophagitis, acute 230

Esophagus 122, 231
Ethambutol 394
Ethmoidal artery 260
  anterior 256
Ethylene glycol 129
Eustachian tube 382
  dysfunction 243
Exacerbate angina 105
Examiner's thumb 39
Excessive crying 174
  common causes of 175
Exogenous inhibition 53
Extra-abdominal diseases 1, 9*t*
Extracorporeal shock wave therapy 344
Extractable nuclear antigen 297
Extraocular movements 131
Extraocular muscle involvement 270
Extrapyramidal symptoms 667
Extrasystoles 538
Eye
  abnormalities 131
  movement, rapid 285
  problems 262

F

Facial artery 260
Facial muscle 504
Facial nerve
  cells 526
  neurinoma 74
  palsy 72
    pathophysiology of 72
    prevalence of idiopathic 72
Facial paralysis, idiopathic 72
Facial swelling 279
Falciparum malaria 442
Famciclovir 529
Familial mediterranean fever 19
Fasciitis, necrotizing 475
Fat
  embolism 236
  necrosis, traumatic 80
Fatigability 146
Fatigue 27, 284
  causes of 288*t*
Febrile convulsion 153
Febrile seizure
  complex 154
  simple 153
  treatment of 158
Fecal impaction 138, 139

Femur fracture 513
Fentanyl 562
Ferguson hemorrhoidectomy 367
Ferrous sulfate 231
Fever 126, 152, 243, 244, 294
　evaluation for 303*fc*
　history of 155
　pathophysiology of 296*fc*
　relapsing 300
　types of 294
　without localizing signs 299
Fiber supplements 140
Fiberoptic bronchoscopy 361
Fibrin clot formation 53
Fibrinogen 62
　degradation products 61
　disorders 52
　　congenital 54
　level, measurement of 61
Fibroadenoma 80
Fibula fracture, distal 41
Fibular compression test 39
Fine-needle
　aspiration cytology 81, 327, 492
　biopsy 328
Finger and nail problems 307
Finger dislocation 307
Finger nail 245
　avulsion 310
Finsterer study table 73
Fire smoke, toxicity of 619
First aid 500
Fissure 20
Fissurectomy 26
Fissure-in-ano, etiology of 24
Fistula 20
Fitz-Hugh-Curtis syndrome 2
Flaccid blisters 598
Flail chest 512
Flexion 132
　contracture 310
Fluconazole 524, 612
Fluctuation test 113
Fluid
　administration 176
　ascites, accumulation of 45
　imbalance 12
　restoration 89, 496
　wave test 457
Flu-like syndrome 165
Fluorescent bulbs 184
Fluoroquinolones 388
Focal motor seizures 142

Focal myositis 502
Focal nonmotor seizure 142
Focal seizures 142
Foley's catheterization 352, 354
Folic acid deficiency 29
Follicular hyperplasia 486
Folliculitis 600
　clinical features 600
　deep 601
　etiology 600
　superficial 600
　treatment 601
Food
　allergy, mediated 19
　borne infections 666
　lodgment, long-term 194
　types of 230
Football sign 17
Foreign body 236, 242, 253, 636
　aspiration 164, 175
　intraocular 265
　suspected 171
　underneath nail 313
Foreskin score, etractability of 546
Formaldehyde 619
Fosphenytoin 149
Fracture
　Allman classification of 119*f*
　mid-clavicle 121
　of distal third 119
　of medial third 119
Fresh frozen plasma 63, 64, 67, 362
　indications for 65*b*
Friedreich's ataxia 318
Frostbite 605
　clinical features 605
　pathophysiology 605
　risk factors 605
　treatment 606
Functional disorders 19
Fungal debris 246
Fungal infection 165, 295
　chronic 300
Fungus culture 360
Furious rabies, stages of 566
Fusobacterium 626

G

Gabapentin 469
Gait abnormalities 316, 321
　types of 317
Gait disorders, classification of 316, 316*t*

Gallbladder
　disease 18
　palpable enlarged 444
Gallstone ileus 84
Gamma-aminobutyric acid 375
　receptors 149
Gastric antral vascular ectasia 345
Gastric cancer, causes of advanced stage 46
Gastric varices 495
Gastritis, chemical 18
Gastroenteritis 13, 16, 18
Gastroesophageal reflux 156, 164, 175
　disease 18, 165, 172, 237, 377, 626
　symptoms of 165
Gastrointestinal bleeding 11
　risk of 49
Gastrointestinal blood loss 19
Gastrointestinal conditions 101
Gastrointestinal diseases 674
Gastrointestinal reflux 163
Gastrointestinal system 543
Genetic
　defects, inherited 28
　disorders 176
　syndromes 156
Genital trauma 519
Genitourinary injuries 519
Genitourinary tract symptoms 19
Giant cell arteritis 295
Gianturco steel coils 362
Gilbert's syndrome 441, 443
Gingiva 522
Gingivitis
　catarrhalis 331
　desquamative 333
　fibromatosa 332
　necroticans ulcerosa 332
Ginkgo biloba 182
Glans penis 549
Glanzmann's thrombasthenia 56
Glanzmann's thrombocytopenia 54
Glasgow coma
　scale 123, 130, 131*t*, 134, 135
　score 241*f*
Glaucoma emergencies 273
Glenohumeral joint 593
Glenoid fossa 595
Global vaccine action plan 407
Globe injury, closed 267
Globins, structurally abnormal 28

Glucagon 45
Glucocorticoids 668
Glucose-6-phosphate
    dehydrogenase 445
    deficiency 28
Glue n-butyl cyanoacrylate 361
Glutathione synthetase deficiency 28
Glycerin 22
Glycolytic enzyme deficiencies 28
Goiter 280, 323
Gonadotropin-releasing hormone 362
Gonococcemia 455
Goodpasture's syndrome 358
Gout 455, 458
Gouty arthritis 455
Gram stain 360
Gram-positive bacillus 389
Granulation tissue 478
Granulomatous
    disease 29
    inflammation 486
    thyroiditis 324
Graves' disease 280, 324, 326, 327
Guaiac-positive stool 20
Guillain-Barré syndrome 74, 236, 237, 319, 320
Gum disorders 330
Gum hyperplasia 331
Gut brain 19
Gut obstruction 666
Gynecomastia 82, 496

H

Hair loss 326
Hallucination 146
Hampton's hump 106
Hand muscles, intrinsic 502
Hansen's disease 74
Hard palate 522f
Harlequin color change 577, 577f
Hartmann's procedure 92
Hashimoto's disease 324, 327
Head injury 152
    evidence of 38
Head trauma 74, 129, 130, 156, 375, 517
Headache 19, 38, 130, 369, 387
    disorders 370t
    history, previous 371
    mild 278
    tension-type 370

Head-to-toe examination 180
Healthcare professionals 404, 406
Healthy sleep, rules of quality of 291f
Hearing 254
    aid 245
    loss 251, 254
Heart
    beating 530
    defects, congenital 357
    disease 669
        congenital 115, 117, 177, 183, 184
        cyanotic congenital 112
    failure 46, 105, 282, 478, 540
    murmurs 114
    rate, assess 259
Heartburn 8, 100
Heat cramps 334, 335
Heat edema 334, 336
Heat exhaustion 334, 337
Heat illness 334
    drugs contributing to 340b
    investigations for 335, 335b
    risk factors for 335, 335b
    symptoms of 334t
    types of 334t, 335
Heat rash 334, 336
Heat syncope 334, 336
Heat tetany 334, 336
Heatstroke 334, 338
Hectic fever 300
Helicobacter pylori
    infection 18
    stool 21
Hemarthrosis 61
    presence of 57
    traumatic 449
Hematemesis 8, 15, 345, 355, 496
Hematochezia 15
Hematogenous pathway 46
Hematologic disease
    spectrum of 52
    symptoms of 586
Hematoma 21, 471
Hematopoietic neoplasms, primary 29
Hematuria 348
    causes of 349t
    evaluation of 353fc
    glomerular 352
    nonglomerular 352
Heme, types of 187
Hemiparesis 132

Hemiplegic gait 317
Hemiptera 423
Hemoconcentration 6
Hemoglobin 27, 33, 182, 346
    abnormal 182, 185
    classification on 31
    deoxygenated 182
    electrophoresis 31
    greenish derivative of 182
    H disease 32
    levels 30t
    synthesis, deficiencies affecting 28
Hemoglobinopathy 412
Hemolysis 443, 444
    chemical 68
Hemolytic anemia 300
Hemolytic disease 28
Hemolytic reaction 68
Hemolytic uremic syndrome 13, 28, 62
Hemophilia 54, 204, 205, 257, 455
    A 52, 61, 66, 69
    B 52
Haemophilus influenzae 247, 305, 387, 409, 412
Hemoptysis 113, 168, 282, 355, 355t, 358, 362
    etiology of 357
    grading of 356t
    minor 355
Hemorrhage 94, 129
    cause of internal 511
    external 513
    intracranial 65, 66, 69, 151
    intraocular 163
    postpartum 33
    subarachnoid 129, 131, 133, 371
Hemorrhagic shock 442
Hemorrhagic stroke 317
Hemorrhoidectomy
    complications of 368
    excisional 367
    stapled 368
Hemorrhoids 139, 365, 368
    classification of 365
    external 365
    internal 365
Hemosiderin 183
Hemostasis
    defect mechanism, classification on 53t
    disorders 52
    primary 53

process, pathophysiology of 53
secondary 53
Hemothorax 119, 122
Hemotympanum 130
Henoch-Schönlein purpura 16, 302, 591
Heparin 52, 474
 unfractionated 261
Hepatic encephalopathy 45, 132
Hepatic failure, fulminant 442
Hepatic jaundice 443
 causes of 441t
Hepatic metastasis 49
Hepatic veins 45
Hepatitis 397
 A 298, 396, 418
  vaccine 411
  virus 396
 B 397, 409, 417, 418, 422, 505
  immune globulin 398
  surface antigen of 398
  vaccine 411, 413, 414
  vaccines, vaccination of 398t
  virus 397
 C serologies 505
 chronic active 112
Hepatoblastoma 303
Hepatocellular dysfunction 441
Hepatocellular injury 447
Hepatocellular liver disease 29
 severe 28
Hepatopulmonary syndrome 237
Hereditary afibrinogenemia 54
Hereditary bleeding disorders 53
Hereditary elliptocytosis 28
Hereditary spastic paraparesis 317
Hereditary spherocytosis 28, 32
Hernia 13, 21
 strangulated 3, 6
Herpes labialis 527fc
 causes of 526fc
 pathophysiology of 527
Herpes simplex 73, 74
 virus 24
Herpes skin test 528
Herpes zoster 74, 101, 103, 393, 606
 clinical features 606
 etiopathogenesis 606
 management 607
 ophthalmicus 606
 oticus 606
 rule out of 75
 treatment 607
 viruses 73

Hexokinase deficiency 28
Hiatal hernia 18
Hiccup 374
 bout 374
Hinge joint 464
Hip muscles 502
Hirschsprung's disease 13, 15, 16, 17
Histamine 18
Histiocytosis 303
 malignant 295
 X 75
Hodgkin's disease 490
Hodgkin's lymphoma 289
Homan's test 471
 positive 471
Homeostasis, abnormal 52
Homonymous hemianopia 131
Hormonal changes 330
Hormonal disorder 78
Hormonal influences 94
Hormone replacement therapy 80
Horn cells, anterior 503
Hot fluids 384
Human immunodeficiency virus 24, 163, 280, 286, 295, 300, 371, 411, 471, 487, 549, 586, 609
 infection 74
Human papillomavirus 393, 410, 422, 549, 610
 vaccine 419, 421
Human tetanus immunoglobulin,
 dose of 639
Human tissues, invasion of 433
Humoral intraosseous access 514f
Huntington's disease 321
Hydatid cyst 357, 363
Hydatid torsion 590
Hydration 136
 status 14
Hydro-air levels, presence of 6
Hydrocephalus 129, 133, 152, 375
Hydrocortisone 602
Hydrogen
 cyanide 618
 sulfide 182
Hydrophobia 402, 565
Hydrotherapy 305
Hydroxocobalamin 621, 624
Hyperbaric oxygen therapy 476, 621, 622
Hyperbilirubinemia
 congenital 443
 conjugated 441
 unconjugated 441

Hypercalcemia 129, 494
Hypercapnia 129
Hypercarbia 582
Hyperfibrinolysis 56
Hyperglycemia 129
Hyperkalemia 494
Hypermobile joint syndrome,
 benign 456
Hypermotility syndrome 449
Hypernatremia 129
Hyperparathyroidism 502
Hyperphosphatemia 494
Hyperplastic candidiasis 522f
Hyperprothrombinemia 54
Hypersplenism 52, 56
Hypersynchronous discharges,
 uncontrolled 141
Hypertension 20, 104
 portal 15, 45, 46, 444
Hypertensive encephalopathy 129
Hyperthermia 128, 129
 exercise-induced 296
Hyperthyroidism 296, 320, 679
Hypertrophic cardiomyopathy 144
Hypertrophic osteoarthropathy 112
Hypertrophic pulmonary
 osteoarthritis 113
Hypertrophied papilla 24
Hyperuricemia 457
Hyperventilation 136, 379
 cause of 379
 physiological effects of 379
 symptoms of 379, 380t
Hypoalbuminemia 540
Hypocalcemia 138, 494, 500
Hypochondrium pain
 left 2
 right 2
Hypoglycemia 129, 130, 144, 152
Hypogonadism
 primary 82
 secondary 82
Hypomagnesemic muscle 500
Hyponatremia 129
Hypoproteinemia 282, 469
Hypotension 101, 130, 302
 cause 134
Hypothalamic-pituitary-thyroid
 axis 325f
Hypothermia 129, 130, 183
Hypothyroidism 21, 78, 129, 137, 138, 320
Hypoventilation 582
 syndromes 182

Hypovolemia 85
Hypovolemic shock 183
Hypoxia 112, 129, 130, 384
Hypoxic encephalopathy 132

I

Iatrogenic pulmonary rupture 363
Ibuprofen 306
Ice fomentation 462
Ichthyotic scales 578
Icterus 105
   prolonged 114
Idiopathic scrotal edema, acute 591
Idiopathic syndrome 72
Idiopathic thrombocytopenic
   purpura, acute 68
Ileus
   functional 8
   paralytic 83, 89
Illiac fossa pain
   left 2
   right 2
Illicit drug 104
Illness symptoms, severe 479
Immersion injuries, suggestive of 178
Immune
   hemolytic anemia 32
   system disorder 74
   thrombocytopenic purpura 54
Immune-deficiency syndromes 24
Immune-mediated injury 29
Immunization 152, 422
   passive 568
   pre-exposure 568
Immunodeficiency diseases 25, 248
Immunoglobulin E 19, 171
Immunohistochemistry tests 81
Immunosuppressive diseases 475
Impacted tooth 242
Imperforate hymen 19
Impetigo 607
   clinical features 607
   etiology 607
   treatment 607
Implant
   bleeding after 205
   placement 204
Incisional biopsy 81
Incontinentia pigmenti 576, 576*f*
Infantile colic 16, 175
   affects 177
   diagnosing 180

Infection 154, 169, 470, 487, 591
   anaerobic 169
   cases of suspected 171
   dermatophyte 612
   enteroviral 300
   extra-abdominal 14
   illness, signs of 144
   localized 174
   mycobacterial 490
   respiratory 176
   symptoms of 155
   unusual 295
   viral 184, 240
Infectious disease, recent 73
Infectious mononucleosis 303, 625, 626*f*
Inferior vena cava 240, 241*f*
Inflammation
   acute 490
   signs of 456
   chronic 455
   low-grade of 455
Inflammatory bowel
   disease 2, 16, 18, 22, 84, 86, 112, 114, 117, 138
   family history of 19
Inflammatory diseases 300
Inflammatory joint disease 321
Inflammatory obstructive disease 163
Influenza 74, 387, 422
   vaccine 410
      inactivated 418
Inframammary crease 80
Inguinal hernia 586
   large 591
   obstructed 13, 15, 16
Inhalation, management of victims of 618
Initiate diuretic therapy 49
Insect bite 175, 423, 439*fc*
Insomnia 94, 375
Inspiratory stridor 632
Intensive care unit 134, 358, 438
   pediatric 179
Intercostal muscle 162
Interdental gingiva 196
Intermittent fever 300
International League against Epilepsy 142, 142*f*
Interphalangeal dorsal dislocation, classification of proximal 308*fc*
Interphalangeal joint

   distal 455
   proximal 309*fc*
Interstitial fluid 45
Interstitial lung disease 112, 164, 172, 183, 237
   severe 181
Intestinal *Candida albicans* 602
Intestinal ischemia 4, 9
Intestinal obstruction 1, 13, 15-17, 667
   causes of 5
   suspicion of 10, 12
Intestinal occlusion, causes of 6*t*
Intimal tears 362
Intra-abdominal
   disorders 1
   injuries 583
   mass 14
   pressure 163
Intracranial neoplasms 375
Intracranial pathway, longest 72
Intracranial pressure 130, 175
Intractable hiccups 374
   causes of 375*b*
Intraductal papillomas 78
Intranasal instillation 149
Intranasal lidocaine 373
Intranasal steroids 172
Intraocular pressure 373
Intraocular steroids 279
Intraparenchymal hemorrhage 129
Intrapulmonary shunts 183
Intrathoracic injuries 122
Intravenous
   access 176
   diazepam 160
   equipment 559
   fluid 16, 500
   fosphenytoin 160
   immunoglobulins 600
   ketamine 563
   levetiracetam 160
   lorazepam 159, 160
   midazolam 159
   narcotics 368
   phenobarbital 160
   phenytoin 159
   secure 158
   valproic acid 160
Invasive ductal carcinoma 79
Invasive mycetoma 357
Iodine
   deficiency 324
   radioactive 328

Ipsilateral pontine infarction 74
Iris injuries 269
Iron 675
    binding capacity, total 31
    defficiency anemia 34
    deficiency 29
        anemia 28, 32
    sequestration, inflammation-mediated 29
    supplements 137
Irrigation impairment, presence of 83
Irritability, general 193
Irritable bowel syndrome 2, 18, 19, 137
Irritant 245
    diaper dermatitis 573*f*
Irritating gases 619
Irritation, chemical 170
Isabgol 366
Ischemia 6, 14, 83, 85, 87
    and eventually necrosis 85
    and subsequent necrosis 5
    stimulate visceral pain fibers 14
Ischemic colitis 5, 84
Isobutyl-2-cyanoacrylate 362
Isolated axillary lymphadenopathy 77
Isoniazid 151, 394
Isoptera 423
Isotonic fluid 89
Itching 245
Itraconazole 612
Itraconazole solution 524

J

Janeway lesions 114
Japanese encephalitis 401, 409, 418
    vaccine 411, 416
    virus 401
Jaundice 114, 440, 496
    causes of posthepatic 441*t*
    differential diagnosis of 446*fc*
    duration of 443
    management of 446*fc*
    mild 442
    recurrent 443
    types of 440*f*
Jaw dislocation 448
Jerky nystagmus, abnormal 653
Joint
    capsule, shortened 36
    complex 464

    deformity of 37
    disease, degenerative 466
    hypermobility syndrome 456
    instability, risk of 37
    muscle-dependent 593
    related conditions 38
    structure 456
    swelling 20, 456
Joint pain 453, 462, 471
    acute 454
    asymmetric 455
    causes of 458*t*
    chronic 454
    clinical history 453
    distribution of 455
    evaluation of 457
    examination of 456
    involvement of number of 455
    laboratory tests 457
    location of 454, 455
    past medical history 455
    physical examination 456
    role of surgery 463
    symmetric 455
    treatment 461
    worsening factor 455
Jugular venous pressure 105
Juvenile idiopathic arthritis 302, 455

K

Kala-azar 303
Kaposi sarcoma 312
Kawasaki disease 300, 302
Keratic precipitates 273
Ketamine 562, 563
    intramuscular 563
Ketoconazole 281
Ketofol 562, 563
Kidney
    disease, chronic 374, 499
    function test 146
    injury, acute 69
Klebsiella 357, 600
    pneumoniae 586
Kleiger test 38-40
Knee
    dislocation of 465
    injuries 466
    locked 466
    stability 464
    swelling 465
Knee joint 457, 466
    clinical examination of 465

Knee problems 464
    anatomy of 464
Kocher's leverage technique 594
Kyphoscoliosis 237

L

Lactate dehydrogenase 297, 491, 505
Lactulose 22
Lamellar laceration 265
Lamotrigine 598
Langerhans cell histiocytosis 300
Lansoprazole 22
Laparoscopic management 90
Laparoscopic surgeries 14
Laparotomy 90
Large bowel
    obstruction, red flags of 86*b*
    red flags of 86
Laryngeal edema 236
Laryngeal lesion, benign 661, 663
Laryngeal tumor, benign 657, 658, 660
Laryngitis 242, 657, 658, 659, 660, 662
Laryngomalacia 636
Laryngospasm 236
Laryngotracheitis 632
Laryngotracheomalacia 172
Larynx, surgery on 231
Lassar's paste 602
Laxatives 366
Lead poisoning 19, 28
Leduc technique 476
Leg pain, acute 468
Legionella 357
    pneumonia 240
Legionellosis 295
Lemierre's syndrome 629
Lepidoptera 423
Lepirudin 61
Leprosy 74
Leptospirosis 295, 300
Lethal agents 618
Leukemia 24, 74, 295, 300, 303, 332, 609
    acute 29, 490
    inhibitory factor-m 300
Leukocytosis 5
Levetiracetam 149
Levine's sign 104, 105
Levodopa 675
Levothyroxine replacement 328

Lichen planus 230
Lid lacerations 265
Lidocaine 378
Life-threatening 68, 174
   bleeding, locations of 513*b*
   conditions 8
   thoracic injuries 512*t*
Ligament
   of treitz 496
   previously injured 36
Lignocaine 314
Limb
   asymmetry 144
   coldness of affected 37
   neurovascular damage of 38
Limb-girdle involvement 502
Lincosamides 630
Lindane cream 609
Linezolid 74, 475
Lip licking 142
Lipoprotein, high-density 672
Liquid albumin 48
Lithium 318
Live attenuated influenza vaccine 411
Liver
   biopsy 445
   cancer 397
   cirrhosis 45, 397
   disorders 441
   failure 397
   function test 10, 21, 133, 146, 297, 335, 376, 460
   transplantation 49
Liver disease 54, 56, 62, 358, 496
   advanced 45
   chronic 29, 54, 57, 412, 469, 499
   end-stage 443
   progression of 46
   sever 66
   signs of 62
Lobar pneumonia 165
Local wound 424
   care 436
Locoregional treatment 80
Lovibond's angle 113, 114
Low back pain 481, 483*t*, 484
   causes of 481, 481*t*
   diagnostic imaging 482
   evaluation of 481
   laboratory tests 482
   management of 483
   treatment for 483*t*

Low molecular weight heparin 61
Lower extremity pain 468
   causes 468
   clinical presentation 470
   evaluation 470
   pathophysiology 469
Lower extremity ulcers 476
   causes 476
   clinical presentation 478
   evaluation 477
   history 477
   pathophysiology 477
   treatment 479
Lower limb fracture 321
Lower lobe pneumonia 16
Lumbar pain
   left 2
   right 2
Lumbar puncture 65, 133, 135, 157, 372
Lumpiness 79
Lung
   cancer 112
      primary 164
   carcinoma 114
   chronic infections of 165
   contusions 122
   function test 172
   injury, transfusion-related acute 68
   point 240
   sliding 240
   varcinoma of 281
Lung disease
   chronic obstructive 183
   drug-induced 236
   immunologic 358
   occupational 237
   severe chronic 171
   suppurative 171
Lung elastic recoil 162
   reduced 162
Lupus anticoagulants 59
Lupus erythematosus 295
Lupus like syndrome 456
Lyme disease 295
Lymph 45
   drainage 476
Lymph node 488, 489
   benign 493*t*
   enlarged 486
   group of 485
   malignant 493*t*

   regions 485*f*
   retroauricular 489
Lymphadenitis, acute 486
Lymphadenopathy 105, 280, 443, 485, 491
   causes of 487*t*
      localized 488*t*
   clinical evaluation 486
   etiology 486
   peripheral 491
   treatment of 494
Lymphangitis 476, 604
   clinical approach 604
   etiology 604
   management 605
   treatment 605
Lymphatic capillaries 45
Lymphatic flow 45, 46
Lymphatic vascular system 45
Lymphatic vessels 46
Lymphedema 476, 540
Lymphoma 19, 45, 74, 112, 295, 300, 303, 490
Lymphoproliferative disorders 487

M

Macrolide 388, 389
   therapy 172
Maculopapular skin rash 395
Magnesium 500
   citrate 22
   hydroxide 22
Malabsorption syndrome 680
Malaria 28, 295, 303
   chronic 282
Malarial antigen 297
Malassezia furfur 571
Malignant cells, dissemination of 46
Malignant diseases, history of 73
Malingering 95
Malleolus, medial 40
Mallory-Weiss tear 101, 495
Malnutrition 332, 374
Malrotation 178
Mammography 79
Mandible fracture 449
Mantoux test 171
Markle's sign 4
Mass
   malignant 79
   parotid 75
Massive hemoptysis 356
   management of 363*fc*

Massive hemothorax 512
Massive pleural effusion 236
Mastalgia 77
  etiology of 77
  management of 78
  refractory cases of 78
Mastoiditis 74, 243
Maternal drug ingestion 175
Maternal tetanus 410
Maxilla, instability of 130
McCune-Albright syndrome 576
Mean arterial pressure 135
Mean corpuscular
  hemoglobin 29
  volume 32
Measles 395, 410
  vaccine 415
Meatal stenosis 548
Mechanical causes 342
Mechanical injury, result of 36
Meclizine 655
Mediastinal tumors 165
Medical Research Council 235
Mefenamic acid 306
Megaloblastic anemia 32
Melanin 181
Melanoma 436
Melanotic pigment 183
Melena 3, 15, 289, 495, 496
  causes 495
  clinical features 495
  initial evaluation 496
  management 496
Melkersson-Rosenthal syndrome 75
Membrane lipid abnormalities 28
Meniere's disease 242
Meningeal signs 155
Meningismus 133
Meningitis 129, 152, 177
Meningococcal meningitis 392
Meningococcal vaccines 411
Meningococcemia 392
Meningococcus 392
Menometrorrhagia 61
Menorrhagia, history of 58
Menstrual cramps 19
Menstrual cycle 77
Mental deterioration 3
Mental status, altered 126
Mental stress 146
Mesenteric adenitis 13, 16
Mesenteric artery syndrome,
  superior 84

Mesenteric ischemia 1, 9
  acute 5
  chronic 4
Mesenteric lymphadenitis 16
Mesenteric vessels atherosclerosis 4
Metabolic acidosis 3, 236, 537
Metabolic alkalosis 85
Metabolic causes 666
Metabolic derangements 128
Metabolic disease 74
Metabolic disorders 132, 137, 143
  diffuse 131
Metabolic disturbance 144
Metabolic storage disease 144, 487
Metabolism, inborn errors of 175
Metachlorpromide 79
Metastatic cancer 112, 357
Metastatic carcinoma 490
Metastatic epidural tumor 483
Metastatic infiltration 486
Metastatic neoplasms 29
Metformin 665, 675
Methanol 129
Methemalbumin 181, 182, 186
Methemoglobin 181, 185, 186, 623
Methemoglobinemia 181, 182, 184,
  186, 237
Methicillin 475
  resistant *Staphylococcus aureus*
    476
Methylphenidate 378
Metoclopramide 182, 377, 497
Metronidazole 665
Metyrapone 281
Micafungin 524
Miconazole 612
Microangiopathic hemolytic anemia
  28, 69
Microcalcification, form of 81
Microcytic hypochromic anemia 29
Micrognathia 558, 631
Microlaryngeal surgery 662
Microsporum canis 611
Microvascular thrombi 69
Micturition, painful 598
Midazolam 149, 150, 160, 378, 562,
  563
  buccal 160
  intramuscular 160
Midgut
  structures 14
  volvulus 16, 17
Migraine, abdominal 19

Milch technique 595
Milia 571
Miliaria crystallina 571
Miliaria rubra 571, 571f
Miliary tuberculosis 442
Miller-Fisher syndrome 74
Milligan and Morgan
  hemorrhoidectomy 367
Minimally invasive therapy 551
Miscarriages 395
Mitotane 281
Mitral stenosis 357
Mittelschmerz 16, 19
Moebius syndrome 75
Molecular genetic techniques 492
Molecular weight heparin 474
Mondor's disease 554
Mongolian spots 570, 574, 575f
Monkeypox 404
Monospot test 628
Moraxella catarrhalis 247
Morbillivirus 395
Motor cortex 503
Motor dysfunction 132
  variety of 132
Motor loss 470
Motor neuron disease 319
Motor vehicle
  collision 96
  traffic 123
Mucociliary function, enhances 169
Mucoid 252
Mucolytics 172, 173
Mucopurulent conjunctivitis 262
Mucosa 367
  buccal 522
  nasal 198
Mucosal ring 230
Mucous membrane 598
  pale 57
Mucus production, excessive 169
Müllerian and Wolffian ducts 590
Multifocal myoclonus 132
Multinodular goiter 326
Multiple ribs, fracture of 579
Multiple trauma 508
  management of 508
  primary survey 510, 510b
  secondary survey 515
  treatment 517
Multisystem organ dysfunction 69
Mumps 395, 410
  vaccine 416

Murmur 105
Muscle
 atrophy, beneficial role in 507
 biopsy 506
 diagnosis of 473
 diseases, progressive 504
 disorders, primary 502
 group wasting, individual 504
 hematoma 61
 pain 502
 relaxants 368
 spasm 95
 tone 503
Muscle cramp 499, 502
 causes of 499
 clinical presentation 499
 etiology 499
 investigations 500
 management 500
 risk factors 499
Muscle wasting 501, 502
 clinical evaluation 502
 diseases 504
 distal 504
 field of 506
 pathophysiology 501
 proximal 504
 treatment 506
 types of 504t
Muscle weakness 505
 localization of 505t
Muscular dystrophy 320
Musculoskeletal causes 101
Musculoskeletal injuries 42, 43, 519
Musculoskeletal syndromes 102
Mushroom poisoning 283
Mustard oil like urine 443
Myalgia 387
Myasthenia gravis 74, 231, 237, 502, 657
Myasthenic crisis 236
Mycobacterium 586
 tuberculosis 394
Mycoplasma 626
 pneumoniae 597
Myelodysplasia 29
Myelodysplastic syndrome 32, 295
Myelofibrosis 32
Myelopathy 95
Myeloproliferative disorders 29, 56
Myenteric plexus 83
Myocardial infarction 9, 104, 134, 184, 382
 acute 9, 99, 102, 240

Myocarditis 184
Myoclonic jerking 153
Myopathic gait 320
Myostatin inhibition 507
Myotonia 502
Myotonic dystrophy 320
Myringotomy 248, 249
Myxedema 49, 469

N

N-acetylcysteine 590
Nafcillin 476
Nail
 avulsion 311fc
 of hands, clubbing of all 115f
 root dislocation 311
Nail bed 184
 ecchymosis 312
 hematoma 312
 injury 311
 laceration 313
Naloxone 445
Nasal cavity 256
Nasal congestion 175
Nasal packing
 anterior 260
 posterior 260
Nasal secretions, clearing of 172
Nasal spray 387
Nasal vasoconstrictors 248
Nasogastric decompression 16
Nasogastric lavage 497
Nasogastric tube 6, 11, 89, 256
 placement 90
Nasopharyngeal aspirate 171
Natriuretic peptide, B-type 46, 48, 239
Nausea 19, 126, 132, 146, 664
Neck
 lymphadenopathy 79
 muscle 504
 pain of 243
 space infection, deep 177
 stiffness 95
 trauma 517
 zones of 517f
Necrotic tissue 478, 480
Necrotic venom 434
Negri bodies 565
Neisseria
 gonorrhoeae 586, 626
 meningitidis 392

Neodymium-doped yttrium aluminum garnet 361
Neomycin 246
Neonatal skin lesions, benign 571
Neoplasm 84, 143, 152, 230
Nephrolithiasis 2, 351
Nephrotic syndrome 49
Nerve
 compression 499
 conduction velocity, slowing of 506
 diseases, peripheral 320
 entrapment 321
 ganglion, trigeminal 526
 peripheral 503
Nervous stress 375
Nervous system 177
 peripheral 505
Neuralgia 200
 trigeminal 242
Neurinoma 74
Neuroblastoma 300
Neurocirculatory asthenia 531
Neurocutaneous syndrome 154
Neurodevelopmental disorders 171
Neurofibromas 576
Neurofibromatosis 574, 576f
Neurohormonal system, activity of 46
Neurologic cause 342
Neurologic disease 162, 657
Neurologic illnesses 675
Neurologic signs 371
Neurologic symptoms 371
Neurological complication 362
Neurological disorder 137, 565
Neurological dysfunction 147
Neurological examination 144
Neurological phase, acute 402
Neurological system 623
Neuromuscular diseases 233, 236
Neuromuscular innervation, transmission of 83
Neuromuscular junction 503
Neuro-ophthalmology emergencies 273
Neuropathic gait 319, 322
Neuropraxia, reversible 73
Neuropsychological assessment 157
Neurosyphilis 375
Neurotoxic venom 434
Neurotoxin 639
Neurovascular damage, distal 40
Neurovascular injuries 121

Nevirapine 598
Nevus flammeus 570, 578, 578f
Nevus simplex 577
New York Heart Association 235
Nicotinamide adenine dinucleotide 182
Nifedipine 378
Night blindness 443
Night cramps 499
Nipple areola complex 82
Nipple discharge 78
Nipple retraction 77, 79
Nitrate-containing foods 182
Nitric oxide 25, 45
 donor 25
Nitrogen dioxide toxicity 358
Nitroglycerine 25, 182
Nitroprusside 182
Nocturnal enuresis 286
Nodular thyroid disease 324
Nonabdominal diseases, attention to 7
Nonaccidental injuries 175, 178
Nonaccidental trauma 177
Nonasthmatic eosinophilic bronchitis 164
Nonbullous impetigo 608t
Nonconvulsive status epilepticus 148, 155
 treatment of 160
Nonheme pigment 184, 187
 suspect deposition of 186
Non-Hodgkin's lymphoma 490
Nonimmune disease 69
Non-neurologic complications 134
Non-noxious stimuli 131
Nonproductive cough 163
Nonreactive pupils 371
Nonserious causes 481
Nonspinal causes 481
Nonsteroidal anti-inflammatory drug 11, 41, 84, 97, 126, 195, 231, 244, 298, 328, 368, 372, 461, 483, 496, 542, 547, 582, 617, 665, 675
 use of 8, 49
Non-ST-segment myocardial infarction 109
Nontransfusion therapy 66
Nontraumatic causes 468
Nontraumatic ocular emergencies 264, 271

Nonvalvular atrial fibrillation, treatment of 61
Normobaric oxygen therapy 621
Normocytic normochromic anemia 29
Nose 244
 blockage 243
 discharge from 243
Noxious stimuli 14, 131
Nucleic acid amplification test 398, 401
Nutritional anemia, pathophysiology of 30fc
Nutritional deficiencies 28, 31
Nystagmus 318
Nystatin 246
 lozenges 524
 suspension 524

O

Obesity 669
Obstipation 86, 87
Obstruction, type of 88
Occipital headache 133
Occlusion, diagnosis for 180
Octreotide 497
Ocular bobbing 131
Ocular congestion 279
Ocular dipping 131
Ocular emergencies, treatment of 275t
Ocular injury, penetrating 264
Ocular muscle 504
Ocular trauma
 classification for 265b, 266t
 new classification for 266
 score 263
Oculocephalic reflex 131, 132
 loss of 131
Oculovestibular reflex 131, 134
Odynophagia 229
Ofloxacin 246
Olanzapine 378
Open globe injury 267
Operation theater 283, 368
Opiates 129, 137
Opioid 287
Opsoclonus 131
Optic neuritis 274
Optic tract 273
Oral
 anticoagulant therapy 52
 anticoagulation, direct 261

antifungals 612
antihistaminics 248
contrast agent 4
hygiene, poor 330
infections 570
polio vaccine 399
poliovirus vaccine 409, 413
problems 520
thrush 525fc
ulcers 20
viscous lidocaine 378
Oral candidiasis 520, 523fc, 573, 573f
 causes 520
 classification of 520, 521t
 clinical presentation 522
 etiology 520
 evaluation 523
 investigations 523
 oral herpes simplex 520
 pathophysiology 520
 primary 521
 red flags 523
 secondary 521
 treatment 524
 types of 522
Oral contraceptive 469, 665
 dose of 80
 pills 79
Oral herpes simplex 525, 528, 529fc
 causes 526
 clinical presentation 526
 etiology 526
 evaluation 527
 investigations 528
 pathophysiology 526
 red flags 526
 treatment 528
Orchiectomy 589
Orchitis 591
Organic disease 21
Organic disorders 18
Orifice, blockage of 424, 438
Oropharyngeal candidiasis, treatment of 524t
Oropharyngeal disorders 230
Oropharyngeal dysphagia 232t
Orthopnea 282
Orthopoxvirus 404
Orthoptera 423
Orthostatic hypotension 25, 322
Oscillation, high-frequency 644
Osmotic laxatives 140

Osteoarthritis 95, 321, 455, 458
  post-traumatic 43
Osteomyelitis 470
Otitic barotrauma 382
Otitis 245
  fungal external 245
  malignant external 74
  media, chronic suppurative 252, 253
  mild external 246
Otitis externa 176, 245, 252, 253
  malignant 253
Otitis media 74, 175, 176, 247, 249
  acute 247, 248
  acute suppurative 243, 252, 253
  chronic 247-249
Otoscopic examination 177, 243, 244, 246, 248
Ottawa ankle rules 41
Ovarian cancer 45, 46
Ovarian cyst 19
Ovarian torsion 13, 16, 175
Overlap syndrome 231
Oxygen
  administration 176
  saturation 181, 183
  supplementation 560
Oxyhemoglobin 181, 185

P

Pain
  acute 265
  analgesia to reduce 248
  character of 103
  colicky nature of 14
  dental 243
  duration of 20, 78
  epigastric 2
  heel 342, 343*fc*
  hypogastric 2
  in percussion 202
  killer agents 373*t*
  location of 20, 104
  muscular 21
  neuralgic 193
  psychogenic 95
  radiation of 104
  referred 14, 193, 198
  sciatic 482
  severe 7, 236
  teething 193
  testicular 19
  timing of 104
  to caries 193
  types of 77
  umbilical 2
Palatine artery, greater 256
Palmar creases 443
Palmar erythema 496
Palpable solid masses 80
Palpable tender abdominal mass 15
Palpitation 58, 326, 530, 532
  arrhythmic causes of 531
  causes 530
  chest pain 532
  clinical presentation 532
  continuous irregular 532
  diarrhea 532
  dyspnea 532
  emergency department with 537*fc*
  etiologies of 530, 531*t*
  evaluation 536
  intermittent 532
  investigations 537
  noncardiac causes of 531
  pathophysiology 532
  physical examination 536
  polyuria 532
  positional 532
  red flags 536
  sweating 532
  syncope 532
  treatment 538
Pancreatic cancer 444
Pancreatic dysfunction 66
Pancreatic mass 442
Pancreatitis 16, 18, 49
  acute 442, 625
  hepatitis myocarditis 14
  severe acute 1
Panduroga 27
Panic attacks 238
Panic disorder 103
Panic syndrome 102
Pantoprazole 22
Papilledema 131, 273, 274
Paracetamol 306
Paracortical hyperplasia 486
Paragonimiasis 357
Paranasal sinuses 256
Paraneoplastic disease 319
Paraphimosis 549, 552
  causes 550
  clinical presentation 550
  etiology 550
  pathophysiology 550
  treatment 550
Parasite 21
Parasitic worms 407
Parasomnias 286
Parenchymal inflammatory processes 165
Parenteral antibiotic treatment 474
Paresthesia 37, 94, 95, 380
  absence of 36
Parietal pain 14
  originates 14
Parietal peritoneum 14, 45, 51
Parkinson's disease 137, 233, 317, 647
Parkinson's syndrome 75
Parkinsonian gait 317, 322
Parotitis 74
Paroxysmal crying 176
Partial thromboplastin time, activated 58, 261
Parvovirus B19 303
  infection 29
Patch
  bluish discoloration 282
  testing 597
Patellar dislocation 466
Patellar fracture 467
  features in 467
Patellar tap test 457
Pectus excavatum 237
Pedal edema 443, 540
  bilateral 543
  causes of 540
  classification of causes of 541*fc*
  etiology 540
  grading of 541*t*
  investigations 543
  management of 543
  pathogenesis 540
  red flags of 540, 541*b*
Pelvic inflammatory disease 11, 16, 19
Pelvic injury 518
Pelvic malignancy 540
Pelvic metastatic deposits 667
Pemberton's sign 326
Penetrate platysma 518*f*
Penicillin 475
  G, intramuscular long-acting 630
  V 630

Penicillinase inhibitors 607
Penile curvature 554
Penile fracture 552
   causes 552
   clinical presentation 553
   epidemiology 552
   etiology 552
   investigations 554
   treatment 554
Penile swelling 553
Pentavalent vaccine 414, 417
Pentobarbital coma 136
Peptic stricture 230
Peptic ulcer 18, 103
   disease 19, 20, 101, 495
Percutaneous cholangiography 445
Perfusion, loss of 85
Perianal skin tag 20
Pericardial disease 237
Pericardial effusion 282
Pericardial rub 105
Pericarditis 102, 388
Periodic limb movement disorder 286
Periodontal pain 193, 198
Periorbital ecchymosis 130
Peristalsis 88
   absence of 88
Peritoneal carcinomatosis 49
Peritoneal cavity 45, 51, 513
Peritoneal dialysis 164
Peritoneal irritation, indicative of 8
Peritoneal tuberculosis 49
Peritonitis, signs of 7
Periumbilical pain 14
   severe 5
Permethrin 609
Pernicious anemia 29
Peroneal tendon syndromes 41
Persistent hiccups 374
Person's overall posture 95
Personal protective equipment 258, 339
Perth-Dundee technique 551
Pertussis 414
Petechiae, presence of 57
Petechial rashes 301
Peyronie's disease 554
Pharmacologic antagonists 559
Pharmacologic therapy 377
Pharyngitis 242, 625
   chronic 625
   management of 629fc

Pharynx 243
Phenazopyridine 182
Phenylbutazone 598
Phenytoin 149, 318, 598
Pheochromocytoma 237
Phimosis 545
   causes 545
   clinical presentation 546
   etiology 545
   evaluation 546
   management of 547
   pathological 545
   physiological 545
   secondary 548
   techniques 548
   treatment 547
Photophobia 19, 598
Phthiraptera 423
Phyllodes tumor 80
Physical activities, decreased 137
Physical hemolysis 68
Physiologic causes 286
Physiologic fatigue 284
Physiological discharge 78
Pierre-Robin syndrome 558
Pigmentation, disorders of 574
Pigments, types of 182t
Pioglitazone 469
Pituitary adenoma 78
Pityrosporum 572
Plantar fascia 343
Plantar flexion 36, 43
Plantar heel pain 344fc
Plasma 513, 519
   enzymes 505
   normal levels of 64
   pooled 59
Plasmapheresis 69, 600
Plasminogen activator inhibitor-1 59
Plasmodium
   falciparum 294
   malariae 294
Platelet 63, 64, 513, 519
   count 61, 62
      normal 205
   derived growth factor 111
   disorder 56
      congenital 54
   dysfunction 54, 56
   function disorders 66
   plug, consolidation of 53
Pleural effusion 45, 184, 240

Pleuritic chest pain 101
Pleuritis 103, 237
Plummer-Vinson syndrome 231
Pneumatic balloon dilation 26
Pneumatosis intestinalis 15, 17
Pneumococcal conjugate vaccine 392
Pneumococcal disease 391
Pneumococcal pneumonia 298
Pneumococcal polysaccharide vaccine 392, 412, 418
Pneumococcal vaccine 414
Pneumococcus 391
Pneumonia 14, 16, 19, 103, 168, 183, 236, 238, 357, 388, 583
Pneumoperitoneum 15, 17, 89
Pneumothorax 119, 122, 175, 184, 236, 238
Polio 399
   vaccine, inactivated 399
Poliomyelitis 300
Poliovirus
   inactivated 422
   vaccine
      fractional inactivated 417
      inactivated 409
Polyarteritis nodosa 19, 300
Polychondritis, relapsing 295
Polycystic ovary syndrome 670
Polycythemia 181, 183
Polyethylene glycol 22, 138
Polymerase chain reaction 72, 297, 393, 402, 404, 528
   real-time 395
Polymorphonuclear leukocyte 472
Polymyalgia rheumatica 95
Polymyositis 295, 320
Polymyxin 246
Polyostotic fibrous dysplasia 576
Polyvinyl alcohol foam 362
Pons tumor 74
Pontine tegmental hemorrhage 74
Porphyria 19
Portal hypertension, initial phase of 47
Port-wine stain 570, 578
Posaconazole 524
Post-concussion
   symptom scale 124
   syndrome 126
Postextubation stridor 637
Post-laparotomy adhesions 6

Postmyringotomy tube 253
Postnasal drip 163
Postpartum hemorrhage, history of 58
Post-thrombolytic therapy 61
Pradaxa 61
Precise neurological examination 371
Preeclampsia 281
Pre-endoscopy barium esophagogram 232
Prefreeze 605
Pregabalin 469
Pregnancy
 and children, immunization in 407
 test 21
 vaccination in 409
Prehepatic jaundice 443
Pressure ulcers, treatment of 480
Primary lump, extent of 80
Prinzmetal angina 100
Procalcitonin 171
Proctoscopy 25
Profile sign 113
Profound symptoms, absence of 184
Progestin-only pill 278
Projectile vomiting 666
Prolactinemia 78
Promethazine hydrochloride 655
Properdin 411
Prophylaxis
 postexposure 402, 403, 403*t*, 405, 568
 pre-exposure 403, 569
Propofol 160, 562, 563
Prostacyclins 45
Prostaglandin 18, 112
Prostatic hypertrophy 351
Prostatitis 351
Proteus mirabilis 586
Proteus vulgaris 245
Prothrombin complex concentrate 63, 66
Proton pump inhibitor 22, 346
Proven phyllodes tumors 81
Pruritic eruptions 175
Pruritus 114, 252
Pseudogout 458
Pseudogynecomastia 82
Pseudohemoptysis 355
Pseudo-locking, causes of 466

Pseudomonas
 aeruginosa 245
 species 604
Pseudoseizures 156
Psoas sign 21
Psoriasis 245
Psoriatic arthritis 455
Psychiatric causes 530
Psychiatric disorder, diagnosis of 530
Psychiatric features 145
Psychiatric origin 530
Psychiatry diseases 675
Psychogenic dysphagia 231
Psychogenic unresponsiveness 132
Psychological stress 100
Psyllium 25
Puberphonia 657, 659, 660
Pulmonary angiogram 185
Pulmonary arteriovenous 112 malformation 237, 357
Pulmonary artery
 catheterization 358
 pseudoaneurysm 357
Pulmonary conditions 101
Pulmonary contusion 239
Pulmonary disease 162
 chronic obstructive 104, 236-238
Pulmonary edema 134, 238
Pulmonary embolism 102, 109, 110, 144, 184, 236, 238, 357
Pulmonary fibrosis 163
Pulmonary hemosiderosis, idiopathic 358
Pulmonary hypertension 101, 102, 357
Pulmonary infections 114
Pulmonary injuries 119
Pulmonary interstitial disease 168
Pulmonary renal syndrome 358
Pulmonary thromboembolism 385
 chronic 237
Pulmonary tuberculosis 112, 164, 168, 679
Pulmonary tumors 237
Pulmonary vascular diseases 357
Pulmonary veno-occlusive disease 357
Pulp 196
 lacerations 313
Pulpitis
 irreversible 195
 reversible 194

Pulsatile mass 9
Pulse
 oximeter measures 185
 oximetry 133, 136, 239, 560
 peripheral 105
Pupillary presentations 131
Pupillary responses 131
Purpura 443
Purpuric rash 130
Purulent 252
 debris 245
 expectoration, presence of 169
Pyelonephritis 2, 351
Pyloric stenosis 177
Pyrazinamide 394
Pyrexia 362
Pyruvate kinase deficiency 28

Q

QT prolongation 667
Quadriceps muscle weakness 505
Quartan fever 294
Quinidine 231
Quinine 500

R

Rabies 565
 dumb 402
 encephalitic 402
 exposure categories 568*t*
 immunoglobulin 568
 paralytic 402, 566
 pathophysiology of 566, 566*fc*
 prevention of 568
 prophylaxis 565
  etiology 565
  host factors 565
 vaccine 412, 421
 virus 569
Radiculopathy 95
Rading system 37
Ramsay-Hunt syndrome 74, 607
Range of motion 36, 95, 456
Raynaud's disease 282
Raynaud's phenomenon 183
Rectal diazepam 160
Rectal examination, digital 25, 366
Rectal gas, paucity of 15, 17
Rectal prolapse 139
Rectorrhagia 3
Rectosigmoid tumors 84

Rectum 137
　collapse of 163
　lower, examination of 139
Recurrent intrahepatic cholestasis, benign 441, 443
Red blood cell 63, 205, 348, 513, 519, 620
　packed 63, 67
Red cell
　aplasia, pure 29
　destruction 28, 32
　indices 31
　infections of 28
　production, decreased 28
　progenitors, infections of 29
　total circulating 27
Red currant jelly stools 15
Red eye, acute 371
Red flag signs 180
Reflex sympathetic dystrophy 43
Reflux esophagitis 374
Refractory ascites 49
　treatment of 49
Reiter's syndrome 454, 455
Remittent fever 300
Renal cell carcinoma 295
Renal colic, diagnosis of 10
Renal disease 52, 56, 82
　signs of end-stage 57
Renal failure 29
　acute 49, 494
　chronic 237
Renal function test 145, 297, 376
Renal impairment, severe 11
Renin-angiotensin-aldosterone 46
Respiration, normal 579
Respiratory distress syndrome, acute 236, 183, 238, 619
Respiratory examination 170
Respiratory failure 583
　hypercarbia 537
Respiratory manifestations 399
Respiratory rate 477
Respiratory system 167, 543
　specific 170
Respiratory tract infection
　acute 168
　upper 167
Respiratory viruses 171
Restlessness 126
Restrictive lung disease 163
Resuscitation, secondary survey with 516b

Reticular activating system 128
Reticulocyte count 31
Retinal injuries 270
Retinal vein occlusion, branch 274, 276
Retroareolar area 82
Retrognathia 558
Retroperitoneal injuries 518
Retroperitoneum 513
Reye's syndrome 306
Rhabdoviridae family virus 565
Rheumatoid arthritis 29, 295, 300, 455, 458
Rheumatoid factor 460
Rhinorrhea 130
Rhinoscopy, anterior 259
Rib fracture 119, 579
　causes 579
　clinical presentation 580
　complications 582
　evaluation and management 582fc
　lower 579
　management 581
　multiple 579
　　right-sided 581f
　pathophysiology 579
　red flag signs 580
　single 579
Ribonucleic acid 395, 565
　mumps virus 395
Rickettsia prowazeki 437
Rickettsial diseases 303
Rickettsiosis 295
Rifampicin 445
Rifampin 394
Rifapentine 394
Rigler's sign 15, 17
Rituximab 69
Road traffic
　accident 276
　injuries 264
Rockall scoring 346b
Rolling sign 553
Romberg's sign 318
Rosiglitazone 469
Rotation test, external 38, 39, 40f
Rotatory nystagmus 653
Rotavirus 415, 422
　vaccine 409, 415
Roth spots 114
Rotor's syndrome 441
Rubber band ligation 367

Rubella 395, 410
　syndrome, congenital 416
　vaccine 416
Rubivirus 395
Ruling out fracture 38
Runny nose 387
Rupture Baker's cyst 468

S

Saline 22
Saliva 565
Salmon patch 577
Salmonella
　enterica 400
　species 400
　typhi 400, 420
Sarcoidosis 75, 164, 295, 302, 303, 442, 455, 679
Sarcopenia geriatric syndrome 674
Sarcoptes scabiei 438, 573
Scabies 608
　clinical features 609
　diagnosis 609
　etiopathogenesis 608
　infantile 573, 575f
　treatment of 609, 609t
Schamroth's sign 113
Schistosoma haematobium 351
Scleroderma 138, 231, 303
Sclerosis, multiple 137, 231, 317, 318, 375, 657
Sclerotherapy 366
Scrotum
　acute 584
　anatomy of 585f
Scrub typhus 295
Seborrheic dermatitis 245, 572, 572f
Second-line therapy 160
Sedation
　airway assessment procedures for 557
　and analgesia, emergency equipment for 559b
　completion of 561
　management 561
　pharmacologic agents for 562t
　procedural 556
　types of 557t
Sedative overdose 130
Sedoanalgesia 474
Seizure 95, 141, 147, 155, 161, 183
　active 148t
　attack 156

causes of drug-induced 151
classification of 141
differential diagnosis of 145t
episode of 141
family history of 143, 155
generalized 142
  motor 142
  nonmotor 143, 147
manifestations 157
neonatal 155
post-traumatic 151
precipitants 143
provoked 152t
stop 161
treatment of neonatal 158
types of 142f, 155
unprovoked 152t
worsening 157
Sensorium, altered 183
Sensory
  ataxia 318
  gait 320, 322
Sepsis 129
Septic arthritis 454, 455, 458, 463, 470, 474
Septic fever 300
Septic shock 15
Serial seizures 150
Serious life-threatening signs 14
Serogroup B meningococcal vaccines 411
Serological testing 445, 505, 628
Seronegative spondyloarthritis 455
Seronegative spondyloarthropathies 459
Serotonin 18
  reuptake inhibitor, selective 665
Serous 252
Sertaconazole 612
Serum
  amylase 376
  ascites albumin gradient 48
    differential diagnosis of 49t
  biochemical tests 445, 628
  blood sugar levels 146
  calcium 146, 376, 667
  electrolytes 146, 376
  iron, determination of 31
  lactate 88
  magnesium 146
  prolactin test 146
Sexually transmitted
  disease 411
  infections 24

Shallow breathing 380
Shallow mandibular fossa 449
Shock, signs of 7
Shoulder
  girdle 502
  joint 593
  spica 595
Shoulder dislocation 593
  anterior 593
  inferior 593
  mechanism of injury 593
  nonoperative treatment 594
  post reduction care 595
  posterior 593
  radiologic studies 594
  signs 593
  symptoms 593
  types of 593
Shunt
  anatomic 183
  right-to-left 183
Sickle cell
  anemia 32
  beta thalassemia 32
  crisis 16
  disease 19, 28, 175, 412
  trait 32
Sickness, decompression 383
Sideroblastic anemia 29, 32
Sigmoid colon, examination of 139
Sigmoid volvulus 84
Sigmoidoscopy 139
Sinus hyperplasia 486
Sinusitis 242, 279, 626
Siphonaptera 423
Sjögren's syndrome 74, 455, 457
Skin
  and excreta, contact between 602
  and mucosa, parts of 184
  attachment 424
  changes 20
  clammy 31
  color
    evaluate 8
    normal 181
  coloration, blue 181
  darkening 443
  dry 326
  examination 144
  necrosis 555
  pigmentation 442
  problems 596
  splitting 546

tests 171
thickening 79
Skinfold thickness 676, 677t
Sleep
  apnea, obstructive 164, 237, 669
  disturb 442
Sleep deprivation 670
  and fatigue 143
Sleep disorders 284, 286
  specific treatment for 292
Small bowel
  obstruction 83, 85t, 89
    red flags of 86b
  red flags of 86
Smallpox 404
Smoke
  inhalation of 618
  poisoning 624
Smoking cessation 670
Snake
  bites 283
  venom 28
Sodium restriction 51
Sodium tetradecyl sulphate 366
Sodium valproate 149
Soft tissue traumas 474
Solbiati index 491, 492
Solitary nodule 324
Somnolence 126
Sorbitol 22
Sore throat 395, 625
  causes 625
  complications 628
  etiology 625
  investigations 628
  red flags 627
  treatment 629
Sounds, abnormal 105
Spasmodic dysphonia 657-659, 661, 663
Spasmodic jerks 644
Spasms 502
Spastic esophageal disease 231
Speech issues 146
Spermatic cord torsion 586
Sphenopalatine artery 256
Spherocytosis 300
Sphincter tone 15
Sphincterotomy
  chemical 25, 26
  partial 26
Spider angioma 496
Spinal cord injuries 137

Spinal infarct 317
Spinal nerve roots 503
Spinal spondylosis 317
Spinal stenosis 482
Spinal tumor 317
Spinocerebellar ataxia 318
Splanchnic vasodilation 47
Splenectomy 68, 412
Splenic dysfunction 412
Sporadic crying 176
Sport concussion assessment tool 125
Sport-related injuries 93
Sprain, symptoms for 500
Sputum 171
Squamous cell cancer 436
Squeeze test 38, 39, 40f
Stable angina 100
Stapedius muscle fibers 73
Staphylococcal scalded skin syndrome 608
Staphylococcus 4, 357
  aureus 245, 247, 416, 462, 474, 664
Status epilepticus 141, 150, 154
  protocol of 150
  treatment of 150, 159
Steatorrhea, cause of 66
Sternocleidomastoid 641
Steroids 279, 469
  topical 547
Stevens-Johnson syndrome, risk of 598t
Stevens-Johnson syndrome 598, 599, 599t
  clinical approach 597
  etiopathogenesis 597
  management 599
  prognosis 599
  treatment 599
Stiff neck 126
Stilbestrol 554
Stool guaiac test 21
Stool softeners 25, 366
Stork bite 577
Strain, symptoms for 500
Strawberry hemangioma 578f
Strenuous physical activity 43
Streptococcal pharyngitis 14, 172, 626f
Streptococcus 4, 462
  pneumoniae 247, 305, 391
  pyogenes 607, 627
Streptokinase 554

Stress 143
  risk of 94
Stricturing diseases 233
Stridor 631, 638fc
  acquired 633
    causes of 633t
  causes 632
  congenital 633
    causes of 633t
  investigations 635
  pathophysiology 631
  treatment 636
  types of 632t
Stroke 231, 647
  diagnosis of 655
ST-segment elevation myocardial infarction 105, 109
Stye 280
Subclavian steal syndrome 652
Subconjunctival hemorrhage 268, 268f
Subdural hematoma 129
Subhyaloid hemorrhage 131
Submandibular glands autonomic system 73
Submucosal hemorrhoids 367
Subtalar joint, chronic instability of 42
Subungual ecchymosis 311
Subungual hematoma 311
Sulfadiazine 598
Sulfamethoxazole 475, 476
Sulfasalazine 182, 598
SulfHb
  forms 182
  produces cyanosis 183
Sulfhemoglobin 181, 186
Sulfhemoglobinemia 181, 184
Sulfonamides 182
Sumatriptan overdose 182
Superior vena cava syndrome 494
Supraclavicular lymphadenopathy 489
Supraclavicular node 80
Supraglottic growth 242
Suprapubic tenderness 20
Sweat test 171
Sweating, excessive 326
Swelling 37, 95
Swimmer's ear 245
Sydenham's chorea 321
Sympathetic nervous system 46
Symptomatology, complicated 90
Syncopal attack 25

Syncope 58, 101, 156, 163
Syndesmotic ligament 37
Synovial fluid analysis 460, 461t
Syphillis 74
Syringomyelia 317, 375
Systemic antibiotics 480
Systemic corticosteroids 600, 607
Systemic disease 138, 320, 371, 591
Systemic disorders 183, 502
Systemic embolization 362
Systemic fever 470
Systemic illness, signs of 144
Systemic infection 471
  history of 143
Systemic inflammatory response syndrome 88
Systemic lupus erythematosus 29, 54, 56, 74, 286, 300, 358, 455
Systemic neuromuscular diseases 162
Systemic toxic syndrome 5
Systemic toxicity of inhaled gases 620
Systolic dysfunction 106

T

T cell lymphoma 609
Tabes dorsalis 320
Tachycardia 666
  bleeding causes 8
  supraventricular 533f, 538
  ventricular 534f, 538
Tachyphylaxis 25
Tachypnea 183
Taghaandan maneuver 552
Takayasu arteritis 295
Talar tilt test 38, 39f
Talofibular ligament
  anterior 37
  injury, posterior 37
Tamoxifen 82
Tardive dyskinesia 667
Tau protein 125
Tecovirimat 404
Temperature variation, normal 294
Temporomandibular joint 193, 448
Tendon reflexes, deep 132, 144
Tendonitis 41
Tensile limits 36
Tension 14
  pneumothorax 512
Terbinafine 612
Terminal duct, excision of 79

Testicular artery 584
Testicular parenchyma 589
Testicular perfusion 588
Testicular torsion 13, 15, 16, 175, 588, 589
  neonatal 590
  pathophysiology of 586f
Testicular tumors hypothyroidism 82
Tetanospasmin 639
Tetanus 237, 390
  boosters 640
  high-risk 639
  neonatal 410
  prone wound 639, 640
  prophylaxis 639, 640t
  toxoid 410, 414, 417
    vaccine 410
Tetracycline 231, 388, 475
Tetralogy of Fallot 184
Thalassemia 29, 204-206
  syndromes 28
Theophylline 675
Therapeutic bronchoscopy 168
Therapeutic endoscopy 498
Therapeutic paracentesis 49
Thermoregulatory disorders 296
Thiacetazone 598
Thiazolidinediones 469
Third nerve palsy 371
Thoracic cavity 513
Thoracic trauma 518
Thorax 177
Throat
  culture 628
  pain 243
Thrombocytopenia 48, 53, 69, 257, 358
  heparin-induced 63
Thrombocytopenic purpura, idiopathic 68
Thromboembolic occlusion, acute 5
Thrombogenic foams 260
Thrombolytic therapy 474
Thrombophlebitis 470
Thrombotic thrombocytopenic purpura 28, 54, 56, 62, 65, 68, 237
Thyroid
  acropathy 112
  autoantibodies 327
  cytopathology 327t
  disorders 237, 282, 499
  dysfunction 342

gland 326
  position of 323f
  neoplasm 324
  nodules, management of 329fc
  nuclear scan 327
  stimulating hormone 323
  ultrasound 327
Thyroiditis 242
  subacute 324
Thyroxine, free 21
Tibial arteries, posterior 41
Tibiofibular ligaments 39
Ticlopidine 474
Tinea corporis 611
  clinical features 612
  etiopathogenesis 611
  management 612
  treatment 612
Tinea cruris 612
  clinical features 613
  etiology 612
  treatment 613
Tinea pedis 613, 614t
  etiopathogenesis 613
Tinnitus 94, 249, 252, 254
Tissue
  diagnosis 81, 492
  Doppler 110
  extraction 182
  of oxygen 182
Tobacco 104
  exposure 170
Todd's paralysis 144
Toe nail avulsion 310
Tongue 522
Tonic component 644
Tonic seizures 156
Tonic-clonic seizures 150
Tonsillar enlargement, chronic 164
Tonsillitis 242
Tonsils, inflamed 243
Tooth extraction, single 204
Toothache 193
Torsion 589
Torticollis 95, 641
  acquired 643
  causes 642
  congenital 642, 643, 644
  differential diagnosis 645
  etiology 642
  investigations 644
  nondystonic 642
  physical examination 644
  physical therapy 645
  primary 642, 643

  secondary 642, 643
  treatment of 645, 646fc
  types of presentations of 641f
Toxic epidermal necrolysis 598
Toxic ingestion 154, 175
Toxic nodular goiter 326
Toxic substance ingestion 143
Toxicology screen 146, 160
Toxin 666
  and drugs 144
Toxocarosis 74
Toxoplasmosis 303
Trachea 122
  position of 105
Tracheitis 636
Tracheobronchial tree injury 512
Tracheobronchitis 165
Tracheomalacia 164
Traffic accident, neck injury after 511f
Tragal tenderness 245, 254
Tragulizers, large dose of 79
Tranexamic acid 66
Transbronchial lung biopsy 358
Transbronchial needle aspiration 358, 492
Transcoelomic spread 46
Transfusing platelet, indications for 65b
Transfusion reaction 28
  symptoms 68
Transfusion therapy 66
Transient pustular melanosis 571, 572f
Transjugular intrahepatic shunt 49
Transthoracic needle aspiration 358
Transverse myelitis 317
Trauma 13, 16, 154, 174, 469, 481, 591
  abdominal 518
  crepitation, history of 471
  deaths, timing distribution of 509f
  history of 155
  mechanical 28
  pain to 193, 195
  repetitive physical 28
Traumatic brain injury, mild 123
Traumatic injuries, evidence of 144
Tremor 647
  classification 647
  clinical features 647
  drug-induced 648
  drugs useful in essential 649
  dystonic 648

epidemiology 647
essential 647, 649*t*
etiological classification 647
evaluation of 648
flapping 443
intention 647
intentional 318
kinetic 647
neurological cause of 648
neuropathic 648
orthostatic 648
Parkinson's 648
postural 647
psychogenic 648
resting 647
treatment 649
Wilson's 648
Trendelenburg's sign positive 320
Treponema pallidum 626
Trichophyton
   mentagrophytes 611
   rubrum 611
Tricuspid endocarditis 357
Triglyceride 297
Trimethoprim 475, 476
Trismus 449, 558
   presence of 177
Troponin elevation, causes of 107*f*
Troponin, high-sensitivity 106
Trypsin 554
Tuberculin sensitivity 171
Tuberculin test 297
Tuberculosis 114, 165, 171, 286, 295, 300, 302, 303, 394
   infection, latent 394
Tuberculous meningitis 74
Tumor 6
   benign 78
   diagnosis
      of benign 473
      of malignant 473
   necrosis factor-α 300, 501, 590
Tunica albuginea 553, 584
Tympanic membrane 243
Typhoid 400
   conjugate vaccine 420
   fever 295
   vaccination for 298
   vaccine 419
Tzanck smear 528

U

Ubiquitin-proteasome system 501
Ulcer 468, 471
   bacterial corneal 272

corneal 272
diabetic neuropathic 478
duodenal 374
gastric 104
multiple superficial 24
pressure 478
syphilitic 24
Unbound bilirubin 442*f*
Unknown origin, fever of 295, 299
Upper airway
   cough syndrome 163, 164
   viral infection of 163
Upper gastrointestinal
   bleeding 345*b*, 497*f*
   malignancy 495
Urate-lowering therapy 461
Urea 96, 335
   breath test 21
Ureaplasma urealyticum 586
Uremia 129, 130, 666
Ureteral trauma 519
Ureteropelvic junction obstruction 19, 351
Urethra 552
   posterior 519
Urethral injury 553
Uric acid nephropathy 494
Uridine-diphosphate glucuronosyltransferase 441
Urinary catheter 11
Urinary incontinence 139
Urinary retention 139
Urinary stool incontinence 470
Urinary symptoms 20
Urinary tract
   anomalies, congenital 549
   congenital 549
   infection 10, 11, 14, 16, 178, 546, 591
   symptoms, lower 591
Urine
   analysis 146, 360
   causes
      of brown color 350*t*
      of red color 350*t*
   cola-colored 442, 443
   culture 304
   routine 297
Urolithiasis 19
Urticaria 614
   acute 616
   causes of 615, 615*t*
   chronic 616
   classification 614
   clinical features 615
   contact 617

ordinary spontaneous 614
physical 614, 615, 617
pigmentosa 576, 576*f*
treatment of 617, 617*fc*
types
   of acute 616*t*
   of chronic 616*t*
vasculitis 616, 617
Uveitis 272

V

Vaccination, historical aspect of 408
Vaccine
   and immunization, global alliance for 409
   inactivated 397
   vial monitor 422
Vaccinia virus vaccine 404
Vagina, collapse of 163
Valacyclovir 529
Valsalva maneuver 231
Valvular heart disease 236, 237
Vancomycin 475
   linezolid-tigecycline-colistin 280
Variceal hemorrhage 45
Varicella 393, 410
   vaccine 421
   zoster virus 303, 421
Varicoceles 585
Variola 404
Vascular abnormalities 53
Vascular ectasias 345
Vascular emergencies 274
Vascular endothelial growth factor 111
Vascular ischemia 73
Vascular malformations 577
Vascular stasis 605
Vasculitis 19
Vaso-occlusive crisis 175
Venous blood gas 135
Venous insufficiency 470
Venous thromboembolism 385
Venous ulcers, treatment of 479
Ventilation
   monitoring 560
   perfusion
      mismatch 183
      scan 241*f*
Ventricular extrasytolic bigeminism 533*f*
Vertigo 94, 254, 650
   causes of 650*t*, 654, 656
   central 652*t*

etiology 650
evaluation 651
management 655
pathophysiology 650
peripheral 652t
red flags 651
severe 132
Vessels bleeding, large 61
Vestibulo-ocular reflex 651
Veterinary surgeon 424, 438
Vibrio cholerae 420
Vigorous sexual intercourse 554
Viral arthritis 455
Viral conjunctivitis 262
Viral diseases 597
Viral fever 295
Viral hepatitis 295
Virchow's node 231, 489
Virus isolation 567
Viscera, abdominal 1
Visceral pain
  fibers 14
  occurs 14
Visceral peritoneum 45, 51
Visible injury 95
Visible internal sphincter muscles 24
Vision
  blurred 371
  doubling of 265
Visual disturbances 384
Visual field test 274
Vital signs 244
  abnormal 3
  assess 158
Vitamin
  B complex 500
  B$_{12}$ 291, 623, 673
  E 500
    supplements 78
  K 66, 362, 445
    antagonists 261
    deficiency 52, 54, 56
    malabsorption 62
Vitreous hemorrhage 270, 276
Vocal cord
  carcinoma 658, 660, 661, 663
  cyst 658f
  dysfunction 237, 637
  lesion, benign 657-660, 662
  leukoplakia 659f
  nodule 660
  papilloma 659f
  paralysis 636, 657-659, 661, 663
  polyp 658f, 660

Vodder technique 476
Voice
  hoarseness of 326, 627
  professional 657, 659
Voice disorders 657
  etiology 657
  pathophysiology 657
  red flags 660
  treatment 662
Voice therapy
  direct 662
  indirect 662
Voluntary functions 128
Volvulus 178
Vomit, subjective feeling to 664
Vomiting 19, 38, 95, 126, 130, 664, 666
  chronic 667
  etiology of 664t
  management of acute 667
Vomitus
  old blood in 231
  prevent aspiration of 17
von Willebrand
  disease 52-54, 56, 204, 205, 358
  factor 59
Voriconazole 524

W

Wakefulness, absence of 128
Wallerian degeneration 73
Warfarin 62, 474
  ingestion 62
  therapy 66
Warts 610
  clinical approach 610
  common 610
  etiology 610
  management 611
  plantar 610
Wax
  impaction 251
  visualization of 251
Wegener's granulomatosis 358
Weight gain 669
  behavior modification 672
  complications 670
  dietary therapy 672
  drug therapy 672
  etiology 669
  investigations 671
  pathophysiology 669
  red flags 671
  treatment 672

Weight loss 231, 375, 674, 679fc
  assessment of 677
  causes of 675t, 679t
  clinical feature 676
  drugs 675
  etiology 674
  investigations 678
  involuntary 19
  medications leading to 675b
  pathophysiology 675
  red flag signs 677
  treatment 678
Wernicke encephalopathy 129, 130
Westermark's sign 106
Whiplash associated disorder 93, 97t
Whiplash injury 93, 94, 98fc
  acute 94
  chronic 94
  subacute 94
Whirlpool sign 17, 89
White blood cell 4, 304, 436
White papules 233
Whitehead's hemorrhoidectomy 368
Wilms tumor 300
Wilson's disease 321, 441, 445
Wisdom tooth eruption, pain to 193, 197
Wiskott-Aldrich syndrome 56
World Health Organization 27, 262, 277, 325, 369, 407
Worm infestation 680
Worsening pain, rapidly 95
Wound
  management of 568
  types of 640t
Wrist pivot method 452f
Wryneck 641
Wuchereria bancrofti 604

X

Xanthoma 105, 443

Y

Yellow fever 398, 437
  vaccine 412
  virus 398

Z

Zenker's diverticulum 232, 233
Zika virus 437

EU GSPR Authorised Reprsentative
Logos Europe, 9 rue Nicolas Poussin
1700, La Rochelle, France
Phone: +33 (0) 6 67 93 73 78
E-mail: contact@logoseurope.eu

www.ingramcontent.com/pod-product-compliance
Ingram Content Group UK Ltd.
Pitfield, Milton Keynes, MK11 3LW, UK
UKHW051846210426
5322IPUK00019B/281